MRI of the Knee

Second Edition

Editors

Peter L. Munk, M.D., C.M., F.R.C.P.C.
Associate Professor
Department of Radiology
University of British Columbia
Department of Diagnostic Imaging
British Columbia Cancer Agency
Vancouver Cancer Center
Vancouver, British Columbia, Canada

Clyde A. Helms, M.D.
Professor
Department of Radiology
Duke University Medical Center
Durham, North Carolina

Lippincott - Raven
PUBLISHERS
Philadelphia • New York

Printed in the United States of America

9 8 7 6 5 4 3 2 1

Library of Congress Cataloging-in-Publication Data

MRI of the knee / editors, Peter L. Munk, Clyde A. Helms. — 2nd ed.
p. cm.
Includes bibliographical references and index.
ISBN 0-397-51642-8
1. Knee—Magnetic resonance imaging. 2. Knee—Diseases—Diagnosis. I. Munk, Peter L. II. Helms, Clyde A.
[DNLM: 1. Knee—pathology. 2. Magnetic Resonance Imaging—methods. WE 870 M939 1996]
RD561.M75 1996
617.5′82—dc20
DNLM/DLC
for Library of Congress 96-12935

Care has been taken to confirm the acuracy of the information presented and to describe generally accepted practices. However, the authors, editors, and publisher are not responsible for errors or omissions or for any consequences from application of the information in this book and make no warranty, express or implied, with respect to the contents of the publication.

The authors, editors and publisher have exerted every effort to ensure that drug selection and dosage set forth in this text are in accordance with current recommendations and practice at the time of publication. However, in view of ongoing research, changes in government regulations, and the constant flow of information relating to drug therapy and drug reactions, the reader is urged to check the package insert for each drug for any change in indications and dosage and for added warnings and precautions. This is particularly important when the recommended agent is a new or infrequently employed drug.

Some drugs and medical devices presented in this publication have Food and Drug Administration (FDA) clearance for limited use in restricted research settings. It is the responsibility of the health care provider to ascertain the FDA status of each drug or device planned for use in their clinical practice.

To my wife, Alice Maria Chung, and my daughters,
Charlotte Giselle Oiwah Munk, Eleanor Ruth Oiling Munk,
and Sophie Alexis Oiwai Munk.

To my parents, Mr. and Mrs. F. L. Helms.

Contents

Contributing Authors

E. Michel Azouz, M.D., F.R.C.P.C. *Professor, Department of Diagnostic Imaging, University of Toronto, Hospital for Sick Children, 555 University Avenue, Toronto, Ontario, Canada M5G 1X8*

Paul Babyn, M.D. *Associate Professor, Department of Diagnostic Imaging, University of Toronto, Hospital for Sick Children, 555 University Avenue, Toronto, Ontario, Canada M5G 1X8*

Rethy K. Chhem, M.D., F.R.C.P.C. *Associate Professor of Radiology Department of Diagnostic Radiology, McGill University, Montreal General Hospital, 1650 Cedar Avenue, Montreal, Quebec, Canada H3G 1A4*

Douglas G. Connell, M.D. *Associate Professor, University of British Columbia, Department of Radiology, Vancouver Hospital and Health Sciences Centre, 855 West 12th Avenue, Vancouver, British Columbia, Canada V5Z 1M9*

Malcolm M. M. Hayes, F.R.C.P.C., F.R.C.Path., M.B.Ch.B., M.Med.Path. *Clinical Professor of Pathology, University of British Columbia, British Columbia Cancer Agency, 600 West 10th Avenue, Vancouver, British Columbia, Canada V5Z 4E6*

Clyde A. Helms, M.D. *Professor, Department of Radiology, Duke University Medical Center, P.O. Box 3808, Durham, North Carolina 27710*

Dennis L. Janzen, M.D., F.R.C.P.C. *Assistant Professor, University of British Columbia, Department of Radiology, Vancouver Hospital and Health Sciences Centre, 855 West 12th Avenue, Vancouver, British Columbia, Canada V5Z 1M9*

Peter L. Munk, M.D., F.R.C.P.C., C.M. *Associate Professor, Department of Radiology and Department of Diagnostic Imaging, University of British Columbia, British Columbia Cancer Agency, Vancouver Cancer Center, 600 West 10th Avenue, Vancouver, British Columbia, Canada V5Z 4E6*

Peter Y. Poon, M.B.B.S., F.R.C.P.C. *Professor, Department of Radiology, University of British Columbia, Department of Diagnostic Imaging, British Columbia Cancer Agency, 600 West 10th Avenue, Vancouver, British Columbia, Canada V5Z 4E6*

Maximillian F. Reiser, M.D. *Professor and Chairman, Department of Radiology, University of Munich, Munich, Germany*

A. Dale Vellet, F.R.C.P.C., FFRAD.D, MBB.Ch. *Associate Professor, Department of Diagnostic Imaging, University of Calgary, Foothills Hospital, 1403 29th Street, Northwest, Alberta, Canada T2N 2T9*

Preface

A number of changes have been made in the Second Edition to keep it up-to-date. Chapters on the pediatric knee and the postoperative knee have been added. The chapter on technique for knee imaging has been thoroughly revised, and many of the newer pulse sequences are described in greater detail. Some of the pulse sequences, which are not yet widely available on the market such as echo-planar imaging, have been excluded in an effort not to clutter the book with information that is not applicable to most practices. In addition, new illustrations have been added throughout, and the bibliographies have been updated to incorporate the current literature.

We believe these changes help keep *MRI of the Knee* current and useful to readers who seek a book that will give them a good general understanding of knee MRI, as well as those who wish to have a useful reference to help them in day-to-day evaluation of knee MRI in clinical practice.

Acknowledgments

Writing this textbook has made us realize how indebted authors are to a large number of people in the execution of a project.

We are indebted to the Bio-Medical Photography Departments of the Vancouver Hospital and Health Sciences Centre and the British Columbia Cancer Agency, as well as the invaluable contributions from the University of California San Francisco, and University Hospital, University of Western Ontario, for the large volume of excellent work.

Many of the magnetic resonance images could not have been obtained without the efforts of Leonard Tong, head MRI technician at the Vancouver Hospital and Health Sciences Centre, and Karen Kennedy, head technician at the University Hospital in London, Ontario. They often went out of their way to make extra efforts to obtain exceptional quality images. Preparation of the manuscript and figures would have been impossible without the effort and care from Karen Locken and Mark J. Lee. Without them preparation of this project would have been entirely too difficult. I am also greatly indebted to Dr. John Mayo who was invaluable in helping us with details of MR physics for the technique chapter. The encouragement of Drs. Nestor L. Müller and Brian Lentle also made the task much easier.

MRI of the Knee

Second Edition

MRI of the Knee, Second Edition,
edited by P. L. Munk and C. A. Helms.
Lippincott-Raven Publishers, Philadelphia © 1996.

CHAPTER 1

Technique of Magnetic Resonance Imaging of the Knee

Dennis L. Janzen, Peter L. Munk, and Clyde A. Helms

Nuclear magnetic resonance (NMR) was first described in 1946 and was initially used in laboratory investigations of chemical phenomena. In the 1970s it was demonstrated that NMR signals could be spatially localized and thus form the basis of an imaging technique (1). Since that time, magnetic resonance imaging (MRI) has become a vital technique in the assessment of musculoskeletal disease. MRI is now the method of choice for investigation of a wide variety of knee disorders and has largely replaced arthrography and diagnostic arthroscopy (2–5).

MRI is a rapidly evolving technology in which a wide variety of imaging techniques allow many different types of images and tissue contrasts to be obtained. Selection of optimal imaging technique for evaluation of knee disorders may at times be confusing, because of the variety of available methods. In this chapter we outline the physical basis of MRI, the various parameters that must be considered in pulse sequence selection, and our approach to knee MRI technique.

PHYSICAL BASIS OF MRI

Many excellent reviews of this topic are now available (6–9). It is beyond the scope of this book to provide a detailed discussion of magnetic resonance physics. Awareness of basic MRI physics is, however, necessary to understand the clinically important issues of imaging optimization, protocol selection, and image interpretation (10).

Resonance

Clinical MRI is based upon the behavior of hydrogen protons in a static magnetic field. Although other nuclei with an odd number of protons or neutrons (e.g., ^{14}N, ^{31}P, ^{23}Na, and ^{13}C) can be imaged with MRI, the vast majority of clinical imaging is based on hydrogen as hydrogen is plentiful in biological substances and provides a relatively strong MRI signal.

A hydrogen atom consists of a positively charged proton and a negatively charged electron and can be thought of as a tiny bar magnet (a magnetic dipole). When a hydrogen proton is placed in a magnetic field, it tends to align its magnetic field in the direction of the external magnetic field (Bo). Because a proton also has spin, it will not align itself exactly with the magnetic field but will precess around the axis of the magnetic field (Bo) in a fashion similar to that of a spinning top wobbling in the earth's gravitational field. The precession frequency of the hydrogen protons depends on the strength of the magnetic field, as described by the Larmor equation: precession frequency = magnetic field strength (Tesla) × gyromagnetic ratio.

The hydrogen protons, precessing at a known frequency, can be affected by a radiofrequency (RF) pulse tuned to their precession frequency. In the simplest terms, the RF pulse adds energy to the protons; this energy is later emitted as an RF signal, which is the signal used to generate the MRI image. The rate at which the protons return to their equilibrium position is regulated by two constants known as T1 (spin-lattice relaxation time) and T2 (spin-spin relaxation time). Another fundamental concept in MRI is the interaction of moving charges and electromagnetic waves. Any moving electrical charge, including a spinning hydrogen pro-

D. L. Janzen: Department of Radiology, Vancouver Hospital and Health Sciences Center, Vancouver, British Columbia, Canada V5Z 1M9.

P. L. Munk: Department of Diagnostic Imaging, British Columbia Cancer Agency, and Department of Radiology, University of British Columbia, Vancouver, British Columbia, Canada V5Z 4E6.

C. A. Helms: Department of Radiology, Duke University Medical Center, Durham, North Carolina 27710.

ton, induces an electromagnetic field. A continuously varying electromagnetic field, such as that induced by a spinning proton, will produce an alternating current in a wire or coil. This alternating current can be described as a wave function, using parameters of frequency, phase, and amplitude (11). In clinical MRI systems the receiving coil is positioned parallel with the main magnetic field. Thus protons aligned longitudinally with the main magnetic field produce no current in the coil, whereas protons aligned in the transverse plane produce maximal current in the coil.

T1 Decay

The application of a RF pulse to a population of spinning protons results in deflection of the protons' magnetic alignment away from the main longitudinal magnetic field (Bo) axis into the transverse plane. The degree of deflection is dependent on the duration and amplitude of the RF pulse. After the RF pulse ceases, the protons will gradually return to their original alignment with Bo. This gradual longitudinal realignment with Bo is termed *T1 decay* and results from the interaction of the proton with its molecular environment (12). In general, protons attached to large molecules (e.g., in fat) have short T1 relaxation times, because these protons can rapidly exchange energy with surrounding molecules. Pure water has a very long T1 relaxation time because of slow transfer of energy to the environment. With regard to signal induction in a MRI system, protons in the transverse plane produce maximal signal. Because these protons gradually realign with Bo, the signal intensity drops to zero. Thus after a 90° RF pulse, a graph of signal intensity versus time shows initial maximal signal that decays to zero as a result of T1 decay.

T2 Decay

Application of a RF pulse to a group of protons causes all the protons to be in phase with one another in their precession around Bo. After the RF pulse ceases, the protons will gradually lose phase coherence because of local alterations of the magnetic field caused by neighboring nuclei and field inhomogeneities. This loss of phase coherence among a group of protons is described as T2 decay. Substances with homogeneous molecular composition, such as water, will have a long T2 relaxation time, whereas inhomogeneous substances will have a short T2 relaxation time, because of varying magnetic conditions experienced by individual protons (12).

MR Signal Intensity

The intensity of the signal emitted from tissue at any point in time depends on T1 decay, T2 decay, proton density (the number of protons per unit volume of tissue), and motion of the protons in the tissue. These factors can be manipulated to produce MR images emphasizing various features of the tissues. This is the basis for the generation of different types of images using different pulse sequences.

SIGNAL LOCALIZATION

The MRI signal obtained from a volume of tissue is a complex wave that can be described in terms of frequency, phase, and amplitude. The signal from each voxel of tissue is assigned to the correct pixel in the image by the processes of slice selection, frequency encoding, and phase encoding. It is customary to describe the location of MR signals in terms of three axes: the *x*-axis is the transverse horizontal axis, the *y*-axis is the transverse vertical axis, and the *z*-axis is the longitudinal axis of Bo and the magnet bore.

The location of an image slice along the *z*-axis is determined by the effects of a slice selection gradient and a slice-selective RF pulse. The slice selection gradient is applied along the *z*-axis and causes a gradual alteration in the magnetic field strength from the foot end of the patient to the head end. Each location along the *z*-axis thus experiences a slightly different magnetic field strength and has a slightly different Larmor frequency. This situation is analogous to the relationship between the frequency of a piano note and the location of the corresponding piano key. The slice-selective RF pulse is tuned to a range of frequencies that will interact with the protons in the desired slice of tissue. The slice thickness can be altered by changing the range of frequencies in the RF pulse or the steepness of the slice selection gradient.

The location of an MR signal within a transverse slice is determined by frequency encoding and phase encoding. To determine the location along one axis (i.e., the *x*-axis), a frequency-encoding gradient is applied along the *x*-axis that causes the protons on the left-hand side of the slice to precess at a different rate than the protons on the right-hand side of the slice. Thus, the frequency of the RF signal reflects the position of the proton along the *x*-axis. The frequency-encoding gradient is turned on briefly during the collection of the MR signal and is also known as the "readout gradient" (1,6). In most clinical MR systems, the frequency spectrum is divided into 256 segments; thus, the image matrix size in the frequency-encoded direction is 256.

Phase encoding is used to localize the MR signal along the third axis (i.e., the *y*-axis). A magnetic gradient temporarily placed along the *y*-axis causes a slight acceleration of the precessional frequency of the protons. This results in a phase shift of the protons, with the amount of phase shift reflecting the position of a proton along the *y*-axis. When the gradient is removed, the protons return to the original precessional frequency but retain the phase shift caused by the phase-encoding gradient. In clinical imaging systems, a series of phase-encoding steps and signal acquisitions is necessary to localize signals along the *y*-axis, as each phase-encoding step samples the imaged volume at a single spatial frequency. Thus, the number of phase-encoding steps used to compose the image determines the image matrix size and resolution in the phase-encoded direction (1,6,11). Most clinical imaging sequences use 128, 192, or 256 phase-encoding steps to construct an image. The phase-encoding gradient is applied between the excitation pulse sequence and the signal readout.

The MRI signal obtained from a volume of tissue is a complex waveform that contains the tissue signal as well as the frequency-encoded and phase-encoded information that allows the signal to be assigned to the correct pixel in the image. This complex waveform can be described as a sum of many sine and cosine waves of known frequency, amplitude, and phase. A mathematical function known as the Fourier transform is used to convert the complex waveform into a series of waves of specific frequency, phase, and amplitude. The frequency and phase of a particular wave determine its position in the image, and the amplitude (signal intensity) determines the gray-scale intensity assigned to the pixel.

PULSE SEQUENCES

A variety of pulse sequences are available for clinical knee MRI, including spin-echo, fast spin-echo, gradient-echo, and short-tau inversion recovery (STIR) sequences. These sequences have different advantages, disadvantages, and image characteristics.

Spin-Echo Sequences

Spin-echo sequences are composed of a 90° pulse followed by a 180° pulse. The 90° pulse tips the longitudinal magnetic vector into the transverse plane, where the protons begin dephasing relative to one another (T2 relaxation). The 180° pulse rephases the protons, resulting in a signal. The interval between two sequential 90° pulses is known as TR (repetition time), and the time between the 90° pulse and signal acquisition is known as TE (echo time). The time interval between the 90° pulse, and the 180° pulse is TE/2. In spin-echo imaging, tissues with a short T1 relaxation time (e.g., fat, methemoglobin, gadolinium-enhanced tissues) will produce high signal on T1-weighted images. Tissues with a long T2 relaxation time (e.g., fluid, edematous, or cellular tissues) will produce high signal on T2-weighted images (12).

The parameters most important in determining image contrast in spin-echo sequences are TR and TE. By changing these parameters, images may be generated that reflect principally T1, T2, or proton density effects (7,11–14). By changing these parameters, the same anatomic tissues may have markedly different signal characteristics (Fig. 1-1).

To achieve T1 contrast on spin-echo images, both TR and TE should be relatively short. As a general guideline, TR should be 600 ms or less and TE should be 30 ms or less. Although signal intensities seen in the image tend to be controlled primarily by T1 effects, lesser T2 influences are present as well. When TR and TE are lengthened, signal intensities tend to be controlled primarily by T2, with lesser, but usually not negligible, T1 influences as well. When a long TR is selected (greater than 1800 ms), two echoes are generally used. These echoes represent two different values of TE, with the first echo (at TE 30 msec or less) producing a proton-density-weighted image (i.e., 30 ms or less) and the second echo (at TE greater than 50 msec) producing a T2-weighted image (see Fig. 1-4). T1-weighted, T2-weighted, and proton-density-weighted images each demonstrate different properties of the tissues and have certain advantages. T1-weighted images require relatively short imaging times and provide good anatomic detail. Proton density images have good signal-to-noise ratios and good intrinsic contrast, thereby providing crisp anatomic detail. T2-weighted images are excellent for lesion detection because almost all pathologic processes prolong T2 relaxation times, but they have the disadvantages of long imaging times, relatively low signal-to-noise ratios, and greater degradation resulting from patient motion. Spin-echo sequences have been the major pulse sequence in knee MRI, and most of the experience in the literature is based on this technique.

Fast Spin-Echo Sequences

Fast spin-echo imaging is a technique that allows rapid acquisition of images similar to spin-echo images. The pulse sequence consists of a 90° pulse followed by a train of 180° pulses, with a signal acquired after each 180° pulse. The number of 180° pulses in the train is referred to as the ''echo train length'' (ETL) and typically is 4, 8, or 16 (12). Thus, with an ETL of four, four signals are acquired during each TR, and an image can be acquired four times faster than a standard spin-echo image using the same parameters. As the signals are acquired at various TEs, the average TE value of the individual signals is expressed as TE-eff (TE-effective) (13–15). Although fast spin-echo techniques are usually used to acquire T2-weighted images, the echo train can be divided into two data sets, the first half of the echo train forming a proton-density-weighted image, and the latter half forming a T2-weighted image.

The main advantage of fast spin-echo imaging is the rapidity with which T2-weighted images can be acquired. The decreased acquisition time can be used to achieve increased resolution (by increasing the number of phase-encoding steps), to increase signal to noise (by increasing NEX), and to minimize patient motion (by decreasing imaging time) (16). Another feature of fast spin-echo imaging is that the repeated 180° pulses minimize signal loss due to magnetic susceptibility (17). This is an advantage in imaging patients with metallic implants but could reduce the detection of diagnostically important calcifications and hemosiderin deposits. The use of longer echo trains reduces imaging time, but also decreases spatial resolution (Fig. 1-2). The loss of spatial

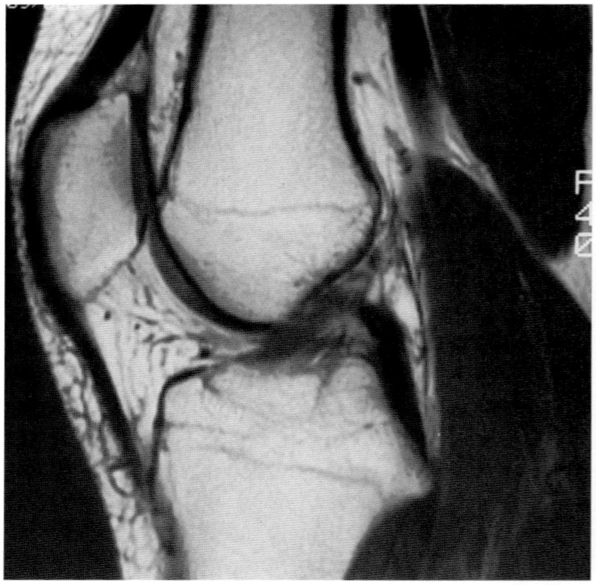

A

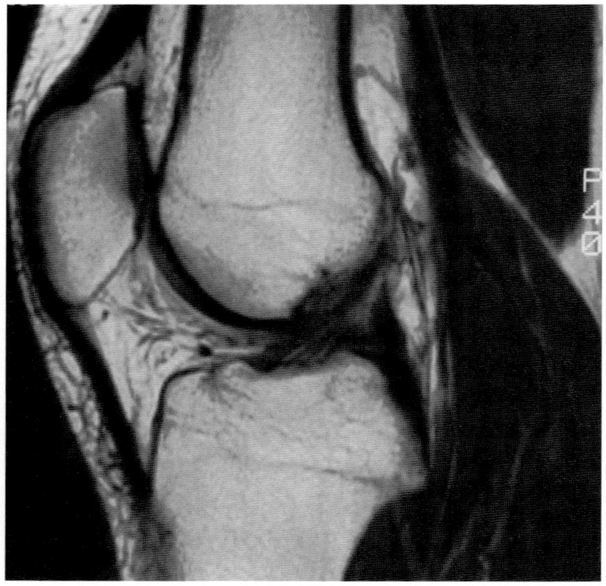

B

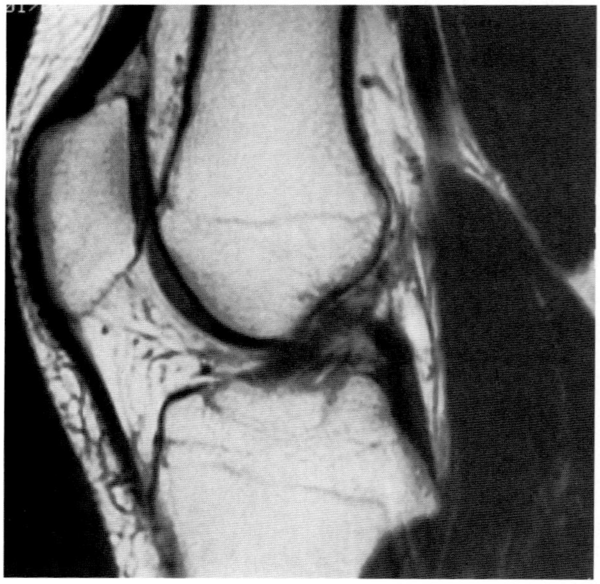

C

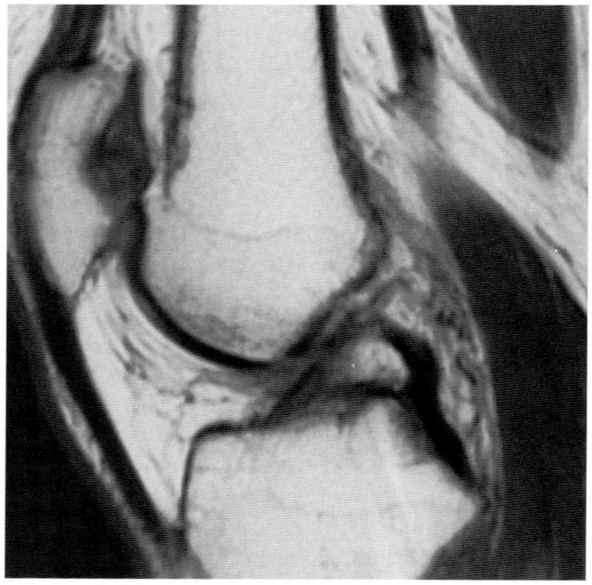

D

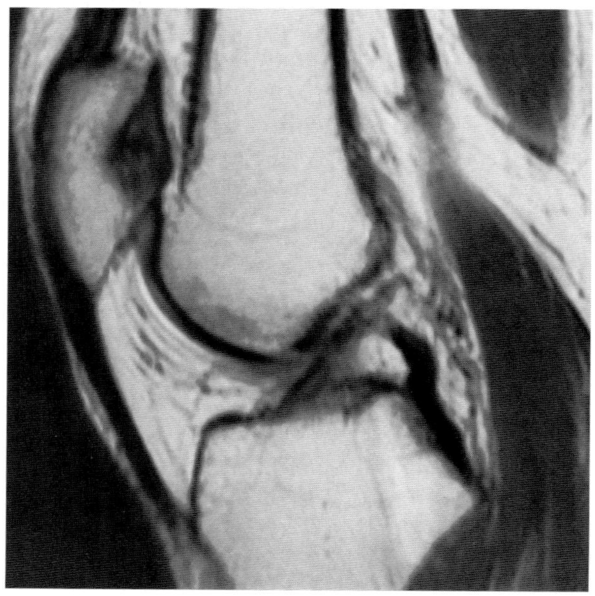

E

FIG. 1-1. Variation of TR and TE in spin-echo sequences. First echo images **(A–E)** have a superior signal-to-noise ratio, and fat is of higher signal compared with second echo images. **A**, TR, 400 ms; TE, 20 ms; **B** TR, 600 ms; TE, 20 ms; **C**, TR, 1200 ms; TE, 20 ms; **D**, TR, 1800 ms; TE, 20 ms; **E**, TR, 2400 ms; TE, 20 ms.

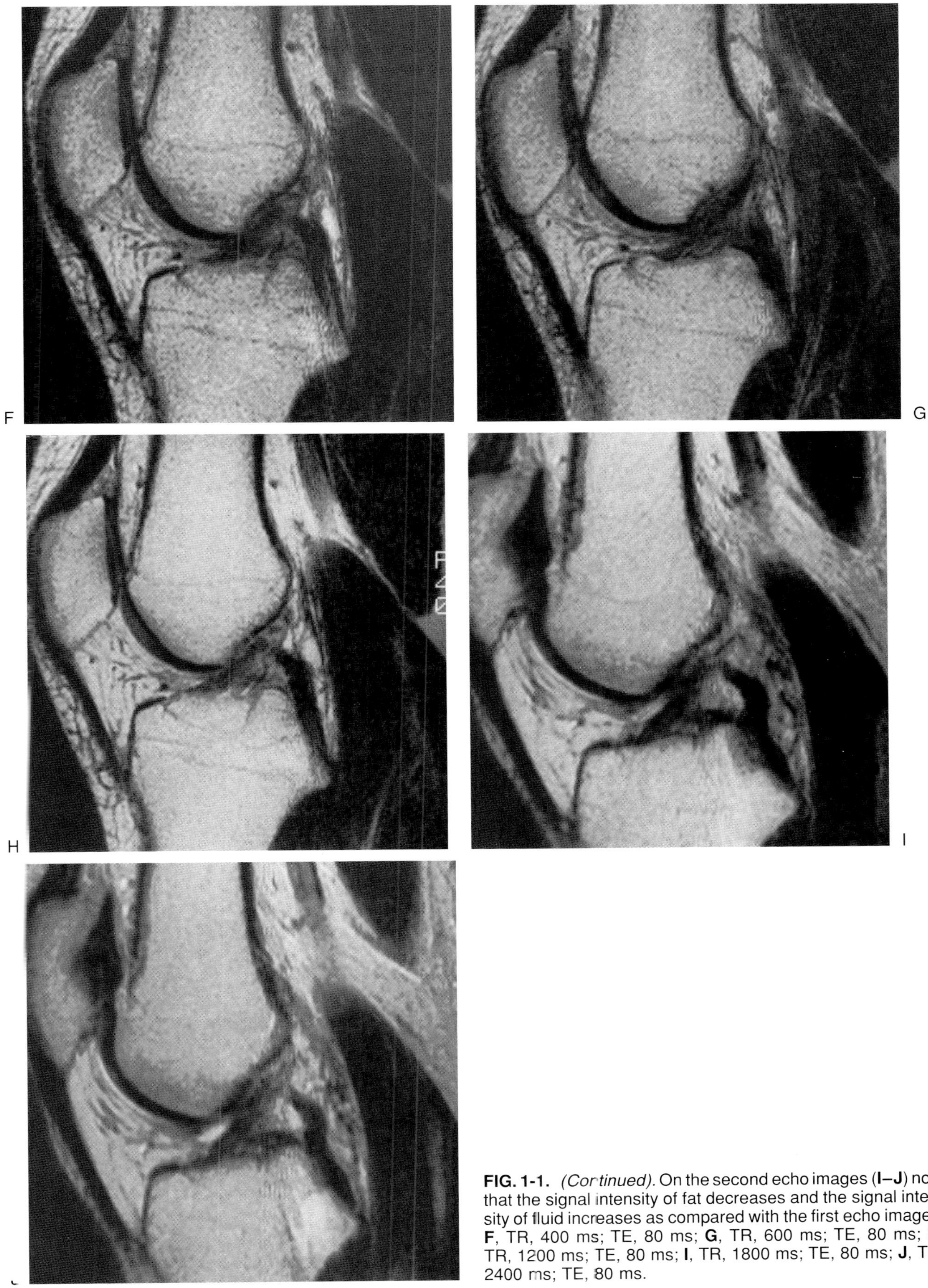

FIG. 1-1. *(Continued).* On the second echo images (**I–J**) note that the signal intensity of fat decreases and the signal intensity of fluid increases as compared with the first echo images. **F**, TR, 400 ms; TE, 80 ms; **G**, TR, 600 ms; TE, 80 ms; **H**, TR, 1200 ms; TE, 80 ms; **I**, TR, 1800 ms; TE, 80 ms; **J**, TR, 2400 ms; TE, 80 ms.

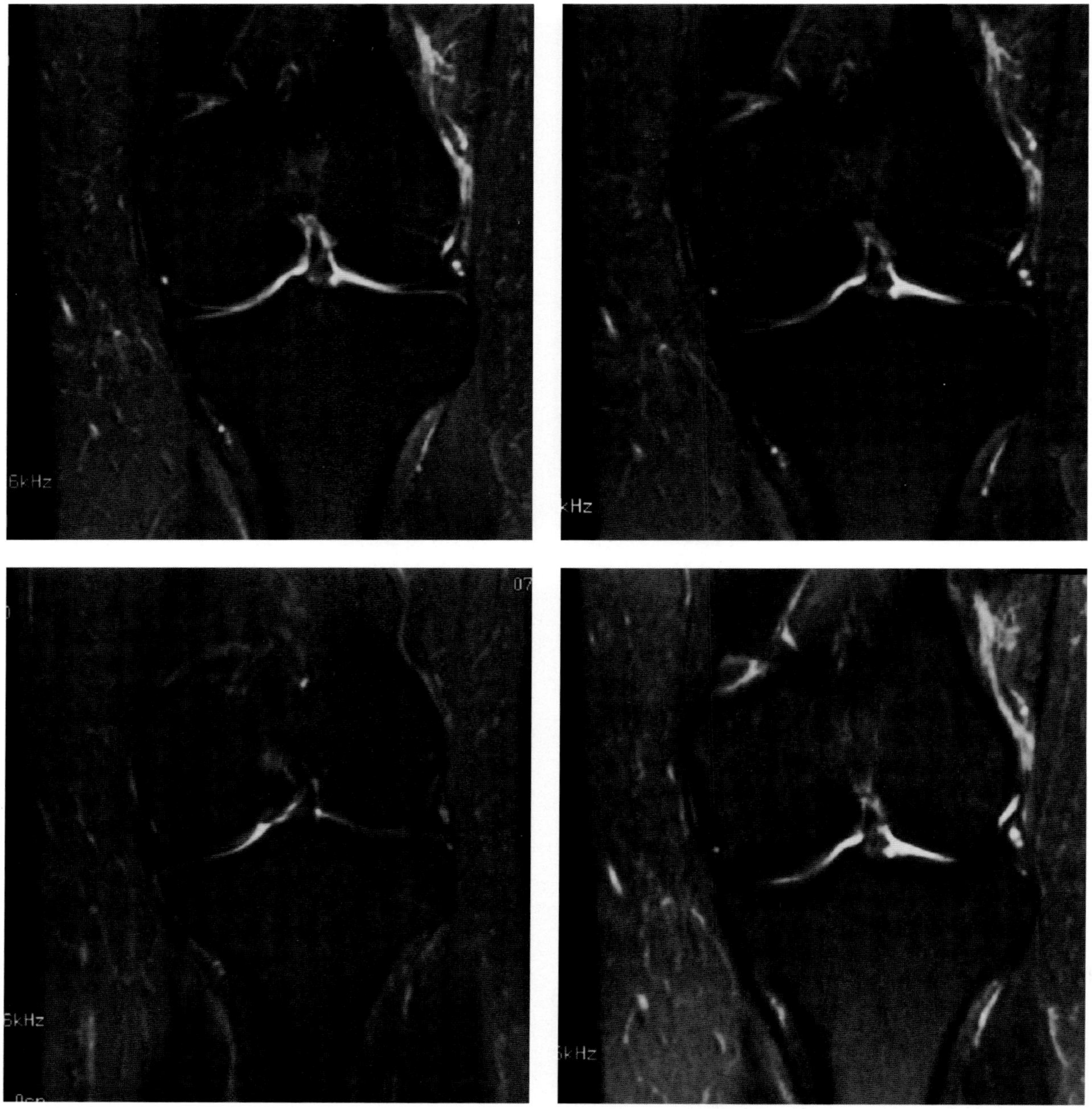

A B C D

FIG. 1-2. Effect of increased echo train length on spatial resolution in fast spin-echo imaging. All images were obtained with TR, 3000 ms; TE, 57–76 ms, and frequency-selective fat saturation. Note the progressive loss of spatial resolution in the phase-encoded direction (supero-inferior) as echo train length increases. **A**, echo train length, 4; **B**, echo train length, 8; **C**, echo train length, 16; **D**, echo train length, 32.

resolution may put fast spin-echo images at a disadvantage compared to conventional spin-echo images for detection of meniscal tears (18).

A disadvantage of fast spin-echo imaging in evaluation of knee disorders is that fat retains high signal intensity on T2-weighted images, thus reducing the conspicuity of fluid and edema. This disadvantage can be overcome by using frequency-selective fat saturation techniques (see later), which do not significantly increase the imaging time. Fast spin-echo imaging with fat saturation is an excellent method of rapidly acquiring T2-weighted images with high conspicuity of bone marrow edema (Fig. 1-3) and fluid around injured soft-tissue structures (Fig. 1-4) (19,20).

Gradient-Echo Sequences

Gradient-echo pulse sequences consist of a slice-selective RF pulse (usually producing less than 90° tip of the protons)

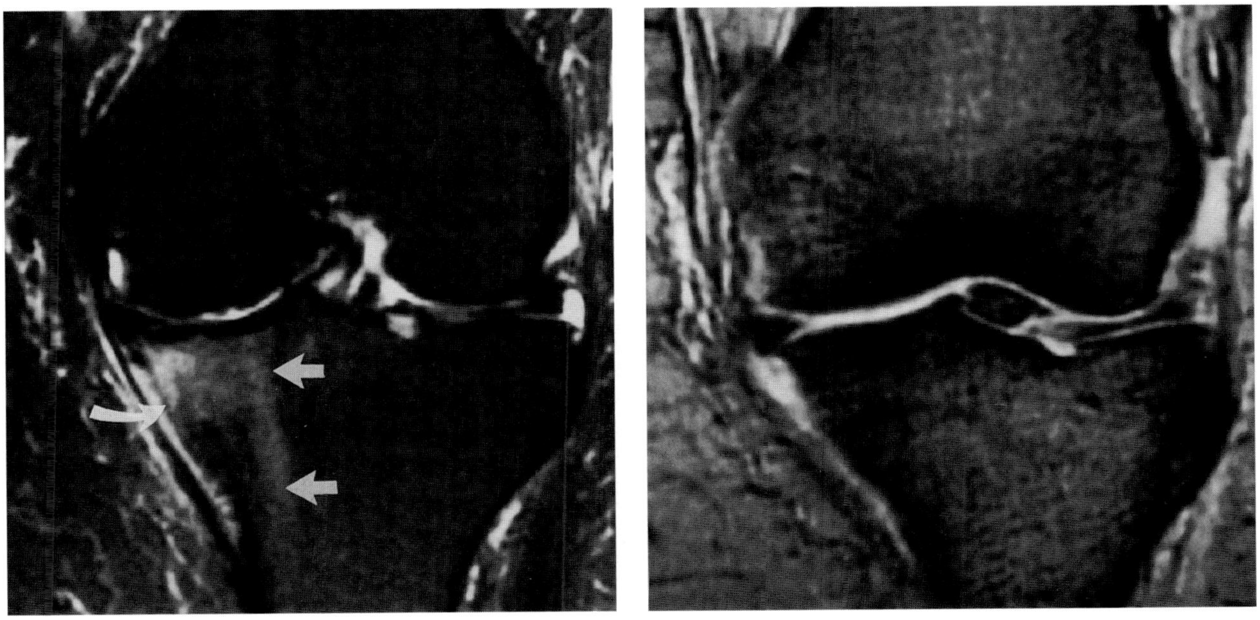

A B

FIG. 1-3. Increased conspicuity of bone marrow edema on **(A)** T2-weighted fat-saturated fast spin-echo images as compared with **(B)** $T2^*$-weighted gradient-echo images. The bone marrow edema in the medial tibial plateau is obvious on the fat-saturated fast spin-echo images *(arrows)* and is not visible on the gradient-echo image. Fluid under collateral ligament (*curved arrow*). The bone marrow edema was due to an insufficiency fracture of the tibial plateau.

followed by a gradient field reversal that refocuses the spins and produces a signal. The main difference between gradient-echo and spin-echo sequences is the absence of a 180° refocusing pulse. Thus, magnetic field inhomogeneities, chemical shifts, and susceptibility gradients will cause signal loss in gradient echo imaging, whereas in spin-echo imaging these static field inhomogeneities are canceled by the 180° pulse. In gradient-echo imaging, proton dephasing (transverse relaxation) is affected by both intrinsic tissue T2 decay and magnetic field inhomogeneities, and is referred to as $T2^*$ decay.

The single most influential parameter in gradient-echo im-

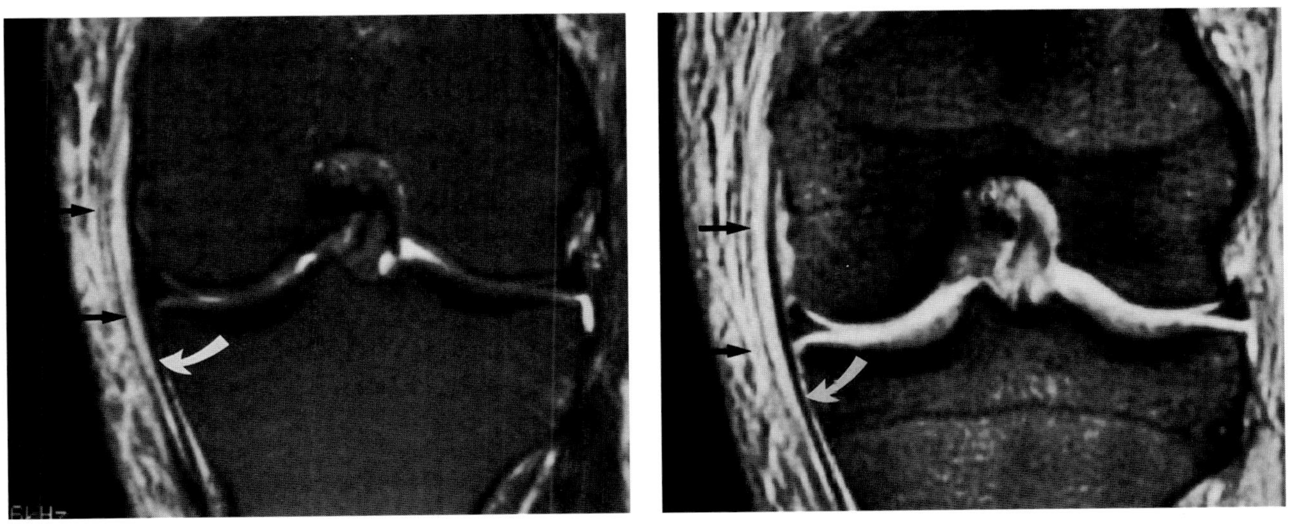

A B

FIG. 1-4. Increased conspicuity of soft-tissue edema on **(A)** T2-weighted fat-saturated fast spin-echo images as compared with **(B)** $T2^*$-weighted gradient echo images. The edema around the disrupted superficial layer *(black arrows)* of the medial collateral ligament is visible on both images but is much more conspicuous in **(A)** because of increased contrast between fluid signal and fat signal. The deep layer of the medial collateral ligament is intact *(curved white arrow)*.

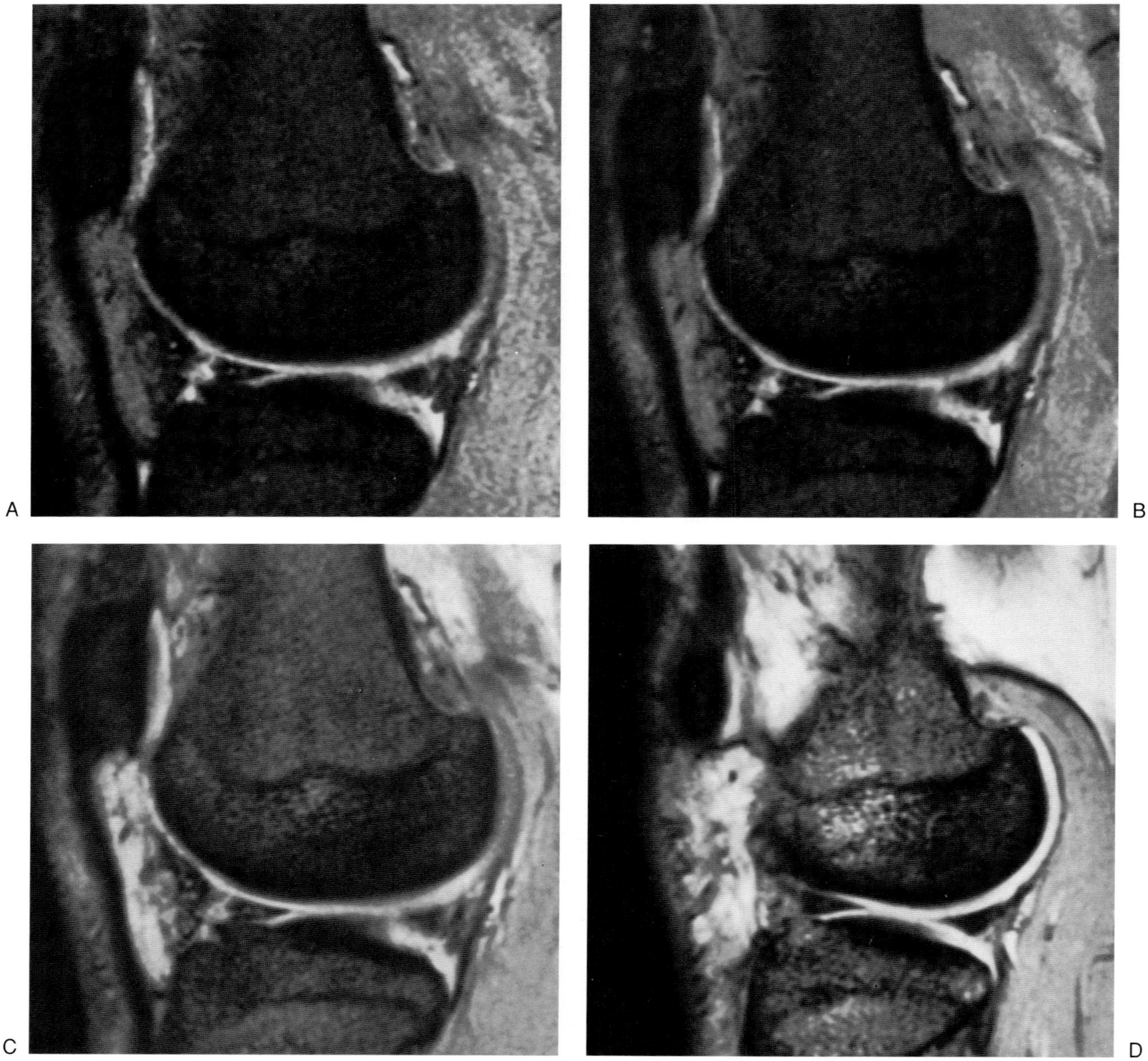

FIG. 1-5. Effect of increasing flip angle on gradient-echo images. Four gradient echo images are shown (TR, 600 ms; TE, 20 ms) with varying flip angles: **A**, 15° ; **B**, 30° ; **C**, 60° ; **D**, 90° . As the flip angle increases, the signal intensity of fat increases relative to that of fluid, indicating increased T1-weighting.

aging is the flip angle (Fig. 1-5). The flip angle, TR, and TE determine the relative T1- versus T2-weighting of a gradient-echo image (21–24). A flip angle near 90°, combined with a long TR (300–500 msec) and a short TE (<15 msec) will provide T1-weighted images. These images provide high contrast between fat and muscle but poor differentiation of bone and cartilage. A small flip angle (10–20°) combined with a long TR (>200 msec) and a long TE (>15 msec) will produce a T2*-weighted image. These images provide excellent visualization of joint fluid (i.e., arthrographic effect); however, fluid and cartilage have similar signal intensity and are difficult to resolve. The signal-to-noise ratio decreases as TE is lengthened and as TR is shortened (Fig. 1-6). Intermediate flip angles provide a middle ground and have been recommended when it is not desirable to emphasize one component over the other (25,26). Thus, intermediate flip angles, ranging from approximately 30 to 40°, permit all components of the knee joint and surrounding tissues to be adequately evaluated, and because the signal-to-noise ratio is relatively good, anatomic detail is largely preserved (24).

The main advantage of gradient-echo techniques is that

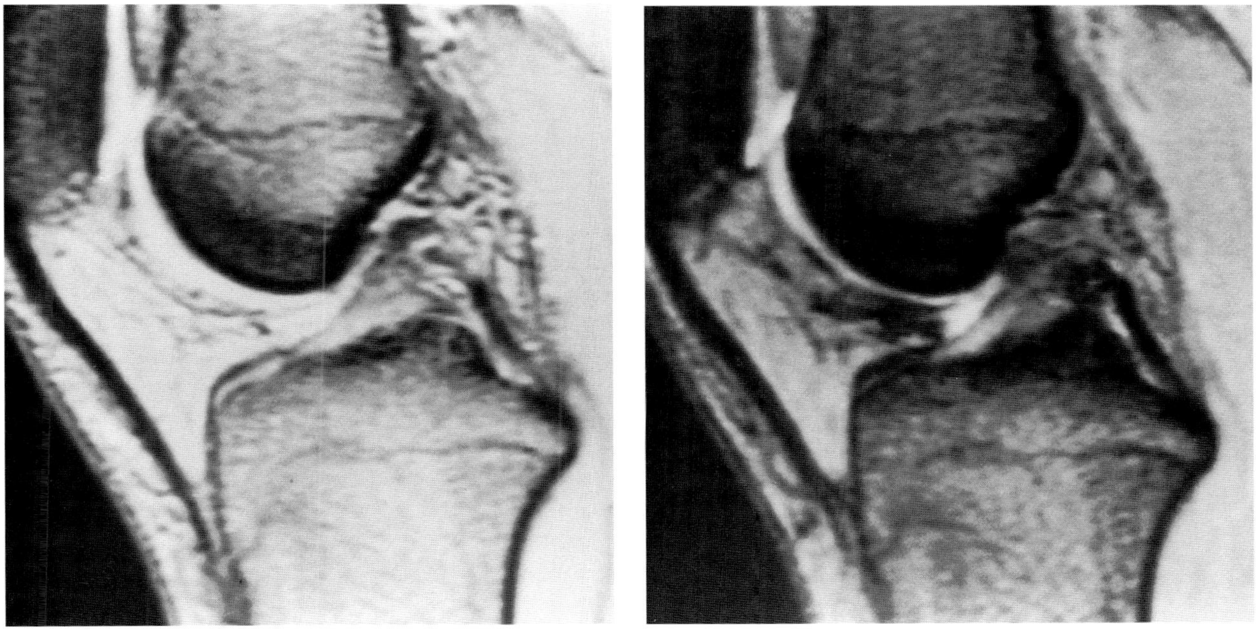

A B

FIG. 1-6. Effect of TR on gradient-echo images. Both images were obtained with a flip angle of 30° and a TE of 13 ms. **(A)** TR, 150 ms; **(B)** TR, 800 ms.

images with T2*-weighting can be acquired more rapidly than is possible with spin-echo T2-weighted sequences. Gradient-echo T2*-weighted sequences are quicker than spin-echo T2-weighted sequences because the TR is much shorter and because the reduced flip angle requires a shorter RF pulse. The rapidity of gradient-echo sequences allows high-resolution, thin-section, or volumetric imaging to be performed in a tolerable amount of time (17–24).

A wide variety of gradient-echo techniques are available, unfortunately the nomenclature and acronyms are not standardized among the MR manufacturers (27). The most useful gradient-echo techniques for evaluation of knee disorders include basic gradient-echo techniques (28), "steady-state" techniques (29–32), and "spoiled gradient-echo" techniques (Table 1-1) (33,34). Basic gradient-echo techniques are primarily used to rapidly acquire images with T2* contrast. In basic gradient-echo imaging, the combination of the TR and flip angle causes the longitudinal magnetization to reach equilibrium; the transverse magnetization decays during the relatively long TR and does not contribute to subsequent signals. Steady-state techniques are characterized by a very short TR (<50 msec) and differ from basic gradient echo in that both the longitudinal and transverse magnetizations are in equilibrium and do contribute to subsequent signals. Spoiled gradient-echo sequences are similar to steady-state sequences but include disruption ("spoiling") of the transverse magnetization after each signal; thus, T1-weighted contrast can be produced.

Although gradient-echo sequences can often replace T2-weighted spin-echo sequences, the images generated are by

TABLE 1-1. *Summary of selected gradient-echo techniques and vendor acryonyms*

Manufacturer	Basic GRE	Steady state	Spoiled GRE
GE Medical Systems (Milwaukee, WI)	MPGR, FS	GRASS	SPGR
Siemens Medical Systems (Iselin, NJ)	FISP		FLASH
Philips Medical Systems (Shelton, CT)	FFE		CE-FFE-T1
Picker International (Highland Hts, OH)	FE, FESUM, FEDIF	FAST	RF-FAST, T1-FAST

Information summarized from Munk PL, Helms CA, Genant HK, Holt RG. Magnetic resonance imaging of the knee: current status, new directions. *Skeletal Radiol* 1989;18:569–577; Elster AD. Gradient-echo MR imaging: techniques and acronyms. *Radiology* 1993;186:1–8.

CE-FFE-T1, contrast-enhanced fast field echo with T1-weighting (Philips); FAST, Fourier acquired steady state (Picker); FE, field echo (Picker); FEDIF, field echo with fat and water signals out of phase (Picker); FESUM, field echo with fat and water signals in phase (Picker); FFE, fast field echo (Philips); FISP, fast imaging with steady-state precession (Siemens); FLASH, fast low-angle shot (Siemens); FS, fast scan (GE, 0.5 T); GRASS, gradient recalled acquisition in the steady state (General Electric); MPGR, multiplanar gradient echo (General Electric, 1.5 T); RF-FAST, RF-spoiled FAST (Picker) SPGR, spoiled GRASS (General Electric); T1-FAST, gradient spoiled FAST with T1 contrast (Picker).

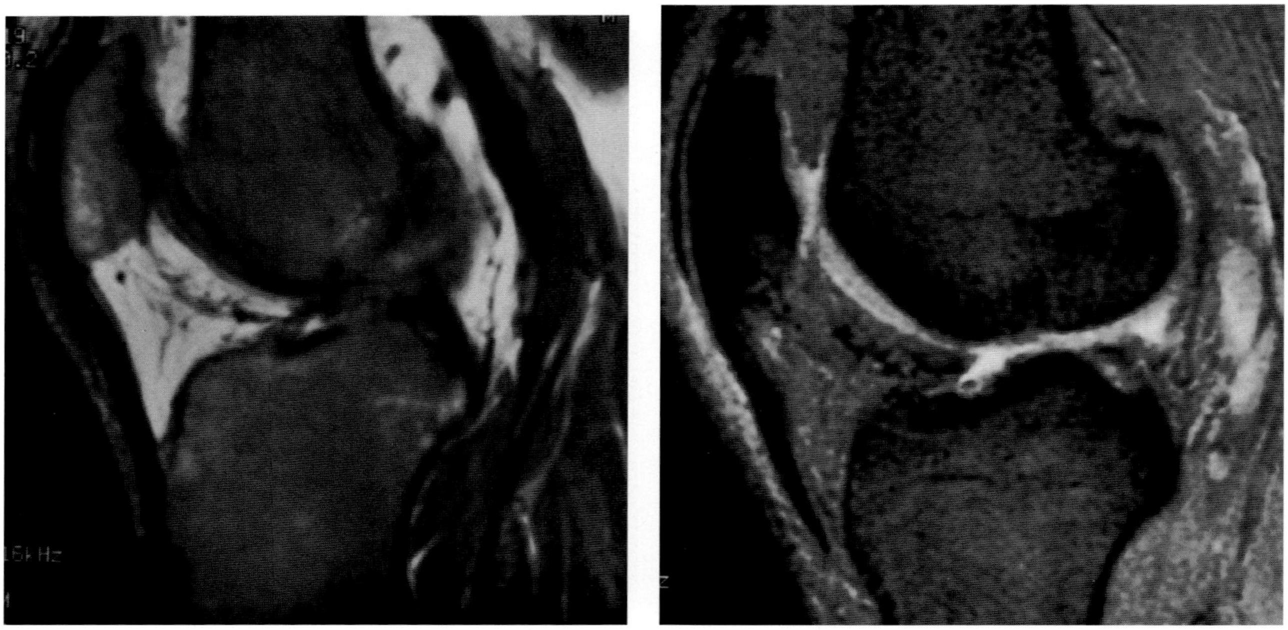

A B

FIG. 1-7. Insensitivity of gradient-echo images to nondestructive bone marrow infiltration. The extensive marrow infiltration due to non-Hodgkin's lymphoma is obvious on a T1-weighted image **(A)** but is not visible on a T2*-weighted gradient-echo image **(B)**.

no means precisely analogous. For instance, on most gradient-echo images, articular cartilage will be of higher signal than on T2-weighted spin-echo images. Corticular bone, normal menisci, and ligaments have low signal on both T2*-weighted gradient-echo and T2-weighted spin-echo images. The appearance of bone marrow on gradient-echo images is complex and depends on the content of trabecular bone within the marrow cavity. Bone trabeculae cause loss of signal on gradient-echo images because of magnetic susceptibility effects; the degree of signal loss correlates with the number of trabeculae per unit volume and is therefore more marked in the epiphyses than in the diaphyses (35). As a result, gradient-echo images are relatively insensitive to nondestructive bone marrow abnormalities such as bone marrow edema, contusion, and infiltration (Figs. 1-4, 1-7, 1-8) (16).

The signal loss caused by magnetic susceptibility makes gradient-echo images particularly useful in detecting calcifications, hemosiderin, and minute metal fragments in tissues. These substances produce signal voids that appear much larger on gradient-echo images than on spin-echo images (''blooming'').

Three-Dimensional Fourier Transform Imaging

Volume Acquisition Imaging

Three-dimensional Fourier transform imaging (3DFT) involves imaging a volume of tissue rather than a slice, as in conventional spin-echo and gradient-echo techniques. In 3DFT imaging the signal is localized by means of frequency encoding in one plane and phase encoding in the other two planes. The major advantage of 3DFT is that very thin image slices (<1 mm) can be acquired without interslice gaps. Also, the volumetric image data can be reformatted for viewing in any plane (including oblique, curved, and angled planes) and are ideally suited to 3D viewing and volumetric quantification. Thus, multiple high-resolution images in any desired plane can be obtained from a single imaging sequence (24,25,32,36–43).

The major disadvantage of 3DFT is the long imaging time. 3DFT techniques are best used with gradient-echo techniques, because the short TR times of these techniques allow 3DFT sequences to be performed in reasonable imaging times (28,30–32,41). Minor disadvantages include increased motion and flow artifacts propagated in both phase-encoded directions.

The ultrathin slices generated with 3-D Fourier transform provide excellent spatial resolution of normal anatomy (Fig. 1-9). Meniscal tears and degeneration are well seen, as are the cruciate ligaments. The menisci and ligaments, which are normally seen as areas of low to virtually absent signal with spin-echo sequences, almost invariably have areas of intermediate to high signal with this technique. Articular cartilage can also be assessed easily, and the patellar cartilage can be well visualized even without the use of axial images because volume averaging does not pose a problem. Fat-saturated spoiled gradient recalled acquisition in the steady state (GRASS) sequences provide excellent depiction of articular cartilage with 3DFT techniques (Fig. 1-10) (24,44). Loose bodies may be identified more readily on

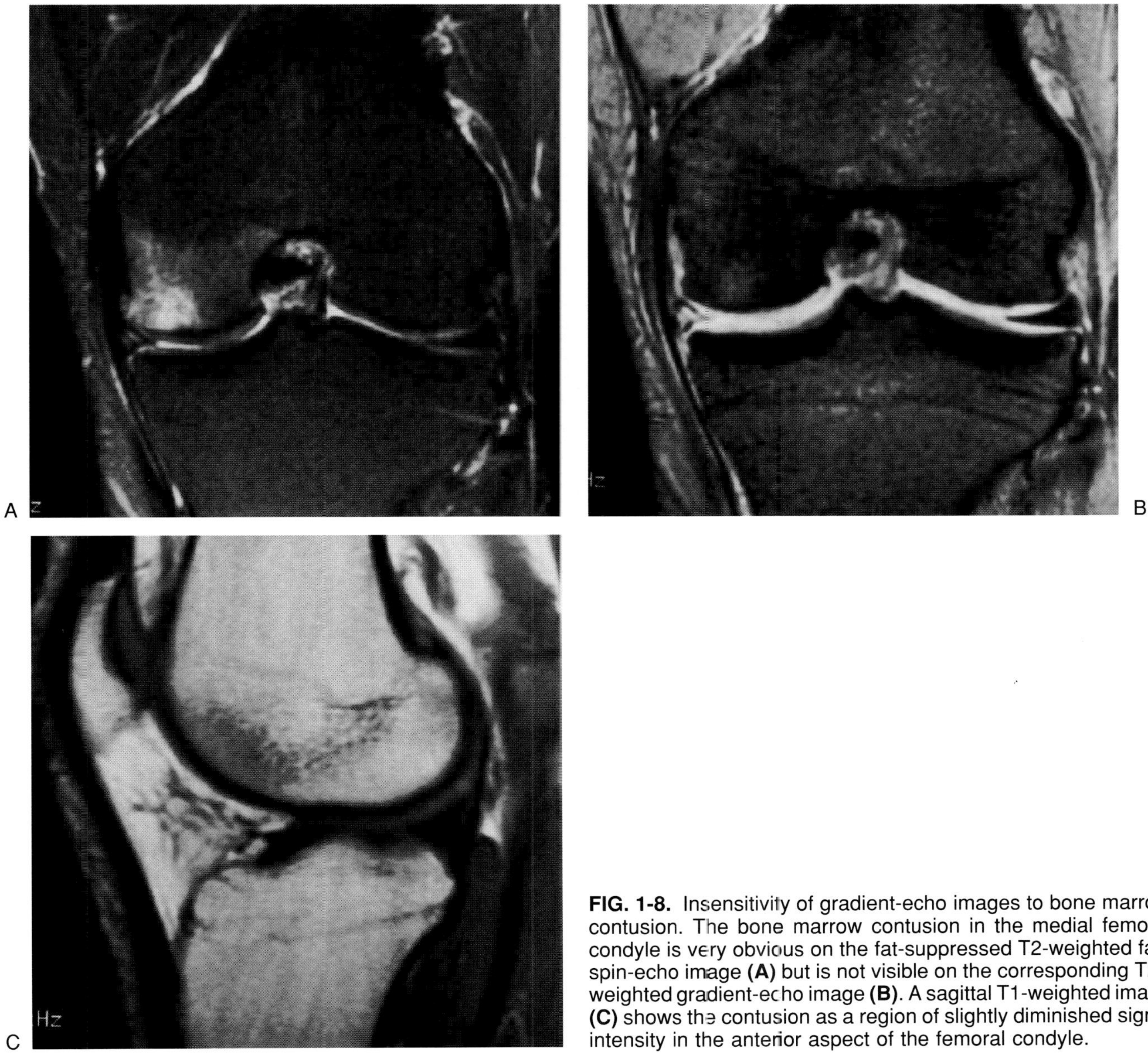

FIG. 1-8. Insensitivity of gradient-echo images to bone marrow contusion. The bone marrow contusion in the medial femoral condyle is very obvious on the fat-suppressed T2-weighted fast spin-echo image **(A)** but is not visible on the corresponding T2*-weighted gradient-echo image **(B)**. A sagittal T1-weighted image **(C)** shows the contusion as a region of slightly diminished signal intensity in the anterior aspect of the femoral condyle.

thin slices than on the thicker slices generally used with conventional sequences.

Short-Tau Inversion Recovery Sequences

Short-tau inversion recovery (STIR) sequences consist of a 180° inverting RF pulse followed by a 90°, 180° pulse sequence as in spin-echo imaging. The time between the inverting pulse and the 90° pulse is known as TI (inversion time). Fat and water protons have different T1 relaxation times; thus, there will be a moment when fat protons have no residual magnetization (null point) and water protons have some magnetization remaining (15). Because the inversion time is designed to correspond to the null point of fat, STIR images result in complete suppression of fat signal. Selection of an inversion time that does not correspond to the null point of fat will result in incomplete fat signal suppression and unusual tissue contrast (Fig. 1-11). The inversion time necessary to correspond to the null point of fat depends on the magnet strength and varies slightly between individuals and within the magnet bore due to minor magnetic field inhomogeneity (45).

Areas of edema or fluid are extremely conspicuous on STIR images because of the suppression of fat signal and the additive T1 and T2 contrast effects. STIR images are most useful in detecting subtle areas of edema in traumatic, neoplastic, or inflammatory conditions. The main disadvantages of STIR sequences are the long imaging time, lower spatial resolution, and poor signal-to-noise ratios (14).

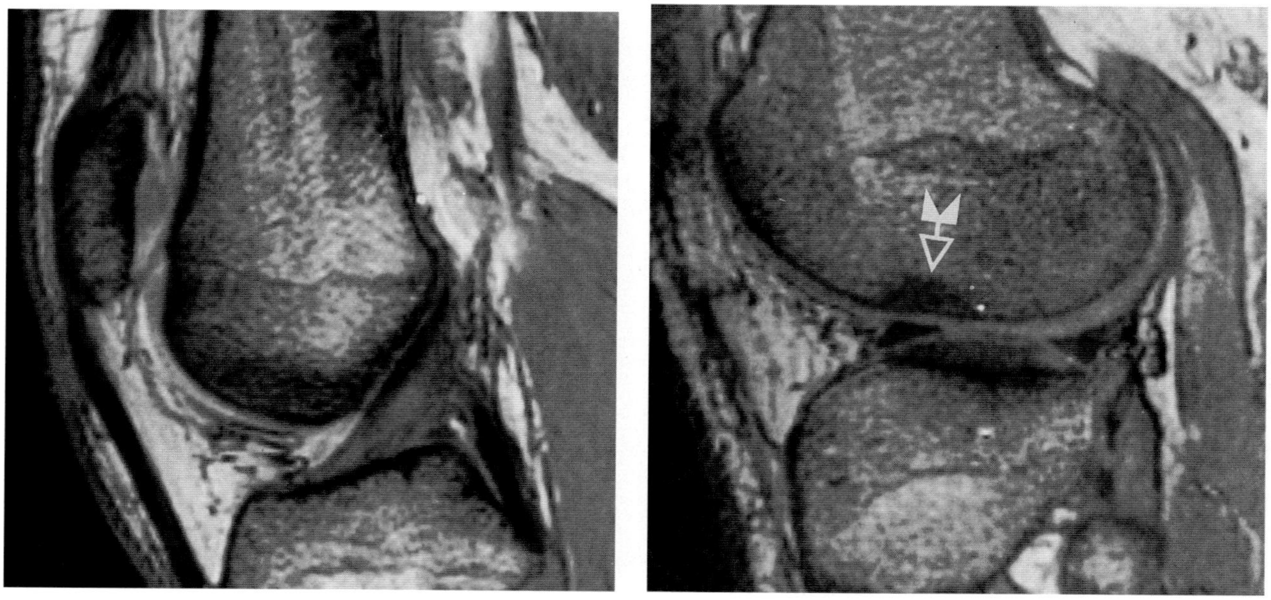

A

B

FIG. 1-9. Volumetric (3-D Fourier transform) imaging. Shown are two sagittal images 2 mm thick through **(A)** the intercondylar notch with excellent demonstration of the anterior cruciate ligament and **(B)** the lateral meniscus. Incidentally seen in **(B)** is a low-signal region *(arrow)* representing a subchondral infraction.

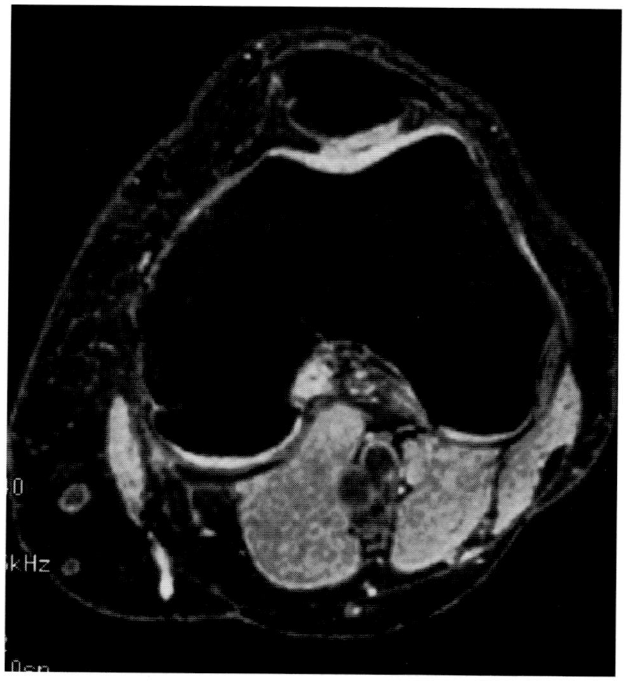

FIG. 1-10. Three-dimensional Fourier transform volumetric imaging of articular cartilage. A 1-mm-thick axial slice shows excellent spatial resolution of patellofemoral articular cartilage. A fat-saturated spoiled GRASS sequence was used with the following parameters: TR, 60 ms; TE, 7 ms; flip angle 40°.

Fast STIR techniques have recently been developed to reduce the long imaging times necessary for STIR imaging. Fast STIR sequences consist of initial 180° (inverting) and 90° pulses, followed by a train of 180° pulses, analogous to fast spin-echo techniques. Fast STIR techniques allow rapid acquisition of images with contrast features similar to STIR and better coverage because more slices can be obtained within the long TR. The disadvantage of fast STIR is a loss of spatial resolution with longer echo trains and shorter imaging times (Fig. 1-12) (46).

FAT-SUPPRESSION TECHNIQUES

Suppression of fat signal is often desirable in knee MR imaging, particularly to make high signal intensity edema and fluid more conspicuous on T2-weighted images as compared to adjacent fat. Fat suppression has been shown to increase the detection of bone marrow contusions (19,20), and it can be used to increase the conspicuousness of gadolinium-enhanced tissues, to prove the presence of fat within lipomatous tumors, and to reduce motion artifacts and chemical-shift artifacts (14,15,47). Fat suppression is particularly valuable with T2-weighed fast spin-echo sequences, as fat retains high signal intensity on these images and is difficult to distinguish from fluid in the absence of fat suppression.

The most commonly available techniques for fat suppression are chemical-shift selective presaturation, phase-contrast methods, and STIR imaging (discussed earlier). Within any magnetic field, fat protons resonate at a slightly different frequency than water protons. The chemical-shift selective

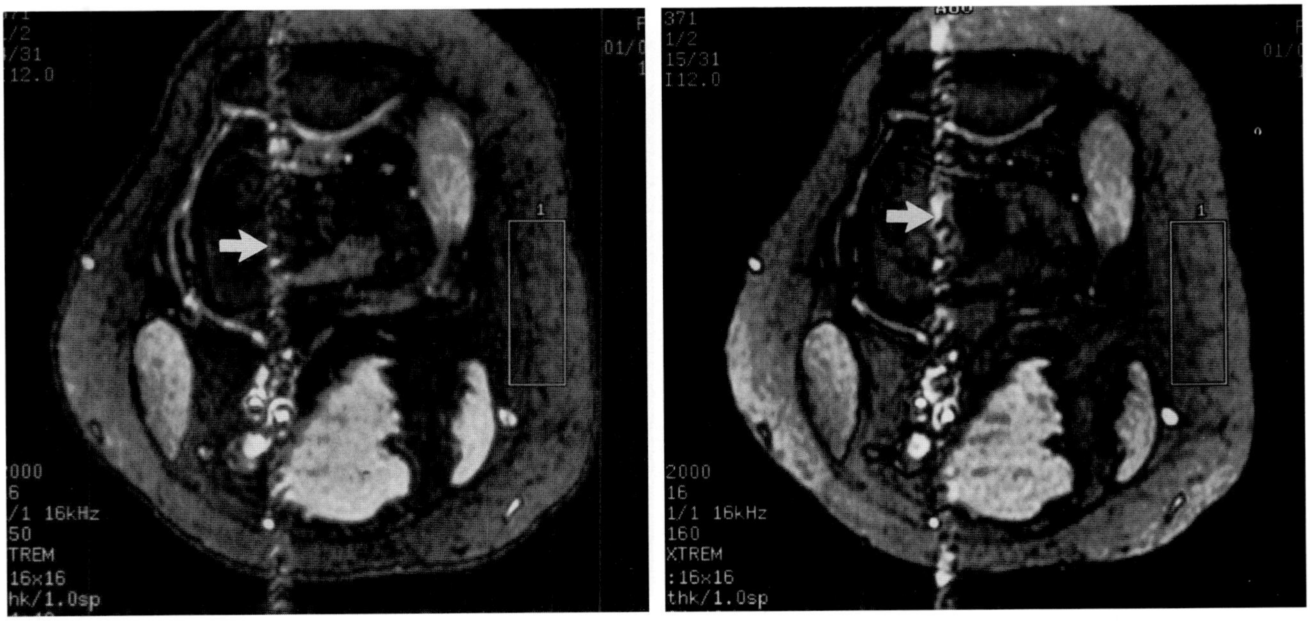

A B

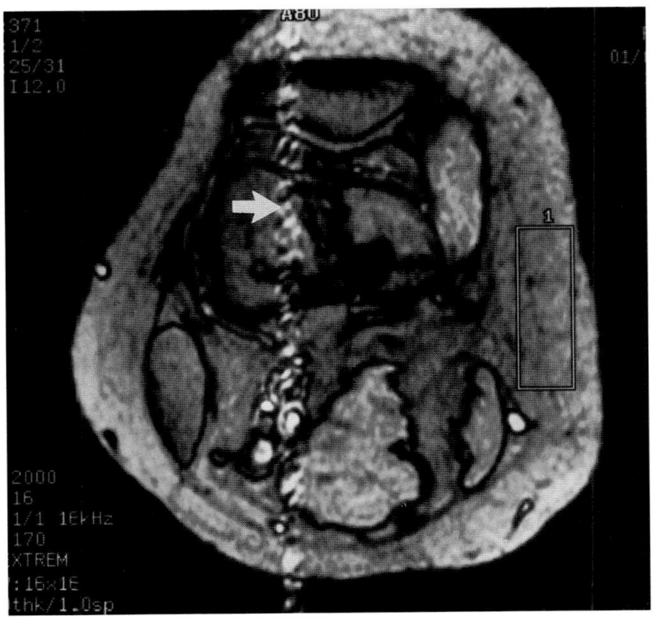

C

FIG. 1-11. Effect of various inversion times on fat signal in STIR imaging. The images were obtained with inversion times of **(A)** 150 ms; **(B)** 160 ms; **(C)** 170 ms. Note that the fat signal is well suppressed in **(A)**, whereas in **(C)**, the signal of fat is nearly equal to that of muscle and fluid. Also note the prominent linear artifact arising from phase encoding misregistration of flow in the popliteal artery *(white arrow)*.

presaturation method uses RF pulses tuned to the resonance frequency of fat protons to saturate the fat protons prior to the imaging pulse sequence. This method requires an extremely uniform magnetic field, because slight field inhomogeneities will alter the expected resonance frequencies of fat protons and water protons, leading to a failure of fat saturation (16). The uniformity of fat suppression can be improved by placing bags of water or kaolin around the body part being imaged (48). Incomplete fat saturation is the major problem encountered with chemical-shift selective presaturation. Other disadvantages of this method are slight increases in imaging time and RF power deposition in the tissues (15).

Phase-contrast techniques are based on sampling the tissue signal at moments when the fat protons and water protons are in phase and out of phase (14). The Dixon technique requires acquisition of two image data sets and postprocessing combination of the data to provide a fat-suppressed image; the disadvantages of this technique are the long imaging times and image misregistration due to patient movement during or between the two imaging sequences. The "chopper" fat-suppression technique acquires tissue signal at a moment when the fat and water protons are out of phase, thus producing a fat-suppressed image. "Chopper" fat-suppression techniques do not increase imaging time and

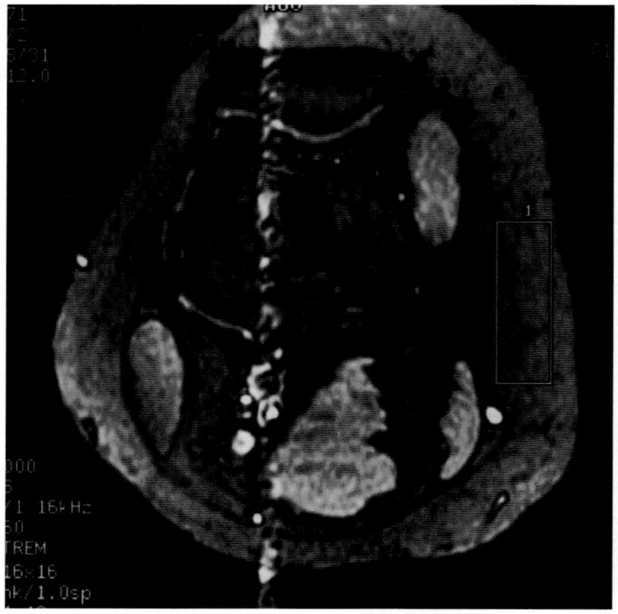
A

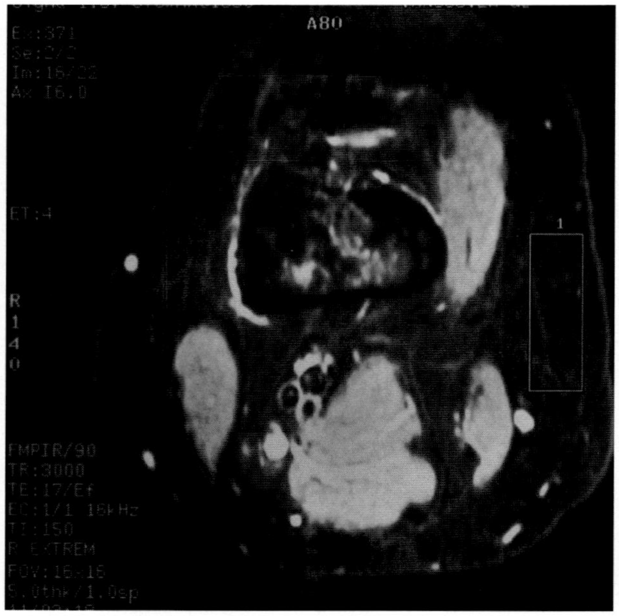
B

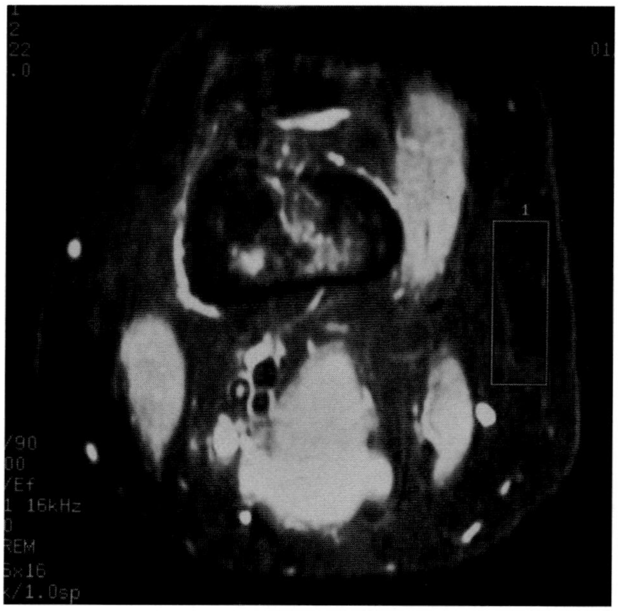
C

FIG. 1-12. The effect of echo train length on spatial resolution in fast STIR imaging: **(A)** standard STIR image; **(B)** fast STIR image with echo train length of four; **(C)** fast STIR image with echo train length of eight. Note that the use of longer echo trains causes a loss of spatial resolution but does not significantly affect the suppression of fat signal.

have been shown to provide good anatomic detail and improved visualization of cartilage, as compared to spin-echo sequences (49).

IMAGING COILS

Imaging coils transmit the RF pulse to the tissue being imaged and receive the RF signal from the patient. Optimal knee MR imaging is currently performed with a circumferential send–receive extremity coil. These coils provide adequate depth penetration, uniform signal intensity across the image, and good signal-to-noise performance. Circumferential knee coils allow a maximal field-of-view of 16–20 cm, which is adequate for complete visualization of most knee abnormalities. Flat surface coils [also termed *local coils* (50)] can be used for high spatial resolution imaging of superficial structures but can only image small volumes of tissue. With flat surface coils, signal drop-off from deeper tissues produces uneven signal intensity across the image (Fig. 1-13). To avoid this problem Helmholtz-type coils, saddle-shaped coils, and circumferential extremity coils were designed to greatly diminish signal drop-off from deeper structures (51–56). The body coil is unsatisfactory as a receiver because of limited signal-to-noise ratios.

Regardless of the type of coil utilized, an interesting and

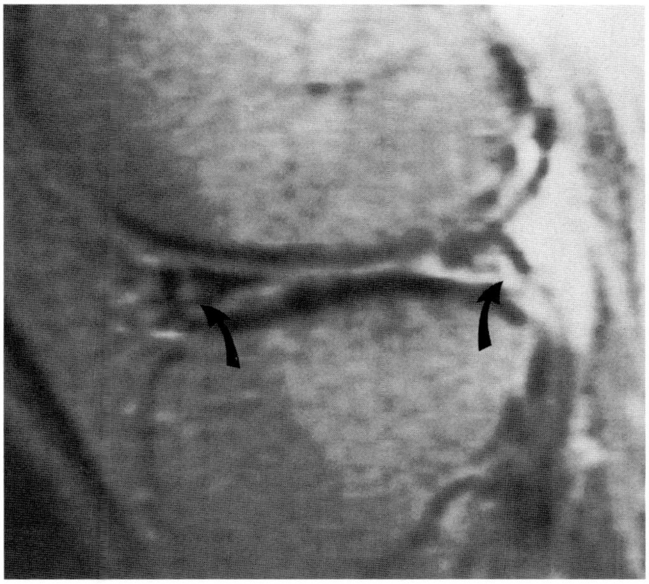

FIG. 1-13. Flat surface coil image. The surface coil has been placed at the posterior aspect of the knee where the signal intensity is greatest. More anteriorly, the signal has dropped off markedly. Incidentally, a bucket-handle tear is present through the lateral meniscus *(arrows)*.

important relationship exists between signal-to-noise ratio and the volume of tissue being imaged by the coil. The coil receives both the MR signal from the tissue (which is primarily dependent on magnet strength, TR, and TE) and randomly fluctuating voltages (noise). The noise arises from random thermal activity in the tissue inducing current in the coil. Coils that image large volumes of tissue receive large amounts of noise and have intrinsically lower signal-to-noise ratios and lower image quality (50,57). Thus, one should use the smallest coil possible to visualize the diagnostically important structures. Recently, "phased-array" coils have been developed; these consist of a group of small surface coils placed around the body. The signals from all the coils are combined to form a single image, which has better signal-to-noise characteristics than an image produced by a single large coil (58). The widespread use of high-field-strength magnets and dedicated extremity coils has allowed considerable improvement in the quality of knee MRI images as compared to use of the body coil for knee imaging.

IMAGING PLANES AND PROTOCOLS

The optimal imaging protocol for any particular case depends on a number of factors, including the clinical problem being investigated, the magnet field strength, the pulse sequences available, and the familiarity of the interpreting radiologist with the appearance of normal and abnormal findings on various imaging sequences. Despite these constraints, standard knee-imaging protocols can be developed that provide excellent depiction of most knee abnormalities in a reasonable amount of imaging time (see Table 1-2). This section will discuss our basic MR imaging protocol for the evaluation of knee trauma.

TABLE 1-2. *Suggested protocols for routine knee imaging*

Protocol	Sagittal	Transverse	Coronal
A	T1 and T2*	T2* or FSE-T2	T2* or FSE-T2
B	PD and T2	T2* or FSE-T2	T2* or FSE-T2

Frequency-selective fat saturation is best used with transverse or coronal FSE sequences. A sagittal 3DFT sequence is optional in both protocols and is used when high-resolution images of cartilage or menisci are desired. STIR sequences are also optional and are most useful in evaluating tumors or inflammatory processes.

The sagittal plane is ideal for evaluating the cruciate ligaments and menisci, as well as the patella, patellar tendon, quadriceps, and quadriceps tendon (Fig. 1-14). The biceps femoris, semimembranosus, semitendinosus, and gastrocnemius muscles and tendons are also visualized. The femoral and tibial hyaline articular cartilage may be assessed; however, partial volume averaging due to the obliquity of the posterior patellar facets makes assessment of the patellar cartilage difficult on sagittal images. Visualization of the entire length of the anterior cruciate ligament on a single image usually requires 5–15° of external rotation of the knee or the use of an oblique sagittal imaging plane (59). The correct obliquity can be determined from a transverse image (60) or from an external stabilization device attached to the patient's leg (61). For optimal evaluation of the menisci and cruciate ligaments in the sagittal plane, two pulse sequences are necessary—namely, a T1- weighted or proton-density-weighted sequence and a T2-weighted or T2*-weighted sequence. The most efficient methods of acquiring the two sagittal sequences are a dual-echo spin-echo sequence providing both proton density and T2-weighted images, or a T1-weighted spin-echo sequence and a T2*-weighted gradient-echo sequence.

The coronal plane is essential in evaluation of the collateral ligaments (Fig. 1-15). It also provides a second look at the menisci and cruciate ligaments, although it is unusual to demonstrate an abnormality of these structures that cannot be detected on sagittal images. Meniscal cysts, particularly small ones, and discoid menisci are possible exceptions to this. The meniscofemoral, meniscotibial, and capsular ligaments; the pes anserinus; and the iliotibial band are best seen in the coronal plane. T2-weighted or T2*-weighted sequences are essential for adequate assessment of the collateral ligaments and are ideal for depicting meniscal cysts and pes anserinus bursitis (62). Fat suppression is helpful, because it increases the conspicuity of edema and fluid collections. T1-weighted coronal images are of very limited value and are not recommended (63).

The transverse plane is usually used as a localizer in programming in sequences in the other planes. It also offers the best view of the patellar cartilage and should be used when

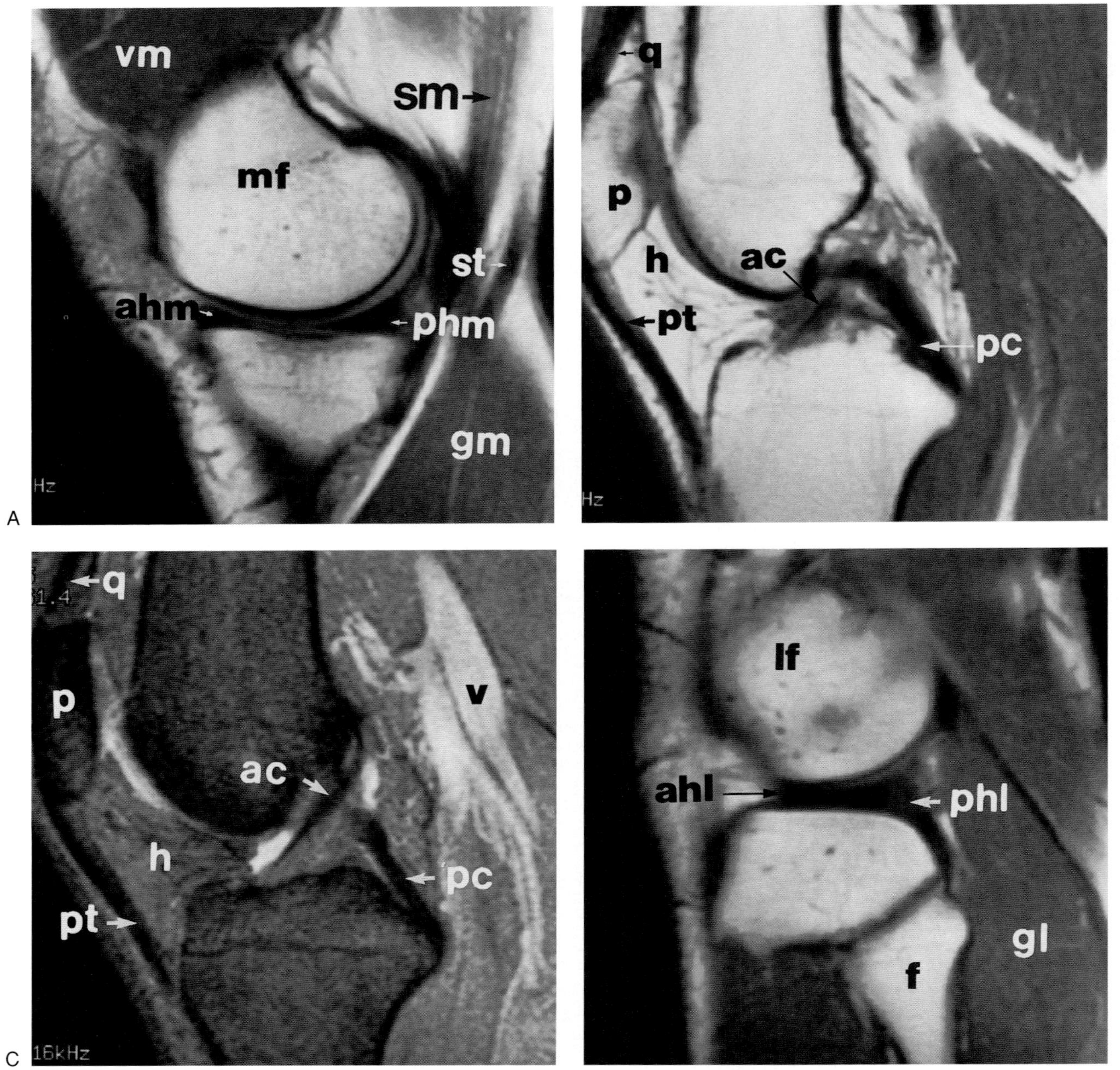

FIG. 1-14. Normal knee anatomy in the sagittal plane. Sagittal images through the medial compartment **(A)**, intercondylar notch **(B,C)**, and lateral compartment **(D)**. Images A, B, and D are T1-weighted; image C is T2*-weighted. ac, anterior cruciate ligament; ahl, anterior horn of lateral meniscus; ahm, anterior horn of medial meniscus; f, fibula; gl, gastrocnemius lateral head; gm, gastrocnemius medial head; h, Hoffa's fat pad; lf,lateral femoral condyle; mf, medial femoral condyle; pt, patellar tendon; p, patella; pc, posterior cruciate ligament; phl, posterior horn lateral meniscus; phm, posterior horn medial meniscus; q, quadriceps tendon; sm, semimembranosus tendon; st, semitendinosus tendon; v, popliteal vessels; vm, vastus medialis.

patellar cartilage abnormalities are suspected (Fig. 1-16). This plane can also be useful in delineating popliteal cysts and their relationship to the muscles of the popliteal fossa. Most centers use T2*-weighted gradient-echo sequences in the transverse plane, because this technique provides excellent depiction of patellar cartilage abnormalities (33,64).

Radial imaging may be used to view the meniscus in radial cross section along its entire length (Fig. 1-17). Although radial imaging exquisitely demonstrates meniscal abnormalities, it has not proved superior to sagittal imaging in detecting meniscal pathology apart from small central tears of questionable clinical significance, and it has the drawback

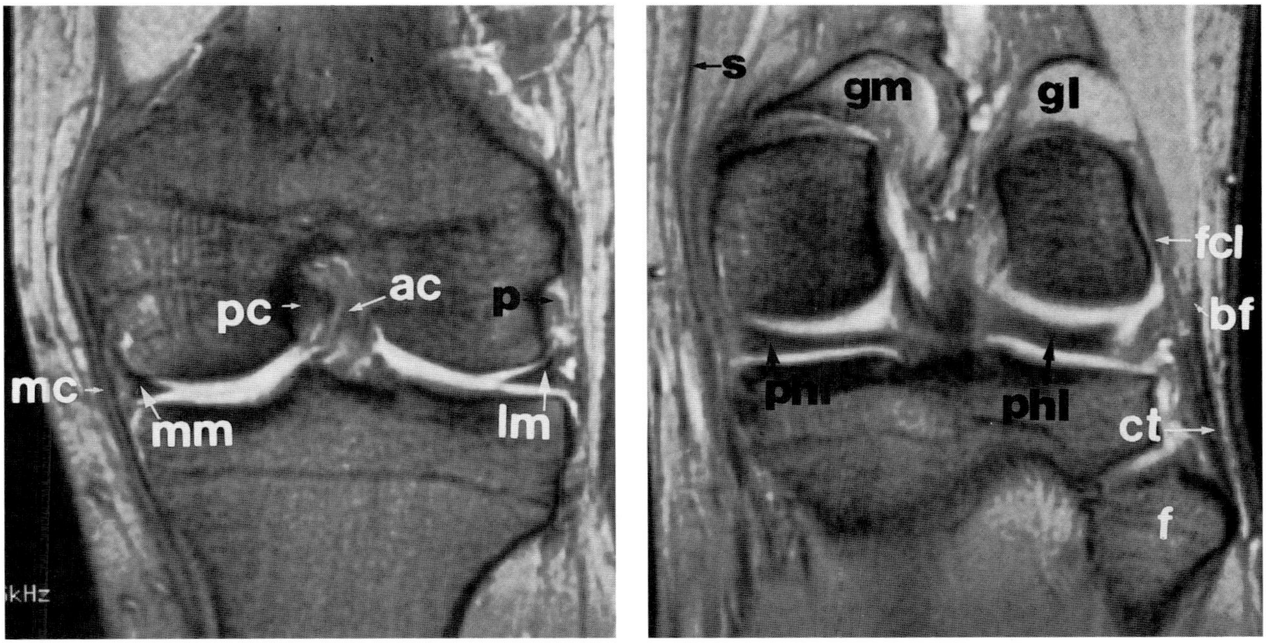

FIG. 1-15. Normal knee anatomy in the coronal plane. Coronal T2*-weighted images through **(A)** the anterior portion of the intercondylar notch, and **(B)** the posterior horns of the menisci. ac, anterior cruciate ligament; bf, biceps femoris tendon; ct, conjoined tendon; f, fibula; fc, fibular collateral ligament; gl, gastrocnemius lateral head; gm, gastrocnemius medial head; lm, lateral meniscus; mc, medial collateral ligament; mm, medial meniscus; p, popliteus tendon; pc, posterior cruciate ligament; phl, posterior horn lateral meniscus; phm, posterior horn medial meniscus; s, sartorius tendon.

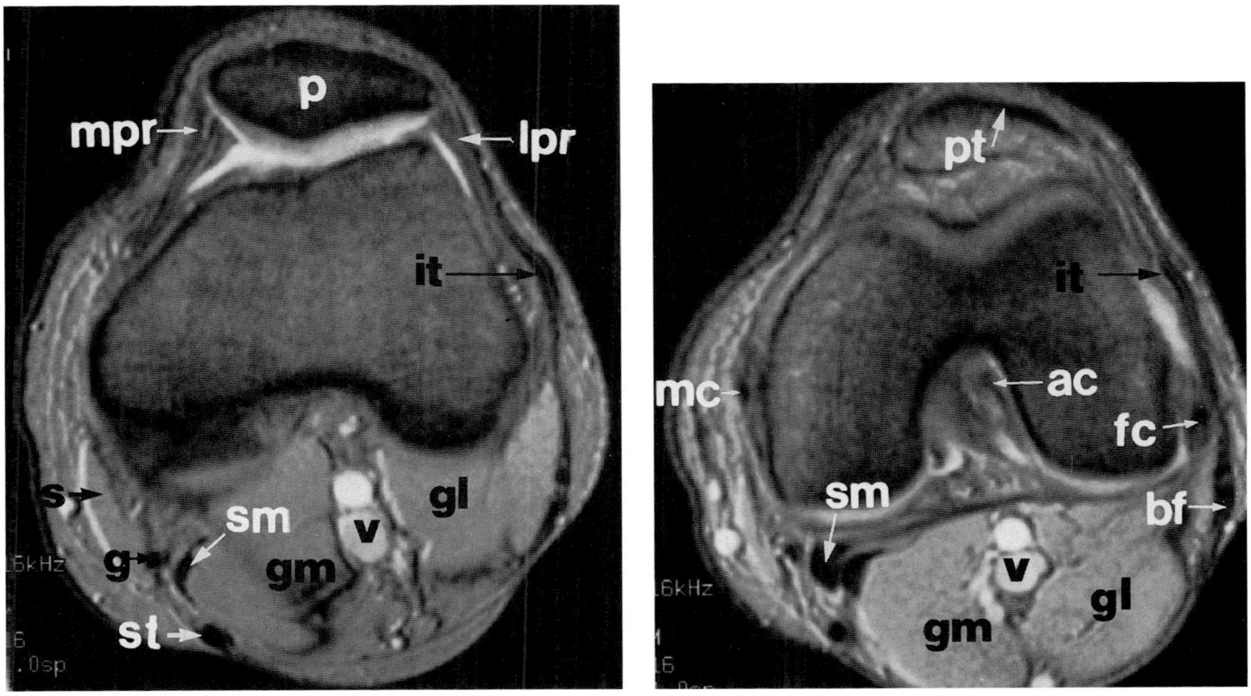

FIG. 1-16. Normal knee anatomy in the transverse plane. Transverse T2*-weighted images through **(A)** the patellofemoral joint and **(B)** the femoral condyles. ac, anterior cruciate ligament; bf, biceps femoris tendon; fc, fibular collateral ligament; g, gracilis; gl, gastrocnemius lateral head; gm, gastrocnemius medial head; it, iliotibial tendon; lpl, lateral patellar retinaculum; mc, medial collateral ligament; mpr, medial patellar retinaculum; p, patella; pt, patellar tendon; s, sartorius; sm, semimembranosus tendon; st, semitendinosus tendon; v, popliteal vessels.

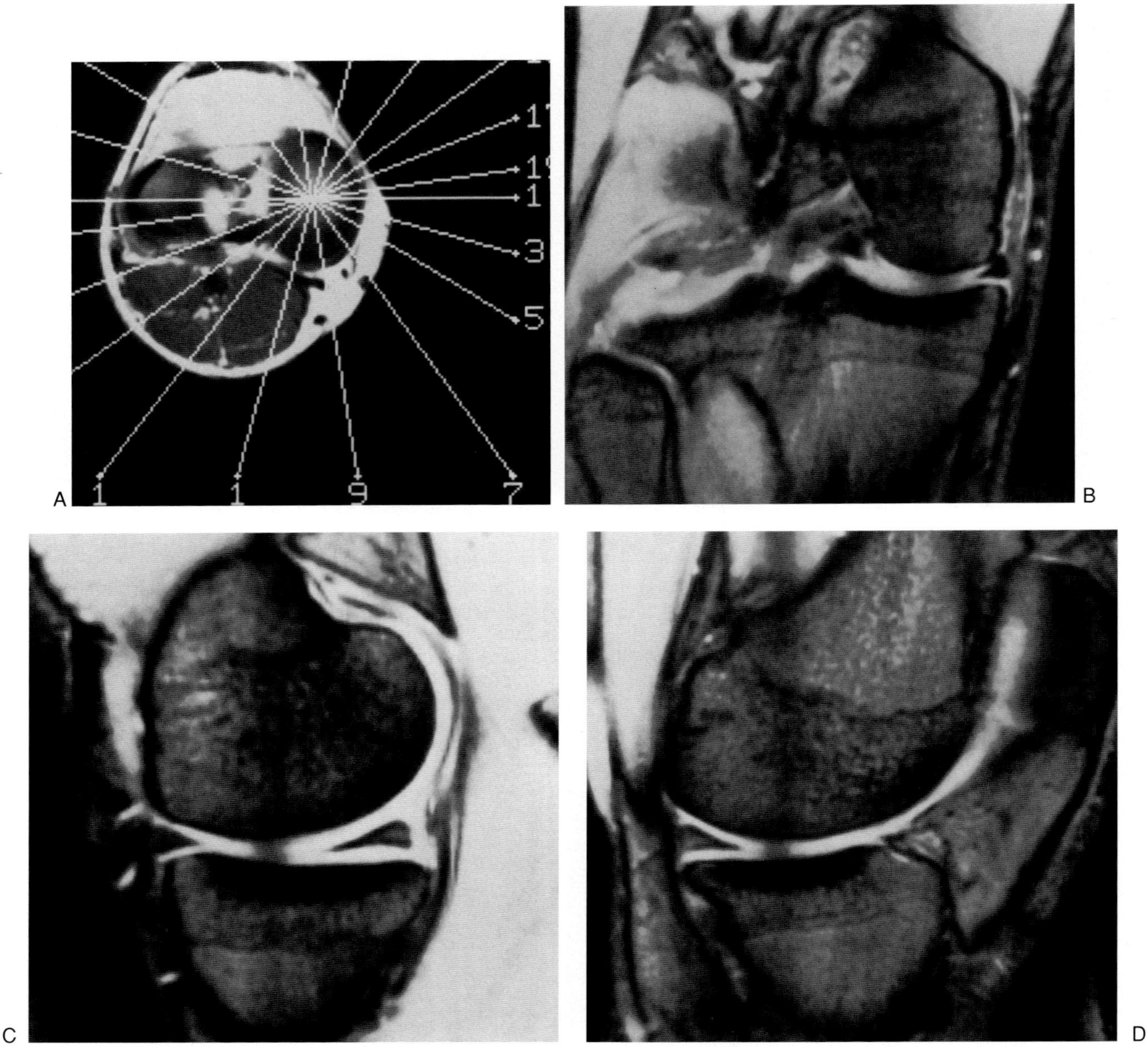

FIG. 1-17. Radial imaging of the knee. **(A)** Radial scout image showing orientation of slices centered at the medial tibial plateau to evaluate the medial meniscus. **(B–F)** Radial images (TR, 500 ms; TE, 19 ms; flip angle 22°) corresponding to slices numbered 17 **(B)**, 11 **(C)**, 7 **(D)**, 5 **(E)**, 1 **(F)**.

of making evaluation of the cruciate ligaments difficult (23,65–68). Thus, most centers rely on sagittal and coronal imaging for meniscal evaluation. If radial sequences are used, separate sequences should be programmed for the lateral and medial menisci, with the axis of rotation being centered at the middle of each tibial plateau. Because one of the characteristic features of images generated with this technique is signal void down the center of the image (representing the location of the axis of rotation), it may be helpful to interleave the sequence because this will partially suppress this artifact. Gradient-echo sequences are preferred for radial imaging; spin-echo sequences may be used but require longer imaging times and have a larger axis of rotation artifact.

A basic concept in the interpretation of knee MR images is that information regarding a particular structure in one should be supplemented with the appearance of the structure in other planes. Evaluation of supplemental imaging planes has been shown to increase the accuracy of assessment of the anterior cruciate ligament (66,67) and menisci (68).

Once the images have been obtained, window levels and widths may be adjusted to best display the structures of inter-

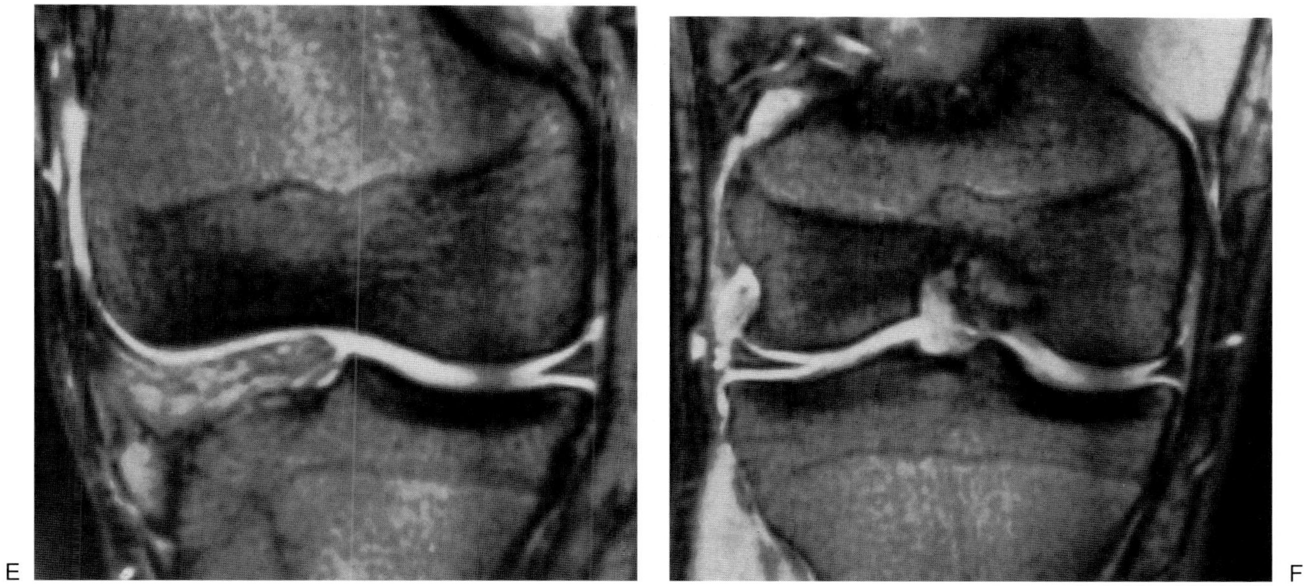

FIG. 1-17. *(Continued).*

est. Many centers use narrow window widths ("meniscal windows") to display meniscal abnormalities, although this technique has not been shown to improve diagnostic accuracy (68). To some degree, selection of window levels and widths is a matter of individual preference and may vary considerably from one institution to the next (Fig. 1-18).

SCAN PARAMETERS

Many of the pulse sequence parameters are variable and operator defined including TR, TE, flip angle, slice thickness, interslice gap, field of view, matrix size, and direction of phase encoding. Specific scan parameter recommenda-

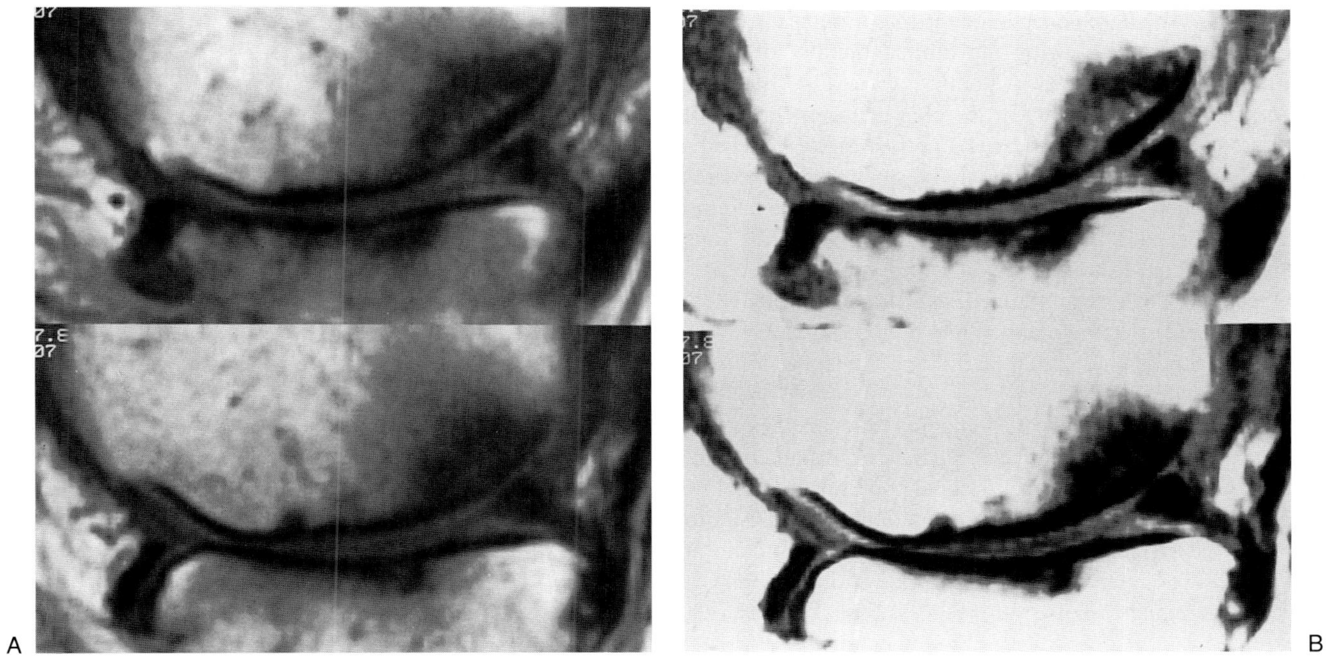

FIG. 1-18. Alteration of display parameters. Both **A** and **B** are the same image, with a much narrower window width ("meniscal windows") in B. In both instances, the meniscal maceration and osteochondral lesion are visible, but they are more obvious in B.

TABLE 1-3. *Typical pulse sequence parameters (at 1.5 T)*

Plane	Slice thickness (mm)	Gap (mm)	TR (msec)	TE (msec)	Flip angle (degrees)	ETL	NEX	MAT
Sagittal T1	4	0–1	800	20	—	—	2	256 × 192
Sagittal T2*	4	0–1	600	20	20–30	—	2	256 × 192
Sagittal 3DFT	0.8–2.0	0	40–50	15–20	20–40	—	1	256 × 256
Sag. PD/T2	4	1	2000	30, 80	—	—	2	256 × 192
Axial T2*	5	0–1	600	20	20–30	—	1	256 × 192
Axial FSE	5	2	2800	90	—	8	1	256 × 192
Coronal T2*	4	0–1	600	20	20–30	—	2	256 × 192
Coronal FSE	5	1–2	2800	40	—	8	2	256 × 192

Frequency-selective fat saturation is best used with axial or coronal FSE sequences. TR, repetition time; TE, echo time; ETL, echo train length; NEX, number of excitations; MAT, matrix size; 3DFT, three-dimensional Fourier transform; FSE, fast spin echo; PD, proton density.

tions for imaging systems operating at 1.5 T are listed in Table 1-3; MR systems operating at other field strengths may require different parameters for optimal imaging. Selection of appropriate scan parameters has significant impact on image quality, imaging time, and diagnostic accuracy (69–72).

The TR will affect the total imaging time, as described by the following formula: imaging time = TR × number of phase-encoding steps × NEX (number of excitations). Pulse sequences with short TR, such as T1-weighted and T2*-weighted gradient-echo sequences therefore have short imaging times. The disadvantage of short TR sequences is that the number of slices available will decrease, and it may be impossible to cover the entire region of interest (25,73,74). This problem may be overcome by using an interleaved sequence, but such a sequence increases the examination time. An alternate technique is to place gaps between the slices, thereby allowing the limited number of slices available to cover a larger anatomic region. The risk is, of course, that an abnormality in the area between slices will be missed if the gaps are too large. For this reason we recommend that the interslice gap should be small enough to provide an adequate number of slices to cover the anatomic region of interest. Other advantages of using interslice gaps is that the signal-to-noise ratio is improved because cross-talk between slices is minimized, and tissue contrast is increased (71,72). Theoretically, a gap of approximately 50% of slice thickness is ideal in maximizing the signal-to-noise ratio and tissue contrast.

The TE has minimal effect on imaging time but does affect image contrast. Long TE images, such as T2-weighted spin-echo sequences, are intrinsically signal poor, resulting in low signal-to-noise images. Multiple excitations can be used to improve the signal-to-noise ratio; however this is done at the expense of increased imaging time. Short TE images have higher signal-to-noise ratios but less tissue contrast (73, 74).

Slice thickness is an important parameter to consider. When very thick slices are utilized, considerable volume averaging may occur, and spatial resolution may be decreased. Thin slices have a lower signal-to-noise ratio, and because each slice examines only a small portion of the region in question, coverage is diminished. This problem may be compensated for by using interleaved sequences, by employing gaps, or by increasing the number of excitations. Very thin slices (i.e., <3 mm) should be avoided with spin-echo sequences and consideration given to 3DFT techniques (75).

Selection of matrix size significantly affects both signal-to-noise ratio and resolution. With a high-field-strength magnet, it is possible to use a matrix routinely of 256 × 256. The use of large matrices increases the amount of imaging time, as the number of phase-encoding steps is equal to the matrix size in the phase-encoded direction. For this reason, matrices of either 256 × 192 or 256 × 128 are often used to reduce imaging time, at the expense of reduced spatial resolution (77). Large matrices also result in a reduced signal-to-noise ratio, because the amount of tissue and signal contained in each voxel is relatively small.

The number of excitations directly affects imaging time and signal-to-noise ratio. Increasing from 1 NEX to 2 NEX results in a 40% increase in signal to noise; increasing from 1 NEX to 4 NEX results in a 200% increase in signal to noise (Fig. 1-19).

As if these were not enough variables to juggle in setting up imaging sequences, the proper field of view must be chosen. When the object to be imaged is larger than the field of view in the phase-encoded direction, aliasing or ''wrap-around artifacts'' may occur (Fig. 1-20). In general, the better the region of interest fills the coil, the better the signal-to-noise ratio will be. In standard knee imaging we have typically found that fields of view of 14–18 cm are adequate (50,55,78).

A final point of note is the importance of proper selection of the direction of phase encoding. Because vascular pulsation artifact is projected in the direction of phase encoding, it is important to determine ahead of time whether this artifact (usually from the popliteal artery) will obscure the area of interest. An example of this would be anteroposterior phase encoding in an axial slice obscuring the patella in a patient being evaluated for chondromalacia (see Fig. 1-11).

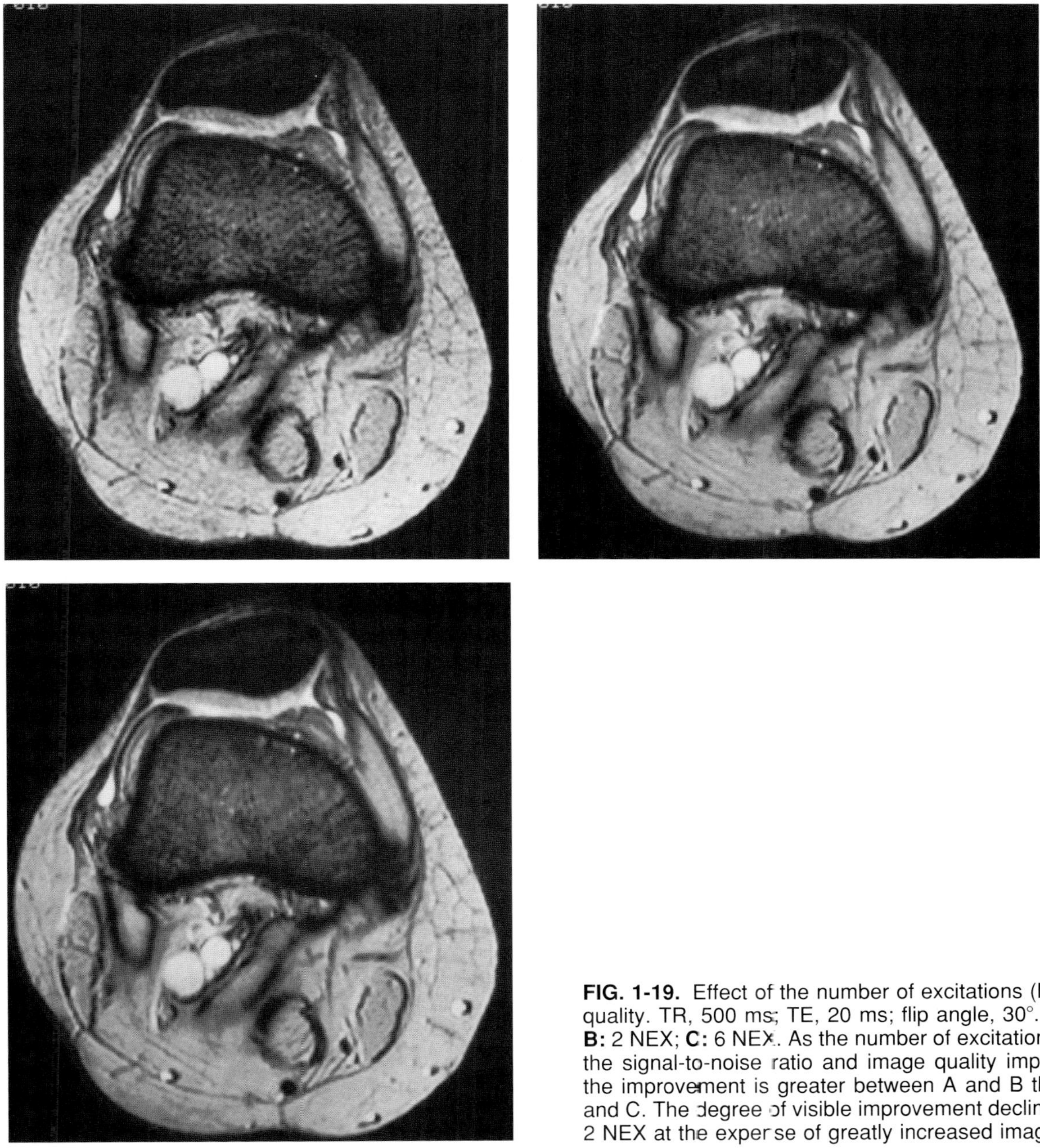

A B C

FIG. 1-19. Effect of the number of excitations (NEX) on image quality. TR, 500 ms; TE, 20 ms; flip angle, 30°. **A:** 0. 75 NEX; **B:** 2 NEX; **C:** 6 NEX. As the number of excitations is increased, the signal-to-noise ratio and image quality improve; however, the improvement is greater between A and B than between B and C. The degree of visible improvement declines rapidly after 2 NEX at the expense of greatly increased imaging time.

SIGNAL CHARACTERISTICS

Regardless of the pulse sequence selected, air, cortical bone, calcification, normal ligaments, tendons, fibrocartilage, and mature scar will be of low signal intensity on all images. Similarly, paramagnetic substances such as deoxyhemoglobin and hemosiderin also produce low signal. Metal produces signal displacement because of to magnetic field distortion and will be seen as a signal void. Substances with high signal intensity on T1-weighted sequences include fat, gadolinium-enhanced tissues, methemoglobin, proteinaceous fluids, and rarely, calcification (25,75–78). Fluid and edema have low signal intensity with T1-weighting and high signal intensity on T2-weighted sequences (75,77,78). Normal striated muscle has an amazingly consistent dark gray appearance on virtually all pulse sequences. High-velocity flow such as that seen in arteries will often produce an area of signal void on spin-echo images; the faster the flow and the more perpendicular to the plane of section, the darker the signal. Flow within blood vessels usually produces high signal on gradient-echo images. The nature of various tissues can usually be determined by assessing the signal characteristics on various pulse sequences.

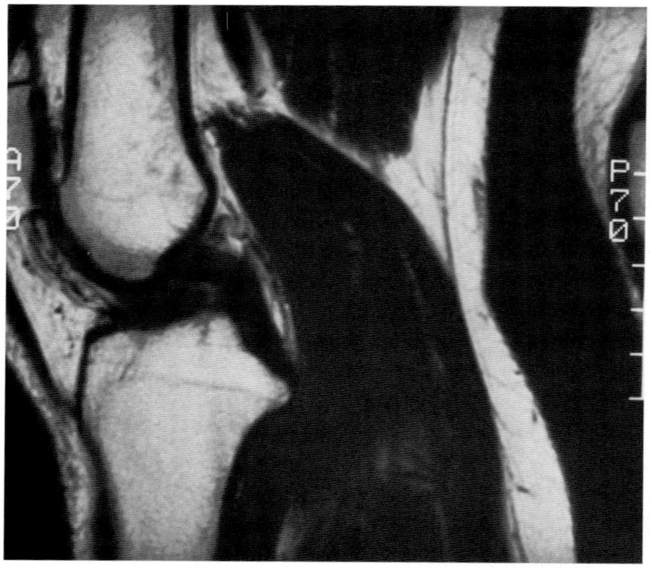

FIG. 1-20. Aliasing artifact. A sagittal T1-weighted image shows a portion of the left side of the image wrapped around to the right side of the image. This artifact can make interpretation difficult if a large portion of the image is aliased, or if the artifact covers a region of diagnostic importance.

PATIENT CONSIDERATIONS

A number of patient-related factors must be considered to ensure safe and optimal MR imaging. If this is not done there is risk of injuring the patient, obtaining inadequate or inappropriate images, or wasting imaging time. All patients who are scheduled for knee MRI should arrive with a brief clinical history because this allows the imaging protocol to be tailored to the areas of clinical concern. Information regarding the possible presence of implanted metallic devices or metallic foreign bodies should routinely be obtained from both the referring physician and the patient (25).

Certain implanted metallic devices are strong contraindications to MRI because the magnetic field may produce movement of the device or induce electrical currents in the device. Cerebral aneurysm clips, cochlear implants, dorsal column stimulators, bone growth stimulators, and automatic cardiac defibrillators are strict contraindications for MRI (79–91). The presence of a cardiac pacemaker is a strong relative contraindication. Should it be absolutely necessary to image a patient with a pacemaker, a physician who is able to insert a temporary transvenous pacer should be present (83–85). Cardiac valve replacements with nonmetallic leaflets are generally believed to be safe, because the forces applied to metal valve ring with each cardiac stroke are greater than the torque imposed by the magnetic field. Valves with metallic leaflets, such as Starr-Edward valves, should be considered unsafe unless information documenting the safety of the specific valve type is available (79,89). A number of documents that report the safety of various medical devices are available (79,92–95).

The presence of an intraorbital metallic foreign body is a contraindication to MR imaging as movement of the metal fragment caused by the magnetic field may produce retinal injury (96). Patients who have a history of possible intraorbital metallic foreign body should have plain radiographs or computed tomography of the orbits to detect or exclude the presence of a foreign body prior to MRI (86,97,98). If the safety of an implanted device within the magnet is unclear or if it is uncertain whether a foreign body is present in the eye, it is wise to err on the side of caution and pursue alternative imaging if possible.

Although the presence of metallic objects will produce a signal void in the area of the object and the immediate surrounding tissues, useful information may still be obtained when appropriate sequences are utilized. Gradient-echo sequences are most susceptible to the effects of adjacent metal and are best avoided in the presence of metallic implants, if possible. With spin-echo imaging, the amount of signal loss increases with increasing TE. Thus, T1- and proton-density-weighted sequences are preferable to T2-weighted sequences. Fast spin-echo sequences are less sensitive to metal-induced artifacts than are spin-echo sequences (17). Metallic objects must be excluded from the magnet area, as the magnetic field may accelerate these objects into the magnet bore (99).

The safety of MRI in pregnant patients has not been definitively established. The Safety Committee of the Society of

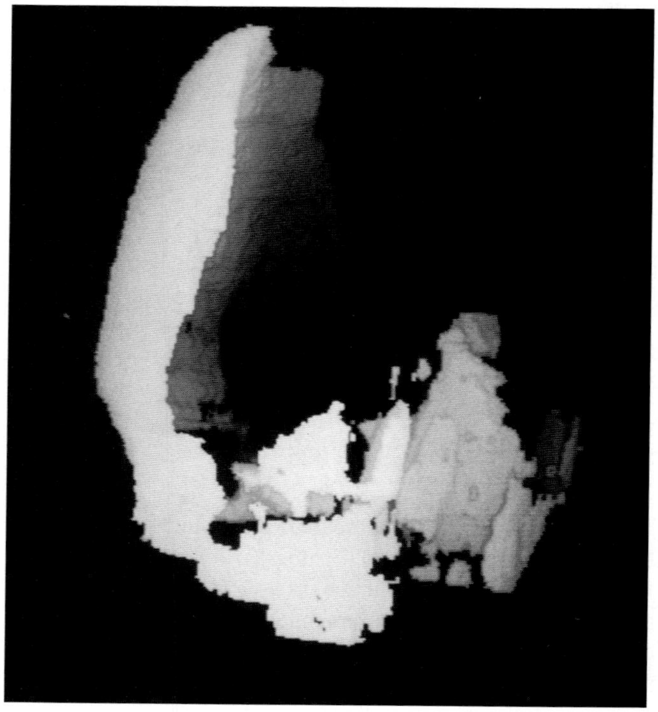

FIG. 1-21. Three-dimensional display. A large joint effusion is displayed as viewed from the posterolateral aspect. (Courtesy of A. Heuck and P. Lang, Berlin, Germany, and H. Genant, San Francisco, California.)

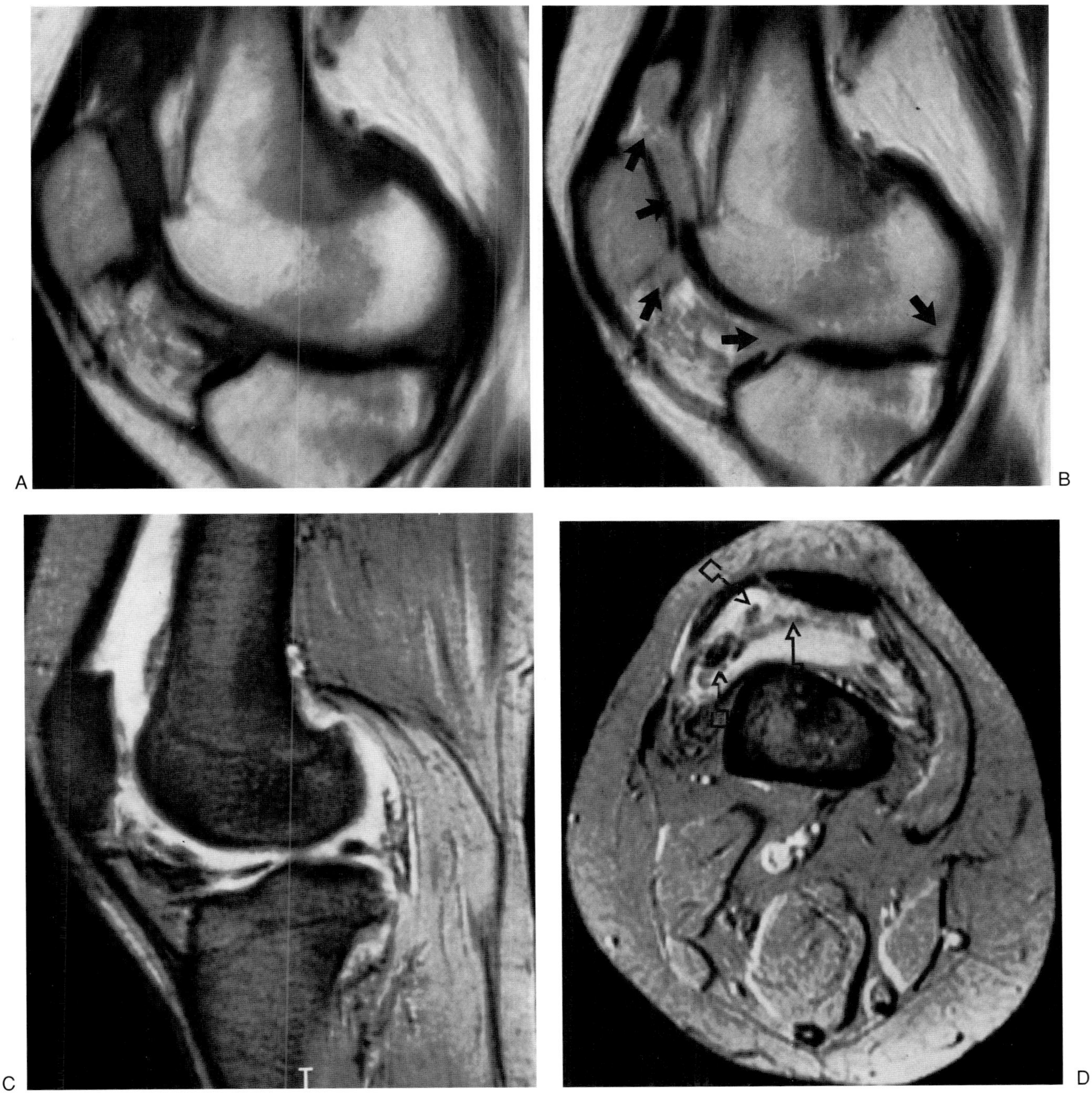

FIG. 1-22. Effect of intravenous gadolinium-DTPA chelate used as a contrast agent. All images are from patients with juvenile rheumatoid arthritis. **(A)** TR, 800 ms; TE, 20 ms. **(B)** TR, 800 ms; TE, 20 ms; following administration of gadolinium-DTPA. The marked enhancement of the pannus *(arrows)* is striking and allows easy differentiation of pannus from joint fluid. **(C)** T2*-weighted image obtained in the same patient (TR, 600 ms; TE, 20 ms; flip angle 20°) shows both pannus and joint fluid as being of high signal. **(D)** T2*-weighted image in a different patient shows low-signal intensity pannus *(curved arrow)* well differentiated from surrounding fluid. The low signal intensity of the pannus in this case is presumably due to fibrosis or hemosiderin deposition.

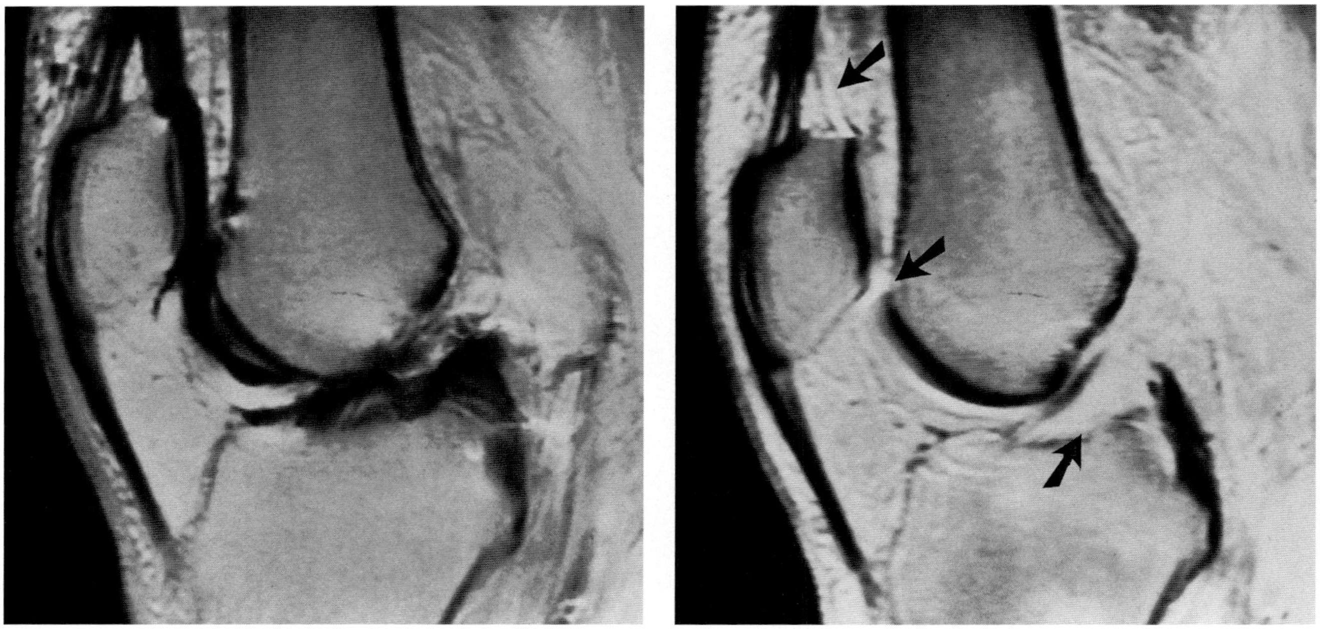

A B

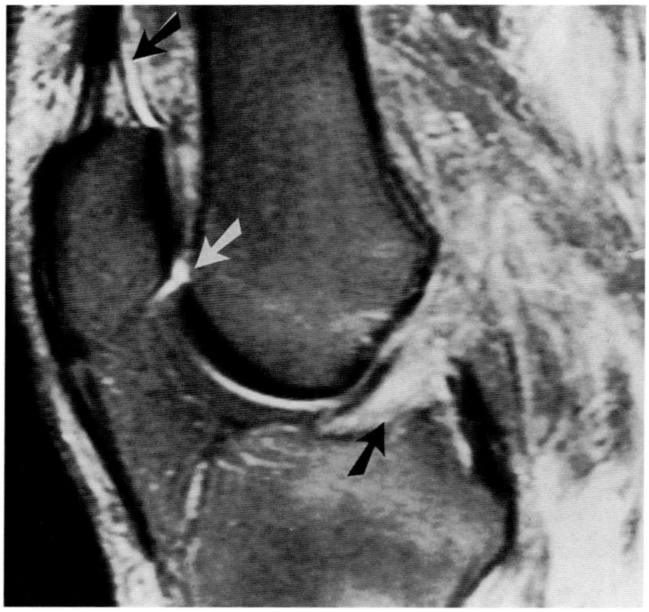

C

FIG. 1-23. Gadolinium-DTPA arthrography. T1-weighted images were obtained **(A)** before and **(B)** after intraarticular injection of gadolinium-DTPA. In B the high signal fluid outlines the synovial and cartilaginous margins of the joint *(arrows)*. **C:** A T2-weighted image obtained prior to gadolinium-DTPA injection also shows high signal intensity of joint fluid, but has lower signal-to-noise ratios and a longer imaging time than the T1-weighted image.

Magnetic Resonance Imaging recommends that "MR imaging may be used in pregnant women if other nonionizing forms of diagnostic imaging are inadequate or if the examination provides important information that would otherwise require exposure to ionizing radiation (e.g., fluoroscopy, CT, etc.). It is recommended that pregnant patients be informed that, to date, there has been no indication that the use of clinical MR imaging during pregnancy has produced deleterious effects. However, as noted by the FDA, the safety of MR imaging in pregnancy has not been proved (100)."

A number of other patient factors must be considered. Patients who are uncomfortable, uncooperative, or claustrophobic may be unable to tolerate long imaging times and an abbreviated examination may be necessary. Careful patient positioning, occasionally including prone positioning, and sedatives may be helpful in alleviating some of these problems (101). Occasionally, despite this, a satisfactory examination cannot be conducted (102,103). Patients should be given earplugs to reduce the ambient noise level within the magnet bore, as the noise produced by the gradient fields can produce anxiety and temporary hearing loss (104,105). Critically ill patients who require close monitoring and life support systems are usually poor candidates for MRI, although equipment suitable for use in the presence of strong

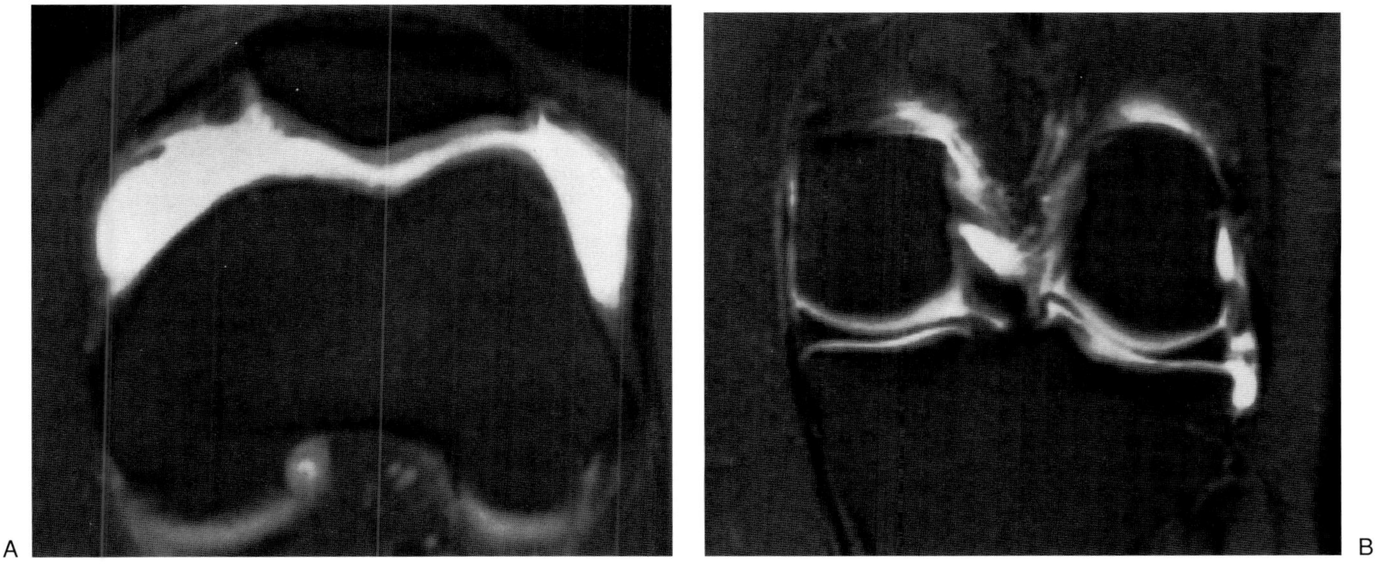

FIG. 1-24. Gadolinium-DTPA arthrography. Fat-suppressed T1-weighted axial (A) and coronal (B) images show excellent depiction of the cartilaginous and meniscal surfaces. Thinning of the medial patellar facet cartilage is is depicted in (A).

magnetic fields is available (106). Respiratory and/or cardiac monitoring should be performed in all patients to avert unforeseen complications.

THREE-DIMENSIONAL RECONSTRUCTION AND DISPLAY

Recent advances in computer software and graphic displays have allowed three-dimensional (3-D) models to be created from standard planar slices in both computed tomography (CT) and MRI. These reconstructions provide an interactive display of complex anatomic structures, and their utility in diagnostic radiology is now being widely investigated (39,107–109). The 3-D reconstruction can be viewed and rotated as a volume, viewed as slices in any desired plane, or used to calculate tissue volumes. High-spatial-resolution 3-D images are typically produced using 3-DFT imaging and gradient-echo techniques. The volume of specific tissues can be determined manually (by tracing the boundaries of the tissue of interest on each slice) or automatically (by defining a range of pixel intensity values representing the tissue of interest) (110,111).

Three-dimensional reconstruction and display have been shown to allow accurate estimation of knee effusion volume (Fig. 1-21; see also color plate 1) (108). Other potential uses of this technique include estimation of knee cartilage volume (44), design of custom prostheses for reconstructive surgery, and computer simulations of surgical procedures.

MAGNETIC RESONANCE CONTRAST AGENTS

MRI contrast agents containing gadolinium chelates produce marked shortening of T1 relaxation times in tissues, resulting in increased signal intensity on T1-weighted images. Precontrast and postcontrast T1-weighted images should be obtained to allow direct visual comparison of the images. Frequency-selective fat suppression can be use to increase the conspicuity of enhancement. Intravenous gadolinium enhancement is most helpful in the clinical situations of infection, tumor, or synovitis (112). Contrast administration has been shown to increase the detection of early bone and soft-tissue infection and to localize the most appropriate site of osteomyelitis for biopsy (113). In tumor evaluation intravenous contrast enhancement is useful to differentiate between tumor and fluid collections such as seromas and hematomas; this is particularly helpful in postoperative cases. Contrast enhancement has also been used to determine tumor viability, response to chemotherapy, and vascularity (113). The contrast enhancement characteristics may be helpful in determining the histologic nature and grade of the tumor (114). In patients with rheumatologic diseases, contrast administration can improve visualization of inflamed synovium and allow differentiation of synovitis from effusion on T1-weighted images (Fig. 1-22) (115–118).

Intra-articular injection of minute amounts of gadolinium chelates can be used to provide MR-arthrographic images (Fig. 1-23). It must be noted that intra-articular use of gadolinium is not yet officially approved by the FDA. This technique allows high contrast between the intra-articular gadolinium solution and adjacent cartilage and meniscal surfaces (Fig. 1-24). In osteochondritis dissecans, MR arthrography improves assessment of the size, depth, and stability of the osteochondral defect (119). In the evaluation of treated meniscal tears, MR arthrography is useful to determine if signal abnormalities on routine MR images represent recurrent tears or persistent signal change at the site of a healed tear (20). Interestingly, intravenously administered gadolinium compounds will diffuse through normal synovium in sufficient quantity to allow MR-arthrographic images to be obtained after intravenous injection (121,122). This allows MR arthrographic images to be performed without the need for intra-articular injection. Maximal intra-articular enhancement in normal knees occurs at 20–30 minutes after injection and can be accelerated by joint exercise. The rate of gadolinium accumulation in the joint is a function of synovial vascularity and permeability; thus, the enhancement rate can be used as an index of synovitis severity.

Many new applications of intravenous and intra-articular contrast enhancement in knee MR imaging are being investigated, and it is likely that contrast-enhanced techniques will be routinely used for a variety of clinical indications in the future.

REFERENCES

1. Balter S. An introduction to the physics of magnetic resonance imaging. *Radiographics* 1987;7:371–383.
2. Ehman RL, Berquist TH, McLeod RA. MR imaging of the musculoskeletal system: a 5 year appraisal. *Radiology* 1988;166:313–320.
3. Crues JV. Joint imaging. Syllabus of the 1988 RSNA categorical course in MR imaging 1988;175–179.
4. Murphy WA. Musculoskeletal system: syllabus of the categorical course in MR imaging 1988;167–174.
5. Sartoris DJ, Resnick D. MR imaging of the musculoskeletal system: current and future status. *AJR* 1987;149:457–467.
6. Fullerton GD. Magnetic resonance imaging signal concepts. *Radiographics* 1987;7:579–596.
7. Merritt CRB. Magnetic resonance imaging—a clinical perspective: imaging quality, safety and risk management. *Radiographics* 1987; 7:1001–1016.
8. Mink JH, Deutsch AL. Magnetic resonance imaging of the knee. *Clin Orthop* 1989;244:29–47.
9. Burk DL, Dalinka MK, Scheibler ML, Cohen EK, Kressel HY. Strategies for musculoskeletal magnetic resonance imaging. *Radiol Clin North Am* 1988;26:653–672.
10. Rubin DA, Kneeland JB. MR imaging of the musculoskeletal system: technical considerations for enhancing imaging quality and diagnostic yield. *AJR* 1994;163:1155–1163.
11. Horowitz AL. *MRI physics for physicians.* New York: Springer-Verlag;1989.
12. Plewes DB. Contrast mechanisms in spin-echo MR imaging. *Radiographics* 1994;14:1389–1404.
13. Constable RT, Anderson AW, Zhong J, Gore JC. Factors influencing contrast in fast spin-echo MR imaging. *Magn Reson Imaging* 1992; 10:497–511.
14. Mirowitz SA. Fast scanning and fat-suppression MR imaging of musculoskeletal disorders. *AJR* 1993;161:1147–1157.
15. Georgy BA, Hesselink JR. MR imaging of the spine: recent advances in pulse sequences and special techniques. *AJR* 1994;162:923–934.
16. Peterfy CG, Linares R, Steinbach LS. Recent advances in magnetic resonance imaging of the musculoskeletal system. *Radiol Clin North Am* 1994;32:291–311.
17. Tartaglino LM, Flanders AE, Vinitski S, Friedman DP. Metallic artifacts on MR images of the postoperative spine: reduction with fast spin-echo techniques. *Radiology* 1994;190:565–569.
18. Rubin DA, Kneeland JB, Listerud J, Underberg-Davis SJ, Dalinka MK. MR diagnosis of meniscal tears of the knee: value of fast spin-echo vs conventional spin-echo pulse sequences. *AJR* 1994;162: 1131–1135.
19. Mirowitz SA, Apicella P, Reinus WR, Hammerman AM. MR imaging of bone marrow lesions: relative conspicuousness on T1-weighted, fat-suppressed T2-weighted, and STIR images. *AJR* 1994;162: 215–221.
20. Kapelov SR, Teresi LM, Bradley WG, et al. Bone contusions of the knee: increased lesion detection with fast spin-echo MR imaging with spectroscopic fat saturation. *Radiology* 1993;189:901–904.
21. Wehrli FW. *Introduction of fast-scan magnetic resonance.* Milwaukee, WI: General Electric Company, 1986.
22. Wehrli FW, Prost JH, Roberts F. The distinguishing properties of gradient recalled acquisition in the steady state (GRASS). *Magn Reson Imaging* 1987;5(suppl 1):105.
23. Wehrli FW. Image contrast in gradient echo sequences. *Magn Reson Imaging* 1990;8(suppl 1):177.
24. Reiser MF, Bongartz G, Erlemann R, et al. Magnetic resonance in cartilaginous lesions of the knee joint with three-dimensional gradient echo imaging. *Skeletal Radiol* 1989;17:465–471.
25. Munk PL, Helms CA, Genant HK, Holt RG. Magnetic resonance imaging of the knee: current status, new directions. *Skeletal Radiol* 1989;18:569–577.
26. Spritzer CE, Vogler JB, Martinez S, et al. MR imaging of the knee: preliminary results with a 3DFT pulse sequence. *AJR* 1988;150: 597–603.
27. Elster AD. Gradient-echo MR imaging: techniques and acronyms. *Radiology* 1993;186:1–8.
28. Reeder JD, Matz SO, Becker L, Andelman SM. MR imaging of the knee in the sagittal projection: comparison of three-dimensional gradient-echo and spin-echo techniques. *AJR* 1989;153:537–540.
29. Harms SE, Flamig DP, Fisher CF, Fulmer JM. New method for fast MR imaging of the knee. *Radiology* 1989;173:743–750.
30. Heron CW, Calvert PT. Three-dimensional gradient-echo MR imaging of the knee: comparison with arthroscopy in 100 patients. *Radiology* 1992;183:839–844.
31. Araki Y, Ootani F, Tsukaguchi I, et al. MR diagnosis of meniscal tears of the knee: value of axial three-dimensional Fourier transformation GRASS images. *AJR* 1992;158:587–590.
32. Solomon SL, Totty WG, Lee JKT. MR imaging of the knee: comparison of three-dimensional FISP and two-dimensional spin-echo pulse sequences. *Radiology* 1989;739–742.
33. Yao L, Sinha S, Seeger LL. MR imaging of joints: analytic optimization of GRE techniques at 1.5 T. *AJR* 1992;158:339–345.
34. Haacke EM, Tkach JA. Fast MR imaging: techniques and clinical applications. *AJR* 1990;155:951–964.
35. Sebag GH, Moore SG. Effect of trabecular bone on the appearance of marrow in gradient-echo imaging of the appendicular skeleton. *Radiology* 1990;174:855–859.
36. Haggar AM, Froelich JW, Hearshen DO, Sadavisan K. Meniscal abnormalities of the knee: 3DFT fast-scan GRASS MR imaging. *AJR* 1988;150:1341–1344.
37. Tyrell RL, Gluckert K, Pathria M, Modic MT. Fast three-dimensional MR imaging of the knee: comparison with arthroscopy. *Radiology* 1988;166:865–872.
38. Runge VM, Wood ML, Kaufman DM, Nelson KL, Traill MR. FLASH: clinical three-dimensional magnetic resonance imaging. *Radiographics* 1988;8:947–965.
39. Djukic S, Stoller D, Steiger P, Genant HK. Three-dimensional Fourier transform MR imaging of the knee with multiplanar reformation. *Radiology* 1989;173(P):356.
40. Harms SE, Flamig DP, Fisher CF, Fulmer JM. New method for fast MR imaging of the knee. *Radiology* 1989;173:743–750.
41. Adam G, Bohndorf K, Drobnitzky, M, Guenther RW. MR imaging of the knee: three-dimensional volume imaging combined with fast processing. *J Comput Assist Tomogr* 1989;13:984–988.
42. Carlson JC, Crooks LE, Ortendahl DA, Kramar DM, Kaufman L. Signal-to-noise ratio and section thickness in two-dimensional versus three-dimensional Fourier transform MR imaging. *Radiology* 1988; 166:266–270.
43. Reeder JD, Mushinsky DL, Keiser RM, O'Donnell TR, Andelman SM. 3D FISP imaging of the knee: value of multiplanar reconstruction. *Magn Reson Imaging* 1990;8(suppl 1):122.
44. Peterfy CG, van Dijke CF, Janzen DL, et al. Quantification of articular cartilage in the knee with pulsed saturation transfer subtraction and fat-suppressed MR imaging: optimization and validation. *Radiology* 1994;192:485–491.
45. Shuman WP, Lambert DT, Patten RM, Baron RL, Tazioli PK. Improved fat suppression in STIR MR imaging: selecting inversion time through spectral display. *Radiology* 1991;178:885–887.
46. Fleckenstein JL, Archer BT, Barker BA, Vaughan JT, Parkey RW,

Peshock RM. Fast short-tau inversion recovery MR imaging. *Radiology* 1991;179:499–504.
47. Semelka RC, Chew W, Hricak H, Tomei E, Higgins CB. Fat-saturation MR imaging of the upper abdomen. *AJR* 1990;155:1111–1116.
48. Smith DK, Wright J. Water bags: an inexpensive method for improving fat suppression in MR imaging of the extremities. *AJR* 1994;162:1252–1253.
49. Totterman S, Weiss LS, Szumowski J, et al. MR fat suppression in the evaluation of normal structures of the knee. *J Comput Assist Tomogr* 1989;13:473–479.
50. Kneeland JB, Hyde JS. High-resolution MR imaging with local coils. *Radiology* 1989;171:1–7.
51. Reiman TH, Heiken JP, Totty WG, Lee JKT. Clinical MR imaging with a Helmholtz-type surface coil. *Radiology* 1988;169:564–566.
52. Kulkarni MV, Patton JA, Price RR. Technical considerations for the use of surface coils in MRI. *AJR* 1986;147:373–378.
53. Carlson JW, Arakawa M, Kaufman L, McCarter BM, George C. Depth-focused radiofrequency coils for MR imaging. *Radiology* 1987;165:251–255.
54. Froncisz W, Jesmanowicz A, Kneeland JB, Hyde JS. Counter rotating current local coils for high-resolution magnetic resonance imaging. *Magn Reson Med* 1986;3:590–603.
55. Kneeland JB, Jesmanowicz A, Froncisz W, Grest TM, Hyde JS. High-resolution MR imaging using loop-gap resonators. *Radiology* 1986;158:247–250.
56. Axel L, Costantini J, Listerud J. Intensity correction in surface-coil MR imaging. *AJR* 1987;148:418–420.
57. Kaufman L, Kramer DM, Crooks LE, Ortendahl DA. Measuring signal-to-noise ratios in MR imaging. *Radiology* 1989;173:265–267.
58. Smith RC, Reinhold C, McCauley TR, et al. Multicoil high-resolution fast spin-echo MR imaging of the female pelvis. *Radiology* 1992;184:671–675.
59. Buckwalter KA, Pennes DR. Anterior cruciate ligament: oblique sagittal MR imaging. *Radiology* 1990;175:276–277.
60. Do-Dai DD, Stracener JC, Youngberg RA. Oblique sagittal MRI of anterior cruciate ligament. *J Comput Assist Tomogr* 1994;18:160–162.
61. Gay SB, Chen NC, Brookeman JR. A device for rotation and stabilization of the knee during MR imaging. *AJR* 1992;158:1173.
62. Munk PL, Helms CA. The Knee. In: Higgins CB, Helms CA, eds. *Magnetic resonance imaging of the body,* 2nd ed. New York: Raven Press, 1992;1097–1119.
63. Forster BB, Helms CA. Importance of routine T2-weighted or T2*-weighted coronal images in magnetic resonance imaging of the knee. *Can Assoc Radiol J* 1994;44:396–398.
64. Recht MP, Kramer J, Marcelis S, et al. Abnormalities of articular cartilage in the knee: analysis of available MR techniques. *Radiology* 1993;187:473–478.
65. Remer EM, Fitzgerald SW, Friedman H, Rogers LF, Hendrix RW, Schafer MF. Anterior cruciate ligament injury: MR imaging diagnosis and patterns of imaging. *Radiographics* 1992;12:901–915.
66. Fitzgerald SW, Remer EM, Friedman H, Rogers LF, Hendrix RW, Schafer MF. MR evaluation of the anterior cruciate ligament: value of supplementing sagittal images with coronal and axial images. *AJR* 1993;160:1233–1237.
67. DeSmet AA, Norris MA, Yandow DR, Quintana FA, Graf BK, Keene JS. MR diagnosis of meniscal tears of the knee: importance of high signal that extends to the surface. *AJR* 1993;161:101–107.
68. Buckwalter KA, Braunstein EM, Janizek DB, Vahey TN. MR imaging of meniscal tears: narrow versus conventional window width photography. *Radiology* 1993;187:827–830.
69. Bradley WG, Tsuruda JS. MR sequence parameter optimization: an algorithmic approach. *AJR* 1987;149:815–823.
70. Mitchell MR, Tarr RW, Conturo TE, Partain CL, James AE. Spin echo technique selection: bare principles for choosing MRI pulse sequence timing intervals. *Radiographics* 1986;6:245–260.
71. Kneeland JB, Shimakarva A, Wehrli FW. Effect of interslice spacing on MR image contrast and study time. *Radiology* 1986;158:819–822.
72. Schwaighofer BW, Yu KK, Mettrey RF. Diagnostic significance of interslice gap and imaging volume in body MR imaging. *AJR* 1989;153:629–632.
73. Felmlee JP, Morin RL, Salutz JR, Lund GB. Magnetic resonance phase encoding: a pictorial essay. *Radiographics* 1989;9:717–722.
74. Pavlicek W. MR instrumentation and image formation. *Radiographics* 1987;7:809–814.
75. Hajek PC, Gylys-Morin VM, Baker LL, Sartoris DJ, Haghighi P, Resnick D. The high signal intensity meniscus of the knee: magnetic resonance evaluation and in vivo correlation. *Invest Radiol* 1987;22:883–890.
76. Flannigan BD, Kursonoglu-Brahme S, Snyder S, Karzel R, Resnick D. MR arthrography of glenohumeral joint instability: comparison with conventional imaging. *Radiology* 1989;173(P):437.
77. Janzen DL, Peterfy CG, Forbes JR, Tirman PFJ, Genant HK. Cystic lesions around the knee joint: MR imaging findings. *AJR* 1994;163:155–161.
78. Hendrick RE, Osborn AG. Introduction to MR imaging. Part II: Pulse sequences and image contrast. Syllabus of the 1988 RSNA categorical course in MR imaging 1988;15–25.
79. Shellock FG. MR imaging of metal implants and materials: a compilation of the literature. *AJR* 1988;151:811–814.
80. Barrafato D, Henkelman RM. Magnetic resonance imaging and surgical clips. *Can J Surg* 1984;27:509–512.
81. Dujovny M, Kossovsky N, Kossowsky R, et al. Aneurysm clip motion during magnetic resonance imaging: in vivo experimental study with metallurgical factor analysis. *Neurosurgery* 1985;17:543–548.
82. New PFJ, Rosen BR, Brady TJ, et al. Potential hazards and artifacts of ferromagnetic and nonferromagnetic surgical and dental devices in nuclear magnetic resonance imaging. *Radiology* 1983;147:139–148.
83. Prato FS, Nicholson RL, Smith M, Drost DJ. Hazards and recommendations for Canadian MR imaging sites. *J Can Assoc Radiol* 1986;37:233–237.
84. Pavlicek W, Geisinger M, Castle L, et al. The effect of nuclear magnetic resonance on patients with cardiac pacemakers. *Radiology* 1983;147:149–153.
85. Fetter J, Aram G, Holmes DR Jr, Gray GE, Hayes DL. The effects of nuclear magnetic resonance images on external and implantable pulse generators. *PACE* 1984;7:720–727.
86. Zhentlin JD, Thompson JT, Shofner RS. The safety of magnetic resonance imaging with intraorbital metallic objects after retinal reattachment or trauma. *Am J Ophthalmol* 1987;103:831.
87. Leon JA, Gabriele OF. Middle ear prosthesis: significance in magnetic resonance imaging. *Magn Reson Imaging* 1987;5:405–406.
88. Teitelbaum GP, Bradley WG, Klein BD. MR imaging artifacts, ferromagnetism, and magnetic torque of intravascular filters, stents, and coils. *Radiology* 1988;166:657–664.
89. Shellock FG, Crues JV. High field strength MR imaging and metallic biomedical implants: an ex vivo evaluation of deflection forces. *AJR* 1988;151:389–392.
90. Klucznik RP, Carrier DA, Pyka R, Haid RW. Placement of a feromagnetic intracerebral aneurysm clip in a magnetic field with a fatal outcome. *Radiology* 1993;187:855–866.
91. Kanal E, Shellock FG. MR imaging of patients with intracranial aneurysm clips. *Radiology* 1993;187:612–614.
92. Kanal E, Shellock FG. Safety considerations in MR imaging. *Radiology* 1990;176:593–606.
93. Shellock FG, Kanal E. *Magnetic resonance: bioeffects, safety, and patient management.* New York: Raven;1994.
94. Shellock FG, Curtis JS. MR imaging and biomedical implants, materials, and devices: an updated review. *Radiology* 1991;180:541–550.
95. Shellock FG, Morisoli S, Kanal E. MR procedures and biomedical implants, materials, and devices: 1993 update. *Radiology* 1993;189:587–599.
96. Kelsey CA, King JN, Keck GM, Chiu MT, Wolfe DM, Orrison WW. Ocular hazard of metallic fragments during MR imaging at 0. 06 T. *Radiology* 1991;180:282–283.
97. Williamson MR, Espinosa MC, Boutin RD, Orison WW Jr, Hart BL, Kelsey CA. Metallic foreign bodies in the orbits of patients undergoing MR imaging: prevalence and value of radiography and CT before MR. *AJR* 1994;162:981–983.
98. Shellock FG, Kanal E. Metallic foreign bodies in the orbits of patients undergoing MR imaging: prevalence and value of radiography and CT before MR. *AJR* 1994;162:985–986.
99. Mani RL. Potential hazard of metal-filled sandbags in MR imaging. *Radiology* 1992;183:286–287.
100. Shellock FG, Kanal E. Policies, guidelines, and recommendations for MR imaging safety and patient management. *J Magn Reson Imaging* 1991;1:97–101.

101. Moss ML, Buongiorno PA, Clancy VA. Intranasal midazolam for claustrophobia in MRI. *J Comput Assist Tomogr* 1993;17:991–992.
102. Quirk ME, Letendre AJ, Ciottone RA, Lingley JE. Evaluation of three psychologic interventions to reduce anxiety during MR imaging. *Radiology* 1989;173:759–762.
103. Quirk ME, Letendre AJ, Ciottone RA, Lingley JE. Anxiety in patients undergoing MR imaging. *Radiology* 1989;170:463–466.
104. Shellock FG, Morisoli SM, Ziarati M. Measurement of acoustic noise during MR imaging: evaluation of six ''worst-case'' pulse sequences. *Radiology* 1994;191:91–93.
105. Brummett RE, Talbot JM, Charuhas P. Potential hearing loss resulting from MR imaging. *Radiology* 1988;169:539–540.
106. Shellock FG, Myers SM, Kimble KJ. Monitoring heart rate and oxygen saturation with a fiber-optic pulse oximeter during MR imaging. *AJR* 1992;158:663–664.
107. Rusinek H, Mourino MR, Firooznia H, Weinreb JC, Chase NE. Volumetric rendering of MR images. *Radiology* 1989;171:269–272.
108. Heuck AF, Steiger P, Stoller DW, Gleur CC, Genant HK. Quantification of knee joint fluid volume by MR imaging and CT using three-dimensional data processing. *J Comput Assist Tomogr* 1989;13:287–293.
109. Smith DK, Berquist TH, An KN, Robb RA, Chao EYS. Validation of three-dimensional reconstruction of knee anatomy: CT vs MR imaging. *J Comput Assist Tomogr* 1989;13:294–301.
110. Vahlensieck M, Lang P, Chan WP, Grampp S, Genant HK. Three-dimensional reconstruction. Part I: applications and technique. *Eur Radiol* 1992;2:503–507.
111. Vahlensieck M, Lang P, Chan WP, Grampp S, Genant HK. Three-dimensional reconstruction. Part II: optimisation of segmentation and rendering of MRI. *Eur Radiol* 1992;2:508–510.
112. Munk PL, Vellet AD. The musculoskeletal system. In: Higgins CB, Helms CA, ed. *Magnetic resonance imaging of the body,* 2nd ed. New York: Raven Press;1992:1381–1389.
113. Schoenberg NY, Beltran J. Contrast enhancement in musculoskeletal imaging: current status. *Radiol Clin North Am* 1994;32:337–352.
114. Erlemann R, Reiser MF, Peters PE, et al. Musculoskeletal neoplasms: static and dynamic Gd-DTPA enhanced imaging. *Radiology* 1989;171:767–773.
115. Kursonoglu-Brahme S, Riccio T, Weisman MH, Resnick D, Zvaifler N, Sanders ME, Fix C. Rheumatoid knee: role of gadopentetate-enhanced MR imaging. *Radiology* 1990;176:831–835.
116. Konig H, Sieper J, Wolf K. Rheumatoid arthritis: evaluation of hypervascular and fibrous pannus with dynamic MR imaging enhanced with Gd-DTPA. *Radiology* 1990;176:473–477.
117. Adam G, Fenke F, Bohndorf F, Gunther RW. MRI of rheumatoid arthritis: assessment with Gd-DTPA enhanced fast imaging. *Magn Reson Imaging* 1990;8(suppl 1):77.
118. Reiser MF, Bongartz GP, Erlemann R, et al. Gadolinium-DTPA in rheumatoid arthritis and related diseases: first results with dynamic magnetic resonance imaging. *Skeletal Radiol* 1989;18:591–598.
119. Kramer J, Stiglbauer R, Engel A, Prayer L, Imhof H. MR contrast arthrography (MRA) in osteochondritis dissecans. *J Comput Assist Tomogr* 1992;16:254–260.
120. Applegate GR, Flannigan BD, Tolin BS, Fox JM, Del Pizzo W. MR diagnosis of recurrent tears in the knee: value of intraarticular contrast material. *AJR* 1993;161:821–825.
121. Winalski CS, Aliabadi P, Wright RJ, Shortkroff S, Sledge CB, Weissman BN. Enhancement of joint fluid with intravenously administered gadopentetate dimeglumine: technique, rationale, and implications. *Radiology* 1993;187:179–185.
122. Drape J, Thelen P, Gay-Depassier P. Silbermann O, Benacerraf R. Intraarticular diffusion of Gd-DOTA after intravenous injection in the knee: MR imaging evaluation. *Radiology* 1993;188:227–234.

MRI of the Knee, Second Edition,
edited by P. L. Munk and C. A. Helms.
Lippincott-Raven Publishers, Philadelphia © 1996.

CHAPTER 2

The Cruciate Ligaments

Peter L. Munk, A. Dale Vellet, Clyde A. Helms, and Dennis L. Janzen

Acute injuries to the cruciate ligaments of the knee are very common, particularly among competitive athletes (1,2). For appropriate therapy to be instituted, accurate assessment of the nature of these injuries is clearly a prerequisite. Experienced clinicians on careful examination will often be able to obtain most of the information required (2,3). However, even an experienced examiner may have difficulty assessing the extent of an injury, especially in the acute setting, even under anesthesia. In this situation patient pain and muscle spasm may prevent adequate examination. It is important to be aware of the extent of ligamentous injury, not only to effect appropriate treatment but also to predict the degree of functional disability that may eventually result. With the advent of magnetic resonance imaging (MRI), a noninvasive technique that is highly accurate in the assessment of cruciate ligament injuries is now available. Where available, MRI has generally replaced diagnostic arthroscopy (4).

ANATOMY, EMBRYOLOGY, AND FUNCTION

The embryologic derivation of the cruciate ligaments is, in many ways, very similar to that of the menisci. Following formation of the limb bud and the mesenchymal condensations that are the precursors of the tibia and femur, an unchondrified mesenchymal blastoma is present between the bone precursors. As this becomes thinned to form a disk, often referred to as the interzone, adjacent mesenchyme invades this area, giving rise to vascular synovial mesenchyme. The cruciate ligaments form within this vascular synovial mesenchyme, usually slightly before the menisci at approximately 5–7 weeks of gestation. The cruciate ligaments appear well before joint cavitation occurs and at all times remain extrasynovial. From their earliest appearance the cruciate ligaments are recognizable, and their morphology changes very little to achieve their final form. As maturation progresses, an increasingly large amount of collagen is deposited and the ligaments become less cellular (5–10).

The cruciate ligaments are extrasynovial structures that are draped by a synovial membrane. On arthroscopy the cruciates can often be seen through the applied synovial membrane, provided blood and synovial thickening do not preclude this.

The Anterior Cruciate

The anterior cruciate ligament is attached to the femur at the posterior aspect of the medial surface of the lateral femoral condyle. This proximal insertion is in the form of a segment of a circle. Its anterior aspect is almost straight and its posterior side is convex. The ligament in an adult has an average length of approximately 38 mm and a width of 11 mm. The ligament runs anteriorly and inferiorly to its tibial attachment, which is a wide, depressed area in front of and lateral to the anterior tibial spine (Fig. 2-1; see also color plate 2). In some individuals the presence of a bony knob may be appreciated that represents the site of insertion of the medial fibers of the anterior cruciate as well as part of the anterior horn of the medial meniscus. This has been called Parson's knob (tuberculum intercondylare tertium) (11). It is a commonly held fallacy that the cruciate ligaments insert on the tibial spines. The tibial insertion is broader than the proximal femoral insertion. The ligament inserts directly into bone, and the tibial insertion is stronger than the femoral insertion. When the anterior cruciate ligament is carefully examined, it is seen to consist of two parts, an anteromedial band and a thicker posterolateral portion. The tibial insertion

P. L. Munk: Department of Diagnostic Imaging, British Columbia Cancer Agency, and Department of Radiology, University of British Columbia, Vancouver, British Columbia, Canada V5Z 4E6.

A. D. Vellet: Department of Diagnostic Imaging, University of Calgary, Foothills Hospital, Alberta, Canada T2N 2T9.

C. A. Helms: Department of Radiology, Duke University Medical Center, Durham, North Carolina 27710.

D. L. Janzen: Department of Radiology, Vancouver Hospital and Health Sciences Center, Vancouver, British Columbia, Canada V5Z 1M9.

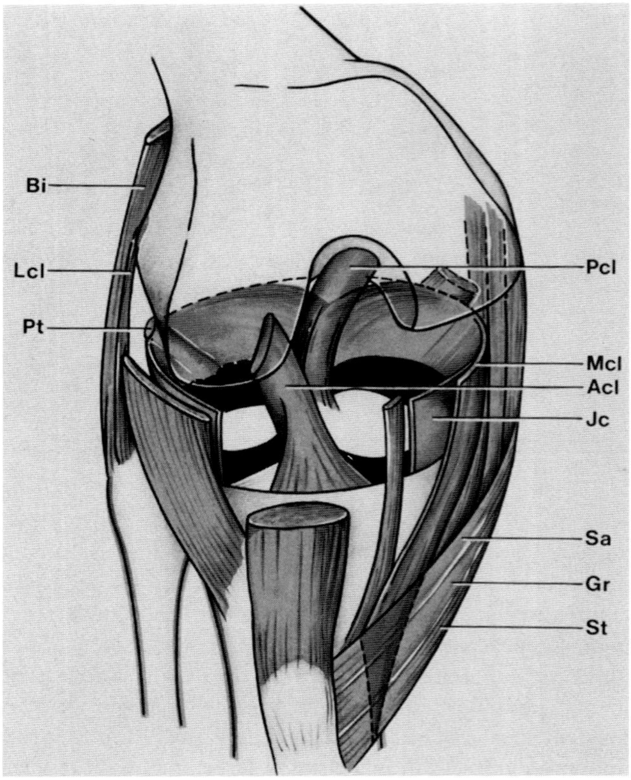

FIG. 2-1. Diagram of the cruciate ligaments. View of the knee from anterior perspective with the joint partially flexed. bi, biceps femoris; lcl, lateral collateral ligament; pt, popliteus tendon; pcl, posterior cruciate ligament; mcl, medial collateral ligament; acl, anterior cruciate ligament; sa, sartorius; gr, gracilis; st, semitendinosus; jc, joint capsule.

consists predominantly of the posterolateral band, which is flared distally (12,13).

The anterior cruciate ligament has several important functions. It resists anterior tibial translation on the femur in flexion and serves to prevent hyperextension and to check internal rotation. In addition, it serves as a secondary knee restraint to both valgus and varus stresses on the knee. When the knee is in extension, the posterolateral band is taut (14–18). However, almost immediately after flexion is initiated, the smaller anteromedial band becomes tight and the posterolateral bulk slackens. Because of this, in flexion it is the anteromedial band that provides the greatest restraint against the anterior displacement of the tibia. Loss of integrity of the anterior cruciate also diminishes position sensation in the lower extremity (19–21).

The Posterior Cruciate

The posterior cruciate ligament is attached to the posterior aspect of the lateral surface of the medial condyle of the femur, and in a fashion similar to the anterior cruciate, the attachment is in the form of a segment of a circle. The upper boundary of the attachment is straight and the lower boundary is convex. The posterior cruciate has an average length of 38 mm and a width of 13 mm. Its middle portion is the narrowest, and it is noted to fan out to a greater extent superiorly than inferiorly. The tibial attachment is in a depression behind the intra-articular upper surface of the tibia (see Fig. 2-1). It usually sends a slip to blend with the posterior horn of the lateral meniscus. It is thicker and stronger than the anterior cruciate ligament and runs in a less oblique plane. It consists of two essentially inseparable parts. An anterior portion forms the bulk of the ligament, with a smaller, variable posterior portion (17,18,22–28).

The role of the posterior cruciate is to prevent posterior displacement of the tibia (it provides 90–95% of the total restraint to posterior displacement) (29,30). Its posterior fibers prevent hyperextension. In flexion the anterior portion is tight and helps to limit hyperflexion. The posterior cruciate resists internal rotation of the tibia by winding around the anterior cruciate ligament. The posterior cruciate thus acts as the dynamic counterpart of the extensor mechanism; therefore, abnormalities of the posterior cruciate ligament can be expected to be reflected in increased stress on the patella, quadriceps, and patellar ligaments as well as increased pressure in the patello-femoral compartment (31). Although some authorities ascribe a relatively unimportant role to the posterior cruciate ligament in knee stability compared with the anterior cruciate ligament, others regard it as the key stabilizer for basic knee function (32–36).

In combination with the other ligaments of the knee and the menisci, the cruciates are involved in a complex synergy that permits knee joint movement. The kinematics of the knee are complex. Flexion and extension of the knee actually consist of a complex combination of knee rolling and gliding that is necessitated by the fact that the condyles are eccentrically curved (Fig. 2-2). The condyles are flatter anteriorly and more spherical posteriorly; in addition, the medial condyle is larger than the lateral. Because of this geometry, early in flexion this action consists mainly of rolling, whereas later in flexion, gliding dominates. When extension occurs, these actions are reversed. To complete extension, the femur rotates inwardly in relation to the tibia. This rotation, the so-called compulsory final rotation, takes place around an axis through the center of the medial femoral condyle. The complex spiral movement of the knee is guided by a mechanism involving the cruciate ligaments in tandem with the menisci (26,37). The interdependence between these structures is reflected in their multiple interconnections, which are discussed in more detail in Chapter 4. The continuity of the ligamentous and meniscal structures has been referred to as the figure-of-eight anatomy.

In considering the action of the cruciate ligaments, it is important to think of them not merely as stays to prevent anteroposterior displacement but, more significantly, as guide ropes to keep the tibia on its winding path when the knee extends and flexes.

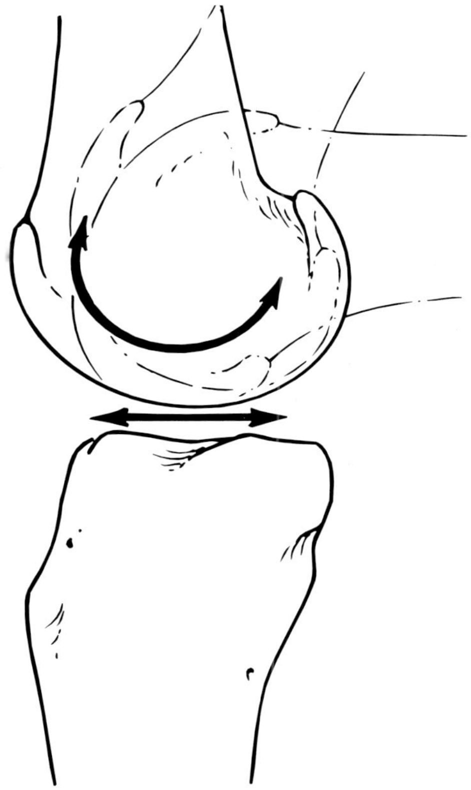

FIG. 2-2. The osseous structures of the knee would be intrinsically unstable (round surface articulating with a flat surface) were it not for a complex mechanism of soft-tissue stabilizers. Knee flexion/extension is a combination of gliding, sliding, and rotation. (Adapted from Hayes CW. *Top Magn Reson Imaging* 1993;5:207–227, with permission.)

MRI APPEARANCE OF THE NORMAL CRUCIATE LIGAMENTS

The Anterior Cruciate

The sagittal and sagittal oblique planes are the best planes to study the anterior cruciate ligament. Even though the anterior cruciate ligament runs in an oblique direction, most individuals, when imaged with the knee extended, rotate the knee externally by approximately 15 to 20°. This places the anterior cruciate ligament approximately in the sagittal plane of imaging. Some institutions choose to employ a brace that immobilizes the knee in this position (38). Generally, the anterior cruciate ligament will be identified on one to three contiguous slices if a 4- or 5-mm-thick section is employed. Some recent work has indicated that the anterior cruciate can be demonstrated to great advantage if 20–30° oblique sagittal images are obtained, especially if T2-weighted images are obtained (39–41) (Fig. 2-3).

With both spin-echo and gradient-echo imaging, the anterior cruciate ligament will be seen to be a band of low signal intensity with striations of intermediate to high signal particularly visible near the attachment points (Fig. 2-4). Often

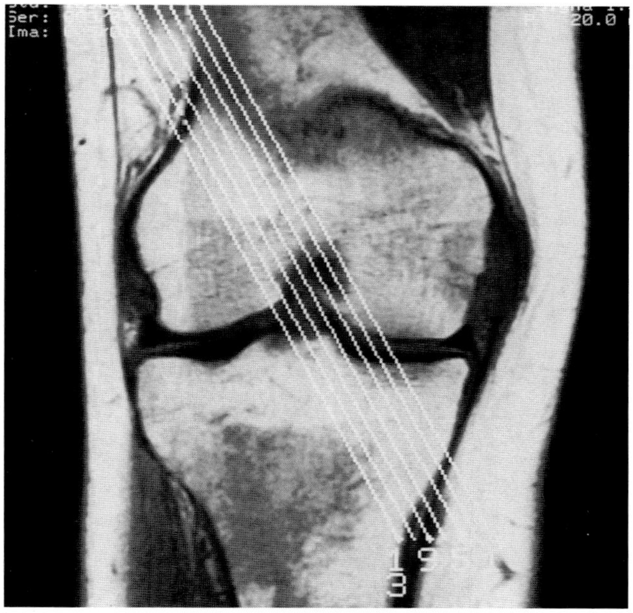

FIG. 2-3. Localizer image for oblique sagittal imaging. Coronal image of any type may be used. Slices are programed through the intercondylar notch along the expected course of the anterior cruciate ligament (superolateral to inferomedial). Methods using axial localizers have also been described.

two bands are identified, especially if oblique images have been obtained. The anterior band is of low signal, with both spin-echo and gradient-echo images. A small amount of fat is sometimes seen as an area of high signal within the anterior band near the tibial insertion on T1-weighted images. The posterior band has a triangular appearance with the apex directed cephalad. It is of low signal on T1-weighted images and of intermediate signal on T2-weighted images. Individual fascicles are seen within both bands near the tibial insertions, especially with T2 weighting (42,43).

The appearance of the anterior cruciate with gradient-echo sequences is of interest because the posterior band is often unidentified because of its intermediate signal intensity when this sequence is used. At times the posterior band may be almost invisible on gradient-echo images, and this could compromise the accuracy of evaluation of partial tears of the anterior cruciate with these sequences. Generally, the distal (tibial) attachment is well seen. The proximal (femoral) attachment is often more indistinct because of volume averaging of the condyle, particularly when thicker sections are utilized (Fig. 2-5). In addition, the ligament is convergent toward its femoral insertion, diminishing our ability to see it because of the smaller volume of tissue. The attachments will be better visualized if thin sections are used (Fig. 2-6). The anterior cruciate ligament may also be identified on coronal images, and once again, in this instance the anterior insertion of the ligament is more easily identified than the posterior femoral insertion (Fig. 2-7).

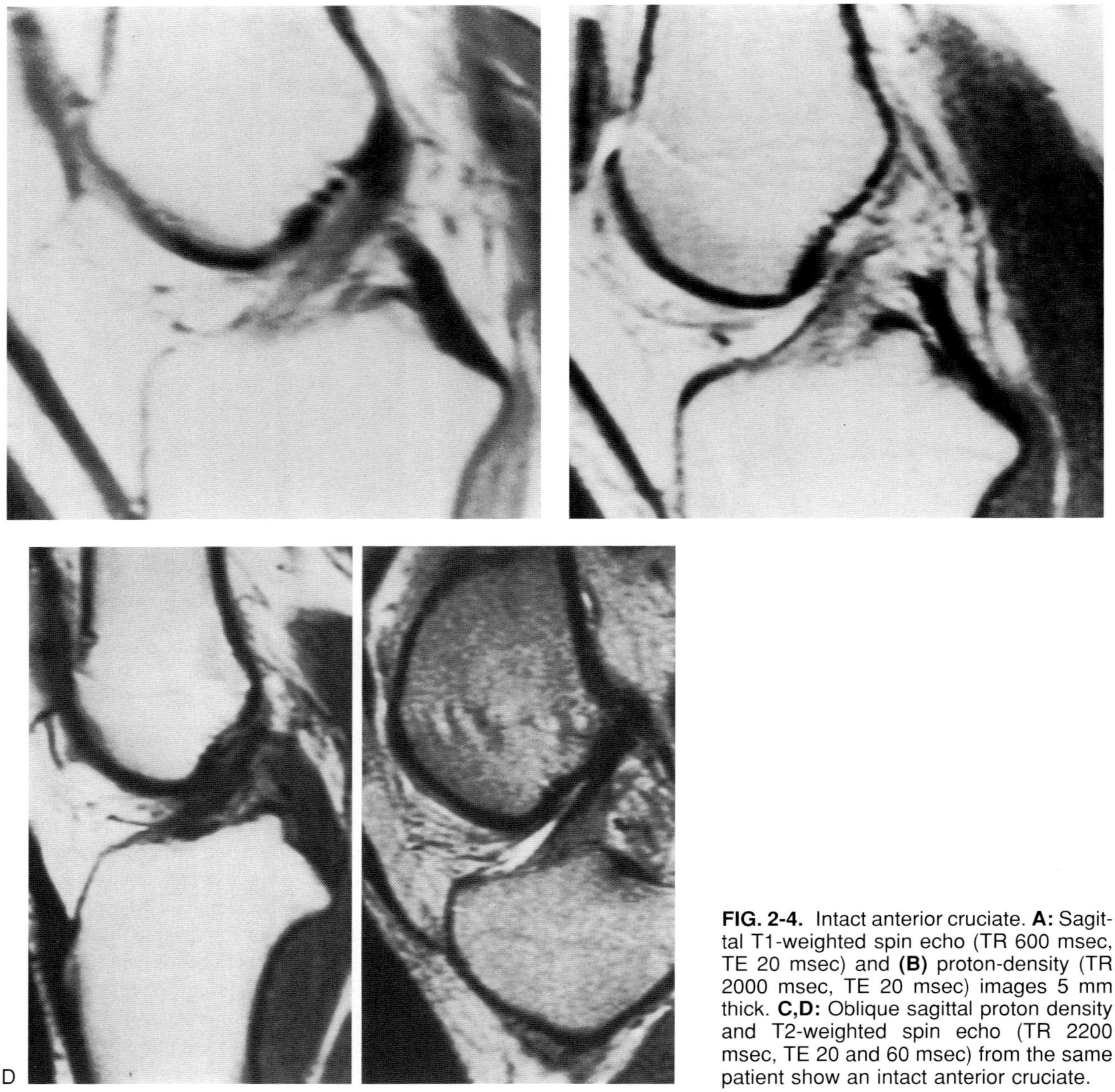

A B C,D

FIG. 2-4. Intact anterior cruciate. **A:** Sagittal T1-weighted spin echo (TR 600 msec, TE 20 msec) and **(B)** proton-density (TR 2000 msec, TE 20 msec) images 5 mm thick. **C,D:** Oblique sagittal proton density and T2-weighted spin echo (TR 2200 msec, TE 20 and 60 msec) from the same patient show an intact anterior cruciate.

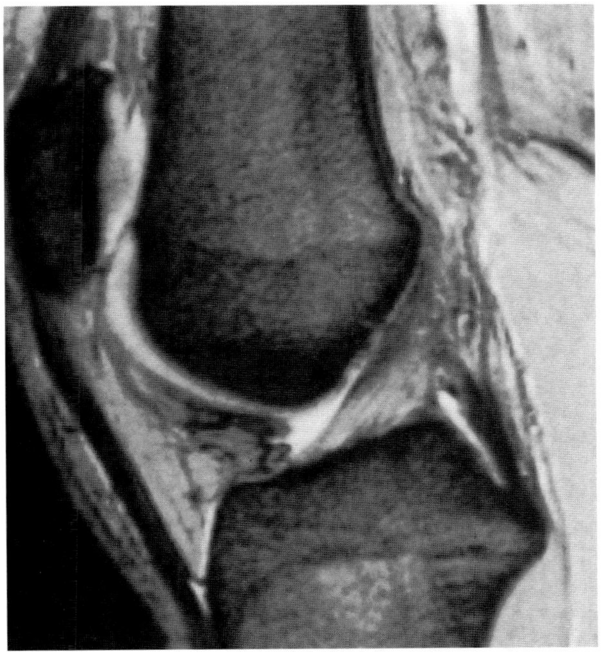

E

FIG. 2-4. *(Continued).* **(E)** Sagittal T2*-weighted gradient-echo MPGR image (TR 400 msec, TE 18 msec, flip angle 30°).

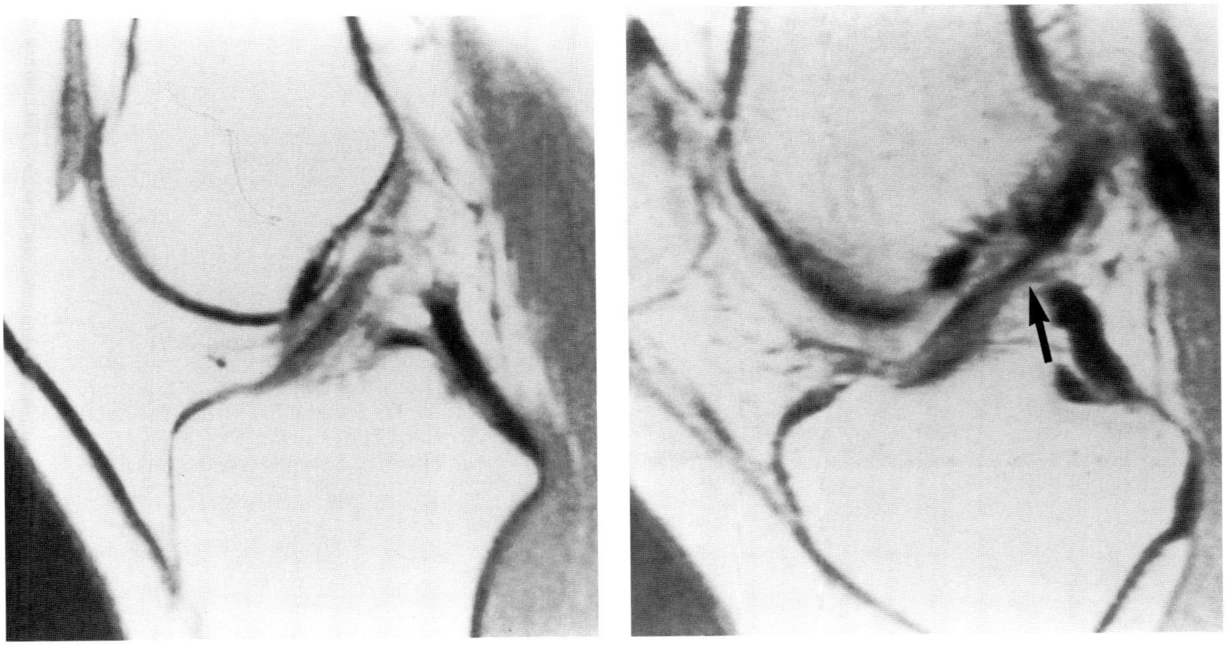

A B

FIG. 2-5. Common variations anterior cruciate appearence. **A:** Sagittal T1-weighted spin echo (TR 800 msec, TE 18 msec) 4 mm thick. The cranial aspect of the ligament appears slightly wispy. This portion of the ligament is usually relatively thin and may also be volume averaged with adjacent femoral condyle surface. **B:** Oblique sagittal proton density spin echo (TR 2200 msec, TE 20 msec). In the extended position the anterior cruciate may be draped over the posterior cruciate giving a bowstrung appearence with slight narrowing *(arrow)*.

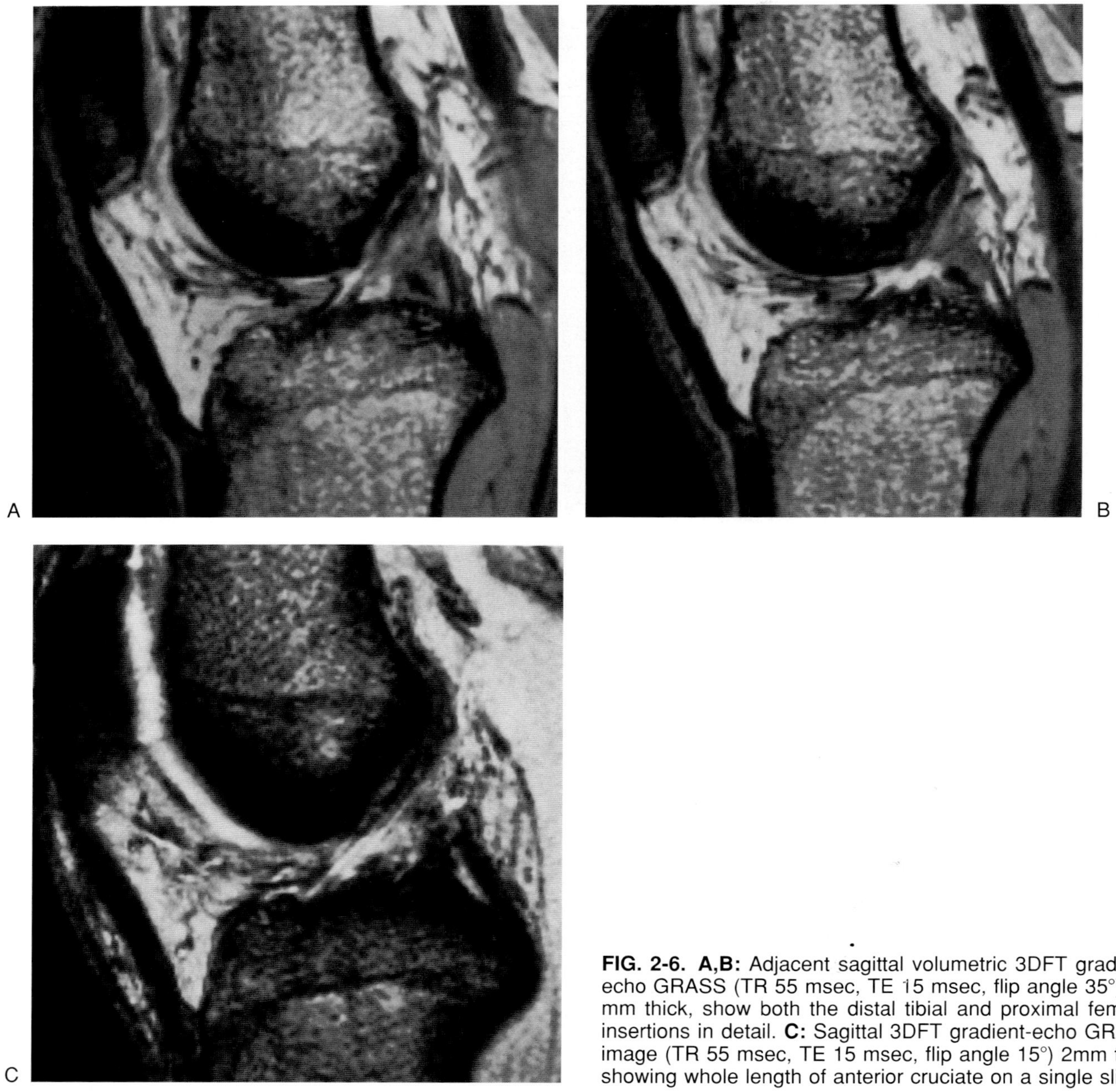

FIG. 2-6. A,B: Adjacent sagittal volumetric 3DFT gradient-echo GRASS (TR 55 msec, TE 15 msec, flip angle 35°) 1.7 mm thick, show both the distal tibial and proximal femoral insertions in detail. **C:** Sagittal 3DFT gradient-echo GRASS image (TR 55 msec, TE 15 msec, flip angle 15°) 2mm thick showing whole length of anterior cruciate on a single slice.

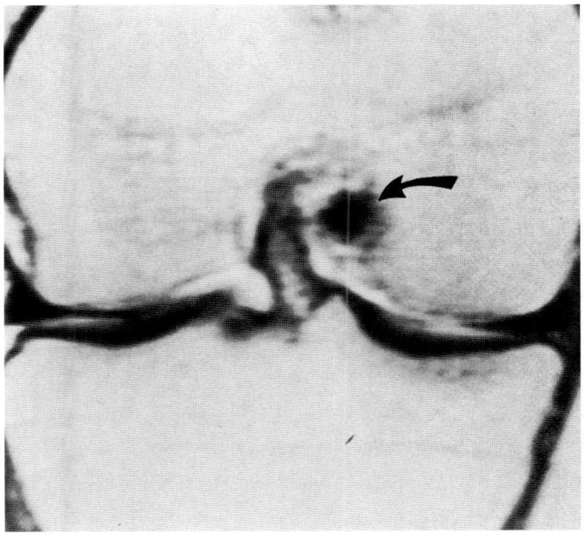

FIG. 2-7. Coronal T1-weighted spin-echo (TR 400 msec, TE 20 msec) image shows the normal appearance of the anterior cruciate insertion. The posterior cruciate is seen adjacent in cross section *(curved arrow).*

The Posterior Cruciate

The posterior cruciate ligament is readily identified as a homogeneously dark structure that, in the extended knee, has a slightly curved configuration near its proximal insertion (Fig. 2-8). With flexion the ligament straightens and becomes taut. Both its proximal and distal insertions are usually well visualized. Unlike the anterior cruciate ligament, no striations are visualized in the normal ligament on spin-echo imaging, except within the ligament immediately adjacent to the femoral insertion, where a small amount of signal may occasionally be seen, especially on T2-weighted images. The difference in signal intensity between the two cruciate ligaments lies in the different fashion in which the fibers are organized. The anterior cruciate has its fibers in a less organized pattern, whereas the fibers of the posterior cruciate are tightly parallel (44).

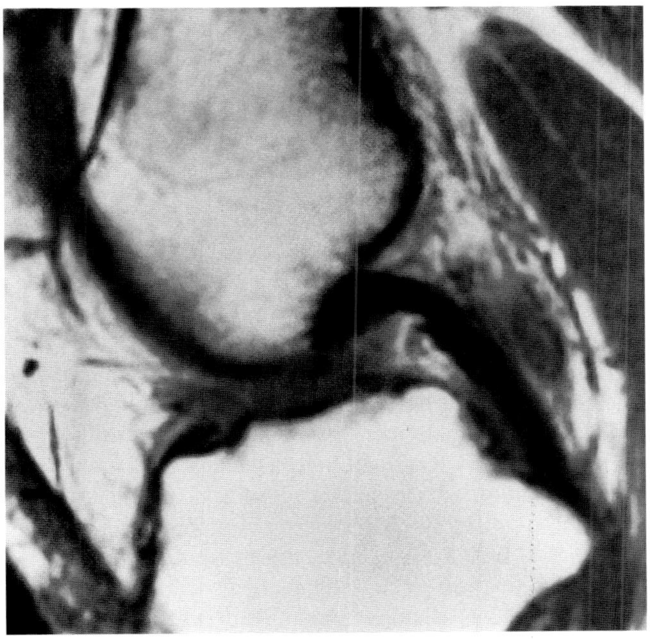

FIG. 2-8. Posterior cruciate ligament. This normal ligament is seen as a curved, uniformly low-signal structure. Sagittal T1-weighted spin echo (TR 600 msec, TE 18 msec).

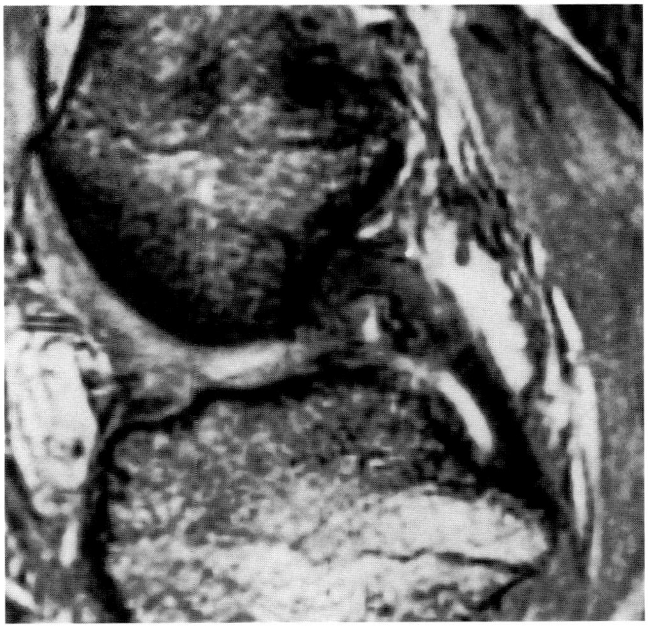

FIG. 2-9. Volumetric imaging of the posterior cruciate. Sagittal 3DFT GRASS (TR 55 msec, TE 15 msec, flip angle 30°), 1.7-mm-thick slice. The ligament is of low signal intensity except for its cranial portion, which has slightly increased signal. This appearance is normal with this technique.

Occasionally with gradient-echo imaging, areas of intermediate to high signal intensity are revealed within the normal ligament (Fig. 2-9). On coronal imaging, the posterior cruciate ligament is easily visualized as an approximately circular or oval structure seen in cross section (see Fig. 2-7). The ligament of Wrisberg, when present, can be identified on both sagittal and coronal images as an oblique band extending from the posterior horn of the lateral meniscus to the medial femoral condyle, seen posterior to the principal portion of the posterior cruciate ligament (Fig. 2-10). The ligament of Humphry runs in a similar plane but anterior to the posterior cruciate. Usually, only one of these meniscofemoral ligaments is present, although on occasion both or neither will be identified (45) (Fig. 2-11). The thickness of these ligaments is extremely variable.

TEARS OF THE CRUCIATE LIGAMENTS

Cruciate ligament injuries are among the most serious injuries suffered by the knee in athletic endeavors. The popula-

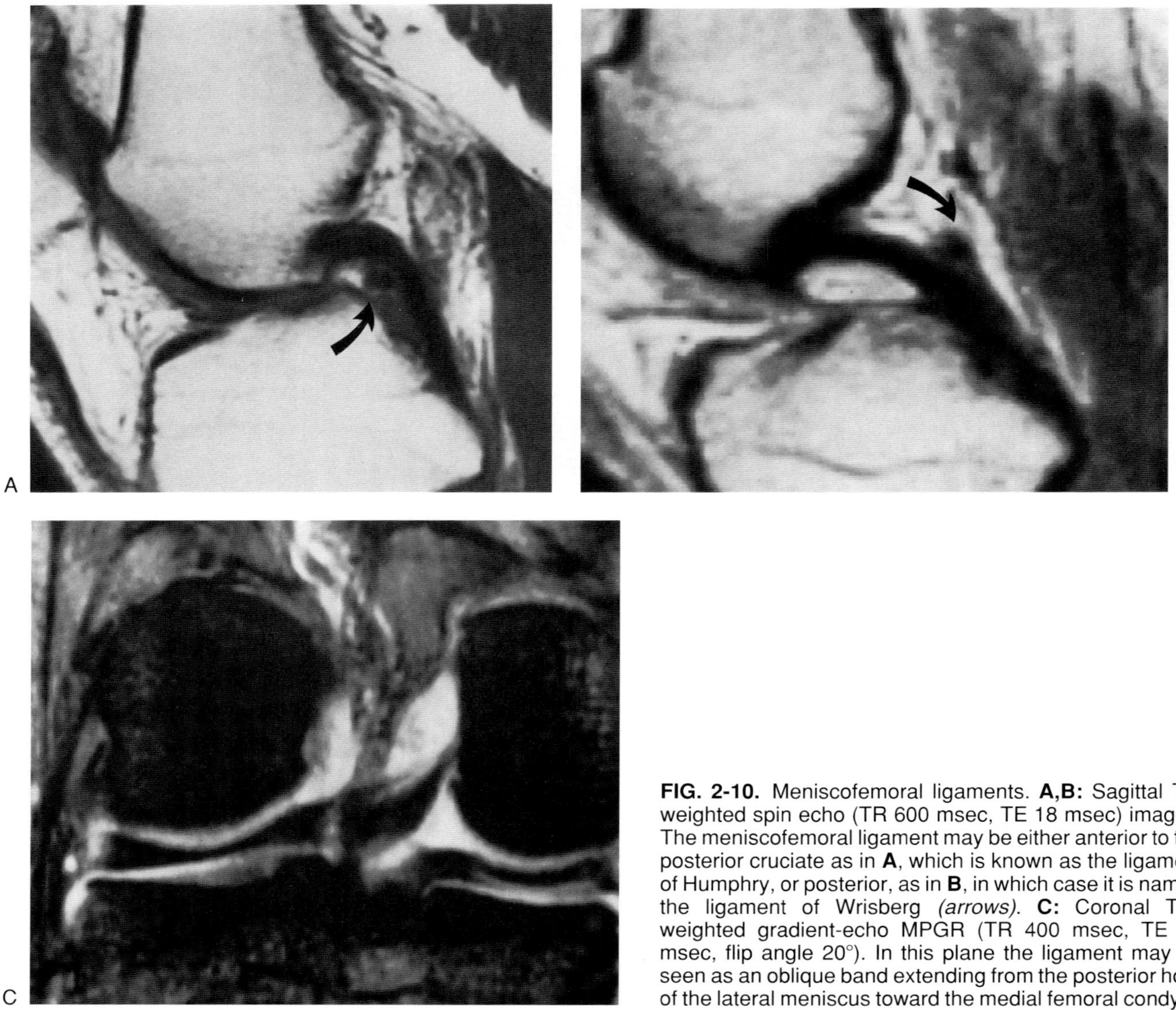

FIG. 2-10. Meniscofemoral ligaments. **A,B:** Sagittal T1-weighted spin echo (TR 600 msec, TE 18 msec) images. The meniscofemoral ligament may be either anterior to the posterior cruciate as in **A**, which is known as the ligament of Humphry, or posterior, as in **B**, in which case it is named the ligament of Wrisberg *(arrows)*. **C:** Coronal T2*-weighted gradient-echo MPGR (TR 400 msec, TE 16 msec, flip angle 20°). In this plane the ligament may be seen as an oblique band extending from the posterior horn of the lateral meniscus toward the medial femoral condyle.

tion at greatest risk includes young males, particularly those engaged in contact sports such as football and rugby. Individuals involved in motor vehicle accidents also can sustain cruciate ligament tears (46). It is important to remember that injuries of the cruciate are often associated with injury to other structures and that these should be sought. History can also be helpful (i.e., complete knee dislocation will in most instances be accompanied by disruption of both cruciates and the collateral ligaments) (47). Although this second group is smaller than the first, their injuries are often severe. In recent years, there has been a considerable controversy over the ideal treatment for cruciate ligament injuries. However, most authorities agree that early, accurate diagnosis is vital.

Imaging Techniques

Because of the frequent difficulty in assessing patients with knee trauma, clinicians have turned to a variety of imaging techniques to help with the assessment of the integrity of the cruciate ligaments. Diagnostic arthrography has been the most widely used. To have the greatest opportunity to identify the anterior cruciate, a double-contrast technique must be utilized (Fig. 2-12). Because the cruciate ligaments are extrasynovial, the radiologist must rely on demonstration of the synovial reflections over the anterior cruciate ligament to demonstrate indirectly the presence of a normal anterior cruciate ligament. Although some investigators have had high accuracy in demonstrating abnormality of the anterior cruciate ligament with arthrography (48–53), most investigators report accuracies of only 50–70%. To maximize the possibility of demonstrating the anterior cruciate ligament in arthrography, the cruciate ligaments should be examined before attempting to demonstrate meniscal lesions, and stress views of the knee should be obtained. Arthrographic demonstration of cruciate ligament pathology is technically demanding and

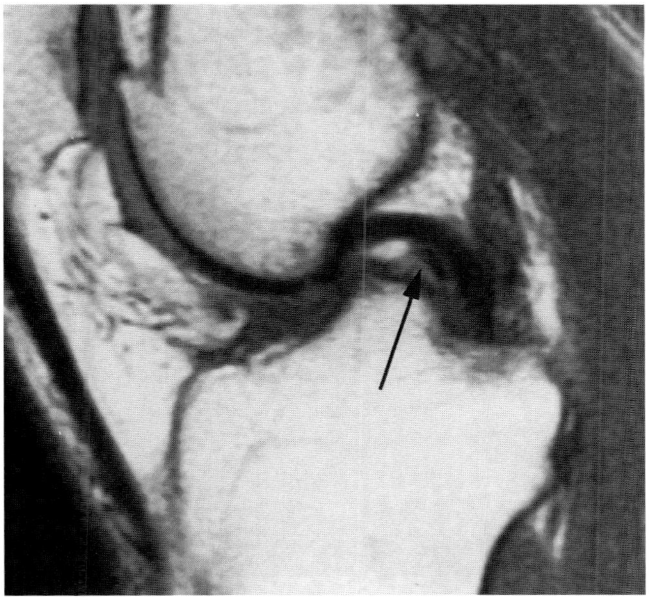

FIG. 2-11. Variability of the meniscofemoral ligaments. Sagittal T1-weighted spin echo (TR 400 msec, TE 16 msec) demonstrates a small, flattened ligament of Humphry *(arrow).*

may be obscured by accompanying torn or peripherally separated menisci and synovial folds (54–56).

Some investigators have used computed tomography (CT) to examine the cruciate ligaments (Fig. 2-13) (57–62). Generally, the posterior cruciate is well visualized by this technique, provided that thin sections (2 mm or less) are utilized. The anterior cruciate ligament is often more difficult to identify. Some authorities state that the presence of joint effusions does not compromise the accuracy of CT of the knee; however, our experience has indicated that this is not always the case. Some investigators have speculated on the potential utility of high-resolution ultrasound for demonstration of cruciate lesions, but it appears that this method does not lend itself readily to demonstration of cruciate ligament tears even in patients with large effusions.

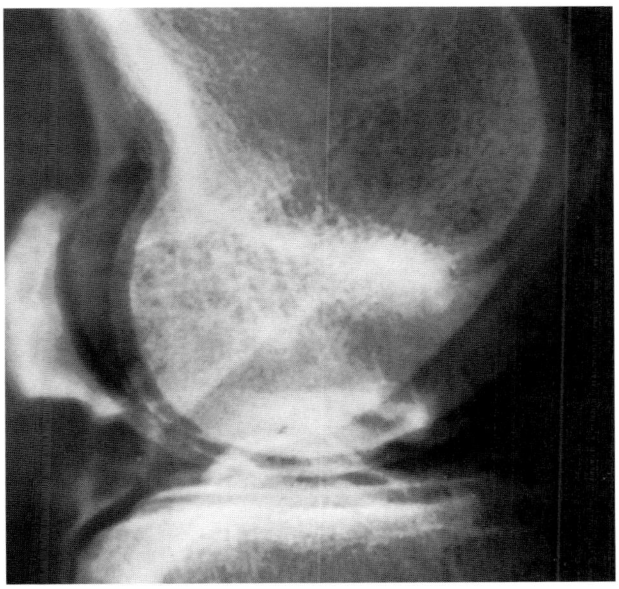

FIG. 2-12. Knee arthrography. On this lateral stress view from a double-contrast knee arthrogram, the normally seen linear synovial reflection is absent, suggesting that the anterior cruciate is torn.

Until the advent of MRI, diagnostic arthroscopy was indisputably the best way for definitively diagnosing cruciate ligament tears (Fig. 2-14; see also color plate 3) (41,63), but there are drawbacks to this technique. It is invasive and requires either general or regional anesthesia. The diagnosis of a torn posterior cruciate ligament usually requires posterior positioning of the arthroscope and/or the use of angled arthroscopes. Many surgeons are uncomfortable with these techniques, so a posterior cruciate tear may be missed. In addition, in patients with chronic hemorrhagic effusions, synovial membrane thickening may occur and obscure the cruciate ligaments, making partial tears especially difficult to diagnose.

Unlike arthrography and arthroscopy, MRI has the advantage of being noninvasive and requires minimal joint manipulation. MRI can examine the cruciate ligaments in the sagittal plane, facilitating demonstration of a tear, whereas CT examines the knee in the axial plane. A number of investigators have advocated the use of nonorthogonal, oblique imaging to better approximate the plane of the anterior cruciate ligament (Fig. 2-15). This may allow improved diagnostic accuracy, especially when the anterior cruciate is not well seen in the usual sagittal plane (39,64).

The Anterior Cruciate

Typically, injury of the anterior cruciate ligament occurs when external rotation and simultaneous valgus movement occur in the flexed knee (37). This mechanism may produce complete or partial tears of the anterior cruciate ligament. Almost invariably, associated tears of collateral ligaments, especially the deep portion of the medial collateral ligament, are present, as well as tears of the menisci. Isolated tears, although unusual, may occur if internal rotation occurs while the knee is in full extension (65). Most often disruption of the anterior cruciate ligament occurs in its midportion (Fig. 2-16), although occasionally the ligament will be avulsed from its femoral insertion (Figs. 2-17 and 2-18). Avulsion from the tibial insertion is much less frequent, and avulsion of a bony fragment may occur (Figs. 2-19 and 2-20) (66). Tibial avulsion is more frequently encountered in children, and periosteal avulsion is rare in both groups. Partial tears (which frequently progress to produce instability) (40) can often be diagnosed, and tears of the posterior band can be differentiated from anterior band tears (Figs. 2-21–2-23). Partial tears may be referred to (especially in the older literature) as "sprains" (67). This differentiation may be of some

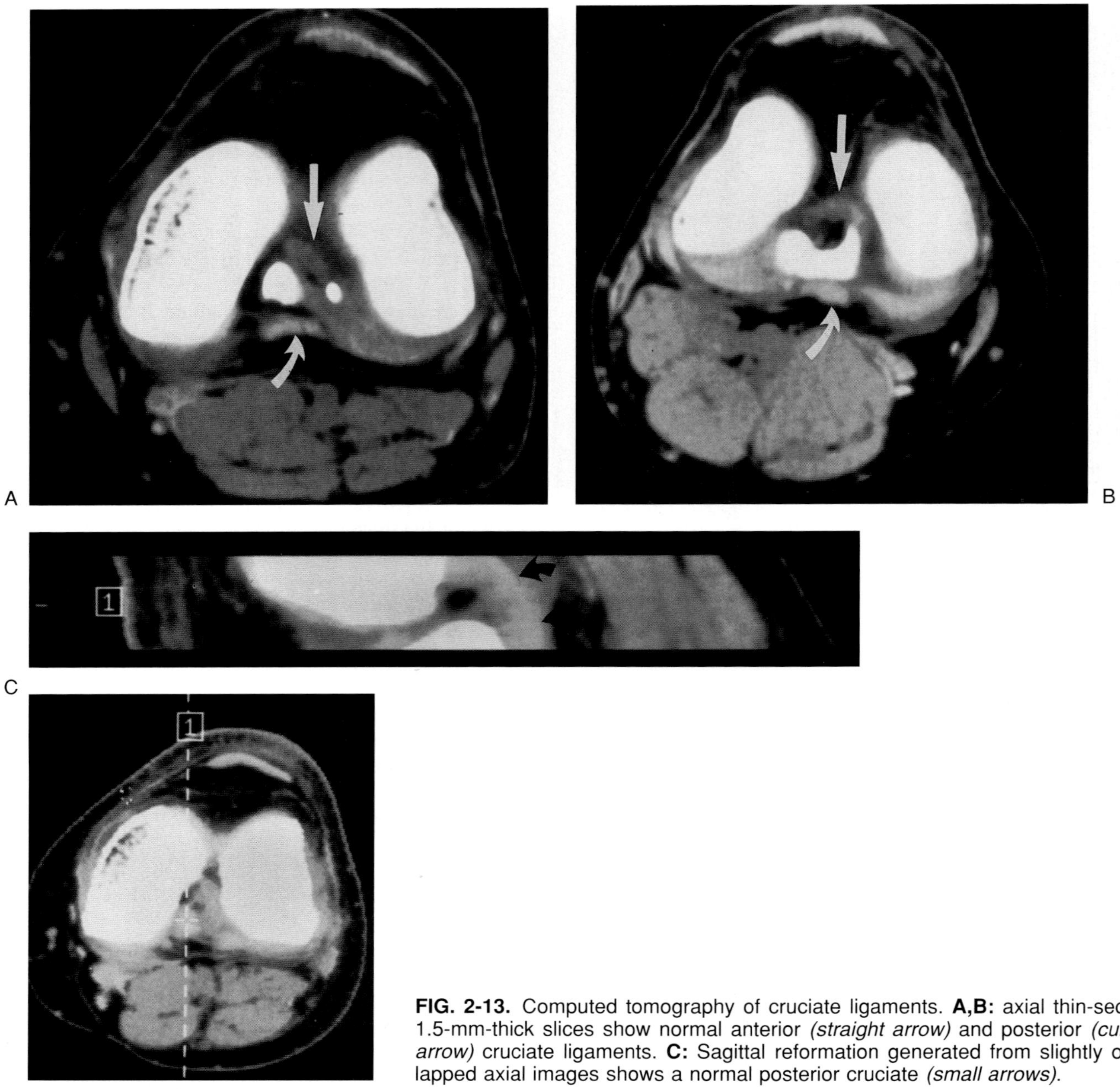

FIG. 2-13. Computed tomography of cruciate ligaments. **A,B:** axial thin-section 1.5-mm-thick slices show normal anterior *(straight arrow)* and posterior *(curved arrow)* cruciate ligaments. **C:** Sagittal reformation generated from slightly overlapped axial images shows a normal posterior cruciate *(small arrows)*.

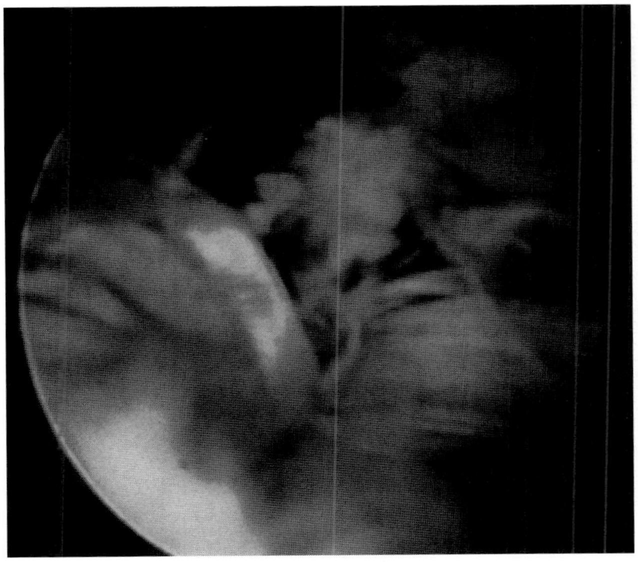

A

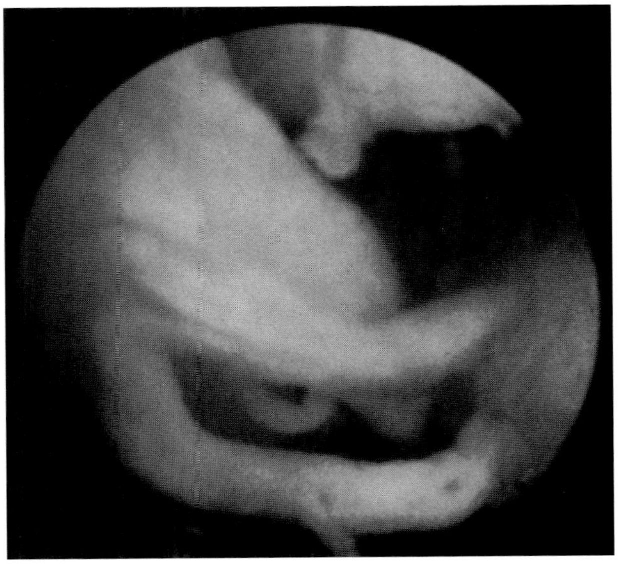

B

FIG. 2-14. Arthroscopic evaluation of anterior cruciate **(A,B)**. Two arthroscopic images of disrupted anterior cruciate ligaments. In **(A)** the torn end is more frayed than in **(B)**.

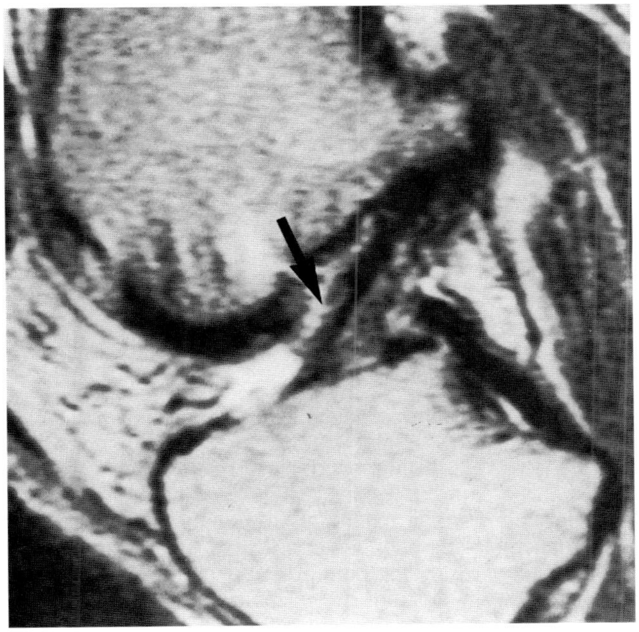

FIG. 2-15. Nonorthogonal anterior cruciate imaging. Oblique sagittal T2-weighted spin echo (TR 2200 msec, TE 80 msec) showing an irregularity of the anterior band *(arrow)* representing a small tear.

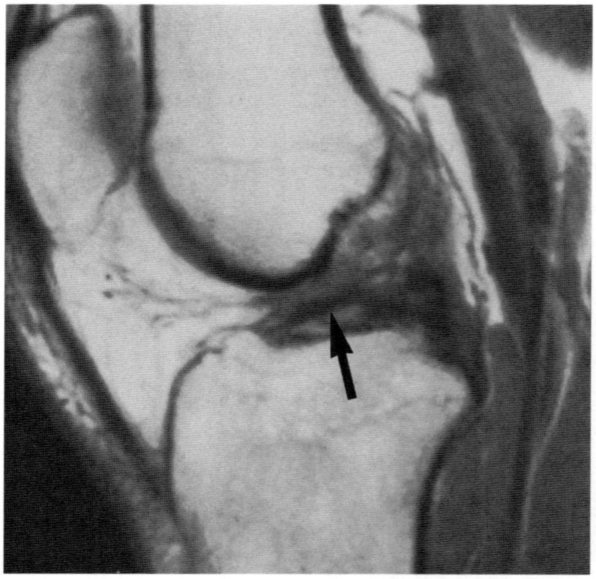

A

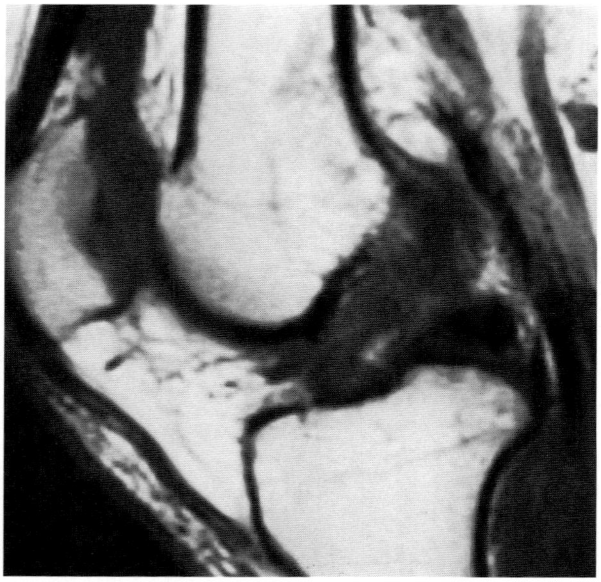

B

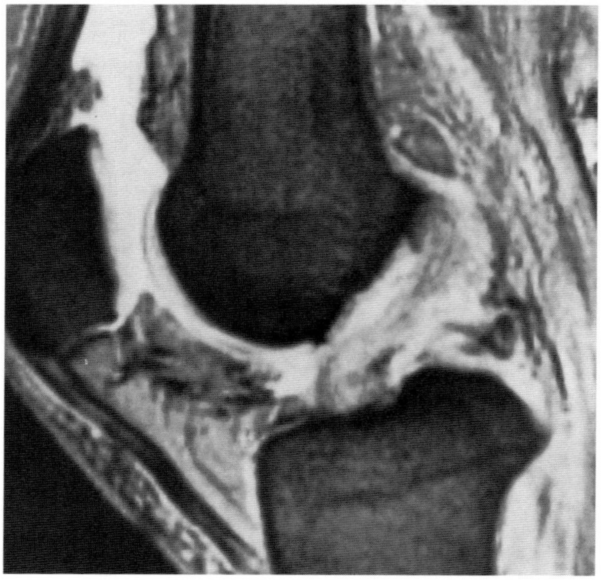

C

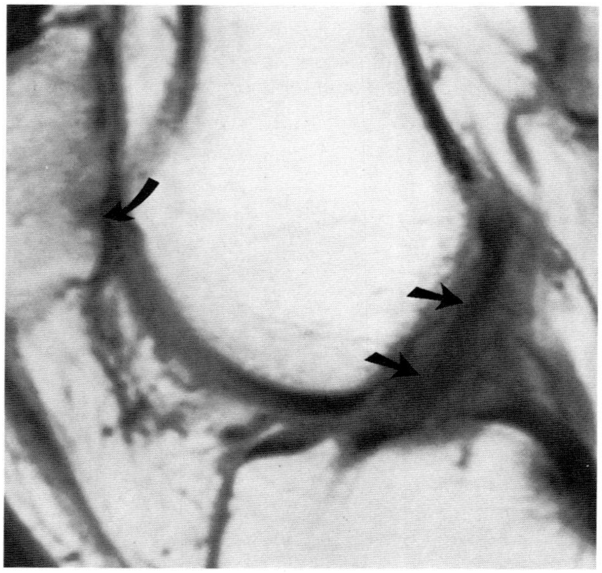

D

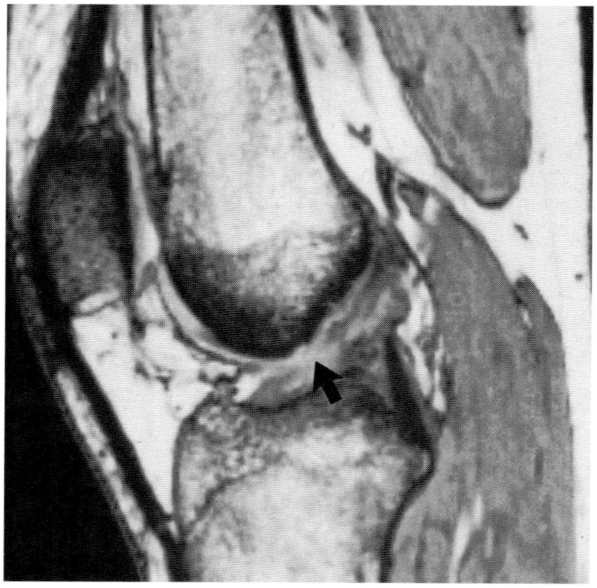

E

FIG. 2-16. Torn anterior cruciate ligament. **A,B:** Sagittal T1-weighted spin-echo images (TR 600 msec, TE 18 msec). Mid-substance tears of the anterior cruciate are often easily appreciated on T1-weighted images, where the ligament is seen to sag dependently *(arrow)* as in **A**. At times a torn cruciate may be difficult to see because of edema and fluid, as shown in **B**. **C:** Sagittal T2*-weighted gradient-echo MPGR (TR 400 msec, TE 18 msec, flip angle 20°). Rapidly acquired gradient-echo images often permit the damaged ligament to be better visualized. The ligament is thick and the high-signal edema/blood outlines the ligament's lower-signal fibers, producing an arthrographic effect. A similar effect can be achieved using spin-echo or fast spin sequences. **D:** Sagittal T1-weighted spin echo (TR 600 msec, TE 18 msec). At times a partially torn ligament may not be appreciated on conventional imaging. *Straight arrows*, anterior band of the anterior cruciate; *curved arrow*, incidental chondromalacia of the patella. **E:** Sagittal T2*-weighted volumetric 3DFT GRASS (TR 55 msec, TE 15 msec, flip angle 30°), from the same patient as **D**. A tear in the anterior band is seen in the anterior band *(arrow)*. (From Munk P. *J Can Assoc Radiol* 1989;40:292-303 used with permission.)

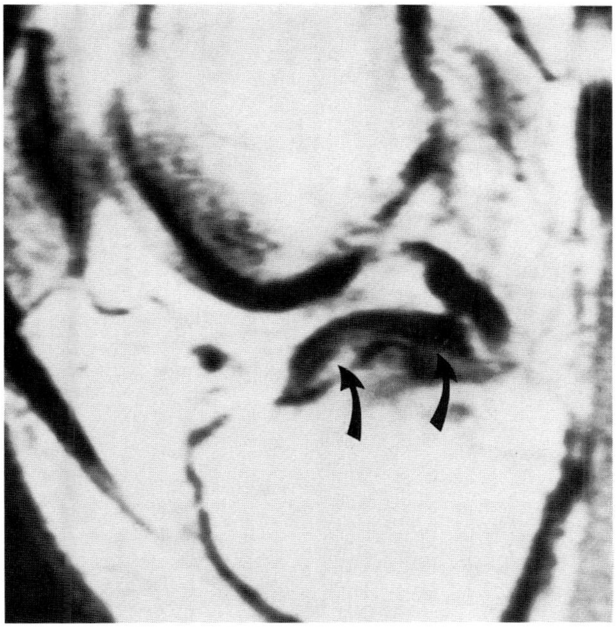

FIG. 2-17. Sagittal T1-weighted spin echo (TR 800 msec, TE 18 msec). Proximal anterior cruciate avulsion from femoral origin. The ligament lies draped inferiorly on the tibial plateau *(arrows)*.

importance in that the anterior band, when torn, more frequently progresses to an unfavorable result (68,69). More often than not, the tear is not a clean one and the anterior cruciate ligament is shredded, making primary repair difficult.

Symptoms are quite variable. The patient may demonstrate immediate instability of the joint with marked pain and hemarthrosis, or in some instances may show symptoms of instability. Clinical examination is often difficult because of patient pain, swelling, joint effusion, and muscular spasm. A large number of clinical maneuvers have been designed to test for integrity of the anterior cruciate ligament (anterior drawer sign, the Lachman maneuver, and pivot shift test, to give a few examples) (2,3,41,70). These are quite accurate in experienced hands and with cooperative patients. Generally speaking, anterior displacement of the tibia of 5 mm or more is a reliable indicator of an abnormal anterior cruciate ligament. This principle has been used with graded stress radiography in making this diagnosis (71). Hemarthrosis is recognized as common (1,72,73).

Both the orthopedic and radiologic literature emphasize the high incidence of associated meniscal tears with tears of the anterior cruciate ligament. Figures vary from 42% to 65% of patients having an associated meniscal tear in the acute situation to 88% of patients who demonstrate tears of the meniscus in the chronic state (over 14 days) (1,2,74–78).

A number of primary and secondary MRI criteria exist for the diagnosis of tears of the anterior cruciate ligament. In the presence of a partial- or full-thickness tear, irregularity or a wavy contour of the anterior margin of the anterior cruciate ligament is often demonstrated on sagittal images (see Fig. 2-16C). In addition, increased signal within the substance of the ligament, presumably representing blood or edema, is present (see Fig. 2-16B). With a complete tear, discontinuity of the fibers will be seen, as well as abnormal orientation of the torn ends (Fig. 2-16A). The angle between the lateral tibial plateau and the anterior cruciate is less than 45° with complete tears (79). Another angle that can be assessed is that between the anterior cruciate and the cortical margin of the intercondylar notch of the femur (Blumenstaat line), which measures more than 15° with complete tears (79). Coronal images show absence of the normal fibers in the intercondylar notch—the "empty notch sign" (80) (Fig. 2-24).

An ancillary or secondary finding consists of anterior displacement of the tibia on the femur, with accompanying bowing of the posterior cruciate ligament. This may result in being able to visualize the whole length of the posterior cruciate on coronal images (81). This is due to anterior displacement of the tibia on the femur. The posterior horn of the lateral meniscus has been used as a marker for tibial translocation on sagittal imaging. If a line is drawn tangential to the posterior cortical margin of the tibia, it should not intersect the meniscus—the "uncovered meniscus sign" (81–84). Probably more useful is the pattern of bone contusions frequently encountered with anterior cruciate tears. Most injuries to the anterior cruciate involve at least part of the force driving the tibia anteriorly to the femur. This results in impaction of the posterior lip of the tibia onto the femoral condyle, usually affecting the lateral compartment (85–90). This produces a classic finding of low-signal subcortical bone marrow in these two areas when viewed on T1-weighted sagittal images (Fig. 2-25). Their presence is accentuated if T2 weighting is used or especially if fat suppression is employed (91). Cartilage and cortex may be fractured or displaced (92). This finding is very suggestive of the presence of an anterior cruciate tear. It is a specific indicator of anterior cruciate pathology but unfortunately is not sensitive (all patients with these contusions have at least a partial tear of the anterior cruciate, but some who have an anterior cruciate tear may not have contusions (about 75–80%) (83,93). Nonetheless, it is probably the most helpful of the ancillary findings for diagnosis of anterior cruciate pathology. The presence of bone contusions is most helpful in the acute and subacute setting(<9 weeks), because they usually resolve. The overlying cartilage may become atrophic and the subcortical bone may be of lower signal than normal, but these findings are subtle in many instances. Cobby and colleagues have noted the presence of an unusually deep lateral femoral notch on lateral knee radiographs in patients with torn anterior cruciates, which may be secondary to the impaction injury that occurs (94). This sign is quite specific, but insensitive (79,81). Although the use of indirect signs of anterior cruciate injury helps alert us to the presence of possible injury because sensitivity is in many instances low, the absence of these signs cannot exclude a tear (79).

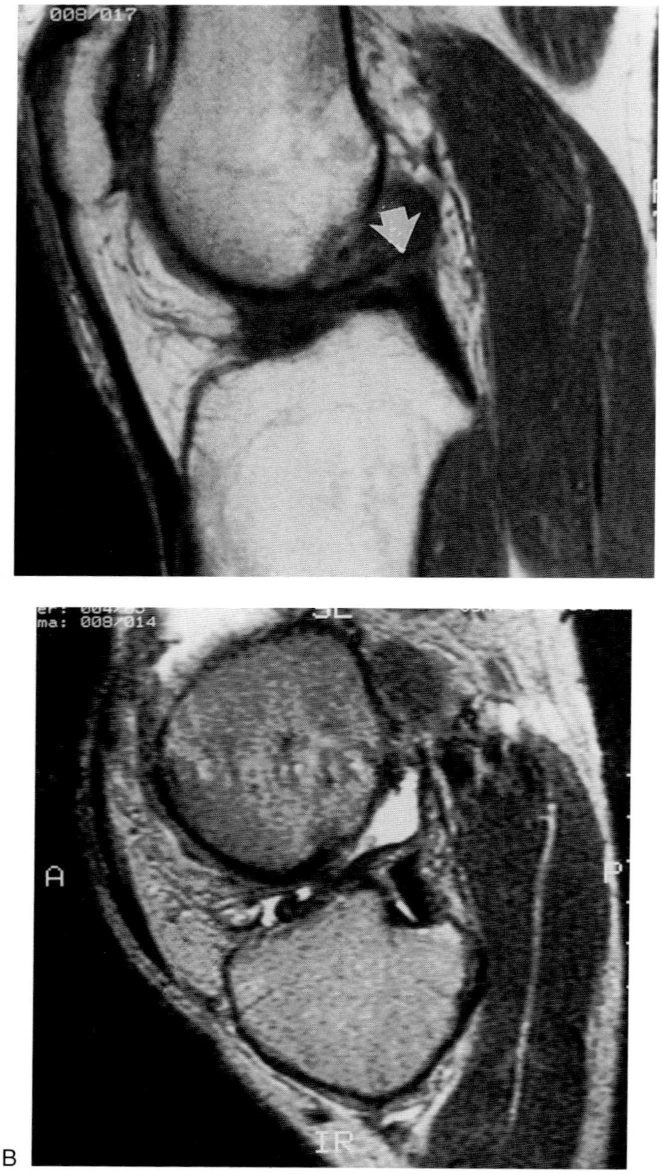

A

B

FIG. 2-18. Proximal ligament avulsion. **A:** Sagittal T1-weighted spin echo (TR 600 msec, TE 18 msec). The avulsed anterior band can be seen as a low-signal structure displaced inferiorly *(arrow)* and surrounded by slightly higher signal edema/blood. **B:** Oblique sagittal T2-weighted spin echo (TR 2200 msec, TE 80 msec) shows the same damaged ligament to greater advantage. The high-signal fluid adjacent to the ligament helps outline the avulsed cranial portion.

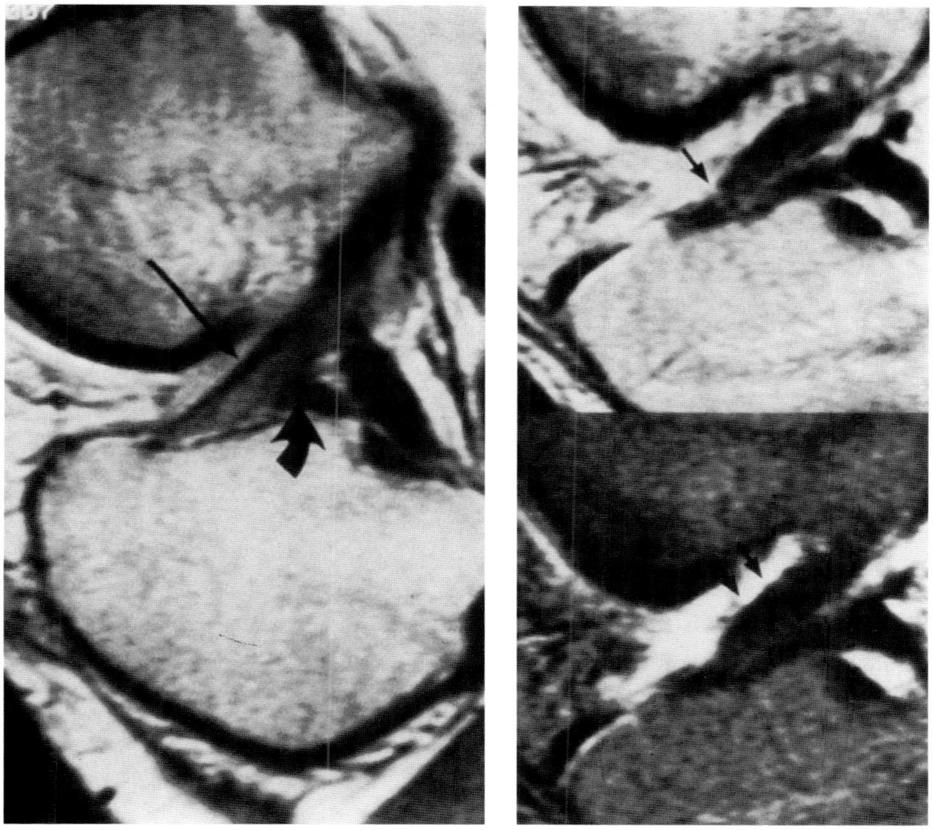

A

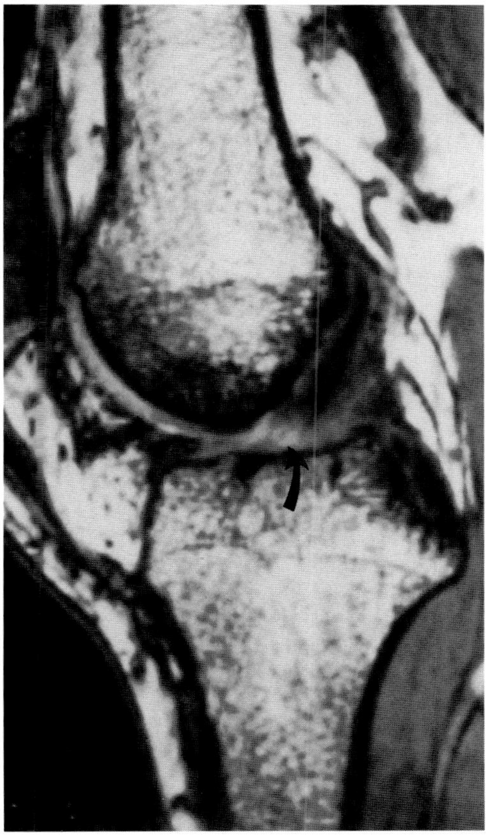

B

FIG. 2-19. Distal anterior cruciate tear. **A:** On the left a normal anterior cruciate is seen. Oblique sagittal proton-density spin echo (TR 2000 msec, TE 20 msec). The anterior band is shown by the *straight arrow*, the posterior band by the *curved arrow*. On the right the proton-density image above and the T2-weighted spin-echo image (TR 2000 msec, TE 80 msec) below show a partially attenuated anterior cruciate ligaments, partly torn from their distal insertion. **B:** Sagittal T2*-weighted 3DFT gradient-echo GRASS (TR 55 msec, TE 15 msec, flip angle 30°) 2-mm-thick image from a different patient shows tear at distal insertion *(curved arrow)*.

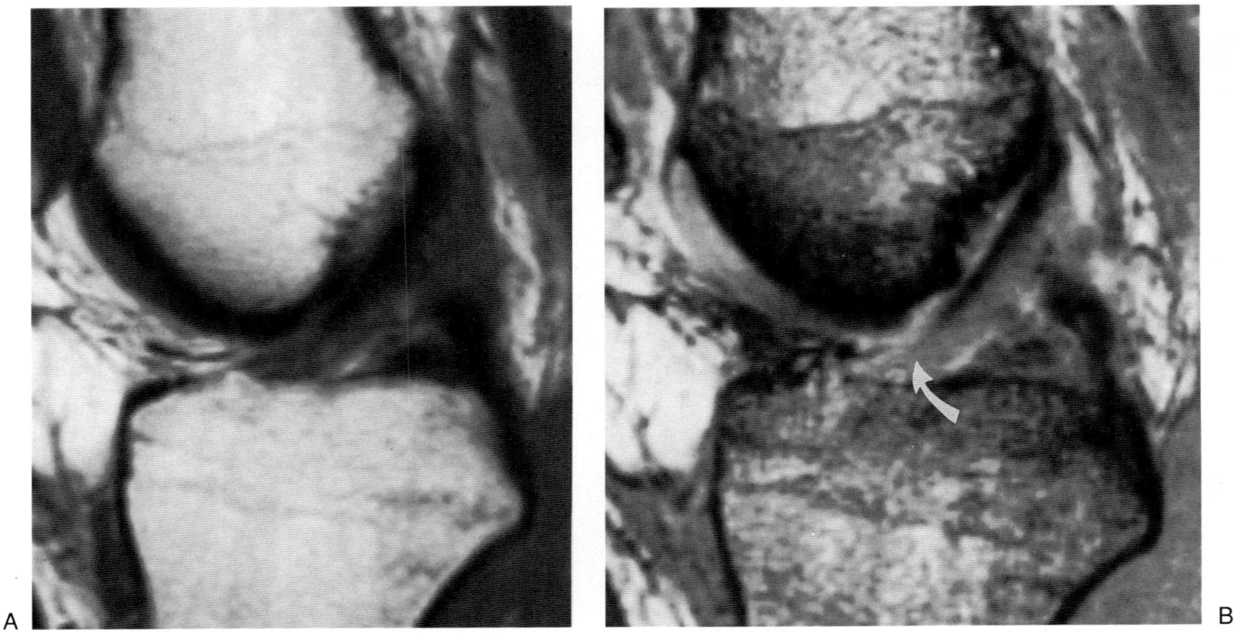

FIG. 2-20. Undisplaced distal anterior cruciate tear. **A:** Sagittal T1-weighted spin-echo (TR 600 msec, TE 18 msec) image with poorly visualized distal portion of the anterior band several weeks after trauma to the knee. **B:** Sagittal T2*-weighted 3DFT gradient-echo GRASS (TR 55 msec, TE 15 msec, flip angle 30°) image from the same patient shows the defect in the caudal aspect of the anterior band with greater clarity *(curved arrow)*.

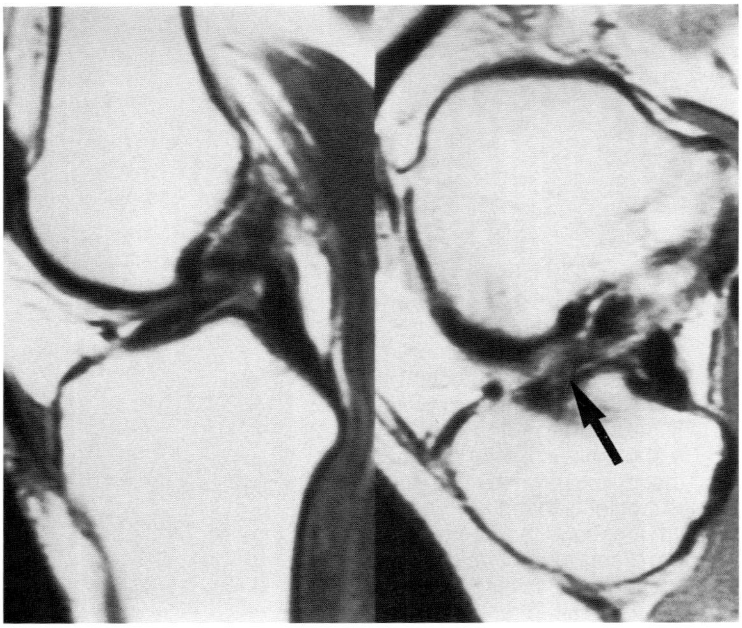

FIG. 2-21. High-grade partial-tear anterior cruciate. On the left a sagittal T1-weighted spin echo-image (TR 800 msec, TE 20 msec) is shown. The partial tear *(arrow)* of the anterior cruciate is better seen on the right oblique sagittal proton density image (TR 2000 msec, TE 60 msec).

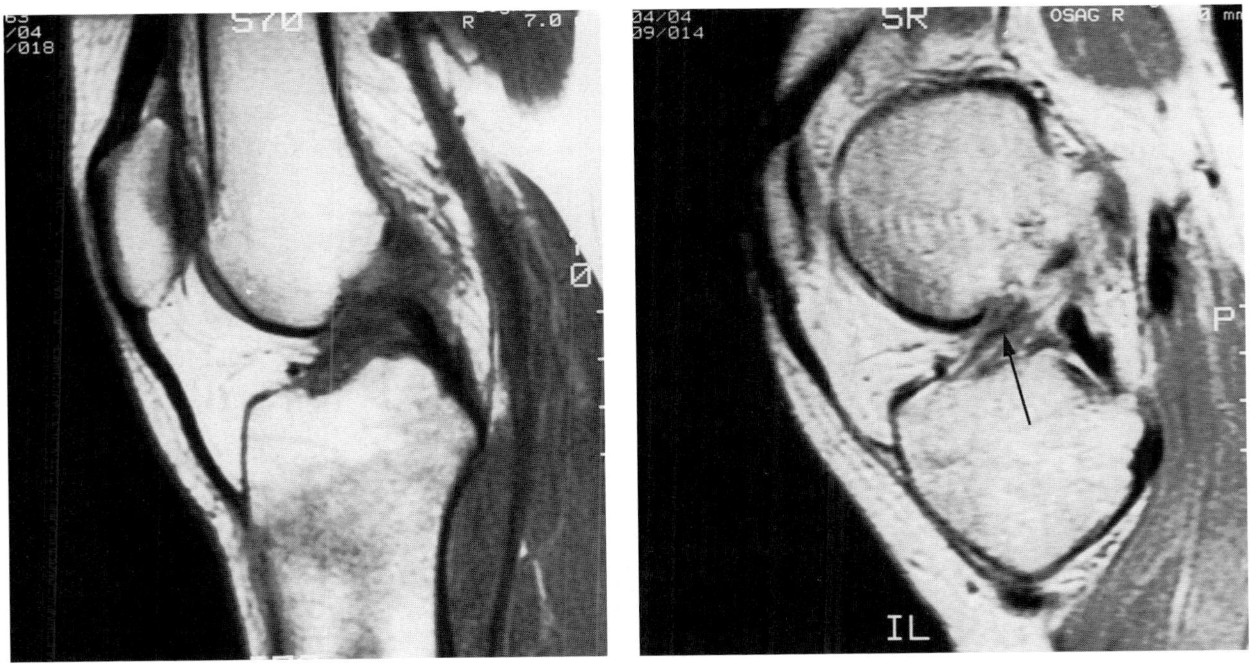

A B

FIG. 2-22. Anterior band partial tear. **A:** Sagittal T1-weighted spin-echo image (TR 600 msec, TE 18 msec). The anterior cruciate is obscured by edema/fluid and a tear must be strongly suspected. **B:** Oblique sagittal T2-weighted spin echo (TR 2000 msec, TE 80 msec) shows the damaged anterior cruciate in much better detail. The anterior band *(arrow)* is seen outlined by fluid and is redundant and displaced slightly inferiorly.

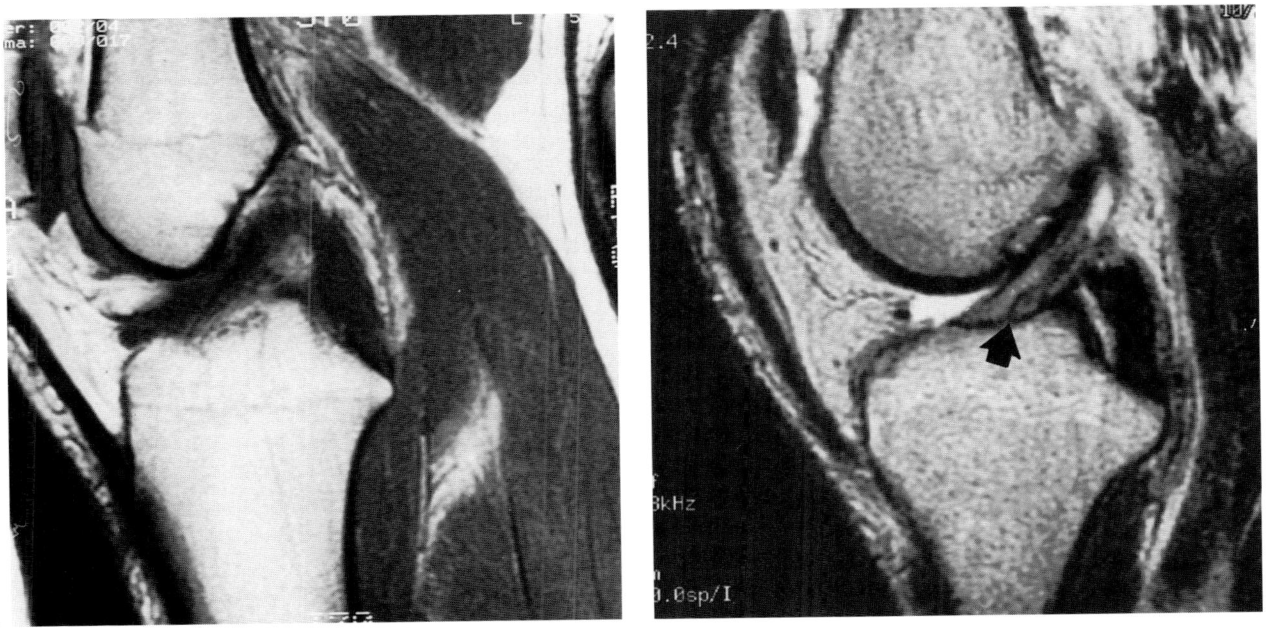

A B

FIG. 2-23. Posterior band partial tear. **A:** Sagittal T1-weighted spin-echo image (TR 600 msec, TE 18 msec). The inferior two-thirds of the anterior cruciate can be visualized, but detail is hazy. **B:** Oblique sagittal T2-weighted spin echo (TR 2000 msec, TE 80 msec). The posterior band fibers *(arrow)* are seen to be redundant/irregular, consistent with a partial tear.

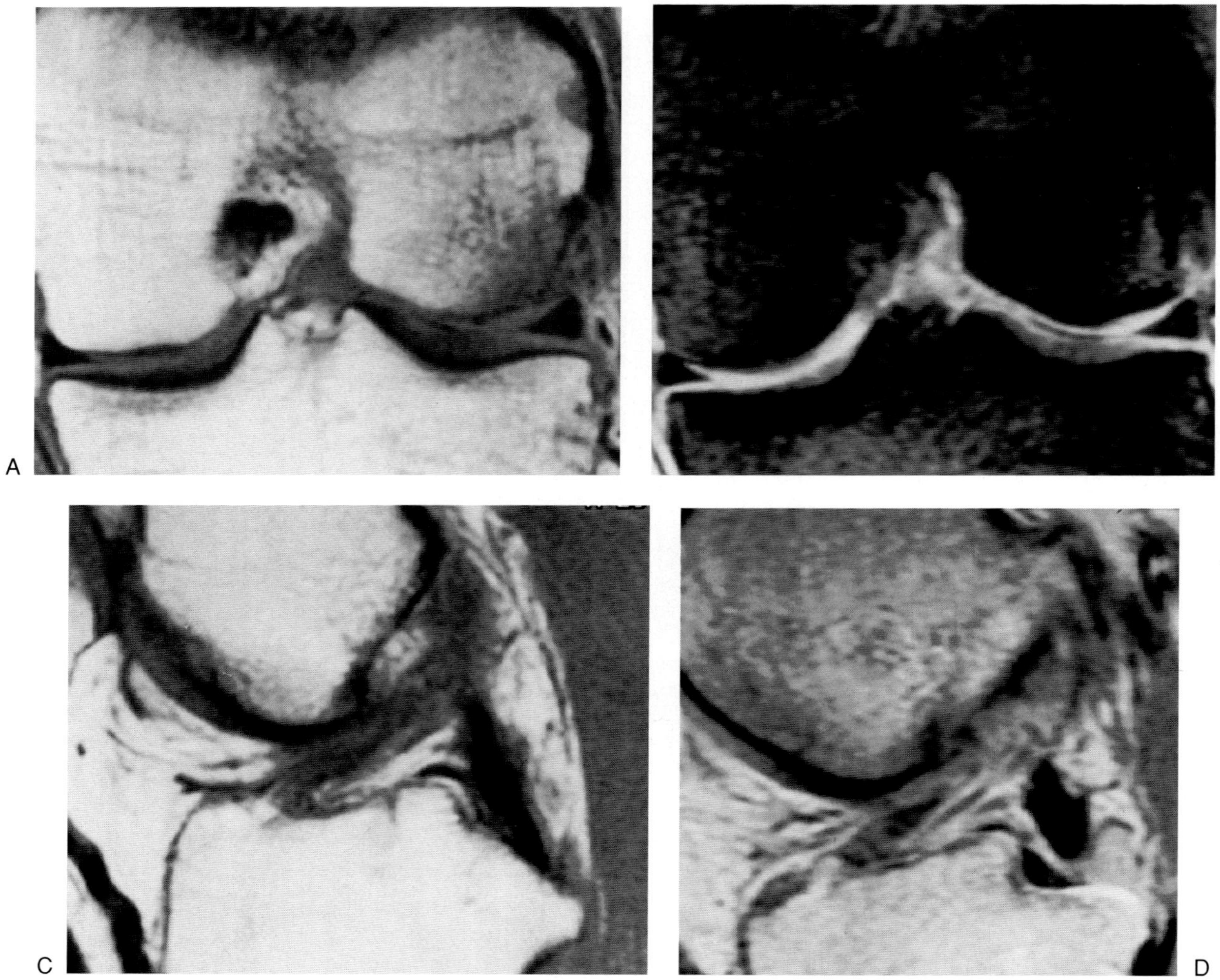

FIG. 2-24. Empty notch sign. **Patient 1: A:** Coronal T1-weighted spin echo image (TR 600 msec, TE 16 msec) through the intercondylar notch shows a hazy area of greyness at the insertion of the anterior cruciate ligament with no distinct fibers visible. **B:** Coronal T2*-weighted gradient-echo MPGR (TR 400 msec, TE 20 msec, flip angle 20°) image shows similar findings with only a few poorly defined low-signal fibers present. **C:** Sagittal T1-weighted spin-echo (TR 500 msec, TE 13 msec) image shows a poorly defined anterior cruciate that is torn and displaced inferiorly. **D:** Oblique sagittal proton density spin echo (TR 2000 msec, TE 30 msec) shows some of the fibers slightly better and confirms the presence of the tear.

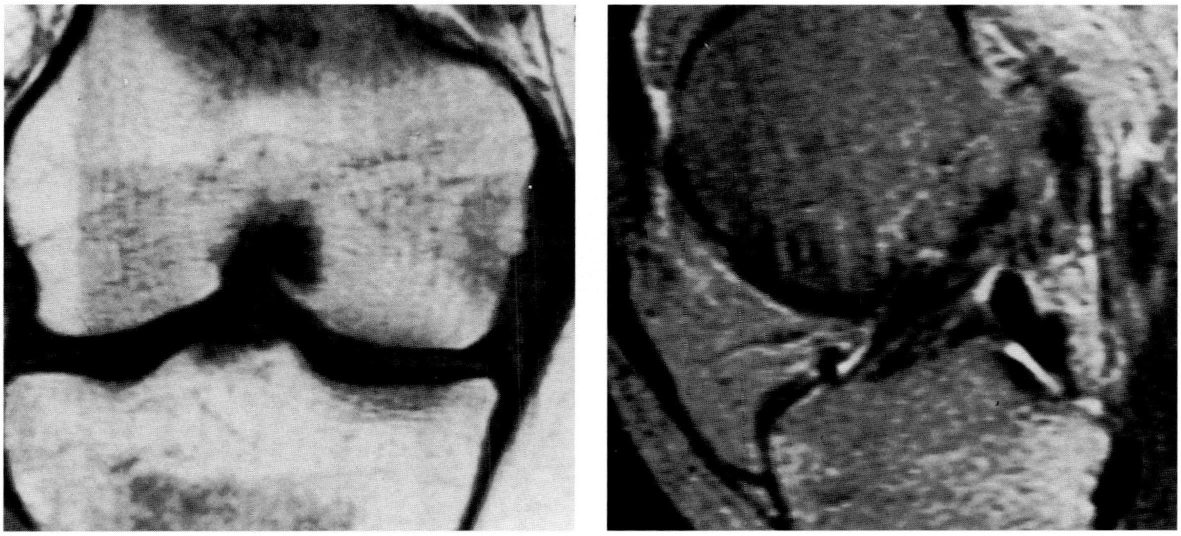

A B

FIG. 2-24. *(Continued).* **Patient 2: A:** Coronal T1-weighted spin-echo (TR 500 msec, TE 20 msec) image also displays an amorphous appearance to the distal anterior cruciate. **B:** Oblique sagittal spin-echo (TR 2500 msec, TE 80 msec) image shows a partial tear of the anterior cruciate with splaying of fibers.

A joint effusion, a common finding in acute cruciate ligament injuries, often obscures the anterior cruciate ligament on T1-weighted spin-echo images. This problem may be circumvented by utilizing either T2-weighted images or gradient-echo T2 images that produce an arthrographic effect, thereby dramatically outlining the anterior cruciate ligament (see Fig. 2-16C).

The Posterior Cruciate

Considerably more force is required to produce a tear of the posterior cruciate ligament than the anterior cruciate (29). The posterior cruciate is thicker and sturdier, measuring 30% larger in cross section (22,30,95). The most common mechanism for producing tears of the posterior cruciate consists of external rotation with a valgus force or internal rotation with a varus force. Occasionally, forceful hyperextension or direct trauma to the upper tibia in flexion, both often occurring in contact sports, will produce a tear in the posterior cruciate (Fig. 2-26) (23,25,26,96,97). The most common site for a tear is the midportion of the ligament (Figs. 2-27 and 2-28) and, less frequently, the femoral insertion (Figs. 2-29 and 2-30). The tibial insertion is very strong, and it is unusual to avulse the ligament distally from its bony insertion (Fig. 2-31). Occasionally, a bony fragment will be avulsed and the ligament will be left intact (Figs. 2-32 and 2-33) (23,97,98). This occurs more commonly at the tibial insertion than at the femoral insertion. When a tibial avulsion occurs, the posterior horn of the adjacent meniscus undergoes detachment or tear. In more than two-thirds of cases, an associated anterior cruciate tear is present, and more than one-half have an associated medial collateral ligament disruption (see Fig. 2-28). When only partial tears of the anterior cruciate are present, usually the posterior band is torn. As with anterior cruciate ligament tears, clinical symptomatology is extremely variable. Many patients demonstrate marked tenderness over the popliteal fossa accompanied by swelling; more than one-half the patients demonstrate a positive posterior drawer sign. Complete tears demonstrate fraying at the site of the tear when seen in the sagittal plane (see Fig. 2-27), whereas incomplete tears are noted as areas of increased signal within the ligament, often accompanied by focal thickening (Fig. 2-34) (99–101). The mere presence of a small focus of increased signal, particularly on T1-weighted images, is not enough to make the diagnosis of a partial tear because this may also be seen in eosinophilic or mucoid degeneration. Some thickening and/or margin irregularity should be present (102). In the coronal plane, a ring of decreased signal may be seen around the posterior cruciate, a finding we refer to as the "halo sign." T2 or T2* images may be helpful in establishing that the posterior cruciate is normal in those instances when T1-weighted images are equivocal (Figs. 2-35–2-38).

Bone contusions may be encountered with posterior cruciate injuries as well. They are usually found at the inferior aspect of the femoral condyle and at the anterior aspect of the tibia, because these injuries have an element of hyperextension. The pattern of bone contusion does not appear to be as characteristic or as common as that seen with anterior cruciate ligament injuries (102).

Accuracy

The accuracy of MRI is high in evaluating the cruciate ligament. Quoted specificities for complete tears range from

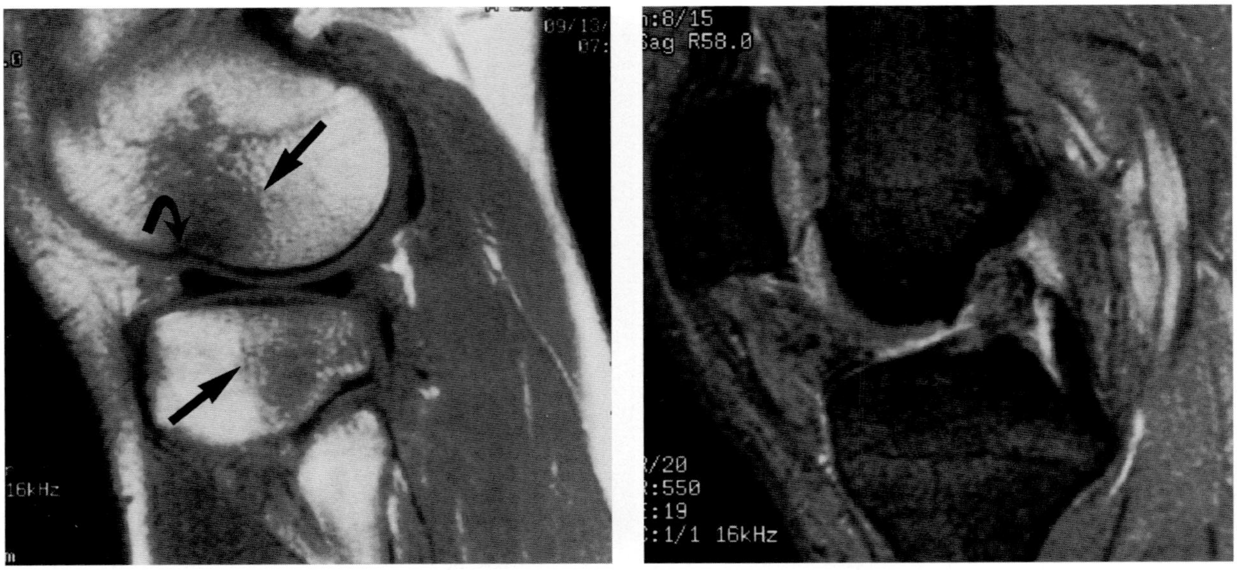

A B

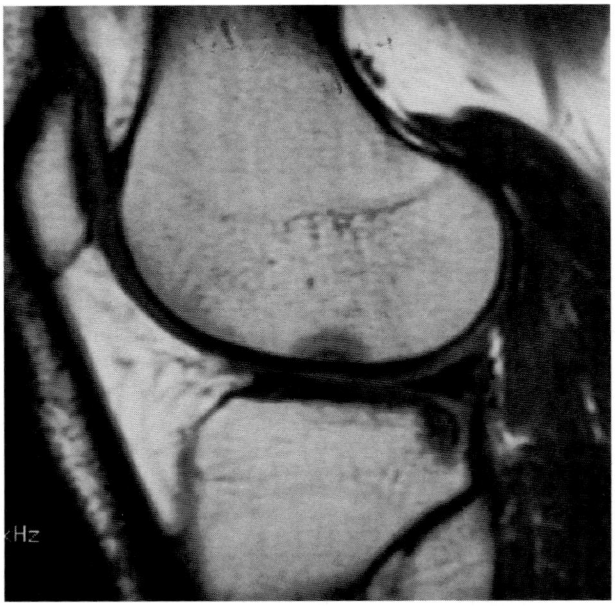

C

FIG. 2-25. Bone contusions. **A:** Sagittal T1-weighted spin-echo image (TR 500 msec, TE 13 msec) from a patient with a complete tear of the anterior cruciate ligament. The areas of edematous/hemorrhagic bone marrow subjacent to the impact sites are seen as zones of diminished signal intensity compared to the bright fat-containing marrow *(arrows)*. An impacted cortical fracture of the femoral condyle *(curved arrow)* is also noted. **B:** Sagittal T2* image showing a torn and inferiorly displaced anterior cruciate. Bone contusions are not seen because of the magnetic susceptibility effect inherent to gradient echo techniques. **C:** Sagittal T1-weighted spin-echo image shows small subchondral contusions at the posterior tibial lip and the femoral condyle. The anterior cruciate was torn.

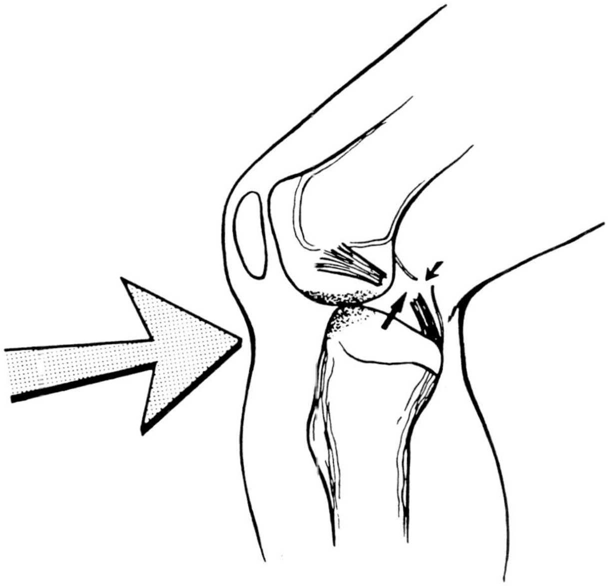

FIG. 2-26. Diagrammatic representation of a common mechanism for posterior cruciate tears. A force *(large arrow)* is applied to the tibia, resulting in posterior displacement (often with hyperextension) of the tibia relative to the femur. Both the posterior cruciate and joint capsule *(small arrows)* become disrupted. (From Sonin A, et al. *Radiology* 1994; 190:455–458 with permission).

A

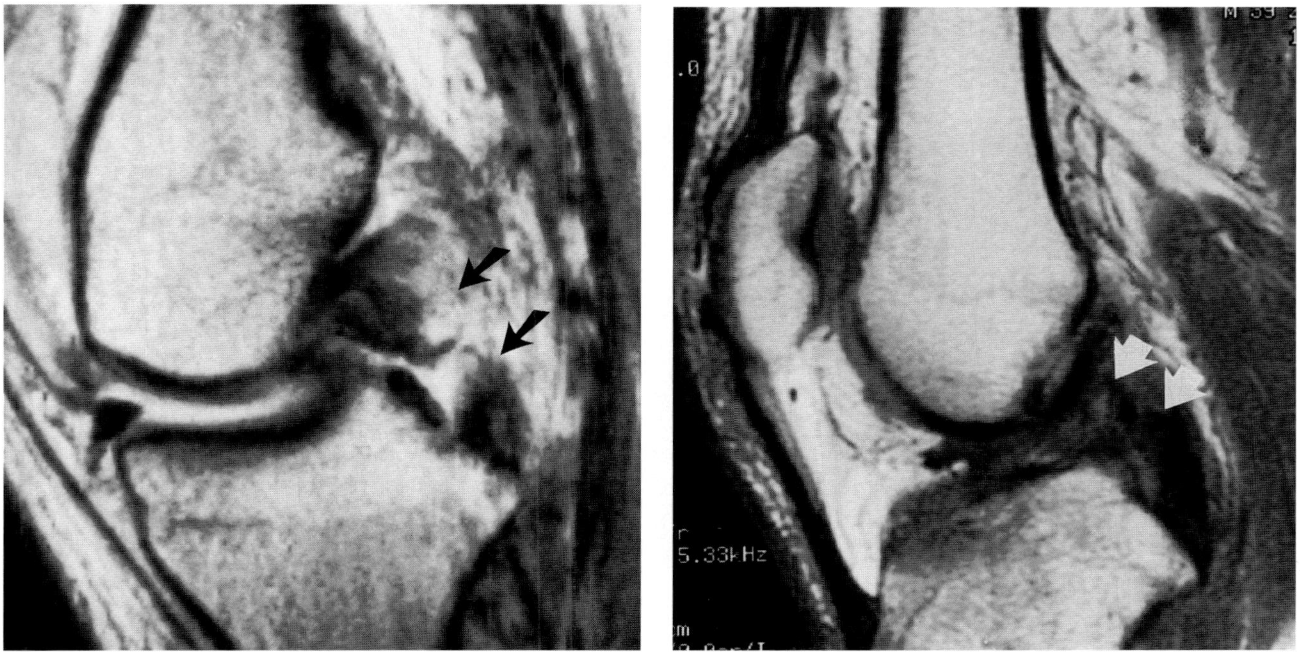

B

FIG. 2-27. Midsubstance disruption of posterior cruciate. **A:** Sagittal proton-density spin echo (TR 2000 msec, TE 20 msec). The whole thickness of the ligament has been torn with the frayed ends being clearly visualized *(arrow)*. (From Munk PL. *J Can Assoc Radiol* 1989;40:296–303, with permission). **B:** Sagittal T1-weighted spin echo (TR 550 msec, TE 15 msec) from a different patient shows a slightly thickened posterior cruciate with increased signal intensity within the substance of the ligament *(arrows)*.

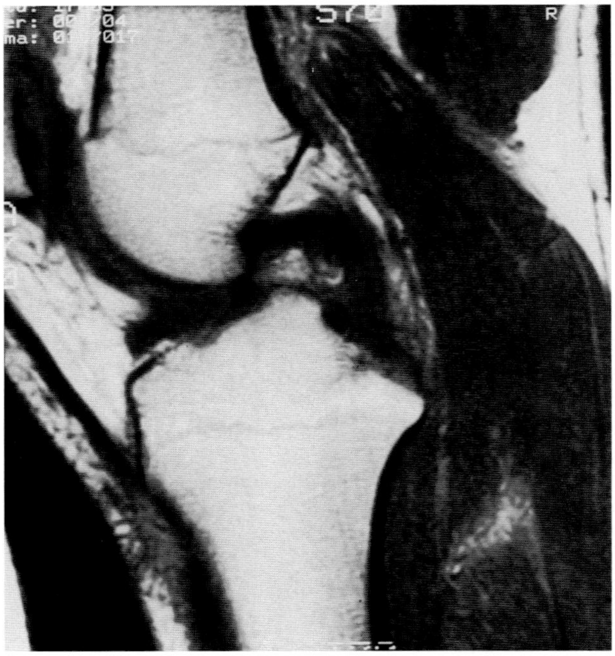

A

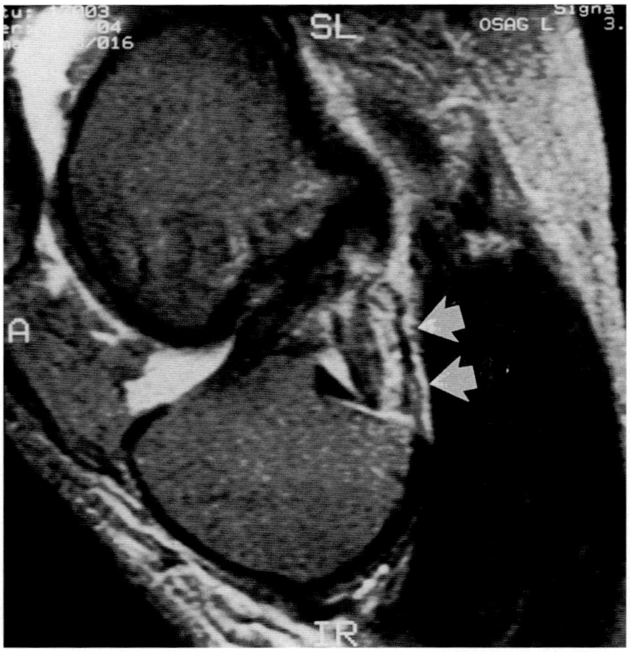

B

FIG. 2-28. Disruption of both cruciate ligaments **(A)** Sagittal T1-weighted spin echo (TR 500 msec, TE 13 msec). Posterior cruciate appears slightly thickened with streaky areas of increased signal intensity. **B:** Oblique sagittal T2-weighted spin echo (TR 2000 msec, TE 80 msec) shows the damaged posterior cruciate to better advantage *(arrows)*. Low-signal fibers are separated by high-signal blood/edema. Note the irregular appearence of the disrupted anterior cruciate.

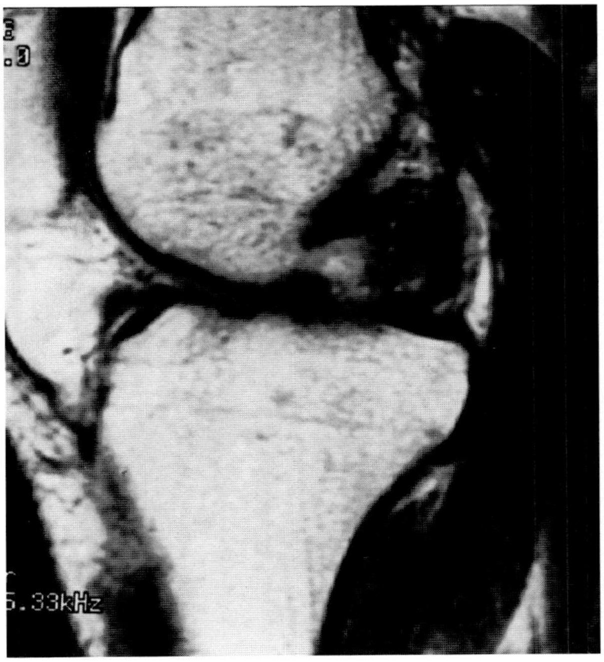

A

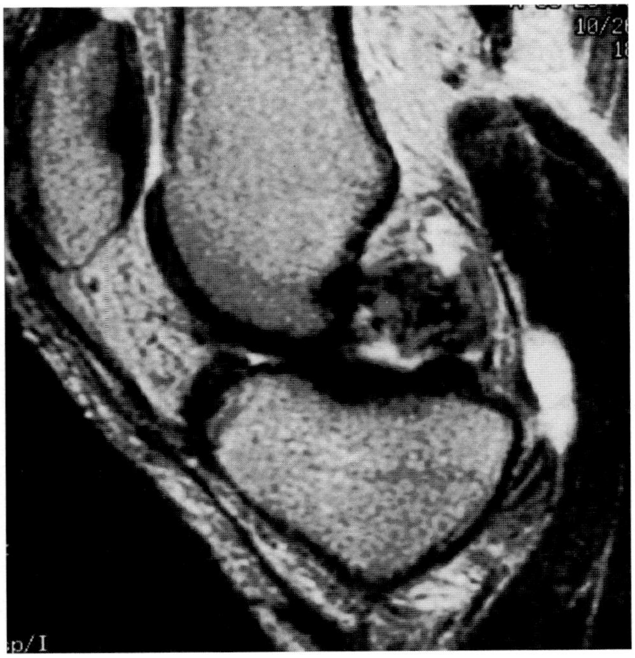

B

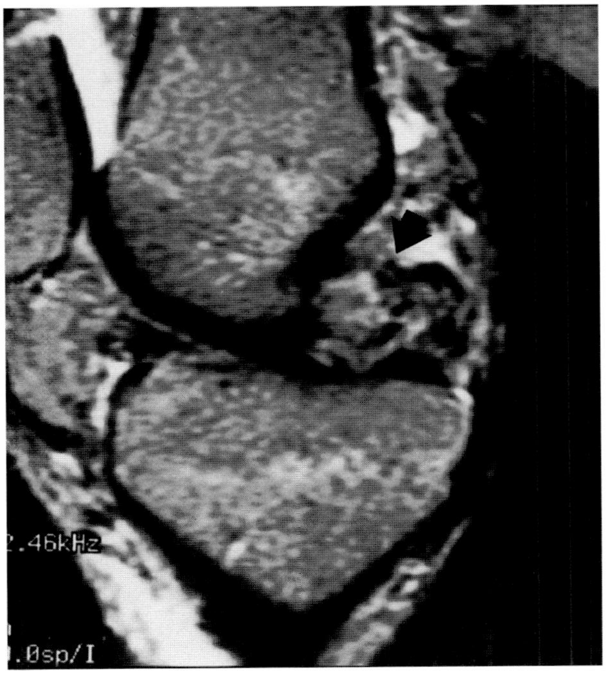

C

FIG. 2-29. Proximal posterior cruciate avulsion. **A:** Sagittal T1-weighted spin echo (TR 500 msec, TE 13 msec) shows a posterior cruciate that is markedly thickened with a globular appearence. **B:** Oblique sagittal T2-weighted image (TR 2000 msec, TE 60 msec) shows the disrupted fibers and edema to advantage and confirms the presence of a tear. **C:** Oblique sagittal T2-weighted image (TR 2200 msec, TE 80 msec) from a different patient. The avulsed cranial portion of the ligament *(arrow)* is seen surrounded by high-signal edema/blood.

A 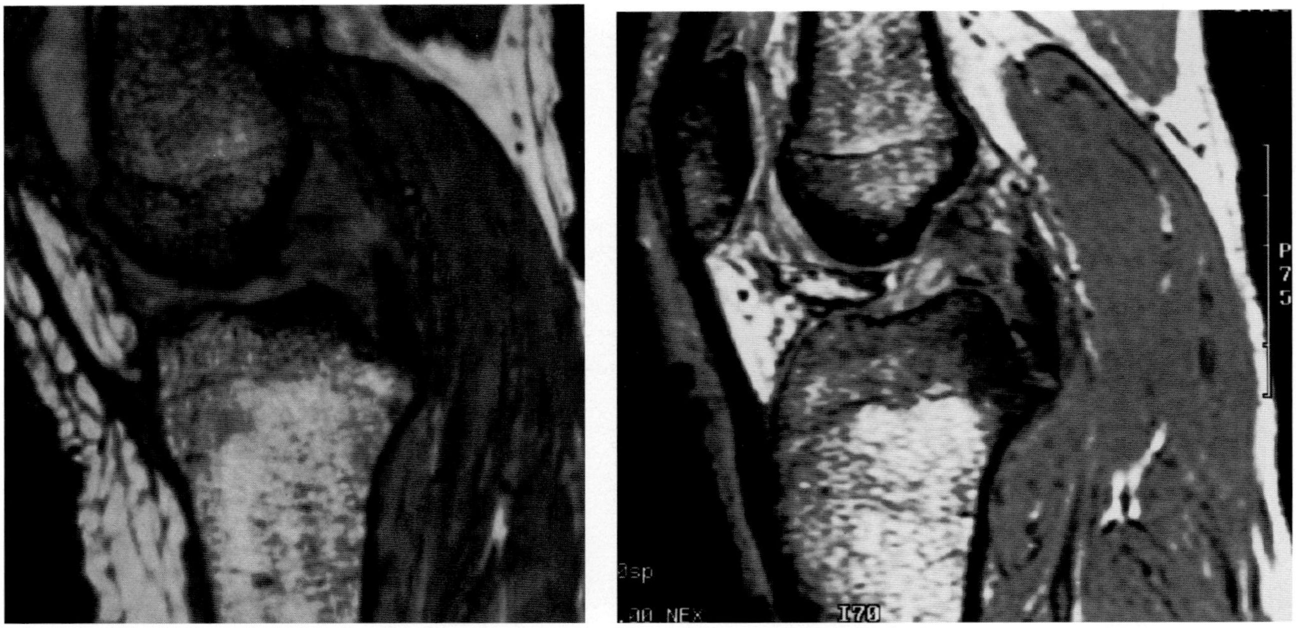 B

FIG. 2-30. A: Sagittal T2*-weighted gradient-echo 3DFT GRASS (TR 55 msec, TE 15 msec, flip angle 30°) shows increased signal in the proximal portion of the ligament, greater than would be expected. **B:** Similar image from a different patient also shows increased signal and irregularity in the proximal fibers.

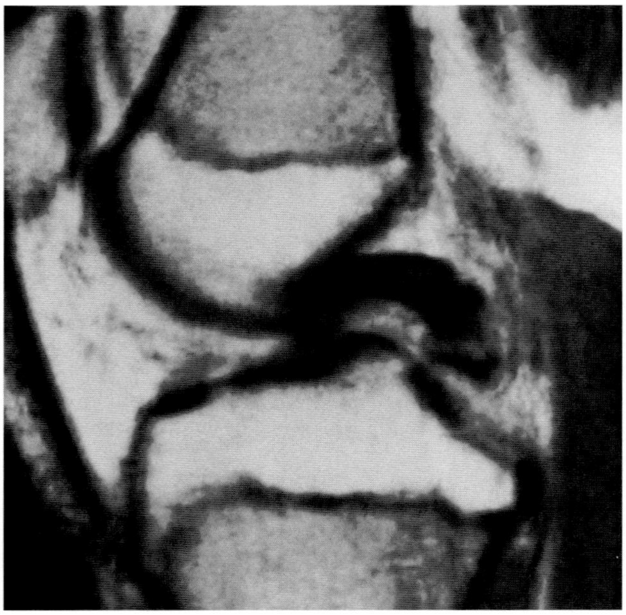

FIG. 2-31. Distal avulsion of the posterior cruciate ligament. Sagittal T1-weighted spin echo (TR 800 msec, TE 18 msec). The distal insertion has been avulsed, in this case not taking a significant bone fragment with it.

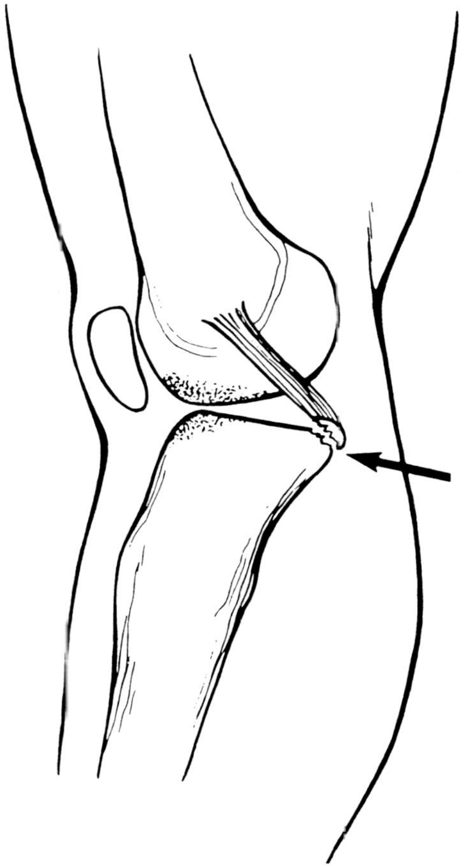

FIG. 2-32. Diagrammatic representation of distal posterior cruciate avulsion injury, usually occurring as part of hyperextension resulting in a bone fragment of variable size being pulled off the posterior lip of the tibia *(arrow)*. The femoral condyle and anterior tibial margin may undergo impaction injury, resulting in "kissing contusions," although this is less common than the contusion pattern seen with anterior cruciate injuries. (From Sonin A, et al. *Radiology* 1994; 190:455–458, with permission.)

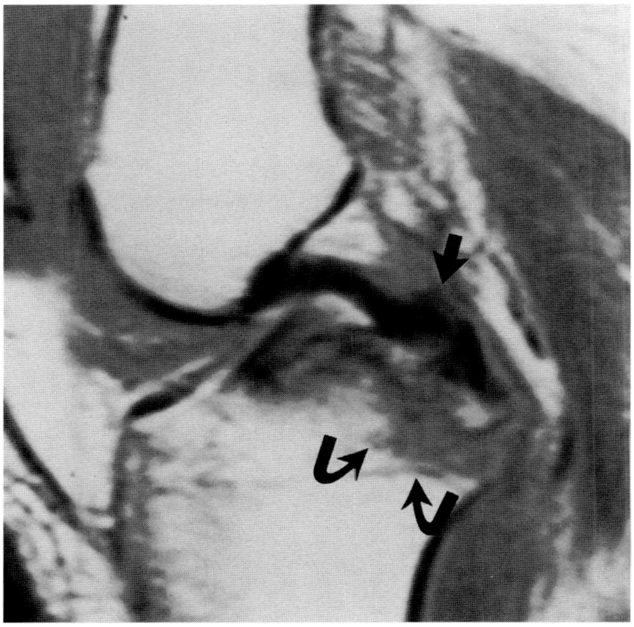

FIG. 2-33. Bone fragment avulsion by posterior cruciate. Sagitta T1-weighted coronal spin-echo image (TR 500 msec, TE 16 msec). The tibial insertion of the posterior cruciate has been avulsed from the posterior tibial lip, taking with it a fragment of bone *(arrow)*. A large region of low signal intensity fills the donor site representing blood and edema *(curved arrows)*.

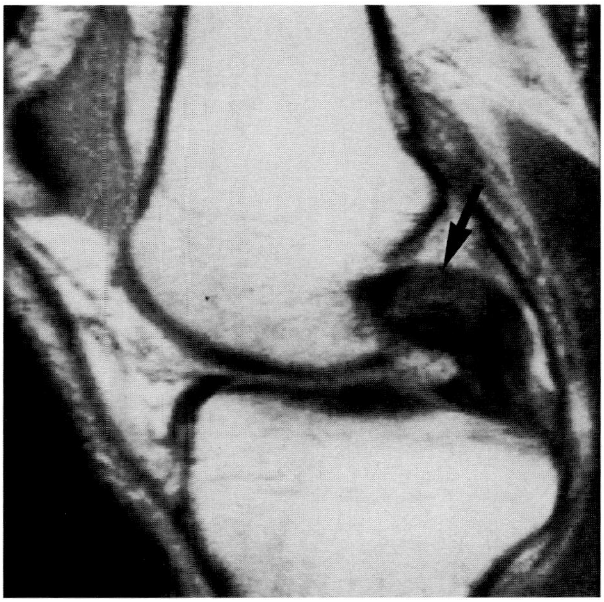

FIG. 2-34. Sagittal T1-weighted spin-echo image (TR 600 msec, TE 20 msec). An area of increased signal intensity is present within the ligament *(arrow)* consistent with an in substance tear. The ligament is also significantly thickened, indicating that this is not a chronic injury.

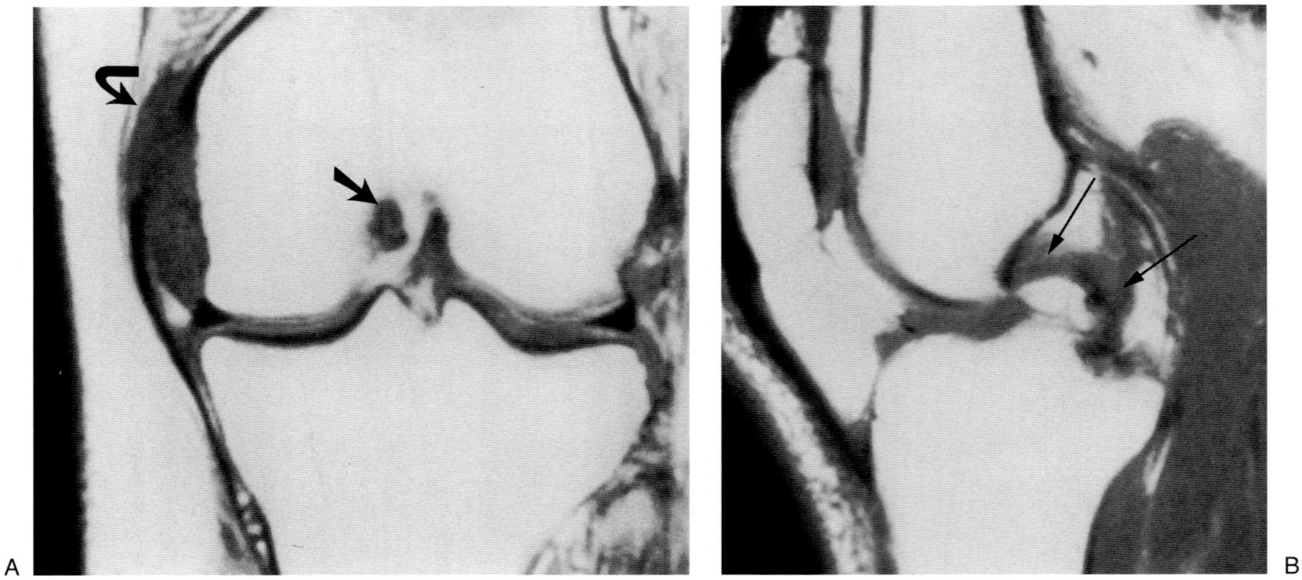

FIG. 2-35. Halo sign, an indicator of posterior cruciate injury. **A:** Coronal T1-weighted spin echo (TR 400 msec, TE 20 msec). The *straight arrow* indicates the posterior cruciate ligament seen in cross section as it curves upward toward its cranial insertion. Rather than being uniformly low signal as normal, an interrupted ring of low signal surrounds a higher-signal core. Note incidental tear of the cranial medial collateral ligament complex *(curved arrow)*. **B:** Sagittal T1-weighted spin-echo (TR 800 msec, TE 20 msec) image from the same patient shows the expected extensive high signal within the posterior cruciate *(arrows)*.

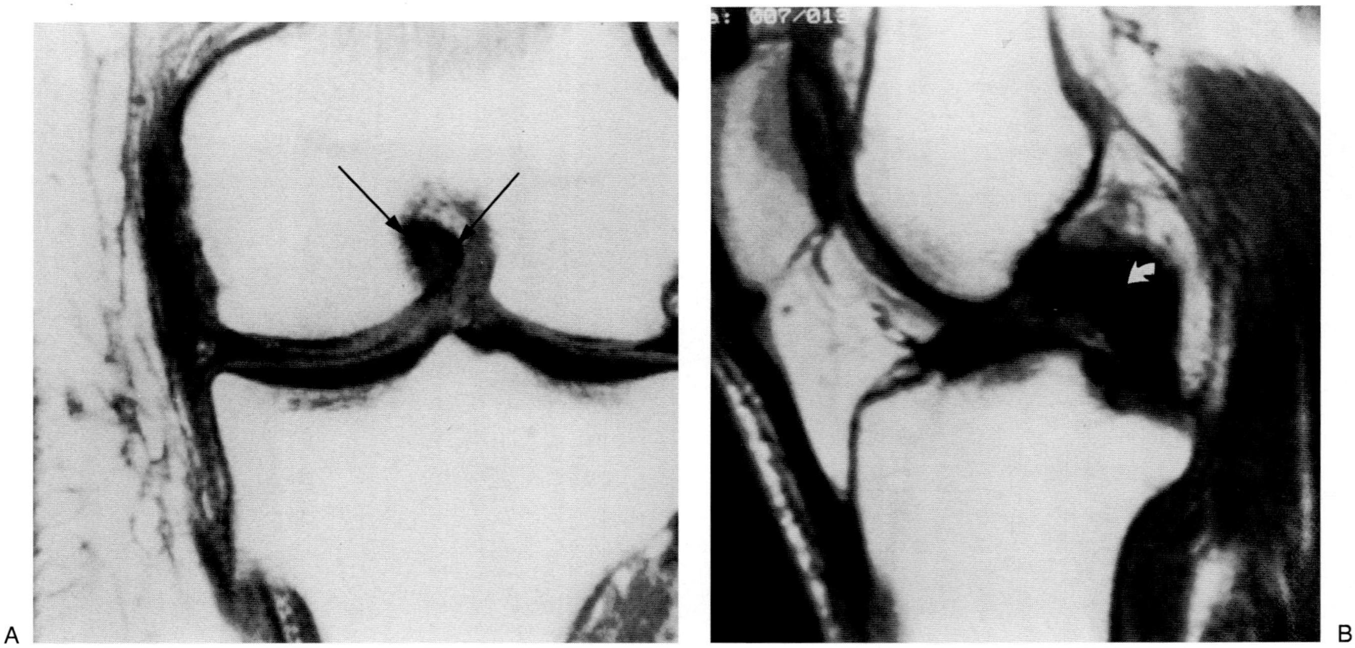

FIG. 2-36. **A:** Coronal T1-weighted spin-echo image (TR 400 msec, TE 15 msec) once again shows a low-signal ring *(arrows)* around a higher-signal core. **B:** Sagittal T1-weighted spin-echo image (TR 500 msec, TE 13 msec) is also abnormal, showing a somewhat thickened ligament, but the high signal intensity is more difficult to appreciate *(small curved arrow)*. The coronal image helps both to detect the posterior cruciate abnormality and to reinforce the diagnosis.

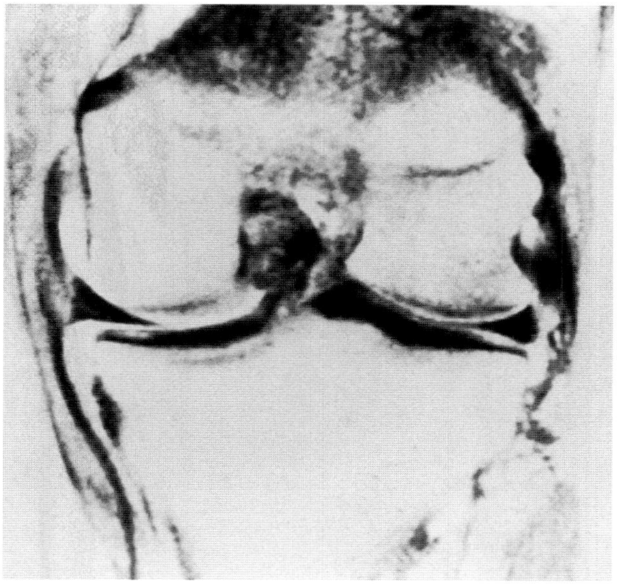

FIG. 2-37. Sagittal T1-weighted spin-echo image (TR 400 msec, TE 20 msec). The posterior cruciate is seen as a poorly marginated, irregular low-signal ring with high-signal-intensity edema/blood within it, consistent with a high-grade in-substance tear.

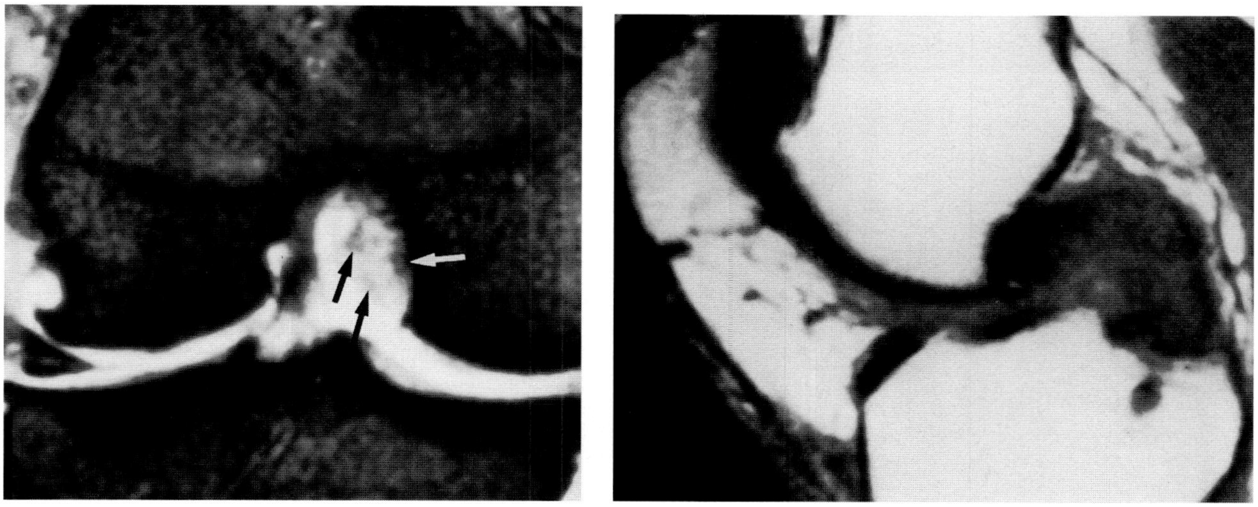

A B

FIG. 2-38. A: Coronal $T2^*$-weighted gradient-echo MPGR (TR 400 msec, TE 13 msec, flip angle 20°). Gradient-echo and T2-weighted sequences will show the edema/blood within the posterior cruciate as high signal intensity, making ligament pathology more obvious in some instances. An interrupted low-signal ring *(arrows)* is seen in this instance. **B:** Sagittal T1-weighted spin-echo image (TR 600 msec, TE 20 msec) from the same patient delineates the extensive injury with marked increase in signal throughout the whole ligament.

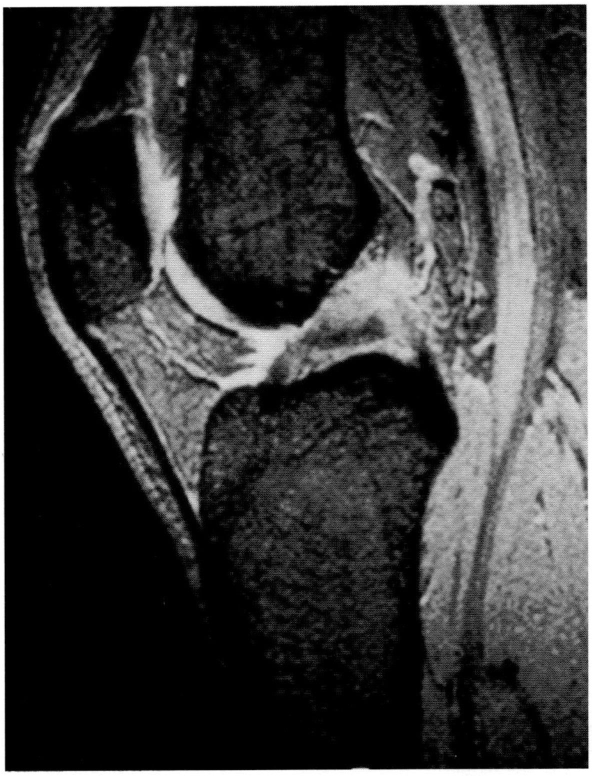

FIG. 2-39. Sagittal T2*-weighted gradient-echo image (TR 400 msec, TE 20 msec, flip angle 20°) from a patient with a chronic anterior cruciate tear that was not reconstructed. The remaining fibers of the ligament are vaguely seen as low-signal structures in the intercondylar notch region.

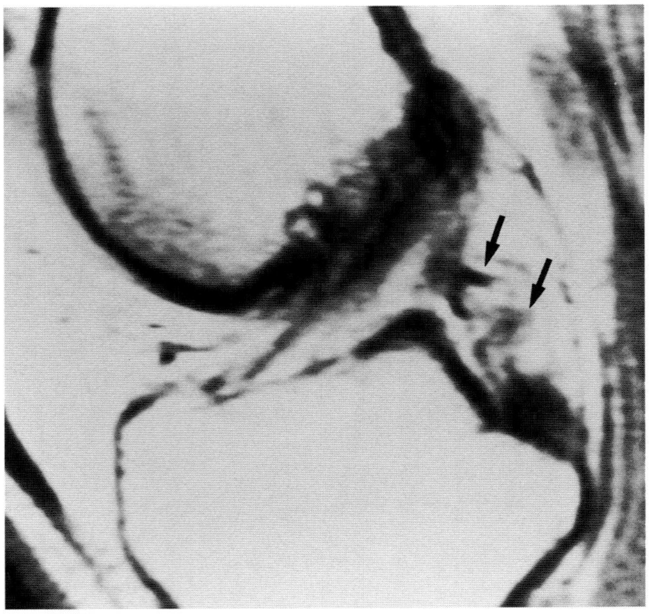

FIG. 2-41. Chronic posterior cruciate ligament tear. Sagittal T1-weighted spin-echo image (TR 600 msec, TE 20 msec) shows only a few crinkled low-signal fibers at the expected location of the ligament *(arrows)*. The ligament is thin and atrophic.

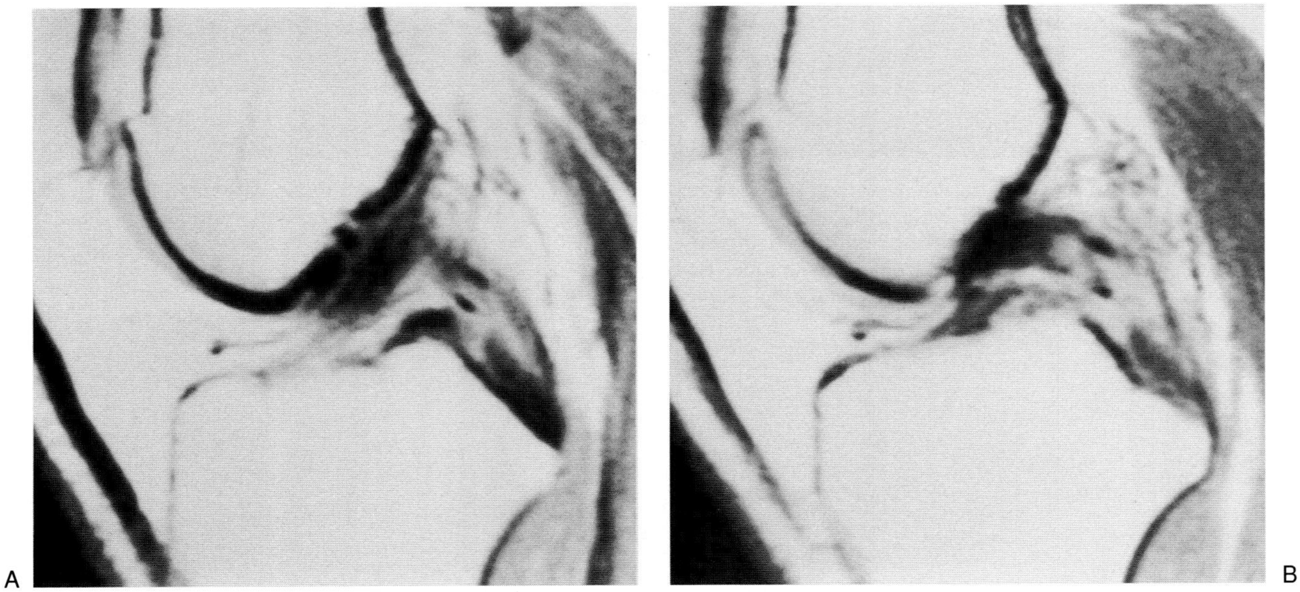

FIG. 2-40. A,B: Adjacent sagittal T1-weighted spin-echo images (TR 600 msec, TE 20 msec) show a chronic high-grade tear of the distal posterior cruciate. High signal intensity replaces most of the caudal part of the ligament, but the ligament is not thickened.

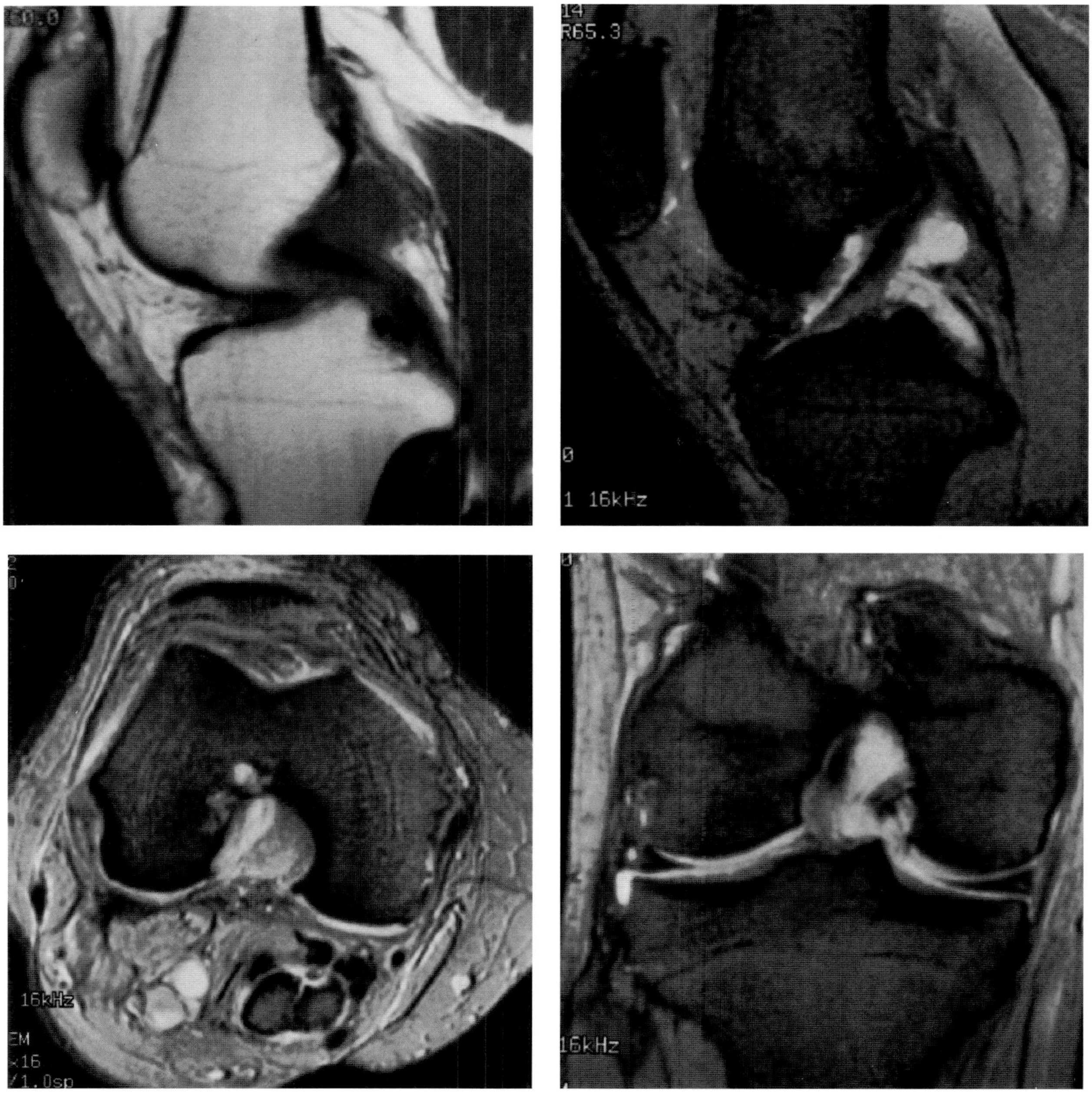

A B C D

FIG. 2-42. **A:** Sagittal T1-weighted image (TR 600, TE 12) demonstrates a soft tissue density immediately cranial to the proximal portion of the posterior cruciate. **B:** Sagittal T2*-weighted gradient echo image (TR 400, TE 20, flip angle 20°) demonstrates a high signal lobulated mass near the cranial aspect of the anterior cruciate, and is also in contact with the posterior cruciate. **C:** Axial gradient echo image (TR 300, TE 12, flip angle 30°) demonstrates displacement of the normal fibers within the intercondylar notch. **D:** Coronal T2*-weighted gradient echo image (TR 400, TE 18, flip angle 30°). This image demonstrates high signal intensity material in the superior aspect of the intercondylar notch causing displacement of the fibers of both the anterior and posterior cruciates. At the time of surgery, this was confirmed to be a cruciate cyst that was likely to have arisen from the posterior cruciate. The posterior cruciate had been injured approximately 2 years before. An origin from the anterior cruciate could not be absolutely excluded.

82% to 100%. Sensitivity in a number of different studies ranges from as low as 61% to as high as 100% (41,103–115). Generally, when T2-weighted or T2* images are utilized, sensitivities improve. In addition, if thinner sections are utilized, the problem of volume averaging is diminished and the ability to pick up cruciate ligament tears, especially partial tears, is greatly enhanced. Although most tears will be readily demonstrated utilizing 4–5-mm-thick conventional T1-weighted spin-echo sequences, the use of T2 or T2* sequences or 3-D Fourier transform thin sections should resolve any doubt in more questionable cases (see Figs. 2-16D and 2-16E).

Mucoid degeneration may occasionally be a cause of false-positive partial tears. In the case of the anterior cruciate, volume averaging from the posterior band could also be misinterpreted as a partial disruption, but this is minimized if oblique sagittal imaging is performed. Chronic complete tears of the anterior cruciate usually result in marked atrophy, and remnants of the ligament may be difficult to demonstrate with MRI or even arthroscopy (Fig. 2-39–2-41). This may result in a false-negative report with MRI. In this setting the torn, fibrotic anterior cruciate may scar to the posterior cruciate, thereby mimicking the normal course and appearance of the anterior cruciate (63,112,116,117). The use of MRI in cases in which the cruciate ligaments are well visualized and clearly normal will, in virtually all cases, eliminate the need for diagnostic arthroscopy.

Occasionally cysts may form around the cruciate ligaments following trauma although congenital origin for these cysts cannot be excluded. These have more frequently been reported with anterior cruciate ligament origins rather than posterior cruciates (Fig. 2-42).

The effect of field strength on the accuracy of knee MRI is unclear (109). The experience of the authors with 1.5-T to 0.5-T units suggests that the imaging quality is similar when comparing middle- and high-field magnets in evaluation of the knee (118).

REFERENCES

1. Maffulli N, Binfield PM, King JB, Good CJ. Acute haemarthrosis of the knee in athletes: a prospective study of 106 cases. *J Bone Joint Surg* 1993;75B:945–949.
2. Zarins B, Adams M. Knee injuries in sports. *New Engl J Med* 1988; 318:950–961.
3. Feagin JA, Cur WW. Isolated tear of the anterior cruciate ligament: 5-year follow-up study. *Am J Sports Med* 1976;4:95–100.
4. Ruwe PA, Wright J, Randall RL, Lynch JK, Jokl P, McCarthy S. Can MR imaging effectively replace diagnostic arthroscopy? *Radiology* 1992;183:335–339.
5. Ellison AE, Berg EE. Embryology, anatomy and function of the anterior cruciate ligament. *Orthop Clin North Am* 1985;16:3–14.
6. Gray DJ, Gardner E. Prenatal development of the human knee and superior tibiofibular joint. *Am J Anat* 1950;86:235–286.
7. O'Rahilly R, Gardner E. The timing and sequence of events in the development of the limbs of the human embryo. *Anat Embryol* 1975; 148:1–23.
8. Gardner E, O'Rahilly R. The early development of the knee joint in staged human embryos. *J Anat* 1968;102:289–299.
9. Sledge CB. Structure, development and function of joints. *Orthop Clin North Am* 1975;6:619–628.
10. Sledge CB, Zaleske DJ. Resnick D, Niwayama G, eds. *Diagnosis of bone and joint disorders,* 2nd ed. Philadelphia: WB Saunders, 1988; 18:604–624.
11. Berg EE. Parsons' knob (tuberculum intercondylare tertium): a guide to tibial anterior cruciate ligament insertion. *Clin Orthop Rel Res* 1993;292:229–231.
12. Horne JG, Parsons CJ. The anterior cruciate ligament: its anatomy and a new method of reconstruction. *Can J Surg* 1977;20:214–220.
13. Odensten M, Gillquist J. Functional anatomy of the anterior cruciate ligament and a rationale for reconstruction. *J Bone Joint Surg* 1985; 67-A:257–262.
14. McLeod WD. The biomechanics and function of the secondary restraints to the anterior cruciate ligament. *Orthop Clin North Am* 1985; 16:165–170.
15. Butler DL, Noyes FR, Grood ES. Ligamentous restraints to anterior-posterior drawer in the human knee. *J Bone Joint Surg* 1980;62A: 259–270.
16. Marans HJ, Jackson RW, Glossop ND, Young MC. Anterior cruciate ligament insufficiency: a dynamic three-dimensional motion analysis. *Am J Sports Med* 1989;17:325–332.
17. Rong G, Wang Y. The role of cruciate ligaments in maintaining knee joint stability. *Clin Orthop* 1987;215:65–71.
18. Girgis FG, Marshall JL, Al Monajem ARS. The cruciate ligament of the knee joint: anatomical, functional and experimental analysis. *Clin Orthop* 1975;106:216–231.
19. Corrigan JP, Cashman WF, Brady MP. Proprioception in the cruciate deficient knee. *J Bone Joint Surg* 1992;74-B:247–250.
20. Beard DJ, Kyberd PJ, Fergusson CM, Dodd CAF. Proprioception after rupture of the anterior cruciate ligament. *J Bone Joint Surg* 1993;75-B:311–315.
21. Brahme SK, Fox JM, Ferkel RD, Friedman MJ, Flannigan BD, Resnick DL. Osteonecrosis of the knee after arthroscopic surgery: diagnosis with MR imaging. *Radiology* 1991;178:851–853.
22. Loos WC, Fox JM, Blazina ME, Del Pizzo W, Friedman MJ. Acute posterior cruciate ligament injuries. *Am J Sports Med* 1981;9:86–92.
23. Barton TM, Torg JS, Das M. Posterior cruciate ligament insufficiency: a review of the literature. *Sports Med* 1984;1:419–430.
24. Cross MJ, Powell JF. Long-term followup of posterior cruciate ligament rupture: a study of 116 cases. *Am J Sports Med* 1984;12: 292–297.
25. Covey DC, Sapega AA. Injuries of the posterior cruciate ligament. *J Bone Joint Surg* 1993;75-A:1376–1386.
26. Kennedy JC, Grainger RW. The posterior cruciate ligament. *J Trauma* 1967;7:367–377.
27. Heller L, Langman J. The menisco-femoral ligaments of the human knee. *J Bone Joint Surg* 1964;46-B:307–313.
28. Van Dommelen BA, Fowler PJ. Anatomy of the posterior cruciate ligament: a review. *Am J Sports Med* 1989;17:24–29.
29. Markolf KL, Wascher DC, Finerman GAM. Direct in vitro measurements of forces in the cruciate ligaments. Part II: the effect of section of the posterolateral structures. *J Bone Joint Surg* 1993;75:387–394.
30. Fu FH, Harner CD, Johnson DL, Miller MD, Woo SL-Y. Biomechanics of knee ligaments. *J Bone Joint Surg* 1993;75-A:1716–1727.
31. Skyhar MJ, Warren RF, Oritz GJ, Schwartz E, Otis JC. The effects of sectioning of the posterior cruciate ligament and the posterolateral complex on the articular contact pressures within the knee. *J Bone Joint Surg* 1993;75-A:694–699.
32. Torg JS, Barton TM, Pavlov H, Stine R. Natural history of the posterior cruciate ligament-deficient knee. *Clin Orthop* 1989;246:208–216.
33. Satku K, Chew CN, Seow H. Posterior cruciate ligament injuries. *Acta Orthop Scand* 1984;55:26–29.
34. Dandy DJ, Pusey RJ. The long-term results of unrepaired tears of the posterior cruciate ligament. *J Bone Joint Surg* 1982;64-B:92–94.
35. Parolie JM, Bergfeld JA. Long-term results of nonoperative treatment of isolated posterior cruciate ligament injuries in the athlete. *Am J Sports Med* 1986;14:35–38.
36. Castle TH, Noyes FR, Grood ES. Posterior tibial subluxation of the posterior cruciate-deficient knee. *Clin Orthop* 1992;284:193–202.
37. Hollister AM, Jatana S, Singh AK, Sullivan WW, Lupichuk AG. The axes of rotation of the knee. *Clin Orthop* 1993;290:259–268.
38. Gay SB, Chen NC, Brookeman JR. A device for rotation and stabilization of the knee during MR imaging. *AJR* 1992;158:1173.
39. Engeler C, Miller S, Ochsner EG. Oblique sagittal MR imaging of the anterior cruciate ligament. *Radiology* 1991;178:890–891.

40. Vellet AD, Marks P, Fowler P, Munro T. Accuracy of nonorthogonal magnetic resonance imaging in acute disruption of the anterior cruciate ligament. *J Arthrosc Rel Surg* 1989;5:287–293.
41. Lee JK, Yao L, Phelps CT, Wirth CR, Czajka J, Lozman J. Anterior cruciate ligament tears: MR imaging compared with arthroscopy and clinical tests. *Radiology* 1988;166:861–864.
42. Munk PL, Vellet AD, Levin MF. MRI evaluation of the knee meniscus. *Australas Radiol* 1993;37:40–46.
43. Munk PL. Magnetic resonance imaging of the knee: an overview. *J Can Assoc Radiol* 1989;40:296–303.
44. Hodler J, Haghighi P, Trudell D, Resnick D. The cruciate ligaments of the knee: correlation between MR appearance and gross and histologic findings in cadaveric specimens. *AJR* 1992;159:357–360.
45. Neuschwander DC, Drez D, Finney TP. Lateral meniscal variant with absence of the posterior coronary ligament. *J Bone Joint Surg* 1992; 74-A:1186–1190.
46. Szalay MJ, Hosking OR, Annear P. Injury of knee ligament associated with ipsilateral femoral shaft fractures and with ipsilateral femoral and tibial shaft fractures. *Injury* 1990;21:398–400.
47. Yu JS, Goodwin D, Salonen D, et al. Complete dislocation of the knee: spectrum of associated soft-tissue injuries depicted by MR imaging. *AJR* 1995;164:135–139.
48. Braunstein EM. Anterior cruciate ligament injuries: a comparison of arthrographic and physical diagnosis. *AJR* 1982;138:423–425.
49. Pavlov H, Warren RF, Sherman MF, Cayea PD. The accuracy of double-contrast arthrographic evaluation of the anterior cruciate ligament. *J Bone Joint Surg* 1983;65A:175–183.
50. Pavlov H, Torg JS. Double contrast arthrographic evaluation of the anterior cruciate ligament. *Radiology* 1978;126:661–665.
51. Pavlov H, Freiberger RH. An easy method to demonstrate the cruciate ligaments by double contrast arthrography. *Radiology* 1978;126: 817–818.
52. Dalinka MK, Gohel VK, Rancier L. Tomography in the evaluation of the anterior cruciate ligament. *Radiology* 1973;108:31–33.
53. Mittler S, Freiberger RH, Harrison-Stubbs M. A method of improving cruciate ligament visualization in double-contrast arthrography. *Radiology* 1972;102:441–442.
54. Dalinka MK, Garofola J. The infrapatellar synovial fold: a cause for confusion in the evaluation of the anterior cruciate ligament. *Am J Roentgenol* 1976;127:589–591.
55. Rijke AM, Tegtmeyer CJ, Weiland DJ, McCue FC. Stress examination of the cruciate ligaments: a radiologic Lachman test. *Radiology* 1987; 165:867–869.
56. Wolfe RD, Dieden JD. Cruciate ligament injury: diagnostic difficulties in the presence of meniscal injury. *Radiology* 1985;157:19–21.
57. Pavlov H, Hirschy JC, Torg JS. Computed tomography of the cruciate ligaments. *Radiology* 1979;132:389–393.
58. Buttner-Janz K, Schellnack K, Rieder T. Noninvasive diagnosis of cruciate ligament damage with particular reference to computed tomography with arthrography. *Am J Sports Med* 1989;17:501–504.
59. Passariello R, Trecco F, De Paulis F, Masciocchi C, Bonanni G, Beomonte Zobel B. CT demonstration of capsuloligamentous lesions of the knee joint. *J Comp Assist Tomogr* 1986;10:450–456.
60. Stoker DJ, Renton P, Fulton A. The value of arthrography in the management of internal derangements of the knee: the first 1000 are the worst? *Clin Radiol* 1981;32:557–566.
61. Pavlov H, Schneider R. Extrameniscal abnormalities as diagnosed by knee arthrography. *Radiol Clin North Am* 1981;19:287–304.
62. Kursunoglu S, Pate D, Resnick D, Andre M, Sartoris D. Computed arthrotomography with multiplanar reformations and three-dimensional image analysis in the evaluation of the cruciate ligaments: preliminary investigation. *J Can Assoc Radiol* 1986;37:153–156.
63. Heron CW, Calvert PT. Three-dimensional gradient-echo MR imaging of the knee: comparison with arthroscopy in 100 patients. *Radiology* 1992;183:839–844.
64. Buckwalter KA, Pennes DR. Anterior cruciate ligament: oblique sagittal MR imaging. *Radiology* 1990;175:276–277.
65. Feagin JA Jr, Lambert KL. Mechanism of injury and pathology of anterior cruciate ligament injuries. *Orthop Clin North Am* 1994;16: 41–45.
66. Lubowitz JH, Grauer JD. Arthroscopic treatment of anterior cruciate ligament avulsion. *Clin Orthop* 1993;294:242–246.
67. Noyes FR, Grood ES, Torzilli PA. The definitions of terms for motion and position of the knee and injuries of ligaments. *J Bone Joint Surg* 1989;71-A:465–475.
68. Remer EM, Fitzgerald SW, Friedman H, Rogers LF, Hendrix RW, Schafer MF. Anterior cruciate ligament injury: MR imaging diagnosis and patterns of injury. *Radiographics* 1992;12:901–913.
69. Fruensgaard S, Johannsen HV. Incomplete ruptures of the anterior cruciate ligament. *J Bone Joint Surg* 1989;71B:526–530.
70. Jensen JE, Conn RR, Hazelrigg G, Hewett JE. Systematic evaluation of acute knee injuries. *Clin Sports Med* 1985;4:295–312.
71. Rijke AM, Goitz HT, McCue FC, Delp JL, Lam D, Southall EP. Graded stress radiography of injured anterior cruciate ligaments. *Invest Radiol* 1994;26:926–933.
72. Keir R, McCarthy SM. Lipohemarthrosis of the knee: MR imaging. *J Comp Assist Tomogr* 1990;14:395–396.
73. Noyes FR, Bassett RW, Grood ES, Butler DL. Arthroscopy in acute traumatic hemarthrosis of the knee: incidence of anterior cruciate tears and other injuries. *J Bone Joint Surg* 1980;62A:687–695.
74. Binfield FM, Maffulli N, King JB. Patterns of meniscal tears associated with anterior cruciate ligament lesions in athletes. *Injury* 1993; 24:557–561.
75. Terry GC, Hughston JC. Associated joint pathology in the anterior cruciate ligament-deficient knee with emphasis on a classification system and injuries to the meniscocapsular ligament-musculotendinous unit complex. *Orthop Clin North Am* 1985;16:29–39.
76. Indelicato PA, Bittar ES. A perspective of lesions associated with ACL insufficiency of the knee. *Clin Orthop* 1985;198:77–80.
77. Ferkel RD, Markolf K, Goodfellow D, et al. Treatment of the anterior cruciate ligament-absent knee with associated meniscal tears. *Clin Orthop* 1994;222:239–248.
78. Staron RB, Haramati N, Feldman F, et al. O'Donoghue's triad: magnetic resonance imaging evidence. *Skeletal Radiol* 1994;23:633–636.
79. Gentili A, Seeger LI, Yao L, Do HM. Anterior cruciate ligament tear: indirect signs at MR imaging. *Radiology* 1994;193:835–840.
80. Fitzgerald SW, Remer EM, Friedman H, Rogers LF, Hendrix RW, Schafer MF. MR evaluation of the anterior cruciate ligament: value of supplementing sagittal images with coronal and axial images. *AJR* 1993;160:1233–1237.
81. Robertson PL, Schweitzer ME, Bartolozzi AR, Ugoni A. Anterior cruciate ligament tears: evaluation of multiple signs with MR imaging. *Radiology* 1994;193:829–834.
82. Boeree NR, Ackroyd CE. Magnetic resonance imaging of anterior cruciate ligament rupture: a new diagnostic sign. *J Bone Joint Surg* 1992;74-B:614–616.
83. Chan WP, Peterfy C, Fritz R, Genant HK. MR diagnosis of complete tears of the anterior cruciate ligament of the knee: importance of anterior subluxation of the tibia. *AJR* 1994;162:355–360.
84. Vahey TN, Hunt JE, Shelbourne KD. Anterior translocation of the tibia at MR imaging: a secondary sign of anterior cruciate ligament tear. *Radiology* 1993;187:817–819.
85. Murphy BJ, Smith RL, Uribe JW, Janecki CJ, Hechtman KS, Mangasarian RA. Bone signal abnormalities in the posterolateral tibia and lateral femoral condyle in complete tears of the anterior cruciate ligament: a specific sign? *Radiology* 1992;182:221–224.
86. Kaplan PA, Walker CW, Kilcoyne RF, Brown DE, Tusek D, Dussault RG. Occult fracture patterns of the knee associated with anterior cruciate ligament tears: assessment with MR imaging. *Radiology* 1992; 183:835–838.
87. Lynch TCP, Crues JV III, Morgan FW, Sheehan WE, Harter LP, Ryu R. Bone abnormalities of the knee: prevalence and significance at MR imaging. *Radiology* 1989;171:761–766.
88. Vellet AD, Marks PH, Fowler PJ, Munro TG. Occult posttraumatic osteochondral lesions of the knee: prevalence, classification, and short-term sequelae evaluated with MR imaging. *Radiology* 1991; 178:271–276.
89. McCauley TR, Moses M, Kier R, Lynch JK, Barton JW, Jokl P. MR diagnosis of tears of anterior cruciate ligament of the knee: importance of ancillary findings. *AJR* 1994;162:115–119.
90. Mink JH, Deutsch AL. Occult cartilage and bone injuries of the knee: detection, classification, and assessment with MR imaging. *Radiology* 1989;198:823–829.
91. Harned EM, Mitchell DG, Burk DL Jr, Vinitski S, Rifkin MD. Bone marrow findings on magnetic resonance images of the knee: accentuation by fat suppression. *Magnet Reson Imaging* 1990;8:27–31.
92. Stallenberg B, Gevenois PA, Sintzoff SA Jr, Matos C, Andrianne Y,

Struyven J. Fracture of the posterior aspect of the lateral tibial plateau: radiographic sign of anterior cruciate ligament tear. *Radiology* 1993; 187:821–825.

93. Tung GA, Davis LM, Wiggins ME, Fadale PD. Tears of the anterior cruciate ligament: primary and secondary signs at MR imaging. *Radiology* 1993;188:661–667.
94. Cobby MJ, Schweitzer ME, Resnick D. The deep lateral femoral notch: an indirect sign of a torn anterior cruciate ligament. *Radiology* 1992;184:855–858.
95. Moore HA, Larson RL. Posterior cruciate ligament injuries: results of early surgical repair. *Am J Sports Med* 1980;8:68–78.
96. Hughston JC, Bowden JA, Andrews JR, Norwood LA. Acute tears of the posterior cruciate ligament: results of operative treatment. *J Bone Joint Surg* 1980;62-A:438–450.
97. Bianchi M. Acute tears of the posterior cruciate ligament: clinical study and results of operative treatment in 27 cases. *Am J Sports Med* 1983;11:308–314.
98. Torisu T. Isolated avulsion fracture of the tibial attachment of the posterior cruciate ligament. *J Bone Joint Surg* 1977;59-A:68–72.
99. Sonin AH, Fitzgerald SW, Friedman H, Hoff FL, Hendrix RW, Rogers LF. Posterior cruciate ligament injury: MR imaging diagnosis and patterns of injury. *Radiology* 1994;190:455–458.
100. Grover JS, Bassett LW, Gross ML, Seeger LL, Finerman GAM. Posterior cruciate ligament: MR imaging. *Radiology* 1990;174:527–530.
101. Clendenin MB, DeLee JC, Heckman JD. Interstitial tears of the posterior cruciate ligament of the knee. *Orthopedics* 1980;3:764–772.
102. Patten RM, Richardson ML, Zink-Brody G, Rolfe BA. Complete vs partial-thickness tears of the posterior cruciate ligament: MR findings. *J Comput Assist Tomogr* 1994;18:793–799.
103. Jackson DW, Jennings LD, Maywood RM. Magnetic resonance imaging of the knee: arthroscopy confirms accuracy of MRI of the knee. *Am J Sports Med* 1988;16:29–38. Abstract.
104. Bellon EM, Keith MW, Coleman PE, Shah ZR. Magnetic resonance imaging of internal derangements of the knee. *Radiographics* 1988; 8:95–118.
105. Mandelbaum BR, Finerman GAM, Reicher MA, et al. Magnetic resonance imaging as a tool for evaluation of traumatic knee injuries: anatomical and pathoanatomical correlations. *Am J Sports Med* 1986; 14:361–370.
106. Fischer SP, Fox JM, DelPizzo W, Friedman MJ, Snyder SJ, Ferkel RD. Accuracy of diagnoses from magnetic resonance imaging of the knee. *J Bone Joint Surg* 1991;73-A:2–10.
107. Reicher MA, Hartzman S, Bassett LW, Mandelbaum B, Duckwiler G, Gold RH. MR imaging of the knee. Part I. Traumatic disorders. *Radiology* 1987;162:547–551.
108. Mink JH, Levy T, Crues JV III. Tears of the anterior cruciate ligament and menisci of the knee: MR imaging evaluation. *Radiology* 1988; 167:769–774.
109. Rothschild PA, Domesek JM, Kaufman L, et al. MR imaging of the knee with a 0.064-T permanent magnet. *Radiology* 1990;175: 775–778.
110. Soloman SL, Totty WG, Lee JKT. MR imaging of the knee: comparison of three-dimensional FISP and two-dimensional spin-echo pulse sequences. *Radiology* 1989;173:739–742.
111. Reeder JD, Matz SO, Becker L, Andelman SM. MR imaging of the knee in the sagittal projection: comparison of three-dimensional gradient-echo and spin-echo sequences. *AJR* 1989;153:537–540.
112. Spritzer CE, Vogler JB, Martinez S, et al. MR imaging of the knee: preliminary results with a 3DFT GRASS pulse sequence. *AJR* 1988; 150:597–603.
113. Tyrrell RL, Gluckert K, Pathria MN, Modic MT. Fast three-dimensional MR imaging of the knee: comparison with arthroscopy. *Radiology* 1988;166:865–872.
114. Gallimore GW, Harms SE. Knee injuries: high-resolution MR imaging. *Radiology* 1986;160:457–461.
115. Griffiths HJ, Detlie T. Imaging of the internal derangement of the knee. *Injury* 1992;4:67–77.
116. Vahey TN, Broome DR, Kays KJ, Shelbourne KD. Acute and chronic tears of the anterior cruciate ligament: differential features at MR imaging. *Radiology* 1991;181:251–253.
117. Harms SE, Flamig DP, Fisher CF, Fulmer JM. New method for fast MR imaging of the knee. *Radiology* 1989;173:743–750.
118. Vellet AD, Lee DH, Munk PL, et al. Anterior cruciate ligament tear: prospective evaluation of diagnostic accuracy of middle- and high-field-strength MR imaging at 1.5 and 0.5 T1. *Radiology* 1995;197: 826–830.

MRI of the Knee, Second Edition,
edited by P. L. Munk and C. A. Helms.
Lippincott-Raven Publishers, Philadelphia © 1996.

CHAPTER 3

The Extensor Mechanism and Patellofemoral Joint

Dennis L. Janzen, Peter L. Munk, and Douglas G. Connell

The extensor mechanism of the knee consists of the quadriceps muscle group, quadriceps tendon, patella, patellar tendon, associated bursae, and the patellofemoral joint. A wide variety of traumatic, degenerative, inflammatory, and congenital abnormalities occur in these structures. Magnetic resonance imaging (MRI) is of particular value in assessing the soft-tissue, cartilaginous, and bony components of the extensor mechanism and patellofemoral joint, and often provides unique and clinically useful information. This chapter will discuss the embryology, anatomy, and MRI features of extensor mechanism and patellofemoral joint abnormalities.

EMBRYOLOGY

The lower limb begins at day 28 of gestation as a mesodermal and ectodermal bud arising from the lateral-caudal aspect of the embryonic plate. The mesodermal component of the limb bud contains three layers. The superficial layer induces and interacts with the ectodermal covering, the intermediate layer forms paraosseous soft tissues, and the deep layer develops into a mesenchymal skeleton (1). From days 37 to 45 the mesenchymal skeleton is transformed into a cartilaginous skeleton in a central-to-peripheral progression within each bone. At day 39 surface features such as the femoral condyles become visible, and the cartilaginous precursor of the patella forms at day 45. By day 47 the cartilaginous skeleton of the leg clearly resembles that of an adult (2). The intermediate mesodermal layer differentiates into periosteum, joint capsule, and myotendinous units. The quadriceps and patellar tendons form during days 42–55 (3,4). During this period of skeletal development, myoblast proliferations form ventral and dorsal muscle masses.

The knee joint structures begin at day 41 as a mass of undifferentiated blastemal cells in the interzone between the femur and the tibia. During this stage of development the knee flexes to 90°. Condensed mesenchyme around the interzone forms the joint capsule. The interzone blastemal cells separate into three layers during days 41–43; the dense superior and inferior layers become articular cartilage, and the vascularized intermediate layer becomes the intracapsular soft-tissue structures (ligaments, menisci, synovium) (1). The menisci, cruciate, and collateral ligaments develop from the interzone blastemal tissue during weeks 8–10. Cavitation of the intermediate layer begins at week 9, resulting in five separate cavities (one femoropatellar, two femoromeniscal, two tibiomeniscal) that coalesce into three cavities (femoropatellar, medial femorotibial, and lateral femorotibial) by 12 weeks, and finally into a single synovial cavity by week 13. Remnants of the synovial partitions between the cavities persist as synovial plicae in 40–80% of adult knees, most commonly in the suprapatellar, infrapatellar, and medial patellar locations (5). Fetal limb movement begins simultaneously with joint cavitation and is necessary for normal development of the knee joint cavity (6,7).

The patellofemoral joint begins at week 9 as a primitive joint plate comprised of the fused patellar and anterior femoral perichondria. Cavitation occurs between the patellar and femoral layers, forming a synovial joint that unites with the remainder of the knee joint by week 13. The suprapatellar bursa forms by week 15 from a superior extension of the patellofemoral synovial cavity. The medial and lateral patellar retinacula develop from thickenings of the adjacent intermediate mesenchymal tissue. The patella undergoes chondrification beginning at day 45, followed by ossification in the postnatal period. The medial and lateral patellar facets are

D. L. Janzen and D. G. Connell: Department of Radiology, Vancouver Hospital and Health Sciences Center, Vancouver, British Columbia, Canada V5Z 1M9.

P. L. Munk: Department of Diagnostic Imaging, British Columbia Cancer Agency, and Department of Radiology, University of British Columbia, Vancouver, British Columbia, Canada V5Z 4E6.

equal in size in the embryonic patella. The adult pattern of lateral facet dominance appears at 23 weeks (3,4,8).

ANATOMY AND BIOMECHANICS

The patella is the largest sesamoid bone in the body. Its function is to protect the extensor mechanism of the knee from friction against subjacent structures, to increase the moment arm of the quadriceps tendon, and to protect the underlying articulation from direct trauma (9,10). Kaufer estimated that a 30% increase in quadriceps muscle strength would be necessary to compensate for absence of the moment arm produced by the patella (11).

The patella is triangular in shape, with the apex pointed inferiorly. The anterior surface of the patella is rounded and is marked by many vascular orifices through which branches of the genicular and recurrent tibial arteries pass. The posterior surface of the patella is composed of a nonarticular surface, which comprises 25% of patellar height, and an articular surface, which comprises 75% of patellar height. The articular surface is divided into medial and lateral facets by the major vertical ridge. The medial and lateral facets are usually subdivided into inferior, middle, and superior facets by small transverse ridges. The inferior, middle, and superior facets successively contact the femoral articular surface during knee flexion. The "odd" facet lies along the medial border of the patella and is separated from the medial facet by the minor vertical ridge (Fig. 3-1) (8,12). The "odd" facet articulates with the medial femoral condyle with knee flexion of greater than 90° (13).

Patellar shape can be classified by the position of the major vertical ridge, as described by Wiberg (14). Type I morphology consists of equal-sized medial and lateral facets; this occurs in approximately 24% of specimens. In type II morphology the lateral facet is larger than the medial facet; this occurs in 57% of specimens. Type III morphology occurs in 19% of specimens and describes a small, steep medial facet and a large, concave lateral facet. Wiberg type III morphology has been associated with patellar instability disorders (8).

The trochlear articular surface of the femur consists of medial and lateral facets separated by a sagittally oriented intercondylar sulcus. The intercondylar sulcus is shallow; thus, the bony patellofemoral articulation is unstable and relies on soft-tissue restraints to prevent patellar subluxation. With the knee in full extension the patella articulates with the prefemoral fat pad in the supratrochlear fossa. During knee flexion the cartilaginous surfaces of the trochlea and patella articulate. Synovium extends from the articular cartilage margins to line the suprapatellar pouch, medial and lateral joint recesses, and infrapatellar (Hoffa's) fat pad.

The patella is held in position by passive (ligamentous) and active (myotendinous) soft-tissue restraints (Fig. 3-2). The major passive restraints are the patellar ligament and the medial and lateral patellar retinacula. The patellar ligament extends from the inferior pole of the patella to the tibial tubercle and measures 2.5–3.0 cm in width, 7 mm in thickness, and 3.5–5.5 cm in length (8). The patellar tendon fibers are continuous with rectus femoris tendon fibers (11). Patellar tendon length is nearly equal to the patellar height; the ratio of patellar tendon length to patellar height is 0.8–1.2 in normal subjects (15). The medial patellar retinaculum aids in prevention of lateral patellar movement. Its fibers are primarily derived from vastus medialis and vastus medialis obliquus muscle fasciae and insert onto the medial margin of the patella and patellar tendon (16). Additional medial

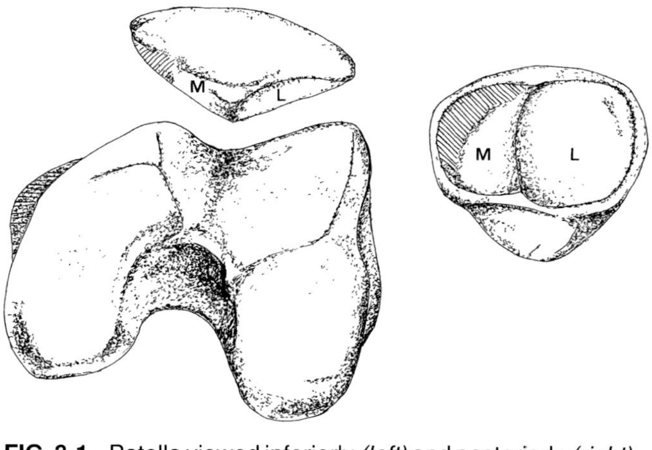

FIG. 3-1. Patella viewed inferiorly *(left)* and posteriorly *(right)*. The medial (M) and lateral (L) facets are labeled. The "odd" or "third" facet arising from the medial aspect of the medial facet is indicated with crosshatching.

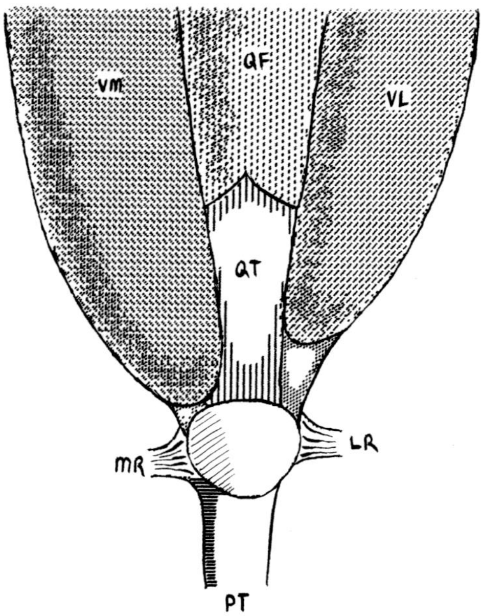

FIG. 3-2. Soft-tissue elements. Schematic illustration of the patellofemoral joint and quadriceps mechanism as viewed from the front. MR, medial retinaculum; LR, lateral retinaculum; PT, patellar tendon; RF, rectus femoris; QT, quadriceps tendon; VL, vastus lateralis; VM, vastus medialis.

fibers are derived from the medial patellofemoral ligament, which is a thickening of the joint capsule extending from the medial femoral epicondyle to the medial patellar margin; these fibers may contribute as much as half the force restraining lateral patellar displacement (8,17). The lateral patellar retinaculum is composed of fibers from the iliotibial tract, vastus lateralis, and vastus lateralis obliquus muscle fasciae that insert onto the lateral margin of the patella and patellar tendon. A thickening of the lateral joint capsule named the lateral epicondylopatellar ligament also prevents medial displacement of the patella (8,16,18).

The quadriceps muscle is composed of four portions, which function as knee extensors and active stabilizers of the patella. The rectus femoris is a long fusiform muscle that arises from the anterior inferior iliac spine and inserts on the anterior aspect of the patella. Some of the rectus femoris tendon fibers continue over the anterior surface of the patella to join the patellar tendon fibers (Fig. 3-3; see also color plate 4). The vastus medialis and vastus lateralis muscles arise from the proximal femoral shaft and insert via the quadriceps tendon onto the superior pole of the patella. Both muscles can be subdivided into proximal longitudinal portions and distal oblique portions; these portions occasionally have separate fascial sheaths. The vastus intermedius muscle arises from the anterior aspect of the upper femur and inserts via the quadriceps tendon into the patella. The articularis genus muscle is located in the deep portion of the vastus intermedius and inserts distally into the joint capsule of the suprapatellar pouch. This small and variably present muscle functions to pull the suprapatellar pouch superiorly during knee extension. The quadriceps muscle group is innervated by the second, third, and fourth lumbar nerve roots. The quadriceps tendon has a laminated appearance, in which rectus femoris fibers compose the superficial layer, vastus medialis and vastus lateralis fibers form the intermediate layer, and vastus intermedius fibers form the deep layer. This arrangement is variable in normal subjects, and blending of the layers usually occurs near the insertion onto the patella (8). The laminar arrangement of the quadriceps tendon can be seen on sagittal MRI images in most normal subjects, which aids in the localization of partial quadriceps tendon tears (19) (Fig. 3-4).

IMAGING TECHNIQUE

The standard pulse sequences and imaging techniques for general evaluation of the knee have been discussed in Chapter 1. This section addresses technical issues relevant to MRI of the patellofemoral joint and extensor mechanism.

The patellofemoral joint cartilage is best evaluated on axial images, because this imaging plane is perpendicular to the cartilage surfaces. T2-weighted spin-echo or T2*-weighted gradient-echo images provide adequate contrast between articular cartilage and adjacent joint fluid to allow visualization of cartilage surface abnormalities (20). Fast spin-echo techniques allow acquisition of high-spatial-resolution T2-weighted images in shorter imaging times than those of conventional spin-echo techniques. This method of evaluating articular cartilage defects has shown good correlation with arthroscopy (21). Optimum spatial resolution and contrast between articular cartilage and adjacent tissues is

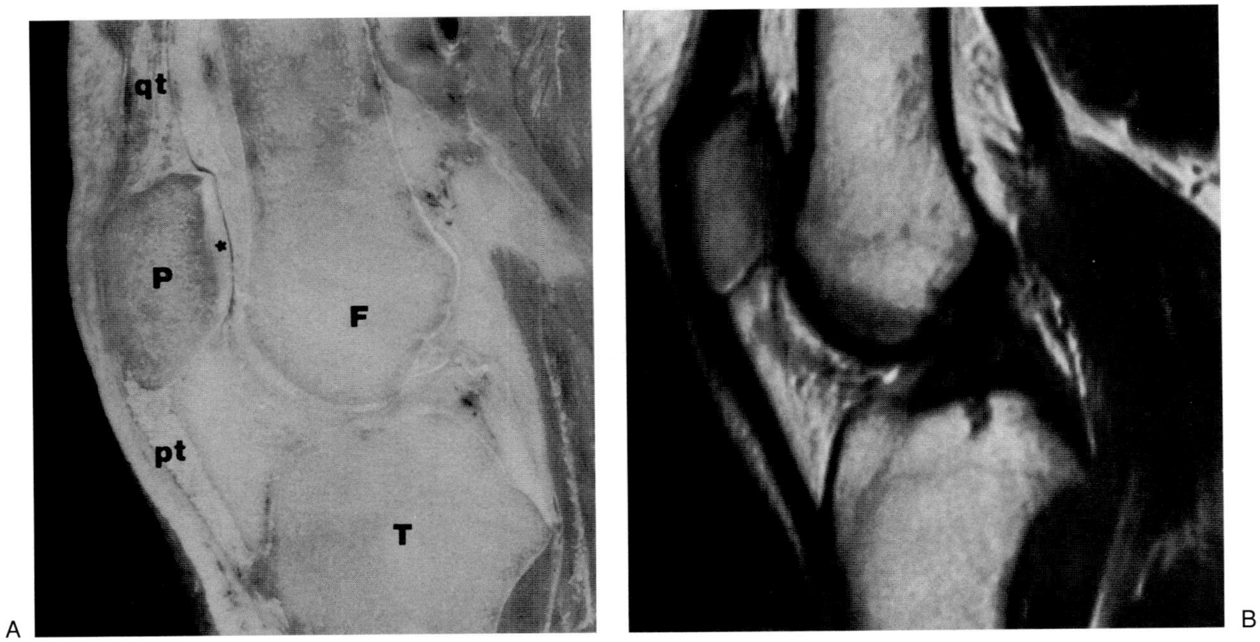

FIG. 3-3. Anatomy of the patellar region. Frozen cadaver sagittal section **(A)** with T2*-weighted image **(B)** at approximately the same level. qt, quadriceps tendon; P, patella; pt, patellar tendon; F, femur; T, tibia.

A 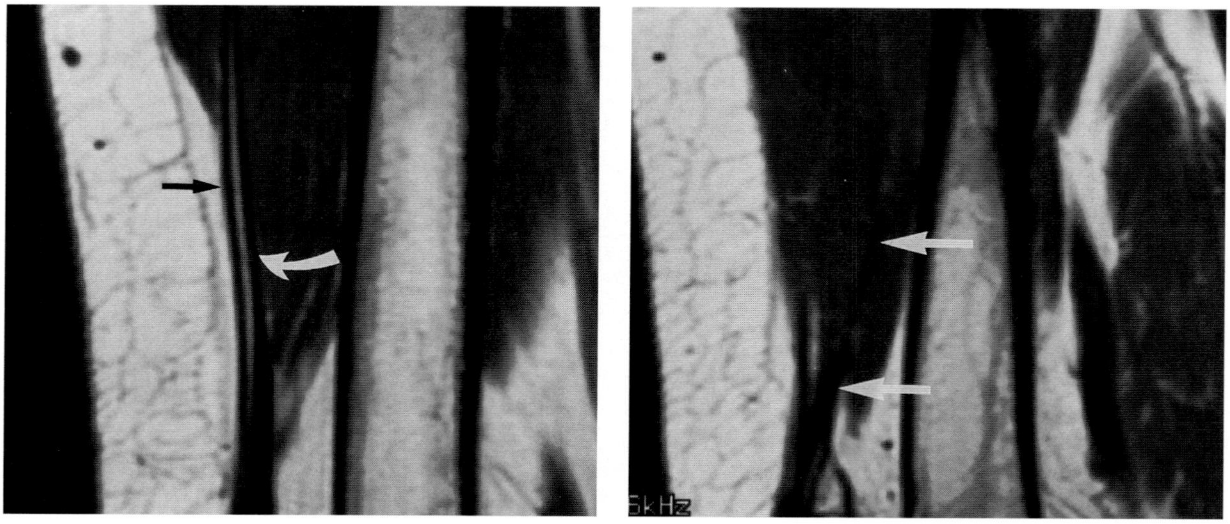 B

FIG. 3-4. The laminar anatomy of the quadriceps tendon. Sagittal T-1-weighted image **(A)** shows the superficial tendon layer *(straight arrow)* arising from the rectus femoris muscle and the intermediate tendon layer *(curved arrow)* arising from the vastus medialis and lateralis muscles. The adjacent T1-weighted sagittal image **(B)** shows the deep tendon layer *(arrows)* arising from the vastus intermedius muscle.

achieved with volumetric fat-suppressed spoiled GRASS (gradient recalled acquisition in the steady state) techniques; a disadvantage of this technique is the relatively long imaging time (22). On high-resolution MRI images, normal articular cartilage has a trilaminar appearance; a low-signal-intensity superficial layer represents a histologic zone of tangential collagen fibers, a high-signal-intensity intermediate layer represents radial collagen fibers, and a low-signal-intensity deep layer represents deep radiate fibers and calcified cartilage (23).

The patellar retinacula are well visualized on axial images (Fig. 3-5). The quadriceps tendon and patellar tendon are best evaluated on T1- and T2-weighted sagittal images; axial images provide an additional cross-sectional demonstration of these structures. Evaluation of quadriceps muscle injuries may require use of a larger field of view and comparison of the abnormal and normal leg for detection of subtle changes in muscle bulk.

Patellar tracking can be evaluated with kinematic MRI (24,25). Axial MRI images are obtained during passive incremental flexion or active knee flexion and are viewed as single-slice images and in a cine-loop format. Active knee motion against resistance provides the most accurate assessment of patellar tracking abnormalities (26,27).

INJURIES OF THE QUADRICEPS TENDON

The quadriceps tendon is usually injured by indirect forces, such as violent quadriceps muscle contraction during a fall, rather than by direct trauma, such as a deep laceration. These injuries are described as partial or complete disruptions. Quadriceps tendon and muscle injuries are usually

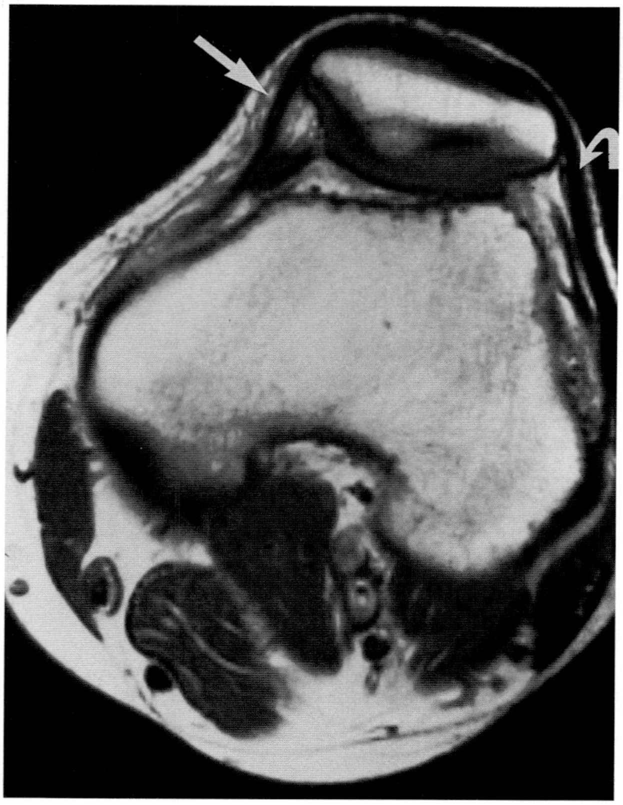

FIG. 3-5. Axial T1-weighted image demonstrates medial *(straight arrow)* and lateral *(curved arrow)* retinacula. The thick patellar cartilage is also well assessed in the axial plane.

incomplete and present with pain, swelling, a variable amount of extensor weakness, and inferior malposition of the patella (patella baja). Early diagnosis and surgical repair of quadriceps tendon tears are necessary to prevent permanent muscle atrophy, fibrosis, and loss of extensor function (28,29).

In the normal young adult the patella is the weakest component of the extensor mechanism and the quadriceps tendon is the strongest. Complete tears of the quadriceps tendon are unusual, unless the tendon has been weakened by degenerative change, systemic disease, or corticosteroid medications (30–32). In patients younger than 40 years, patellar fractures and patellar tendon tears are the most common complete injuries of the extensor mechanism, whereas quadriceps tendon injuries are most common in older patients (29,33).

Plain film, CT (computerized tomography), and ultrasound have all been used with varying success in the diagnosis of quadriceps and patellar tendon abnormalities. Plain films rely on the tendons being outlined by fat to demonstrate their integrity or displacement of the patella with complete tears (34). CT is much more precise but is limited to the axial plane and has poorer soft-tissue contrast than MRI. Ultrasound can be very accurate in skilled hands but is very operator dependent (35).

Quadriceps muscle strains appear as high signal intensity in the periphery of the muscle on T2-weighted and short-tau inversion recovery (STIR) sequences; this signal abnormality correlates with muscle tenderness but may last for many days after resolution of symptoms (36). Acute tears at the myotendinous junction cause edema within the muscle, which appears as muscle enlargement on T1-weighted images and as infiltrating high-signal-intensity edema on T2-weighted images. Complete quadriceps muscle ruptures are unusual but may occur following penetrating trauma or previous vastus lateralis release as a treatment for patellar malalignment (Fig. 3-6). Intramuscular hematomas appear as focal masses with surrounding edema. Intramuscular hematomas usually have high signal intensity on T1-weighted images and T2-weighted images because of the presence of extracellular methemoglobin; this signal pattern has been described in hematomas imaged 2 days to 5 months after injury (37,38).

Quadriceps tendon ruptures occur through the tendinous portion near the superior pole of the patella or at the myotendinous junction (39,40). MRI of acute quadriceps rupture shows discontinuity of the laminated low-signal-intensity tendon surrounded by high signal intensity on T2-weighted images, representing edema and hemorrhage (Fig. 3-7). Recognition of the laminar anatomy of the quadriceps tendon allows localization of partial tears to the rectus femoris tendon (superior layer), vastus medialis and lateralis tendon (intermediate layer), or vastus intermedius tendon (deep layer) (19). The loss of normal quadriceps muscle tension may cause the patellar tendon to appear corrugated or wrinkled on sagittal MRI images; this finding is a useful indicator of quadriceps injury (41). In cases of old quadriceps tendon injury, MRI may be used to assess muscle retraction, muscle atrophy, or fluid collections at the site of rupture (Fig. 3-8).

INJURIES OF THE PATELLAR TENDON

Patellar tendon injuries often occur in young patients during sports-related activities such as jumping, running, or falling. These tears most often occur at the site of tendon insertion on the inferior patellar pole, and occasionally at the tibial tubercle insertion site. In older patients rupture through the midportion of the tendon may occur secondary to degeneration or systemic disease (31,42). Complete patellar tendon tears and transverse patellar fractures present clinically with total loss of extensor function and superior malposition of the patella (patella alta). Partial tears of the patellar tendon present with localized pain in the patellar tendon during and after activity; this condition has been termed *jumper's knee* (43).

Complete tears of the patellar tendon appear on MRI as discontinuity of the tendon, surrounded by hemorrhage and edema (Fig. 3-9). Partial tears or tendinitis usually occur at the superior end of the patellar tendon and produce increased signal within the tendon substance, indistinct tendon margins, and tendon thickening greater than 7 mm (Fig. 3-10). Cystic lesions, granulation tissue, and metaplastic cartilage or heterotopic bone may occur within the substance of a chronic partial patellar ligament tear (Fig. 3-11) (44). A thin vertical band of mildly increased signal is seen posterior to the proximal portion of the patellar tendon in many normal subjects; this should not be misinterpreted as patellar tendinitis (45). Increased signal may also be seen in the patellar tendon when it is aligned at 55° relative to the main magnetic field due to the ''magic-angle'' effect; this is particularly seen in wrinkled patellar tendons (Fig. 3-12) (46,47). Patella alta can be diagnosed on sagittal images if the ratio of the distance between the tibial tuberosity and the inferior patellar pole versus the patellar height exceeds 1.2 (15). Patella alta may result from patellar tendon tears or from congenital variation and is associated with patellar tendon tears, recurrent dislocation of the patella, and patellofemoral pain (48,49).

OSGOOD-SCHLATTER DISEASE

Osgood-Schlatter disease is characterized by focal pain, swelling, and tenderness of the tibial tuberosity in active adolescents. This condition is more common in boys and is bilateral in up to 50% of cases. The etiology is likely repetitive trauma at the tibial attachment of the patellar tendon (50). This condition is treated conservatively with ice, anti-inflammatory medications, and limitation of activity; refractory cases may require excision of bony ossicles and adjacent bursae (51).

Sagittal MRI show enlargement of the distal end of the patellar tendon, increased intratendinous signal, and disten-

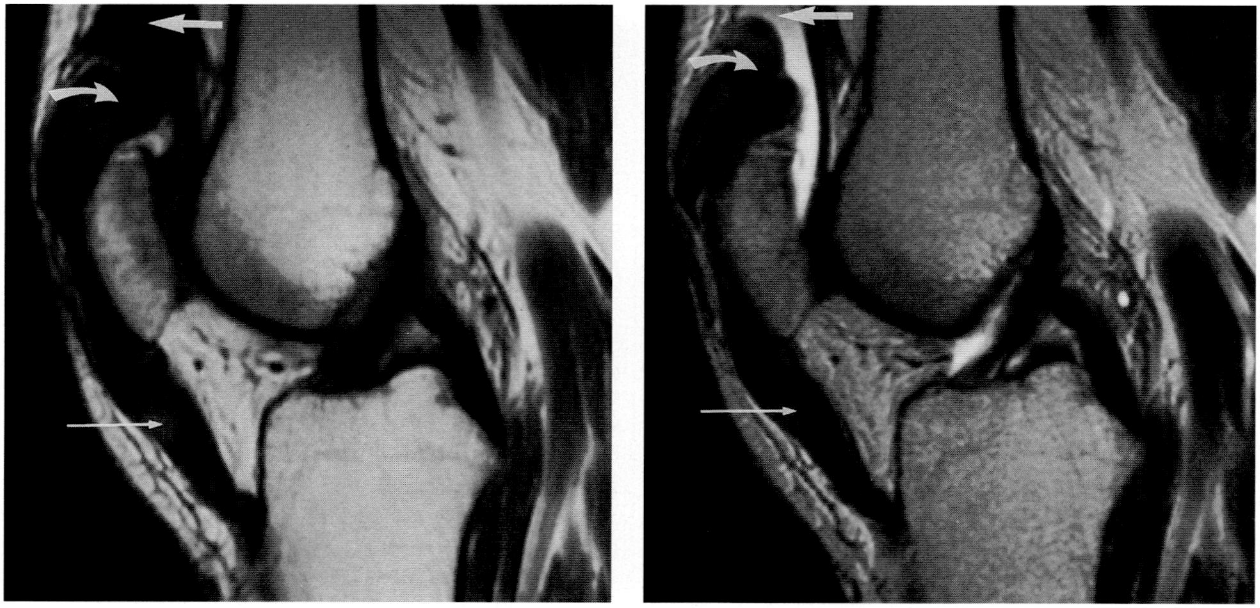

A B

FIG. 3-6. Complete quadriceps muscle rupture. Sagittal T1-weighted **(A)** and T2-weighted **(B)** images show a fluid-filled gap *(arrow)* between the retracted quadriceps tendon *(curved arrow)* and the remainder of the quadriceps muscle. The patella is inferiorly displaced and the patellar tendon *(long arrow)* is thickened due to retraction. (Case courtesy of P. Tirman, San Francisco.)

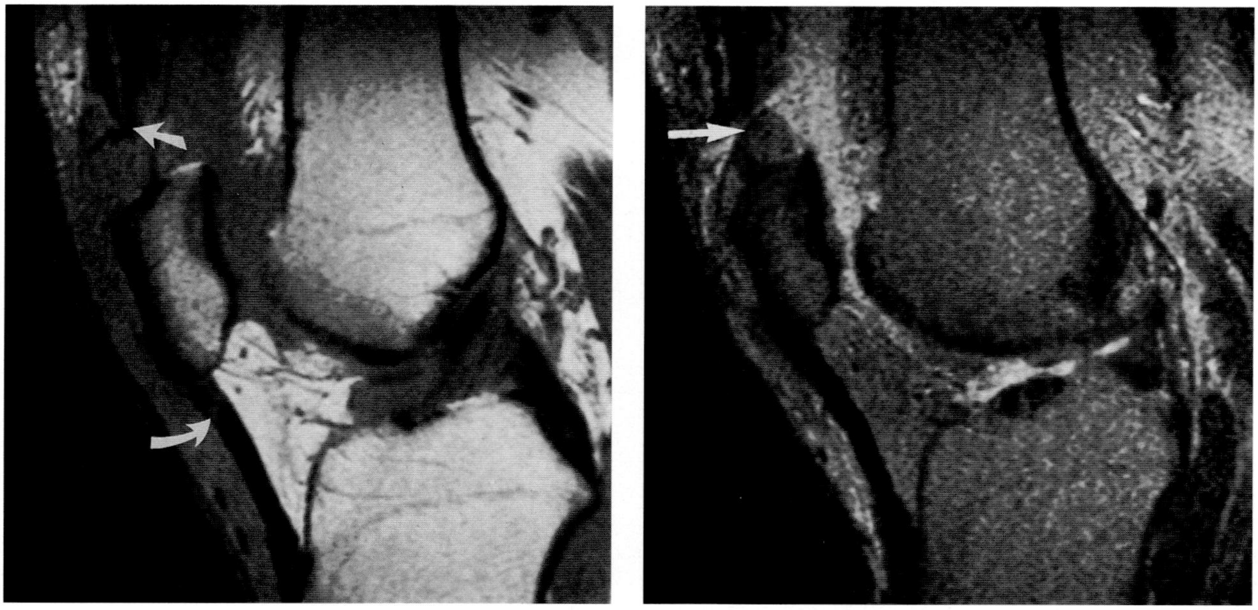

A B

FIG. 3-7. Quadriceps tendon rupture. A sagittal T1-weighted image **(A)** shows discontinuity of the quadriceps tendon layers near the superior pole of the patella *(arrow)*. A small region of increased signal is present in the patellar tendon *(curved arrow)*, because of magic angle effects in a region of tendon buckling. A sagittal T2-weighted image **(B)** shows high-signal-intensity edema and hemorrhage at the site of tendon tear *(arrow)*. (Case courtesy of P. Tirman, San Francisco.)

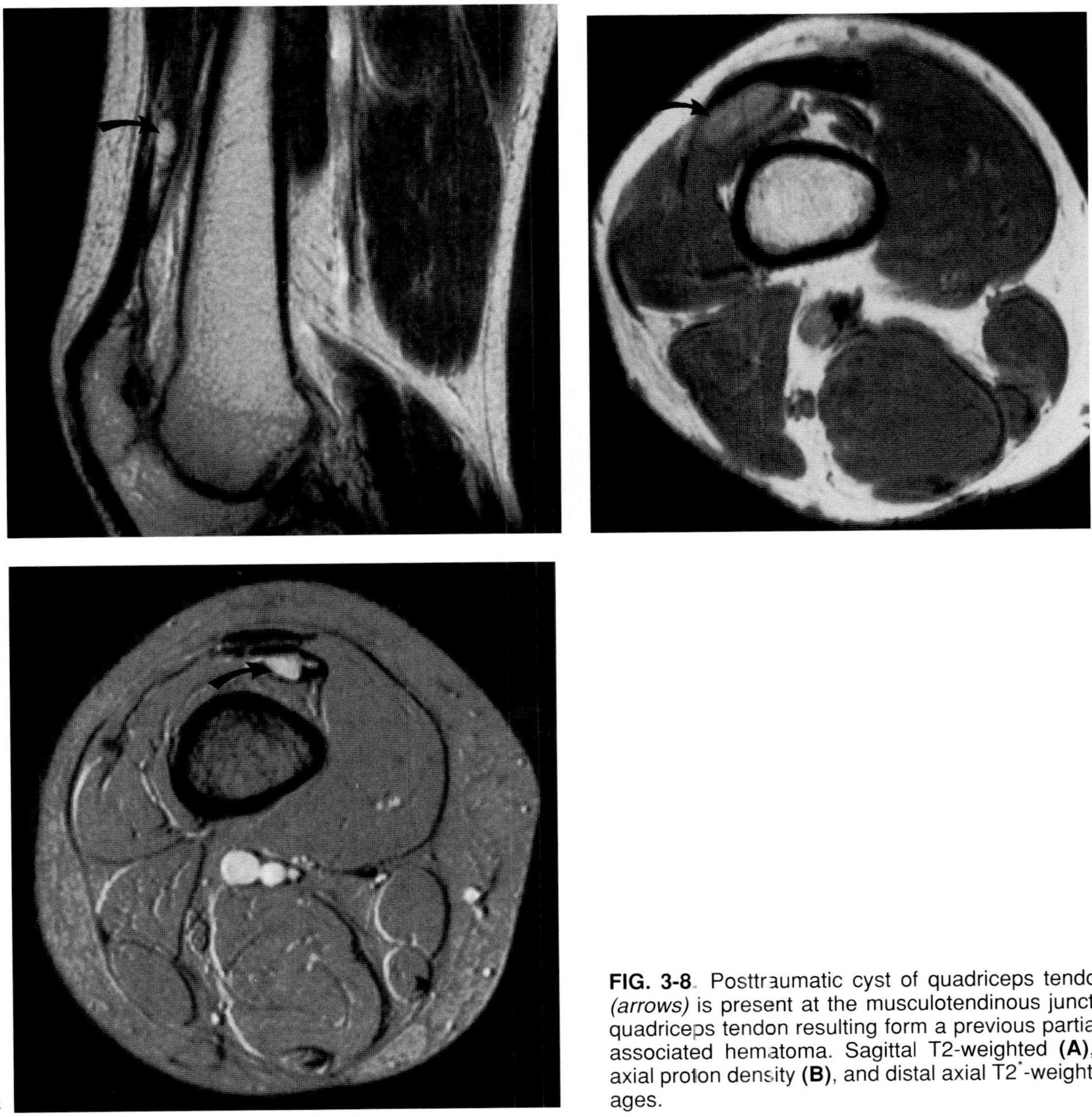

FIG. 3-8. Posttraumatic cyst of quadriceps tendon. A cyst *(arrows)* is present at the musculotendinous junction of the quadriceps tendon resulting form a previous partial tear and associated hematoma. Sagittal T2-weighted **(A)**, proximal axial proton density **(B)**, and distal axial T2*-weighted **(C)** images.

sion of the superficial and deep infrapatellar bursae. These soft-tissue changes are reported to be present in most cases of Osgood-Schlatter disease. Bone marrow edema of the tibial tuberosity is seen in a minority of cases (50,52). MRI, CT, and plain radiographs may show fragmentation of the tibial tuberosity; however, this is not a reliable diagnostic sign because it is often present in asymptomatic subjects (53). Formation of joints between the tibia and ligamentous ossicles has been demonstrated (54).

Sinding-Larsen-Johansson disease is a similar syndrome of focal pain and swelling at the junction of the patellar tendon and the inferior pole of the patella. This condition occurs in active adolescents and probably results from repetitive trauma at the tendo-osseous junction. Radiographs show variable ossification and calcification of the proximal end of the patellar tendon (55).

PERIPATELLAR BURSITIS

The bursae around the patellar tendon reduce friction between the patellar tendon and adjacent structures. The prepatellar bursa is located between the subcutaneous tissues and the patella, the superficial infrapatellar bursa is located between the subcutaneous tissues and the tibial tubercle, and the deep infrapatellar bursa is located between the posterior aspect of the distal patellar tendon and the anterior tibia. Repetitive trauma, hemorrhage, or infection can produce

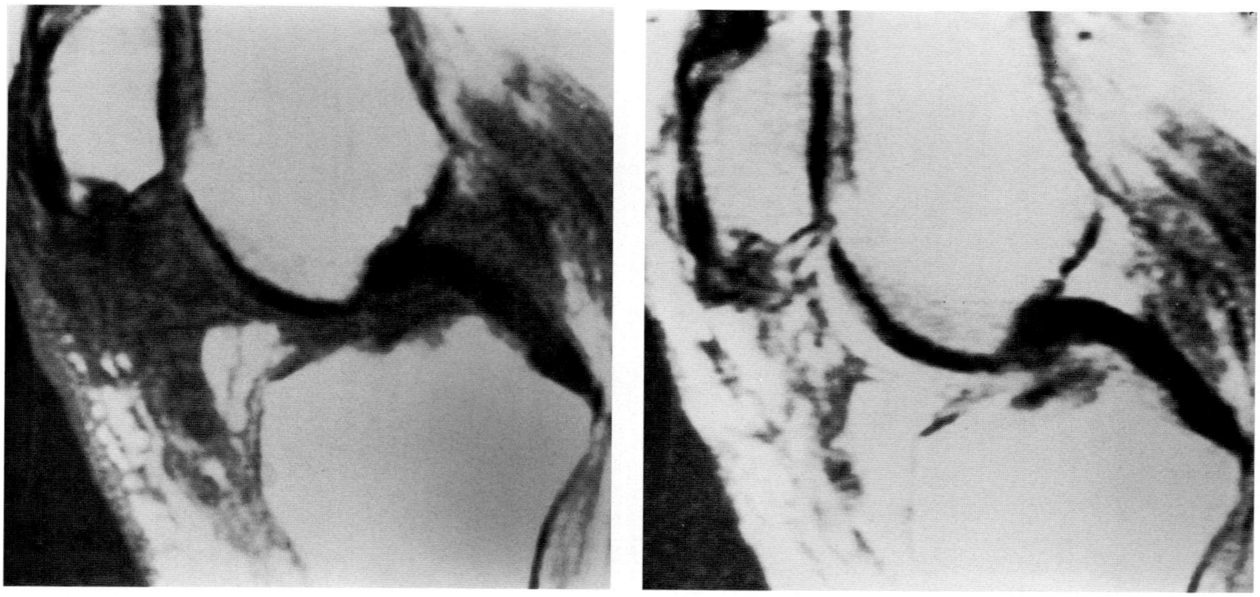

A B

FIG. 3-9. Complete patellar tendon tear. T1-weighted **(A)** and T2-weighted **(B)** sagittal images show complete disruption of the patellar tendon with a large joint effusion. The patella has retracted superiorly (patella alta).

bursitis, which presents clinically with focal pain and swelling.

Prepatellar bursitis ("house-maid's knee") results from chronic trauma, such as occupational or recreational kneeling and crawling. Infectious bursitis results from penetrating trauma and is most commonly due to *Staphylococcus aureus* (56). MRI shows a focal fluid collection between the patellar tendon and the subcutaneous tissues surrounded by edema (Fig. 3-13). Prepatellar bursitis is often hemorrhagic, resulting in an inhomogeneous appearance on MRI images (57,58).

The superficial infrapatellar bursa is an uncommon site of bursitis. MRI imaging shows a focal, ill-defined fluid collection anterior to the tibial tubercle. The deep infrapatellar bursa contains a tiny amount of fluid in asymptomatic patients. Deep infrapatellar bursitis results from overuse of the knee extensor mechanism and is associated with patellar tendonitis, "jumper's knee," and Osgood-Schlatter disease (50,56). MR imaging shows a fluid-filled bursa collection between the anterior tibia and the patellar tendon (Fig. 3-14).

An isolated suprapatellar bursa results from failure of resorption of the suprapatellar plica. Trauma and synovitis cause accumulation of fluid in the bursa. This rare abnormality appears on sagittal MRI images as a focal suprapatellar fluid collection with an intact suprapatellar plica separating the bursa from the knee joint (Fig. 3-15).

PATELLAR DISLOCATION

The patella is held within the femoral trochlea by active muscular restraints, passive ligamentous restraints, and the bony contours of the patellofemoral joint. During knee flexion, valgus, and external rotation of the tibia, strong contraction of the quadriceps generates a lateral displacement force on the patella. This force may exceed the tensile strength of the medial patellar restraints, resulting in rupture of the medial patellar retinaculum, lateral dislocation of the patella, and impaction of the medial patellar facet on the anterior surface of the lateral femoral condyle. A direct impact on the medial aspect of the patella may rarely cause lateral patellar dislocation.

Lateral patellar dislocation is relatively common, accounting for 9–16% of acute hemarthroses in athletes (59,60). The dislocation is usually momentary. Thus, most patients do not recall the dislocation; rather, they present with acute knee pain and hemarthrosis suggestive of cruciate or meniscal injury (61–63). Many anatomic factors predispose to lateral patellar dislocation, including patella alta, genu valgum, external tibial torsion, and patellofemoral dysplasia (16). Medial patellar dislocation is uncommon but typically occurs as a complication of lateral retinacular release or injury (64,65).

A constellation of MRI findings have been described in lateral patellar dislocation: hemarthrosis (82–100% of cases), disruption of the medial patellar retinaculum (82–96% of cases), bone contusion of the anterior aspect of the lateral femoral condyle (81–100% of cases), and chondral or osteochondral fracture of the medial patellar facet (30–64%) (Fig. 3-16) (61–63). Persistent lateral subluxation and lateral tilt of the patella are often present. The bone contusion in the lateral femoral condyle and the edema around the disrupted medial patellar retinaculum are most conspicuous on STIR or fat-saturated T2-weighted fast spin-echo techniques (66–68).

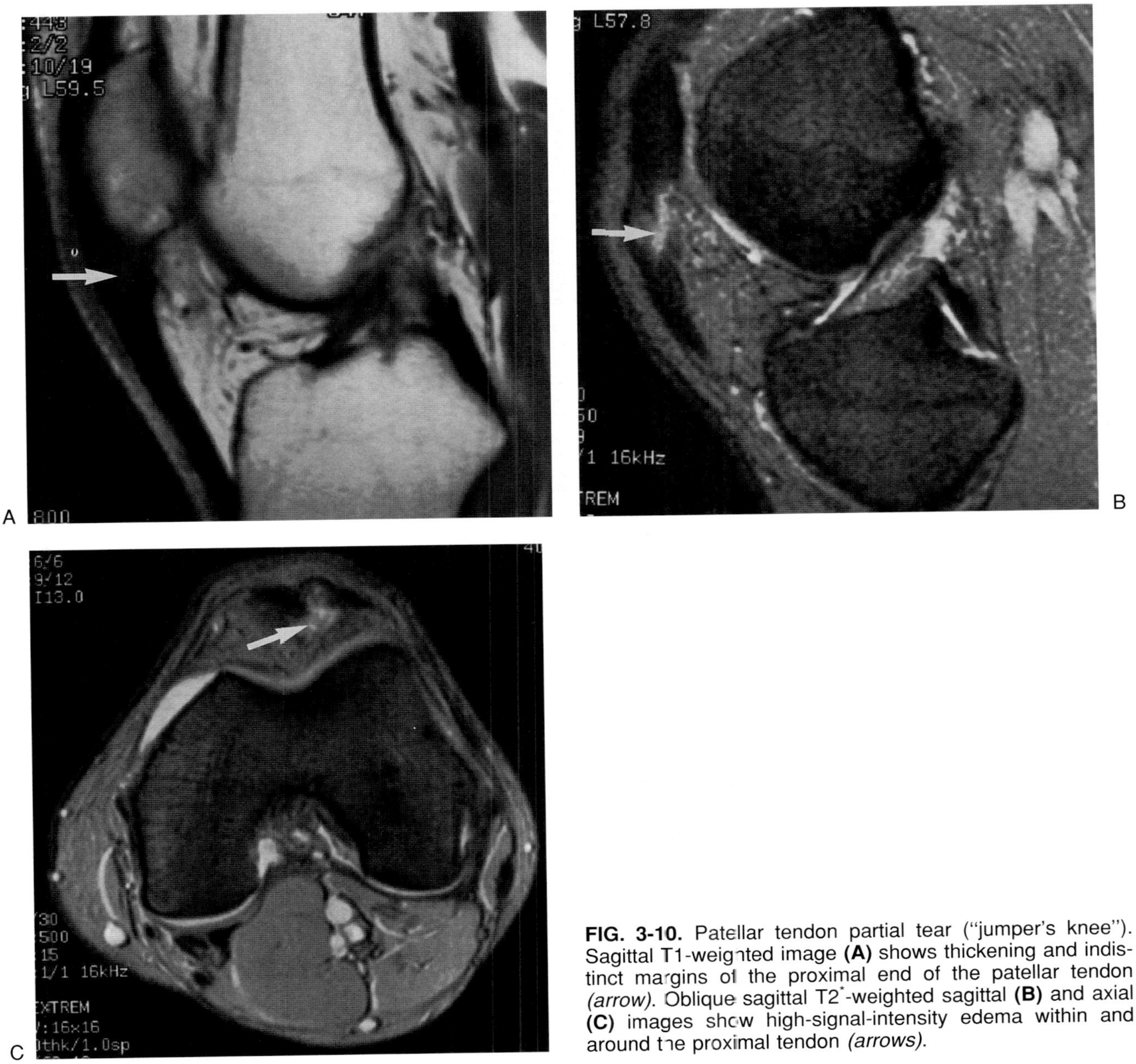

FIG. 3-10. Patellar tendon partial tear ("jumper's knee"). Sagittal T1-weighted image **(A)** shows thickening and indistinct margins of the proximal end of the patellar tendon *(arrow).* Oblique sagittal T2*-weighted sagittal **(B)** and axial **(C)** images show high-signal-intensity edema within and around the proximal tendon *(arrows).*

PATELLAR INSTABILITY AND TRACKING ABNORMALITIES

The position of the patella at rest and during motion depends on patellofemoral bony morphology, passive ligamentous restraints, and active muscular forces. During normal motion the contact area between the patella and the femur follows a complex three-dimensional motion; this distributes the weight-bearing load evenly over the articular surfaces (69). Biomechanical abnormalities of patellar position and motion may result in knee pain from retinacular stress or from secondary patellar cartilage abnormalities (51,70–72). Many plain radiographic methods have been devised to assess patellar position and tracking, attesting to the generally unsatisfactory nature of non-cross-sectional imaging at this site (73). CT has been widely used with considerable success but does not show soft tissue and cartilage as well as MRI. MRI allows excellent visualization of patellofemoral morphology, cartilage abnormalities, and soft-tissue stabilizing structures. Kinematic MRI techniques provide dynamic assessment of patellar tracking abnormalities (24,26,27,74,75).

Patellar Morphology and Position

The morphology of the patellar articular surface has been classified by Wiberg and others (Fig. 3-17) and can be assessed on axial MRI images. The Wiberg classification is

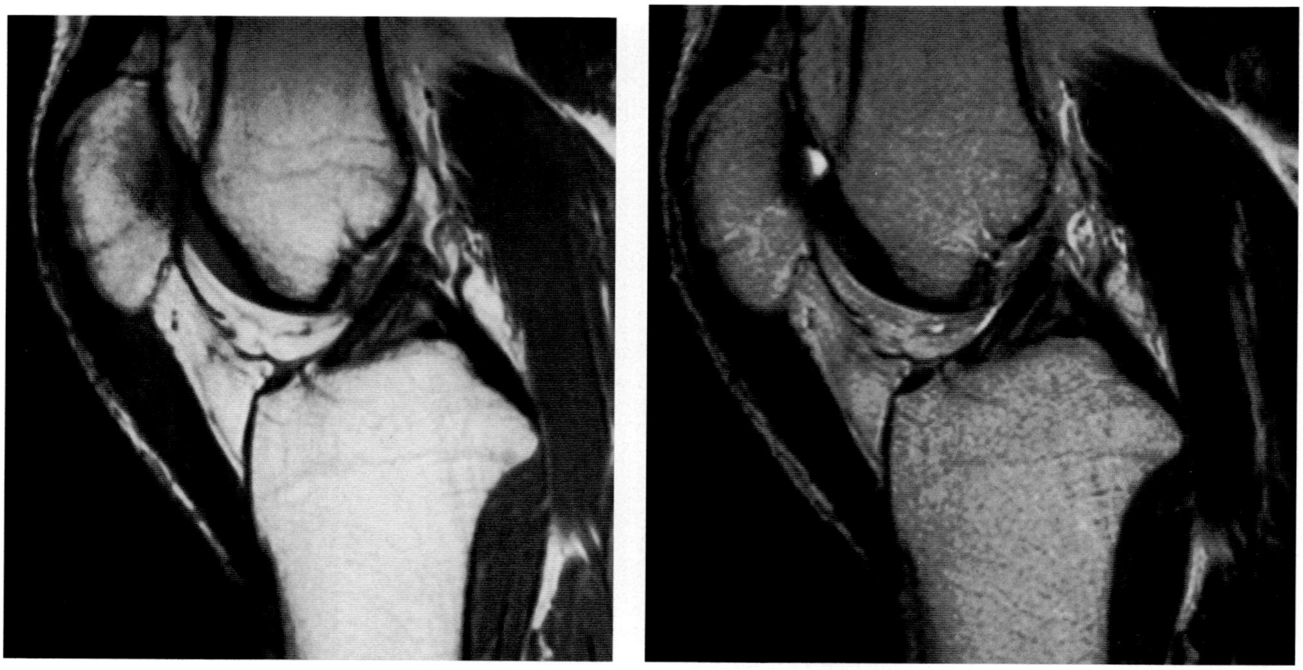

A B

FIG. 3-11. Chronic partial patellar tendon tear. Sagittal T1-weighted **(A)** and T2-weighted **(B)** images show marked diffuse thickening of the patellar tendon with internal increased signal. This represents granulation tissue and fibrosis within the tendon, because of chronic partial tendon tear.

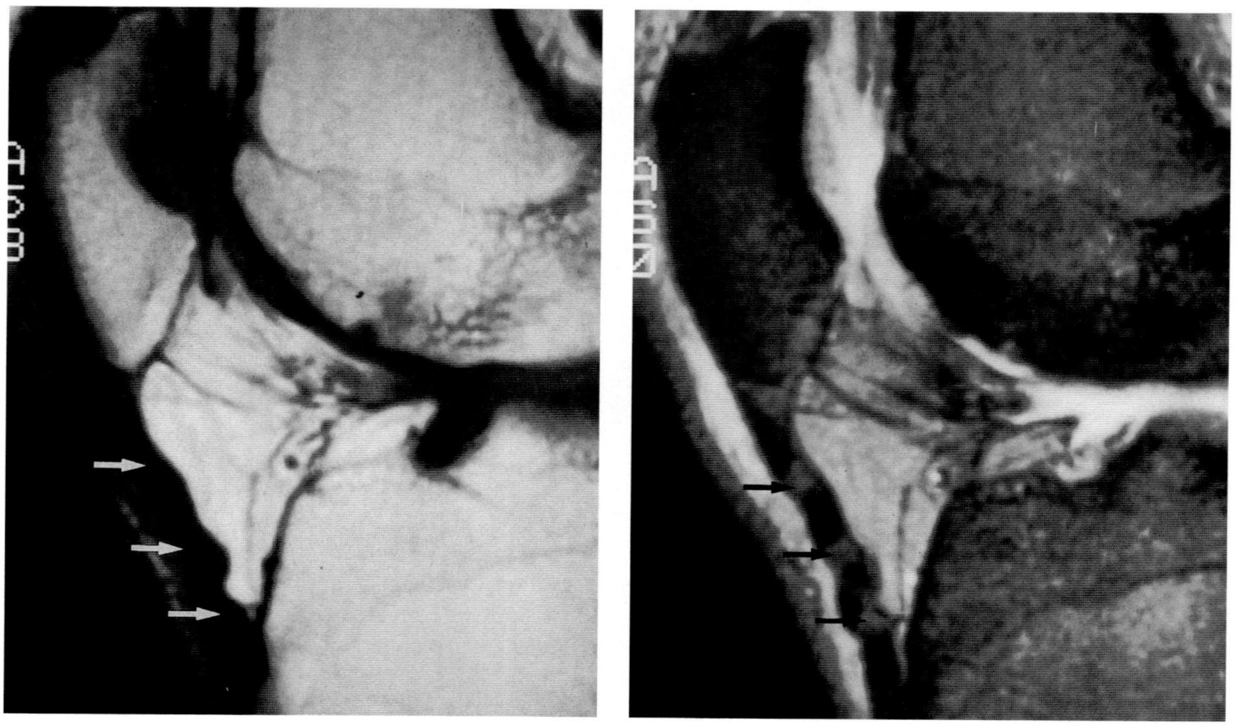

A B

FIG. 3-12. Increased signal in patellar tendon due to tendon wrinkling and "magic-angle" phenomenon. Sagittal T1-weighted **(A)** and $T2^*$-weighted **(B)** images show a wavy contour of the patellar tendon ("wrinkling"), with region of increased signal *(arrows)* in the portions of the tendon oriented near 55° relative to the main magnetic field. This increased signal is due to the magic-angle phenomenon and should not be misinterpreted as a tendon abnormality.

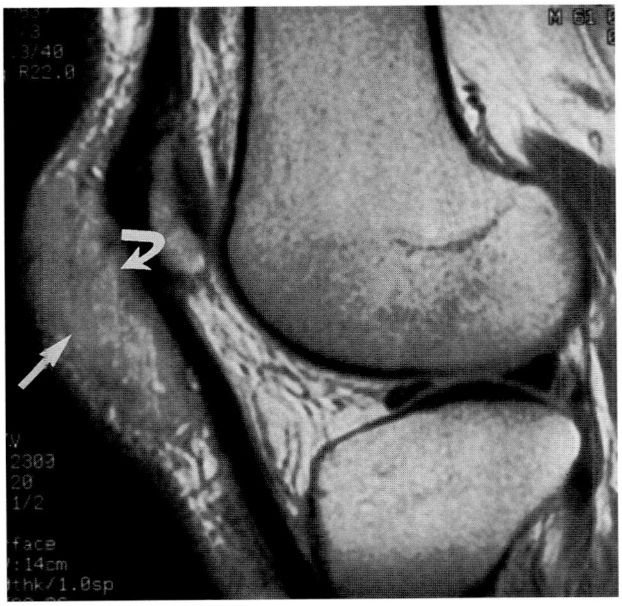

A

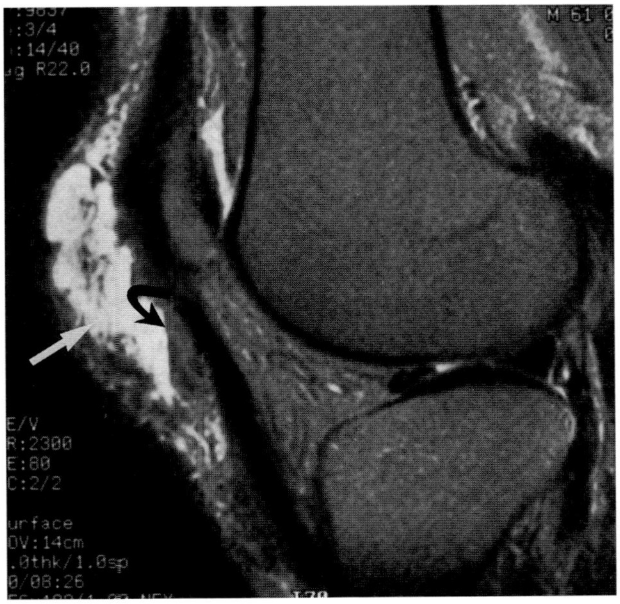

B

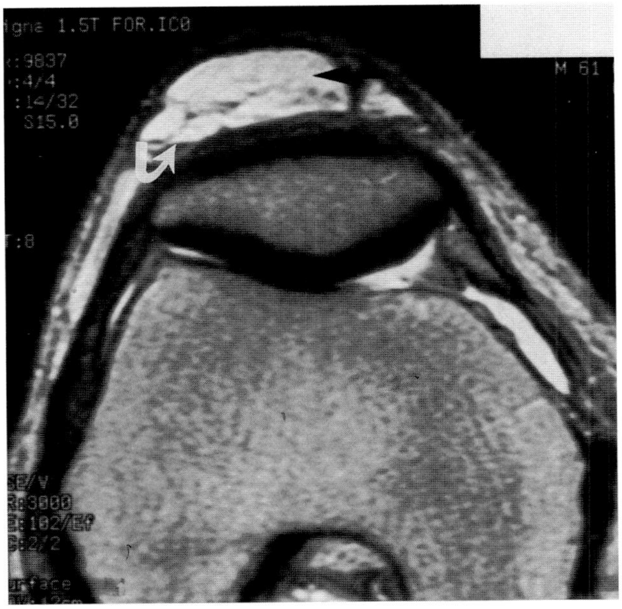

C

FIG. 3-13. Prepatellar bursitis ("housemaid's knee"). Sagittal proton-density-weighted **(A)**, sagittal T2-weighted **(B)**, and axial T2-weighted **(C)** images show a multiloculated fluid collection *(arrows)* superficial to the patella. Some of the loculations contain fluid–fluid levels *(curved arrows)*, typical of hemorrhage or debris within the bursal fluid. (Case courtesy of P. Tirman, San Francisco.)

based on the position of the vertical ridge; in type I the medial and lateral facets are concave and of equal size; in type II the lateral facet is larger than the medial facet; and type III describes a small, convex medial facet and a large, concave lateral facet. Type II is the most common, occurring in 57% of subjects. Types I and II are the most stable, because of the prominent medial ridge. Types III, IV, and V have been associated with patellar instability disorders (8,14,76).

The lateral femoral condyle is normally larger and more protrusive than the medial femoral condyle, providing a bony restraint against lateral patellar displacement. Hypoplasia of the lateral femoral condyle results in a shallow trochlear sulcus, which predisposes to patellar instability (77).

A number of parameters may be used to describe the position of the patella relative to the femur on routine axial MRI images. The most common methods are the patellar tilt angle (the angle between a line parallel to the lateral patellar facet and a line parallel to the posterior aspects of the femoral condyles) and the congruence angle (the angle formed by a line bisecting the trochlear sulcus and a line connecting the patellar apex to the trochlear sulcus). A normal patellar tilt angle is greater than 8°, and a normal congruence angle is $8 \pm 6°$ (25,78). The accuracy of patellar position assessment on routine axial MRI images is limited by the absence of muscle contraction, movement, and loading (79).

On sagittal images, the patellar tendon length should be nearly equal to the height of the patella. Variations of greater

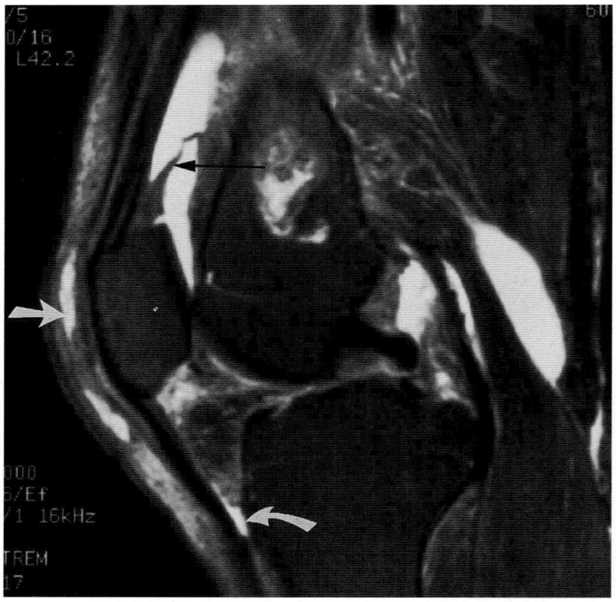

FIG. 3-14. Bursitis and knee joint effusion secondary to gout. A sagittal STIR image shows prepatellar bursitis *(arrow)* and deep infrapatellar bursitis *(curved arrow)*. A large joint effusion is present, distending the suprapatellar recess, which contains a suprapatellar plica *(long arrow)*. A Baker's cyst and a femoral bone infarct are also present.

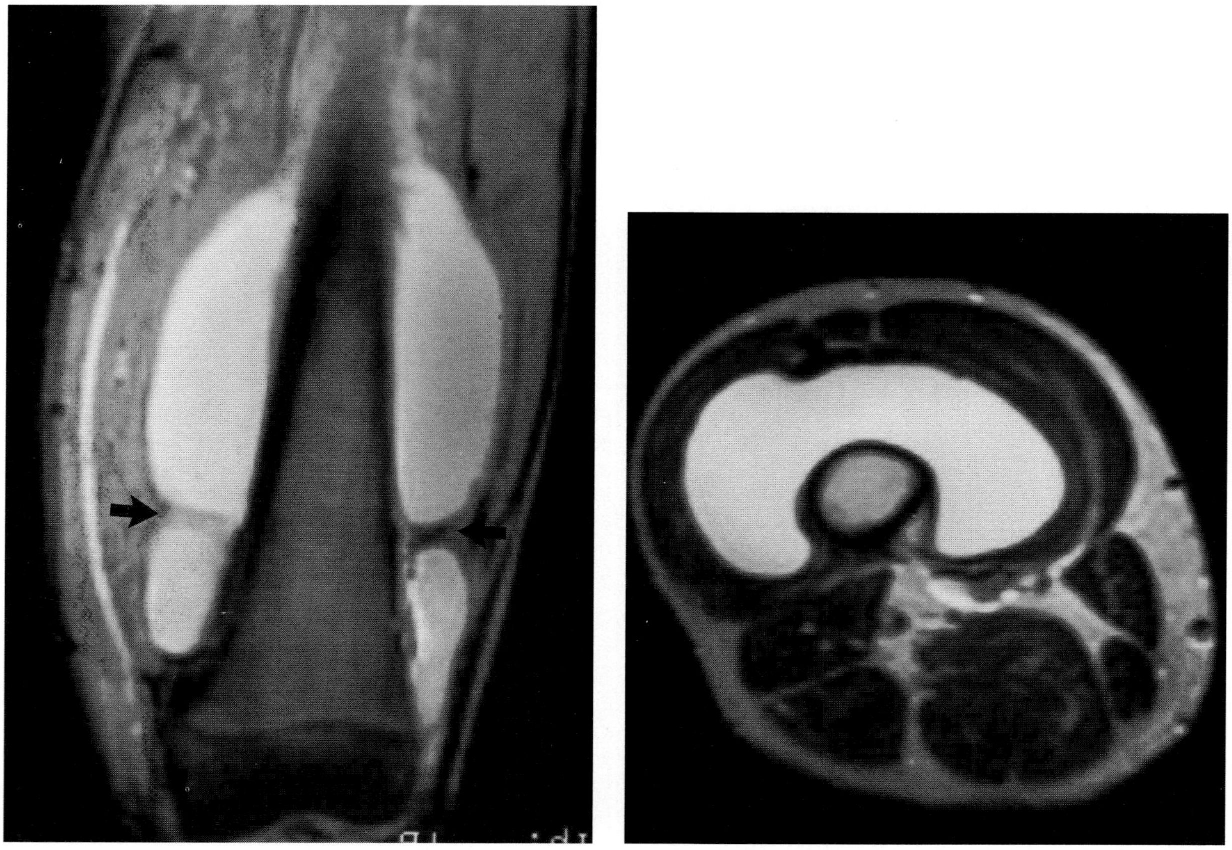

A B

FIG. 3-15. Isolated suprapatellar bursa. Coronal $T2^*$-weighted **(A)** and axial T2-weighted **(B)** images show a complete suprapatellar plica dividing the suprapatellar recess from the remainder of the knee joint. The plica *(arrow)* is outlined by trapped fluid above and joint effusion below.

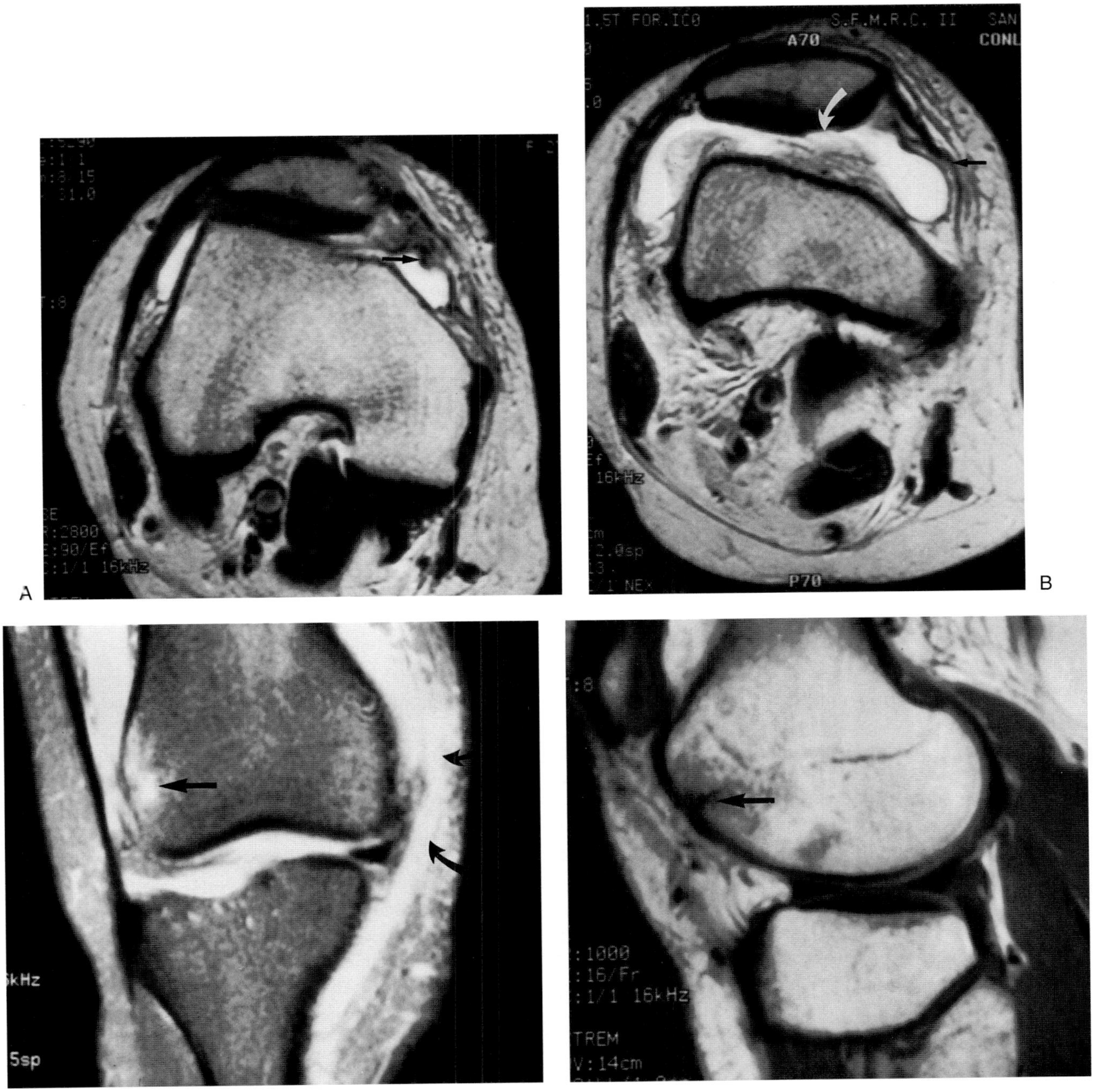

FIG. 3-16. Previous lateral patellar dislocation. Axial T2-weighted images **(A,B)** show disruption and waviness of the medial patellar retinaculum *(arrows)* and a focal chondral fracture of the medial patellar facet *(curved arrow)*. A coronal fat-suppressed T2-weighted image **(C)** shows bone marrow contusion in the anterior aspect of the lateral femoral condyle *(arrow)* and extensive edema around the torn medial patellar retinaculum *(curved arrow)*. A sagittal T1-weighted image **(D)** shows bone marrow contusion in the lateral femoral condyle *(arrow)*. (Case courtesy of P. Tirman, San Francisco.)

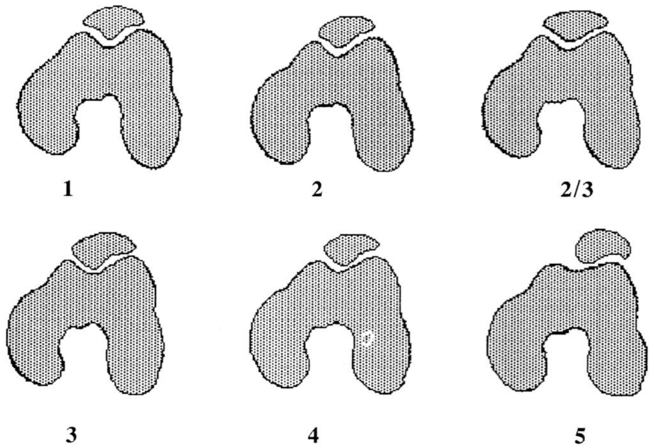

FIG. 3-17. Patellar morphology. Diagrammatic classification of patellar types. (Adapted from Carson WG et al. Patellofemoral disorders: physical and radiographic evaluation. *Clin Orthop* 1984;185:178–186; copyright 1984, JB Lippincott.)

than 20% indicate patella alta (superior position) or patella baja (inferior position). Patellar malposition is associated with patellar dislocation, subluxation, and chondromalacia (15,25,80).

Patellar Tracking Abnormalities

Patients with patellar tracking abnormalities present clinically with anterior knee pain, joint crepitation, and pain on patellofemoral compression. Normal patellar motion during knee flexion is complex, variable, and dependent on many factors, including the nature of the movement (active vs. passive), and the presence of joint loading. During full knee extension, the patella is superolateral to the trochlear surface. At 5–10° of knee flexion the lateral patellar facet contacts the lateral trochlear sulcus. The median vertical ridge should centralize within the trochlear sulcus at 30–45° of passive knee flexion and at 5–30° of active loaded knee flexion (71,81–83).

An excessively lateral position of the patella during full knee extension and early flexion may produce lateral patellofemoral cartilage damage. Chronic lateral tracking may result in shortening of the lateral retinaculum and stretching of the medial restraints. This may lead to a painful compressive arthropathy of the lateral patellar facet termed the *lateral facet syndrome*. Surgical release of the lateral retinaculum is beneficial in most patients who fail to respond to conservative measures. Medial tracking is uncommon but may similarly produce cartilage damage in the medial patellofemoral articulation. Tracking abnormalities are initially treated with conservative measures such as selective muscle strengthening and patellar bracing; surgical treatment with patellar realignment, resurfacing, or patellectomy is reserved for refractory cases (70,75,84).

PATELLOFEMORAL CARTILAGE ABNORMALITIES

A variety of patellofemoral cartilage abnormalities may result from trauma, degeneration, or patellar tracking abnormalities. MRI allows noninvasive assessment of the patellofemoral cartilage based on surface contours and internal signal characteristics. The presence of a knee effusion allows optimum visualization of the cartilage surface on axial and sagittal images.

Normal patellofemoral cartilage has a smooth surface and a trilaminar appearance on high-resolution images. The zones of increased and decreased signal intensity correlate with histologic zones; the low-signal-intensity superficial layer represents tangential collagen fibers, the high-signal-intensity intermediate layer represents radial collagen fibers and proteoglycans, and the low-signal-intensity deep layer is composed of deep radiate fibers and calcified cartilage (23). The signal intensity in the middle zone of radially arranged collagen fibers may be increased by magic-angle effects, if the fibers are positioned at or near 55° to the main magnetic field (40,74). Normal patellar cartilage thickness varies with age, measuring 3 ± 1 mm in subjects less than 20 years old, 4.25 ± 1 mm at 25 years of age, and 3.5 ± 1 mm at 45 years of age (8).

Chondromalacia Patellae

Chondromalacia patellae is defined as pathologic softening or degeneration of the patellar cartilage. This term is also applied to a clinical syndrome of anterior knee pain and joint crepitus in adolescence and young adulthood. The relationship between the pathologic abnormality and the clinical syndrome is not absolute, because some patients with arthroscopically proven chondromalacia patellae have no symptoms and some with the clinical syndrome have normal patellar cartilage. In many cases, chondromalacia patellae is the result of a primary problem of patellar malalignment, tracking abnormality, or overuse. Thus, the term *chondromalacia patellae* is best used as a pathologic description of abnormal cartilage, which may be symptomatic and which may be due to an underlying biomechanical cause (20,25,51,70,85–87). Chondromalacia patellae can be separated histologically into two forms: basal degeneration, which is common in young adults, and superficial degeneration, which is common in older patients and likely is an early manifestation of osteoarthritis. The basal degeneration type of chondromalacia usually does not progress to osteoarthritis, and repair of the cartilage damage may occur via fibrous metaplasia (78). The most common site of chondromalacia is the vertical ridge separating the medial and lateral facets.

Symptomatic chondromalacia patellae is initially treated with conservative measures such as physiotherapy, selective muscle strengthening, and patellar bracing (70). If conservative therapy is unsuccessful, surgical procedures directed at the underlying biomechanical abnormality are considered, including realignment of the patellar tendon, lateral retinacular release, and cartilage debridement. Patellar resurfacing or patellectomy is reserved for chronic debilitating cases (87–90).

Both arthrography and CT arthrography have been used to evaluate the integrity of patellar cartilage (91–94). Defects in the surface of the cartilage can be appreciated with these techniques as well as inhibition of contrast into frayed cartilage. These methods are invasive, and likely less sensitive than MRI in assessment of cartilage abnormalities.

The arthroscopic and MRI appearances of chondromalacia patellae can be graded according to a four-point scale, as proposed by various authors (Table 3-1) (25,85,95,96). Stage I chondromalacia appears as areas of inhomogeneous signal on T1- and T2-weighted images within morphologically normal articular cartilage. Stage I chondromalacia, as defined by arthroscopy, is not reliably diagnosed with MRI, because focal areas of inhomogeneous signal are often seen on MRI images in patients without arthroscopic evidence of chondromalacia. Stage II lesions appear as low-signal-intensity areas that may deform the cartilage surface ("blistering"). Stage III lesions appear as loss of the sharp cartilage margin and/or cartilage thinning. In stage IV lesions the subchondral bone is exposed with focal absence of articular cartilage. Stages II, III, and IV are reliably detected and graded on axial images, with reported accuracies of 70–89% (Fig. 3-18) (22,23,75). Although MRI offers a unique ability to assess cartilage lesions noninvasively, the clinical accuracy and efficacy of MRI versus arthroscopy in evaluation of chondromalacia patellae is not clearly defined at present (97). Experimental studies have also shown that with acutely increased loads across the patellofemoral joint, subchondral bone marrow can show changes consistent with edema/hemorrhage, even though arthroscopy may not be abnormal. Histology usually demonstrates extensive cartilage fissuring (98).

T2*-weighted gradient-echo images are superior to T1-weighted images for assessment of surface contour abnormalities due to the increased contrast between joint fluid and cartilage (20,82 99). The optimal pulse sequence for assessment of cartilage abnormalities is a subject of ongoing research and controversy. MR-arthrography using intra-articular injection of gadolinium complexes and T1-weighted images may be the optimum technique, because this method provides excellent contrast between joint fluid and cartilage, high signal-to-noise images, and relatively short imaging times.

Chondral and Osteochondral Fractures

Chondral and osteochondral fractures in the patellofemoral joint frequently occur during impaction of the patellar cartilage on the lateral femoral condyle during lateral patellar dislocation (16,51–63). Direct blows also may cause chondral or osteochondral fracture, because of impaction of the patella on the femoral condyles. The most common sites of chondral and osteochondral fracture are the medial patellar facet and the lateral femoral condyle (Fig. 3-19) (83). Other injuries are commonly associated with osteochondral fractures; meniscal tears were found in 40% of osteochondral fracture cases in one series (84). A knee joint effusion or lipohemarthrosis is typically seen in acute cases of osteochondral fracture (Fig. 3-20). MRI is of particular value in assessing the cartilaginous surfaces, because size and presence of an osteochondral fracture may be underestimated on plain radiographs and computed tomography. MRI may also demonstrate the dislocated cartilage fragment.

Osteochondritis Dissecans

Osteochondritis dissecans is characterized by a focal cartilage abnormality with necrosis of the subchondral bone. Thinning, fragmentation, ulceration, or detachment of the cartilage may be seen. The underlying bone may also fragment or detach. This condition is likely due to trauma, although other causes—including avascular necrosis, fat emboli, and bone dysplasia—have been suggested (101,102). The most common site of involvement in the knee is the

TABLE 3-1. *MRI and arthroscopic staging of chondromalacia patellae*

Stage	Pathologic findings	MR findings[a]
1	Softening and swelling of articular cartilage	*Surface:* normal *Signal intensity:* normal or focal areas of decreased signal
2	Blistering of cartilage	*Surface:* focal elevation ("blistering") *Signal intensity:* focal areas of decreased signal
3	Surface irregularity and fibrillation not extending to subchondral bone	*Surface:* irregular, with loss of sharp surface margin *Signal intensity:* decreased signal extending to cartilage surface
4	Cartilage erosion with exposure of subchondral bone	*Surface:* absence of cartilage *Signal intensity:* synovial fluid signal extends to subchondral bone

Information derived from Conway WF, Hayes CW, Loughran T, et al. Cross-sectional imaging of the patellofemoral joint and surrounding structures. *Radiographics* 1991;11:195–217; Hodge JC, Ghelman B, O'Brien SJ, Wickiewicz TL. Synovial plicae and chondromalacia patellae: correlation of results of CT arthrography with results of arthroscopy. *Radiology* 1993;186:827–831.

[a] MR signal intensity findings refer to T1-weighted spin-echo images

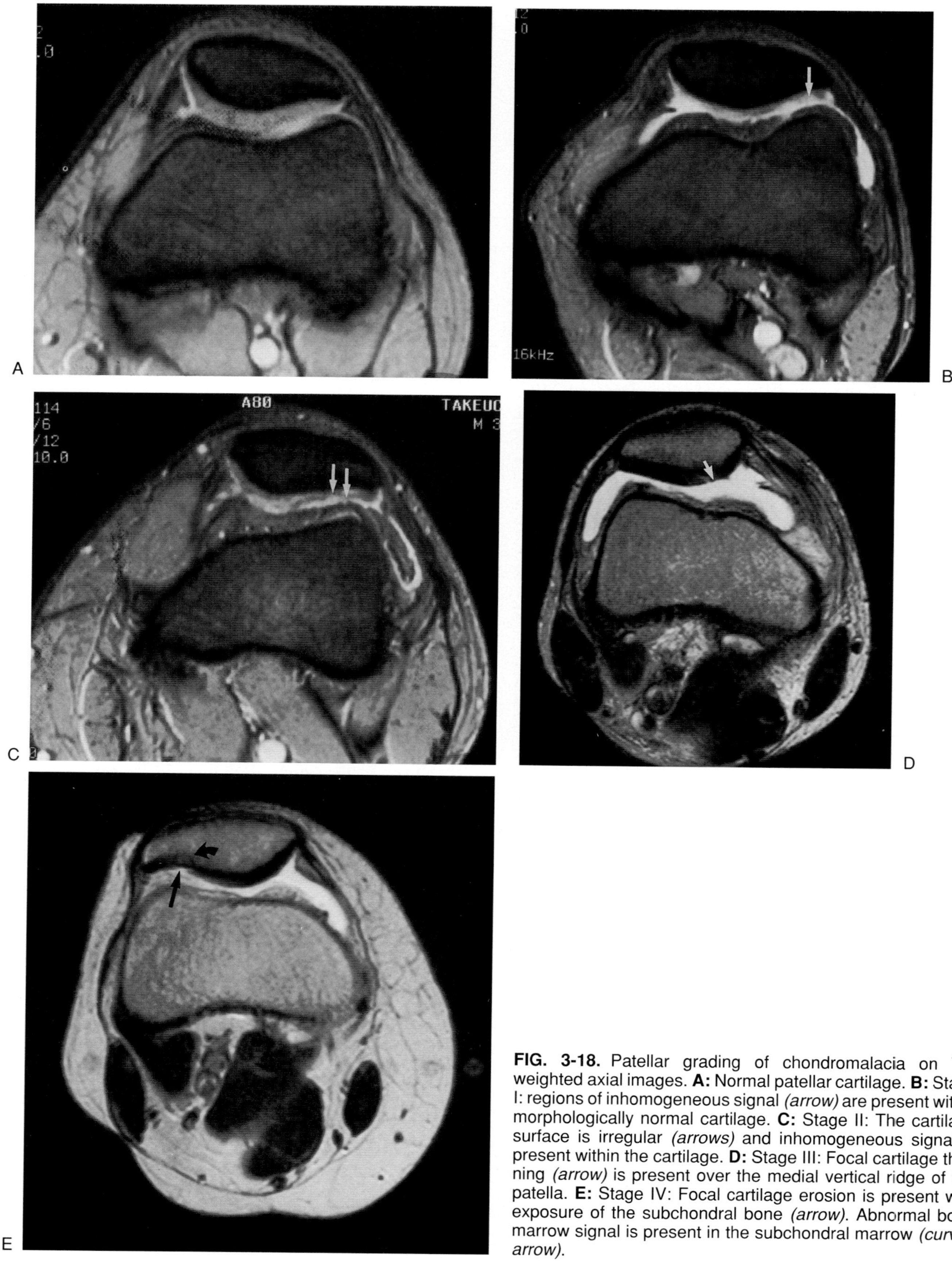

FIG. 3-18. Patellar grading of chondromalacia on T2-weighted axial images. **A:** Normal patellar cartilage. **B:** Stage I: regions of inhomogeneous signal *(arrow)* are present within morphologically normal cartilage. **C:** Stage II: The cartilage surface is irregular *(arrows)* and inhomogeneous signal is present within the cartilage. **D:** Stage III: Focal cartilage thinning *(arrow)* is present over the medial vertical ridge of the patella. **E:** Stage IV: Focal cartilage erosion is present with exposure of the subchondral bone *(arrow)*. Abnormal bone marrow signal is present in the subchondral marrow *(curved arrow)*.

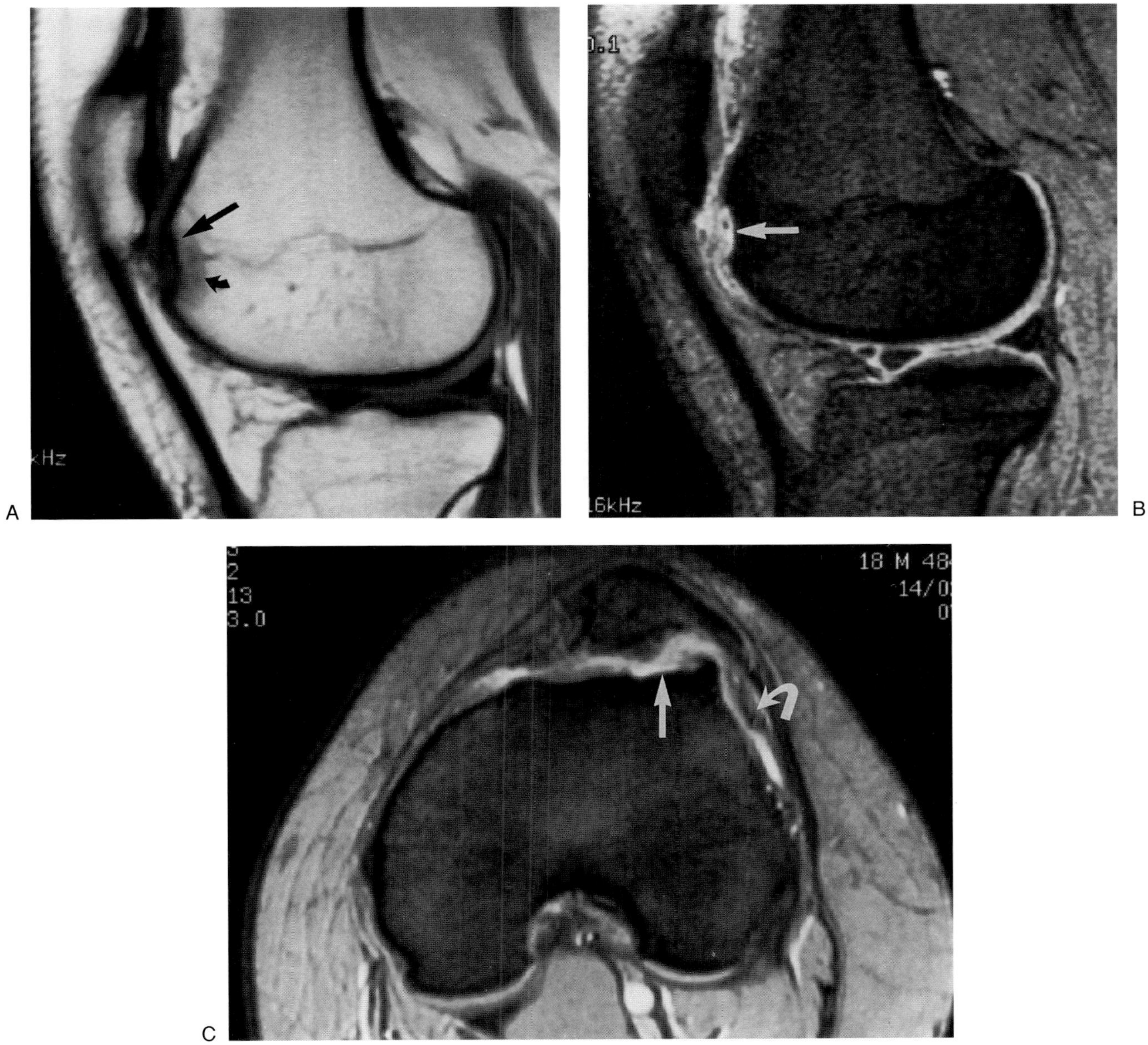

FIG. 3-19. Osteochondral fracture of lateral femoral condyle. Sagittal T1-weighted **(A)**, sagittal T2*-weighted **(B)**, and axial T2*-weighted **(C)** images show a focal osteochondral defect *(arrows)* in the anterior surface of the lateral femoral condyle. A region of subjacent bone marrow edema is present (**A**, *curved arrow*). The displaced osteochondral fragment lies within the lateral aspect of the suprapatellar recess (**C**, *curved arrow*).

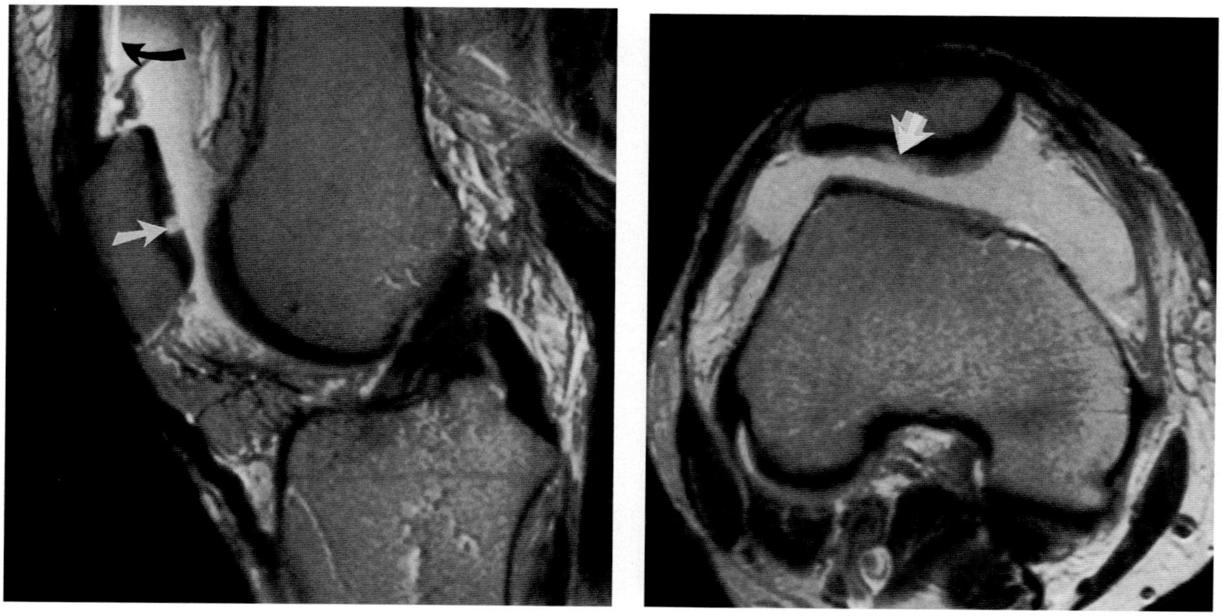

A B

FIG. 3-20. Chondral fracture of patella. Sagittal **(A)** and axial **(B)** T2-weighted images show a focal cartilage fracture *(arrows)* in the lateral patellar facet. A large lipohemarthrosis with a fat–fluid level (**A**, *curved arrow*) is present. The lipohemarthrosis in this case was due to an associated tibial plateau fracture. (Case courtesy of P. Tirman, San Francisco.)

intercondylar aspect of the medial femoral condyle; however, involvement of the patella or femoral trochlear surface is not unusual (103).

Osteochondritis dissecans most commonly occurs in young adults and causes focal pain and joint effusion. The treatment of this condition depends on the stability of the cartilage and bone fragments. Conservative treatment is recommended for stable lesions, whereas partially detached fragments of cartilage or bone should be drilled or pinned. Completely detached fragments should be debrided and removed from the joint (104,105).

On T1-weighted MRI images, osteochondritis dissecans appears as a focal region of diminished signal in the subarticular bone. The overlying cartilage may be intact, thinned, or detached. T2-weighted images are useful to assess the cartilage surface (Fig. 3-21). The presence of high-signal joint fluid partially or completely surrounding the lesion is a reliable sign of fragment instability (Fig. 3-22) (106).

SYNOVIAL PLICAE

Synovial plicae are intra-articular synovial folds that result from incomplete regression of normal embryologic septae (see the preceding section on embryology). Three types of plicae are commonly encountered in normal subjects: the medial patellar plica, the suprapatellar plica, and the infrapatellar plica (ligamentum mucosum) (Fig. 3-23). The medial patellar plica extends along the medial wall of the knee joint from the level of the medial epicondyle to the level of the infrapatellar fat pad. A medial patellar plica is found in 9–50% of normal subjects on arthroscopy or autopsy. The suprapatellar plica lies in the transverse plane between the suprapatellar bursa and the remainder of the knee joint. This plica is present in approximately 20% of subjects and may range in size from a small fold to a nearly complete membrane with a central orifice (see Fig. 3-15). The infrapatellar plica is the most common of the knee joint plicae. This plica is a remnant of the embryologic septum that divided the medial and lateral knee joint compartments. The infrapatellar plica extends from the intercondylar notch to the infrapatellar fat pad and overlies the anterior cruciate ligament. One or more plicae are seen in 40–80% of patients during knee arthroscopy (5,107–112). A lateral patellar plica located along the lateral wall of the knee joint at the level of the patellofemoral joint has been described by a few authors; this is the least common type of plica (86,113).

Although the majority of synovial plicae are asymptomatic, symptoms may be produced by two mechanisms: repetitive trauma to the synovial fold and abnormal compartmentalization of the knee joint (109). The medial patellar plica may extend between the articular surfaces of the medial patellofemoral joint and may be traumatized during joint motion, producing synovitis, hemorrhage, and fibrosis in the plica, ultimately resulting in a markedly thickened fibrous plica. The interposed plica may result in secondary chondromalacia of the medial patellofemoral joint surfaces (86). This pathophysiology produces the "plica syndrome," a clinical syndrome characterized by joint clicking, locking, and anteromedial knee pain (113). The plica syndrome may be difficult to differentiate clinically from more common abnormal-

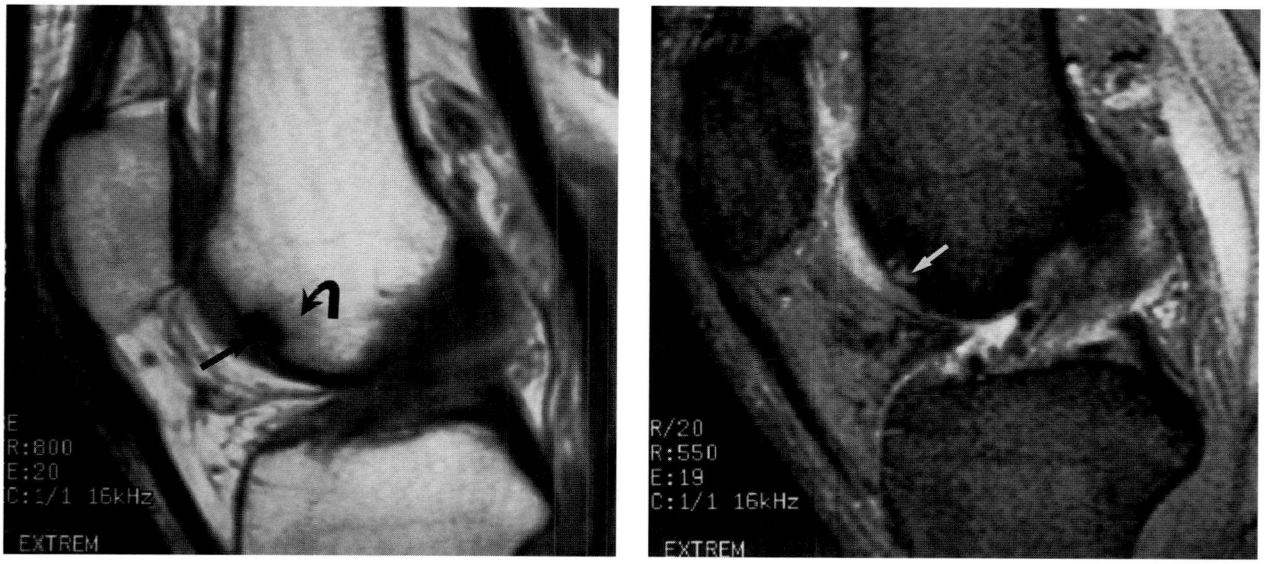

A B

FIG. 3-21. Osteochondritis dissecans of medial femoral condyle. A sagittal T1-weighted image **(A)** shows a focal region of diminished signal in the subchondral bone *(arrow)*, surrounded by bone marrow edema *(curved arrow)*. A T2*-weighted image **(B)** shows a small focus of increased signal within the bone defect, representing edema and granulation tissue within the area of bone necrosis *(arrow)*. The overlying cartilage is intact.

ities such as meniscal tears, patellofemoral instability, loose intra-articular bodies, and chondromalacia patellae. In patients in whom other symptomatic lesions have been excluded, the "plica syndrome" is initially treated with rest, physiotherapy, and anti-inflammatory medications. Arthroscopic resection of the plica is curative in most cases that fail to respond to conservative measures (109,112).

A complete or nearly complete suprapatellar plica may produce symptoms secondary to abnormal compartmentalization of the knee joint (see Fig. 3-15). Joint fluid, synovitis, hemorrhage, or loose bodies may become trapped in the isolated suprapatellar bursa, resulting in painful swelling that interferes with knee flexion (5,109). Rarely, the infrapatellar plica (ligamentum mucosum) may cause complete separa-

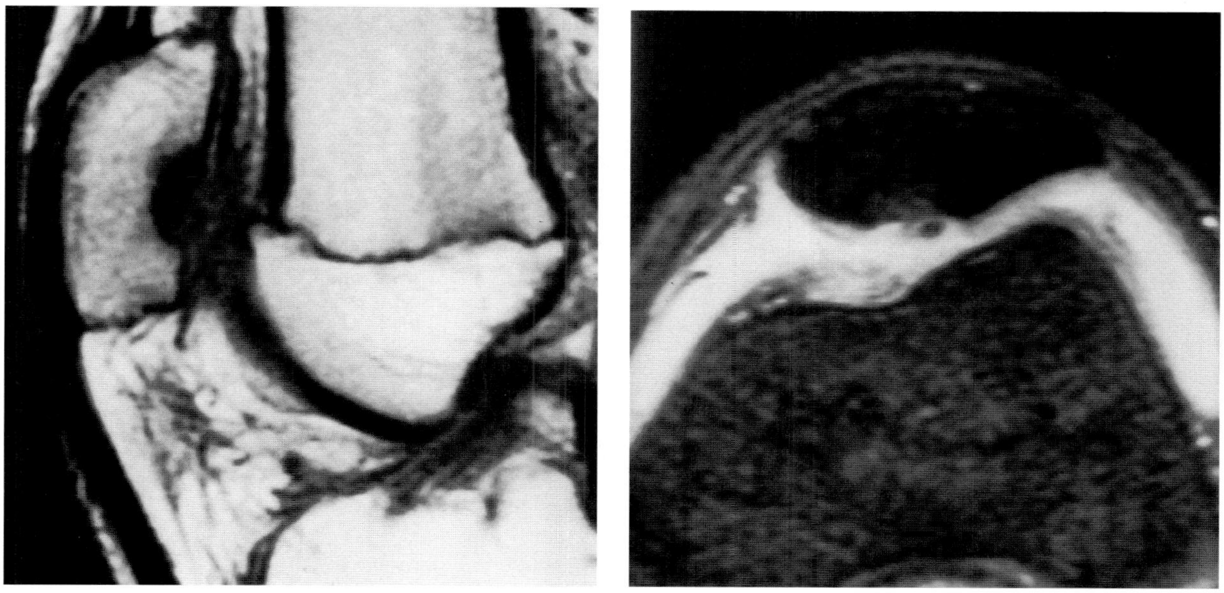

A B

FIG. 3-22. Unstable osteochondritis dissecans of the patella. A sagittal T1-weighted image **(A)** shows focal sclerosis of the patella with irregularity of the overlying cartilage. An axial T2*-weighted image **(B)** shows high signal intensity fluid surrounding an osteochondral fragment. This finding indicates instability of the fragment.

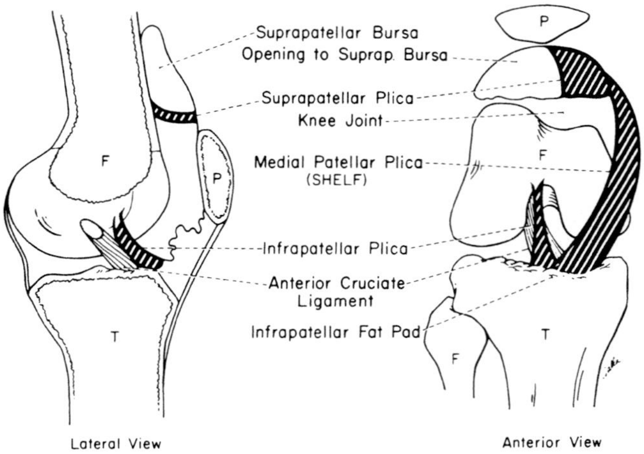

FIG. 3-23. Knee plicae. Diagrammatic representation of the various knee plicae. (From *American Journal of Sports Medicine* 1978;6:218. With permission. Copyright 1978, American Orthopedic Society for Sports Medicine.)

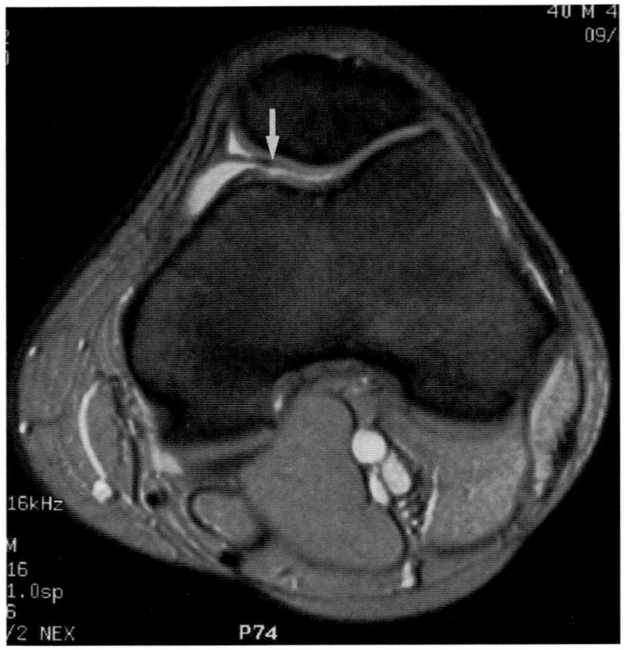

FIG. 3-24. Abnormal medial patellar plica. An axial T2*-weighted image shows a medial patellar plica *(arrow)* interposed between the articular surfaces of the medial patellofemoral joint. A small focus of cartilage thinning is present in the medial trochlear surface.

tion of the knee joint into medial and lateral compartments. This abnormality is usually asymptomatic but causes difficulty in knee arthroscopy or arthrography (113).

Normal plicae appear on MRI images as folds of tissue arising from the wall of the knee joint. Plicae are best seen on T2-weighted images in the presence of joint fluid; the high-signal-intensity fluid will outline the low-signal-intensity plica. Normal plicae are difficult to visualize in the absence of a joint distension, because the synovial fold will be apposed to the joint wall. A normal, asymptomatic medial patellar plica is thin (<5 mm thick) and not interposed into the patellofemoral articulation. Medial patellar plicae that are thickened (>5 mm thick) or interposed in the patellofemoral joint are likely to be symptomatic (Fig. 3-24) (86,106). Suprapatellar and infrapatellar plicae are very unlikely to be symptomatic unless the plica causes complete or near complete compartmentalization of the knee joint. Arthrography (5,107), CT arthrography (86), and sonography are also useful in evaluating synovial plicae (Fig. 3-25).

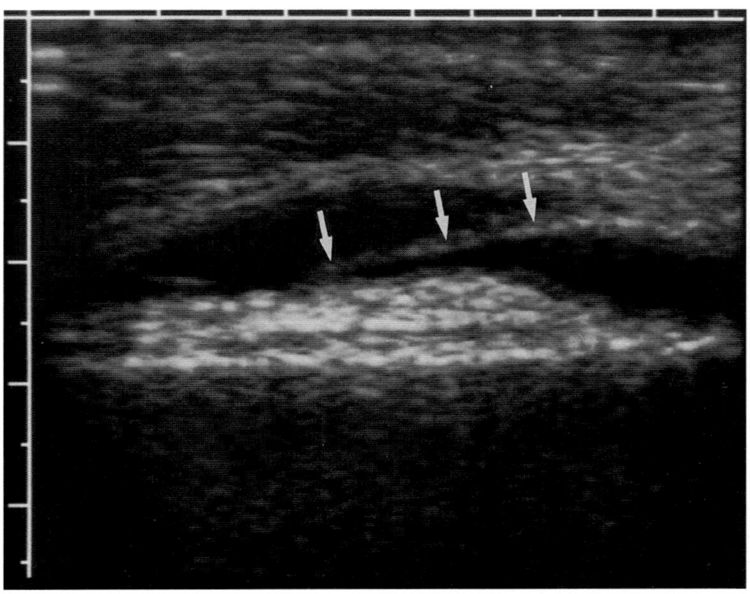

FIG. 3-25. Sonographic demonstration of suprapatellar plica. A longitudinal image through the suprapatellar region shows a normal suprapatellar plica *(arrows)* traversing the fluid-filled suprapatellar recess.

SUMMARY

Routine knee MRI examination provides excellent depiction of the normal and abnormal knee extensor mechanism and patellofemoral joint, and in most cases, a specific accurate diagnosis can be made. Additional imaging techniques such as kinematic MRI, pulse sequences designed to display cartilage, and MRI arthrography have expanded the role of MRI in assessing patellofemoral joint and extensor mechanism abnormalities.

REFERENCES

1. Hosea TM, Tria AJ Jr, Bechler JR. Embryology of the knee. In: Scott WN, ed. *Ligament and extensor mechanism injuries of the knee: diagnosis and treatment.* St Louis: Mosby Year Book, 1991;1–12.
2. Sledge CB. Some morphologic and experimental aspects of limb development. *Clin Orthop* 1966;44:241–248.
3. Walmsley R. The development of the patella. *J Anat* 1940;74: 360–370.
4. Gray DJ, Gardner E. Prenatal development of the human knee and superior tibiofibular joints. *Am J Anat* 1950;86:235–286.
5. Deutsch AL, Resnick D, Dalinka MK, et al. Synovial plicae of the knee. *Radiology* 1981;141:627–634.
6. Pansky B. *Review of medical embryology.* New York: Macmillan, 1982.
7. Moore KL. *The developing human: clinically oriented embryology,* 4th ed. Philadelphia: WB Saunders, 1988.
8. Reider B, Marshall JL, Koslin B, Ring B, Girgis FG. The anterior aspect of the knee joint: an anatomical study. *J Bone Joint Surg Am* 1981;63:351–356.
9. Hungerford DS, Barry M. Biomechanics of the patellofemoral joint. *Clin Orthop* 1979;144:9–15.
10. Carpenter JE, Kasman R, Matthews LS. Fractures of the patella. *J Bone Joint Surg* 1993;75A:1550–1561.
11. Kaufer H. Mechanical function of the patella. *J Bone Joint Surg Am* 1971;53:1551–1560.
12. Main WK, Scott WN. Knee anatomy. In: Scott WN, ed. *Ligament and extensor mechanism injuries of the knee: diagnosis and treatment.* St Louis: Mosby Year Book, 1991;13–32.
13. Goodfellow J, Hungerford DS, Woods C. Patellofemoral joint mechanics and pathology. II. Chondromalacia patellae. *J Bone Joint Surg Br* 1976;58:291–299.
14. Wiberg G. Roentgenographic and anatomic studies of the patellofemoral joint. *Acta Orthop Scand* 1941;12:319–410.
15. Insall J, Salvati E. Patella position in the normal knee joint. *Radiology* 1971;101:101–104.
16. Quinn SF, Brown TR, Demlow TA. MR imaging of patellar retinacular ligament injuries. *J Magn Reson Imaging* 1993;3:843–847.
17. Conaln T, Garth WP, Lemons JE. Evaluation of the medial soft tissue restraints of the extensor mechanism of the knee. *J Bone Joint Surg* 1993;75A:682–693.
18. Fulkerson JP, Gossling HR. Anatomy of the knee joint lateral retinaculum. *Clin Orthop* 1981;153:188–196.
19. Zeiss J, Saddemi SR, Ebraheim NA. MR imaging of the quadriceps tendon: normal layered configuration and its importance in cases of tendon rupture. *AJR* 1992;159:1031–1034.
20. McCauley TR, Kier R, Lynch KL, Jokl P. Chondromalacia patellae: diagnosis with MR imaging. *AJR* 1992;158:101–105.
21. Broderick LS, Turner DA, Renfrew DL, Schnitzer TJ, Huff JP, Harris C. Severity of articular cartilage abnormalities in patients with osteoarthritis: evaluation with fast spin-echo MR vs arthroscopy. *AJR* 1994; 162:99–103.
22. Recht MP, Kramer J, Marcelis S, et al. Abnormalities of articular cartilage in the knee: analysis of available MR techniques. *Radiology* 1993;187:473–478.
23. Modl JM, Sether LA, Haughton VM, Kneeland JB. Articular cartilage: correlation of histologic zones with signal intensity at MR imaging. *Radiology* 1991;181:853–855.
24. Shellock FJ, Mink JH, Deutsch AL, Fox JM. Patellar tracking abnormalities: clinical experience with kinematic imaging in 130 patients. *Radiology* 1989;172:799–804.
25. Conway WF, Hayes CW, Loughran T, et al. Cross-sectional imaging of the patellofemoral joint and surrounding structures. *Radiographics* 1991;11:195–217.
26. Shellock FJ, Mink JH, Deutsch AL, Foo TK, Sullenberger P. Patellofemoral joint: identification of abnormalities with active-movement, "unloaded" versus "loaded" kinematic MR imaging techniques. *Radiology* 1993;188:575–578.
27. Brossmann J, Muhle C, Schroder C, et al. Patellar tracking patterns during active and passive knee extension: evaluation with motion-triggered cine MR imaging. *Radiology* 1993;187:205–212.
28. Ramsey RH, Muller GE. Quadriceps tendon rupture: a diagnostic trap. *Clin Orthop* 1970;70:161–164.
29. Siwek CW, Rao JP. Ruptures of the extensor mechanism of the knee joint. *J Bone Joint Surg Am* 1981;63:932–937.
30. Kricun R, Kricun M, Arangio GA, Salzman GS, Berman AT. Patellar tendon rupture with underlying systemic disease. *AJR* 1980;135: 803–807.
31. Nance EP Jr, Kaye JJ. Injuries of the quadriceps mechanism. *Radiology* 1982;142 301–307.
32. Sherlock DA, Hughes A. Bilateral spontaneous concurrent rupture of the patellar tendon in the absence of associated local or systemic disease. *Clin Orthop* 1988;237:179–183.
33. Keogh P, Shanker SJ, Burke T, O'Connell RJ. Bilateral simultaneous rupture of the quadriceps tendons. *Clin Orthop* 1987;234:139–141.
34. Grogan DP, Carey TP, Leffers D, Ogden JA. Avulsion fractures of the patella. *J Ped Orthop* 1990;10:721–730.
35. Bianchi S, Zwass A, Abdelwahhab IF, Banderali A. Diagnosis of tears of the quadriceps tendon of the knee: value of sonography. *AJR* 1994; 162:1137–1140.
36. Fleckenstein JL, Weatherall PT, Parkey RW, Payne JA, Peshock RM. Sports-related muscle injuries: evaluation with MR imaging. *Radiology* 1989;172 793–798.
37. DeSmet AA. Magnetic resonance findings in skeletal muscle tears. *Skeletal Radiol* 1993;22:479–484.
38. Dooms GC, Fisher MR, Hricak H, Higgins CB. MR imaging of intramuscular hemorrhage. *J Comput Assist Tomgr* 1985;1985:908–911.
39. Newberg A, Wales L. Radiographic diagnosis of quadriceps tendon ruptures. *Radiology* 1977;1977:367–371.
40. Kuivila TE, Brems JJ. Diagnosis of acute rupture of the quadriceps tendon by magnetic resonance imaging. *Clin Orthop* 1991;262: 237–241.
41. Berlin RC, Levinsohn EM, Chrisman H. The wrinkled patellar tendon: an indicator of abnormality in the extensor mechanism of the knee. *Skeletal Radiol* 1991;20:181–185.
42. Splain SH, Ferenz C. Bilateral simultaneous infrapatellar tendon ruptures: support for Davidson's theory. *Orthop Review* 1988;17: 802–805.
43. Kalebo P, Sward L, Karlsson J, Peterson L. Ultrasonography in the detection of partial patellar ligament ruptures (jumper's knee). *Skeletal Radiol* 1991;20:285–289.
44. King JB, Perry DJ, Mourad K, Kumar SJ. Lesions of the patellar ligament. *J Bone Joint Surg Br* 1990;72:46–48.
45. El-Khoury GY, Wira RL, Berbaum KS, Pope TL Jr, Monu JUV. MR imaging of patellar tendinitis. *Radiology* 1992;184:849–854.
46. Erickson SJ, Prost RW, Timins ME. The "magic angle" effect: background physics and clinical relevance. *Radiology* 1993;188:23–25.
47. Erickson SJ, Cox IH, Hyde JS, Carrera GF, Strandt JA, Estkowski LD. Effect of tendon orientation on MR imaging signal intensity: a manifestation of the "magic angle" phenomenon. *Radiology* 1991; 181:389–392.
48. Insall J, Goldberg V, Salvati E. Recurrent dislocation and the high riding patella. *Clin Orthop* 1972;88:67–69.
49. Kannus PA. Long patellar tendon: radiographic sign of patellofemoral pain syndrome—a prospective study. *Radiology* 1992;185:859–863.
50. Rosenberg ZS, Kawelblum M, Cheung YY, Beltran J, Lehman WB, Grant AD. Osgood-Schlatter lesion: fracture or tendonitis? Scintigraphic, CT, and MR imaging features. *Radiology* 1992;185:853–858.
51. Stanitski CL. Anterior knee pain syndromes in the adolescent. *J Bone Joint Surg Am* 1993;75:1407–1416.
52. Hartzman S, Reicher MA, Bassett LW, Duckwiler GR. MR imaging of the knee, Part II: chronic disorders. *Radiology* 1987;162:553–557.
53. Scotti DM, Sadhu VK, Heimberg F, O'Hara AE. Osgood-Schlatter's disease, an emphasis on soft tissue changes in roentgen diagnosis. *Skeletal Radiol* 1979;4:21–25.

54. Hogh J, Lund B. The sequelae of Osgood-Schlatter disease in adults. *Internat Orthop* 1988;12:213–215.
55. Medlar RC, Lyne ED. Sinding-Larsen-Johansson disease: its etiology and natural history. *J Bone Joint Surg Am* 1978;60:1113–1116.
56. Boland AL Jr. Soft tissue injuries of the knee. In: Nicholas JA, ed. The lower extremity and spine in sports medicine. St Louis: CV Mosby, 1986;983–1012.
57. Bellon EM, Sacco DC, Steiger DA, Coleman PE. Magnetic resonance imaging in "housemaid's knee" (prepatellar bursitis). *Magn Reson Imaging* 1987;5:175–177.
58. Janzen DL, Peterfy CG, Forbes JR, Tirman PFJ, Genant HK. Cystic lesions around the knee joint: MR imaging findings. *AJR* 1994;163:155–161.
59. Sperner G, Benedetto KP, Glotzer W. The value of arthroscopy following traumatic patellar dislocation. *Sportverletz Sportschaden* 1988;2:20–24.
60. Neubert M, Steinbruk K. Patellar dislocation in athletes: arthroscopic diagnosis and therapy. *Unfallchirurgie* 1991;94:73–76.
61. Lance E, Deutsch AL, Mink JH. Prior lateral patellar dislocation: MR imaging findings. *Radiology* 1993;189:905–907.
62. Virolainen H, Visuri T, Kuusela T. Acute dislocation of the patella: MR findings. *Radiology* 1993;189:243–246.
63. Kirsch MD, Fitzgerald SW, Friedman H, Rogers LF. Transient lateral patellar dislocation: diagnosis with MR imaging. *AJR* 1993;161:109–113.
64. Hughston J, Deese M. Medial subluxation of the patella as a complication of lateral retinacular release. *Am J Sports Med* 1988;16:383–388.
65. Miller PR, Klein RM, Teitge RA. Medial dislocation of the patella. *Skeletal Radiol* 1991;20:429–431.
66. Kapelov SR, Teresi LM, Bradley WG, et al. Bone contusions of the knee: increased lesion detection with fast spin-echo MR imaging with spectroscopic fat saturation. *Radiology* 1993;189:901–904.
67. Mirowitz SA, Apicella P, Reinus WR, Hammerman AM. MR imaging of bone marrow lesions: relative conspicuousness on T1-weighted, fat-suppressed T2-weighted, and STIR images. *AJR* 1994;162:215–221.
68. Mirowitz SA. Fast scanning and fat-suppression MR imaging of musculoskeletal disorders. *AJR* 1993;161:1147–1157.
69. Rosenberg A, Mikosz RP. Knee biomechanics. In: Scott WN, ed. *Ligament and extensor mechanism injuries of the knee.* St Louis: Mosby Year Book, 1991;33–58.
70. Insall J. Current concepts review: patellar pain. *J Bone Joint Surg Am* 1982;64:147–151.
71. Schutzer SF, Ramsby GR, Fulkerson JP. Computed tomographic classification of patellofemoral pain patients. *Orthop Clin North Am* 1986;17:235–248.
72. Fulkerson JP, Tennant R, Jaivin JS, et al. Histologic evidence of retinacular nerve injury associated with patellofemoral malalignment. *Clin Orthop* 1985;197:196–205.
73. Dowd GSE, Bentley G. Radiographic assessment in patellar instability and chondromalacia patellae. *J Bone Joint Surg* 1986;68B:297–300.
74. Kujala U, Osterman K, Kormano M, Komu M, Chlenzka D. Patellar motion analyzed by magnetic resonance imaging. *Acta Orthop Scand* 1989;60:13–16.
75. Koskinen SK, Hurme M, Kujala U, Kormano M. Effect of lateral release on patellar motion in chondromalacia. *Acta Orthop Scand* 1990;61:311–312.
76. Carson WG, James SL, Larson RL, Singer KM, Winternitz WW. Patellofemoral disorders: physical and radiographic evaluation. Part 2: radiographic evaluation. *Clin Orthop* 1984;185:178–186.
77. Malghem J, Baudouin M. Depth insufficiency of the proximal trochlear groove on lateral radiographs of the knee: relation to patellar dislocation. *Radiology* 1989;170:507–510.
78. Aglietti P, Insall J, Cerulli G. Patellar pain and incongruence. I: measurements of incongruence. *Clin Orthop* 1983;176:217–224.
79. Koskinen SK, Taimela S, Nelimarkka O, Markku K, Kujala UM. Magnetic resonance imaging of patellofemoral relationships. *Skeletal Radiol* 1993;22:403–410.
80. Brattstrom H. Patella alta in non-dislocating knees. *Acta Orthop Scand* 1970;41:578–588.
81. Delgado-Martins H. A study of the position of the patella using computerized tomography. *J Bone Joint Surg Br* 1979;61:443–444.
82. Brossmann J, Muhle C, Bull CC, et al. Evaluation of patellar tracking in patients with suspected patellar malalignment: cine MR imaging vs arthroscopy. *AJR* 1994;162:361–367.
83. Fulkerson JP, Schutzer SF, Ramsby G, et al. Computerized tomography of the patellofemoral joint before and after lateral release or realignment. *Arthroscopy* 1987;3:19–24.
84. Johnson RP. Lateral facet syndrome of the patella: lateral restraint analysis and use of lateral resection. *Clin Orthop* 1986;238:148–157.
85. Hayes CW, Sawyer RW, Conway WF. Patellar cartilage lesions: in vitro detection and staging with MR imaging and pathological correlation. *Radiology* 1990;176:479–483.
86. Hodge JC, Ghelman B, O'Brien SJ, Wickiewicz TL. Synovial plicae and chondromalacia patellae: correlation of results of CT arthrography with results of arthroscopy. *Radiology* 1993;186:827–831.
87. Bentley G. Articular changes in chondromalacia patellae. *J Bone Joint Surg Br* 1985;67:769–774.
88. Christensen F, Soballe K, Snerum L. Treatment of chondromalacia patellae by lateral retinacular release of the patella. *Clin Orthop* 1988;234:145–147.
89. Bentley G. Chondromalacia patellae. *J Bone Joint Surg Am* 1970;52:221–232.
90. Insall J, Falvo KA, Wise DW. Chondromalacia patellae: a prospective study. *J Bone Joint Surg Am* 1976;58:1–8.
91. Boven F, Bellemans M, Gverts J, De Boeck H, Potvliege R. The value of computed tomography in chondromalacia patellae. *Skeletal Radiol* 1982;8:183–185.
92. Horns JW. Single contrast knee arthrography in abnormalities of the articular cartilage. *Radiology* 1972;105:537–540.
93. Angell FL. Fluoroscopic technique of double contrast arthrography of the knee. *Radiol Clin North Am* 1971;9:85–98.
94. Staple TW. Extrameniscal lesions demonstrated by double-contrast arthrography of the knee. *Radiology* 1972;102:311–319.
95. Shahriaree H. Chondromalacia. *Contemp Orthop* 1985;11:27–39.
96. Yulish BS, Montanez J, Goodfellow DB, Bryan PJ, Mulopulos GP, Modic MT. Chondromalacia patellae: assessment with MR imaging. *Radiology* 1987;164:763–766.
97. Hodler J, Resnick D. Chondromalacia patellae. *AJR* 1992;158:106–107.
98. Thompson RC, Vener Mj, Griffiths Hj, Lewis JL, Oegama TR, Wallace L. Scanning electron microscopy and MRI of injuries to the patellofemoral joint after acute transarticular loading. *J Bone Joint Surg* 1993;75A:704–713.
99. Ho C, Cervilla V, Kjellin I, Haghighi P, Amiel D, Resnick D. MRI in assessing cartilage changes in experimental osteoarthritis of the knee. *Invest Radiol* 1992;27:84–90.
100. Gilley JS, Gelman SI, Edson M, Metcalf RW. Chondral fractures of the knee. *Radiology* 1981;138:51–54.
101. Hughston JC, Hergenroeder PT, Courtenay BG. Osteochondritis dissecans of the femoral condyles. *J Bone Joint Surg Am* 1984;66:1340–1348.
102. Cahill,B. Treatment of juvenile osteochondritis dissecans and osteochondritis dissecans of the knee. *Clin Sports Med* 1985;4:367–384.
103. Ghelman B, Shcraft S. Arthrography of the knee. In: Scott WN, ed. *Ligament and extensor mechanism injuries of the knee.* St Louis: Mosby Year Book, 1991;101–120.
104. Ewing JW, Voto SJ. Arthroscopic surgical management of osteochondritis dissecans of the knee. *Arthroscopy* 1988;4:37–40.
105. Thomson NL. Osteochondritis dissecans and osteochondral fragments managed by Herbert compression screw fixation. *Clin Orthop* 1987;224:71–78.
106. De Smet AA, Fisher DR, Graf BK, Lange RH. Osteochondritis dissecans of the knee: value of MR imaging in determining lesion stability and the presence of articular cartilage defects. *AJR* 1990;549–553.
107. Lupi L, Bighi S, Cerve PM, Limone GL, Massari I. Arthrography of the plica syndrome and its significance. *Eur J Radiol* 1990;11:15–18.
108. Patel D. Arthroscopy of the plicae-synovial folds and their significance. *Am J Sports Med* 1978;6:217–225.
109. Tindel NL, Nisonson B. The plica syndrome. *Orthop Clin North Am* 1992;23:613–618.
110. Broom MJ, Fulkerson JP. The plica syndrome: a new perspective. *Orthop Clin North Am* 1986;17:279–281.
111. Apple JS, Martinez S, Hardaker WT, Daffner RH, Gehweiler JA. Synovial plica of the knee. *Skeletal Radiol* 1982;7:251–254.
112. Johnson DP, Eastwood DM, Witherow PJ. Symptomatic synovial plicae of the knee. *J Bone Joint Surg Am* 1993;75:1485–1496.
113. Patel D. Plica as a cause of anterior knee pain. *Orthop Clin North Am* 1986;17:273–277.

MRI of the Knee, Second Edition,
edited by P. L. Munk and C. A. Helms.
Lippincott-Raven Publishers, Philadelphia © 1996.

CHAPTER 4

The Menisci

Peter L. Munk, Clyde A. Helms, Dennis L. Janzen, and A. Dale Vellet

Injuries of the menisci are commonly encountered lesions in orthopedic practice, most frequently seen in men younger than 40 years. The true importance of the meniscus in the functioning of the knee was not appreciated for many years; however, investigations over the past several decades have changed this view. It was once thought that the meniscus could be removed with impunity. Now the attitude in orthopedic circles has changed to the point where meniscus-sparing treatments are employed whenever possible. With this change in the treatment of meniscal abnormalities, an increasingly important role for imaging in the diagnosis and evaluation of meniscal lesions has emerged. Traditionally, arthrography has been the main imaging technique for examining the meniscus. Diagnostic arthroscopy is also widely used and has been generally accepted as the gold standard against which all other methods should be compared. Magnetic resonance imaging, a new noninvasive technique, has now proved to be highly accurate in evaluating the meniscus (1–15).

ANATOMY, EMBRYOLOGY, AND FUNCTION

In human embryos the limb buds appear at approximately 28 days of gestation, and by 38 days, mesenchymal condensations are present. These condensations are the precursors of the tibia and femur. An unchondrified mesenchymal blastoma is present between these bone precursors. It becomes thinned to form a disc, which is usually referred to as the interzone. Adjacent mesenchyme invades this interzone to give rise to the vascular synovial mesenchyme. The menisci are derived from this substance. The menisci are identifiable by 8 weeks of gestation, when they already have their characteristic semilunar configuration. This configuration occurs even before the knee joint cavity has formed (approximately 14 weeks). The menisci at this time are well vascularized, and as gestation progresses, more collagen is laid down and the degree of vascularity slowly diminishes (16–21).

The menisci consist of two semilunar-shaped fibrocartilaginous structures that rest in the surface of the tibial plateau (Fig. 4-1; see also color plate 5). Each meniscus covers approximately the peripheral two-thirds of the corresponding articular surface of the tibia. The peripheral border of each meniscus is a thick structure with a convex margin attached to the capsule of the knee joint. The inner border tapers to a thin free edge. In cross section the semilunar cartilages have an approximately triangular contour. The proximal surface of the meniscus is concave and in contact with the femoral condyles. The distal surface is flat and rests on the tibial plateau (22).

The medial meniscus has the larger radius of the two menisci, and its posterior horn is significantly wider than its anterior horn. The medial meniscus has firm attachments in the region of the posterior intercondylar fossa of the tibia and to the medial collateral ligament. Its anterior attachment is considerably more variable. It is usually firmly attached to the anterior intercondylar fossa, but at times its attachment may be loose. Its tibial attachment is sometimes referred to as the coronary ligament or meniscotibial ligament. Its fibers are difficult to separate from the underlying capsular fibers and collateral ligament fibers. The coronary ligament attaches to the margin of the tibia several millimeters distal to the articular surface and may give rise to a small synovial recess in this area (Fig. 4-2). Posteriorly and medially the meniscus receives part of the insertion of the semimembranosus muscle.

P. L. Munk: Department of Diagnostic Imaging, British Columbia Cancer Agency, and Department of Radiology, University of British Columbia, Vancouver, British Columbia, Canada V5Z 4E6.

C. A. Helms: Department of Radiology, Duke University Medical Center, Durham, North Carolina 27710.

D. L. Janzen: Department of Radiology, Vancouver Hospital and Health Sciences Center, Vancouver, British Columbia, Canada V5Z 1M9.

A. D. Vellet: Department of Diagnostic Imaging, University of Calgary, Foothills Hospital, Alberta, Canada T2N 2T9.

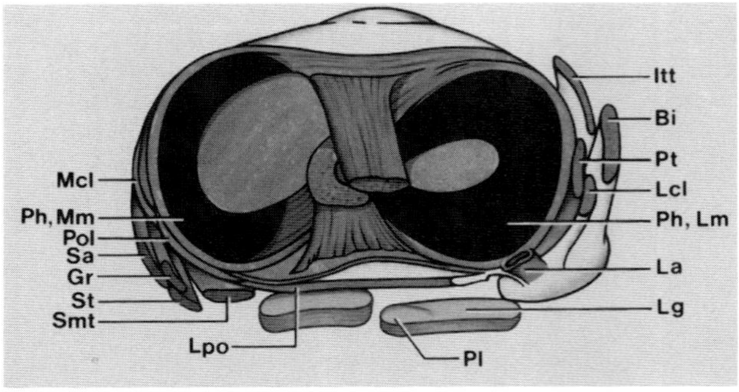

FIG. 4-1. Schematic diagram of the menisci. Mcl, medial collateral ligament; Ph, Mm, posterior horn medial meniscus; Pol, popliteal oblique ligament; Sa, sartorius; Gr, gracilis; St, semitendinosus; Smt, semimembranosus; Lpo, posterior oblique ligament; Pl, popliteus ligament; Lg, lateral head gastrocnemius; La, arcuate ligament; Ph, Lm, posterior horn lateral meniscus; Lcl, lateral collateral ligament; Pt, popliteus tendon; Bi, biceps femoris; Itt, iliotibial tract.

The lateral meniscus is more circular and has a smaller radius than the medial meniscus. It covers a larger portion of the articular surface of the tibia than its partner. The anterior horn of the meniscus is also attached to the intercondylar fossa, just laterally and posteriorly to the anterior cruciate ligament. The posterior horn is attached to the intercondylar fossa immediately anterior to the posterior end of the medial meniscus. At its posterior horn a ligament is present that stretches from the meniscus to the medial condyle of the femur, running immediately posterior to the posterior cruciate ligament. This is known as the ligament of Wrisberg, sometimes also referred to as the accessory posterior cruciate bundle. A more inconstant ligament, the ligament of Humphry, runs in a similar direction but immediately anterior to the posterior cruciate ligament. Together these are called the meniscofemoral ligaments (Fig. 4-3). Their size varies considerably. The ligament of Humphry may measure up to one-third of the diameter of the adjacent posterior cruciate ligament; the ligament of Wrisberg may measure as much as one-half of that diameter. One or both may be absent. The role of the meniscofemoral ligaments is unclear, but they may balance the action of the popliteus muscle by drawing the lateral meniscus medially and anteriorly in knee flexion. Only in about 3–20% of knees examined in autopsy specimens are both ligaments present in the same joint. There is a groove at the posterolateral aspect of the lateral meniscus that actually extends through the substance of the meniscus and accommodates the bursa and tendon of the popliteus muscle. This groove or tunnel through the meniscus runs from the posteroinferior aspect of the meniscus in a superior and anterior direction (Fig. 4-4). The collateral ligaments have no firm attachment to the lateral meniscus (23–25).

The anterior horns of the menisci are attached to one another by the transverse ligament, sometimes known as the ligament of Winslow or transverse geniculate ligament. The transverse ligament lies behind Hoffa's fat pad and anterior to the joint capsule (Fig. 4-5). Its thickness is extremely variable, and it may be completely absent. Barkow's ligament is another ligamentous attachment between the menisci that connects the posterior horn of the lateral meniscus to the anterior horn of the medial meniscus. In addition, firm attachments exist between the anterior cruciate ligament and the medial meniscus. The interrelationship of the menisci with these various ligaments illustrates the interdependence

A

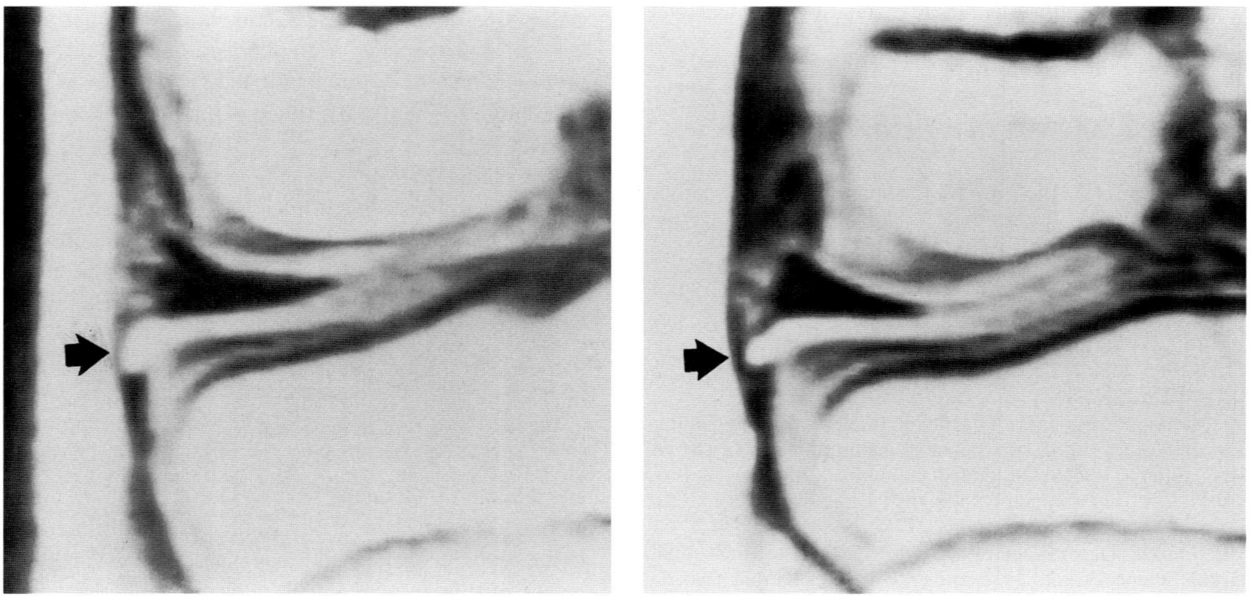

B

FIG. 4-2. Meniscotibial ligament. **A,B:** Coronal T1-weighted spin-echo (TR 400 msec, TE 20 msec) adjacent images show the thin ligament connecting the ligament with the proximal tibia *(arrows)*.

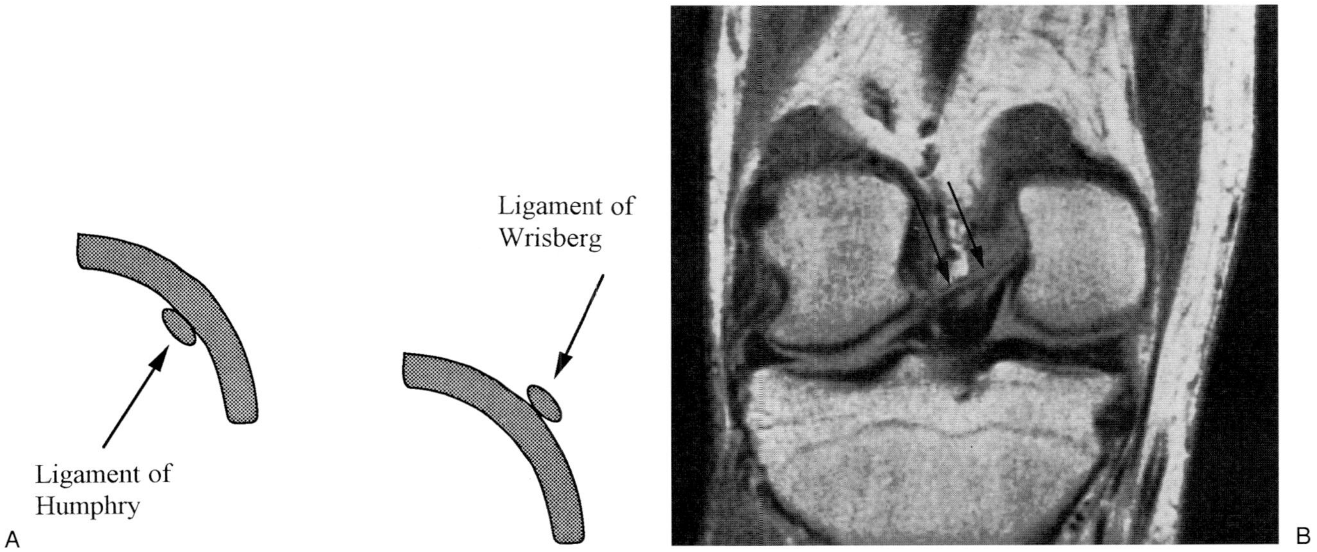

FIG. 4-3. Meniscofemoral ligaments. **A:** Diagrammatic representation of the position of the meniscofemoral ligaments relative to the posterior cruciate ligament as seen on sagittal images. **B:** Coronal T1-weighted spin-echo image (TR 400 msec, TE 20 msec) demonstrates the course of a meniscofemoral ligament *(arrows)* as it passes from the posterior horn of the lateral meniscus to the lateral aspect of the medial femoral condyle. (From Munk PL. *Canadian Association of Radiologists Journal* 1989; 40:263–303. With permission).

of these structures in regulating the complex movements of the knee joint (26).

The menisci have several important functions. Their contribution to the stability of the knee joint has until recent years been underestimated. The menisci function as spacers, deepening the knee joint and improving congruity between the tibia and the femoral condyles (27–32). This point is better appreciated when the anterior cruciate ligament is disrupted. When this occurs the anteroposterior stability of the knee is largely dependent on the menisci, particularly the medial meniscus. Because of this, performing meniscectomy in patients with untreated anterior cruciate ligament tears will create a grossly unstable joint (33). Removal of the menisci markedly increases rotary instability of the knee (34). The menisci also function as shock absorbers and load transmitters. When a load is placed on the knee joint, the menisci are elongated and are pushed outward. The fibers of the meniscus run in parallel bundles along the long axis, which allows them to resist these circumferential tensions better. Thus, the menisci help dissipate a vertical compressive load by converting a significant portion into circumferential stresses (35–38).

When a load is transmitted through the knee joint in full extension, the medial meniscus will take approximately 60% of the load transmitted through the medial side of the joint, and the lateral meniscus may take as much as 70% (28,39).

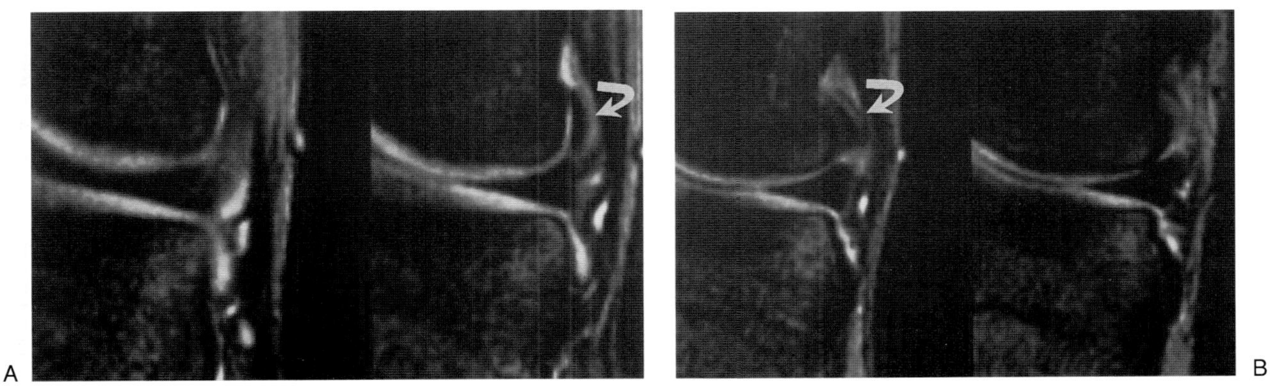

FIG. 4-4. Popliteus tendon. **A,B:** Series of coronal T2-weighted gradient-echo MPGR images (TR 400 msec, TE 16 msec, flip angle 20°) showing the popliteus tendon as it traverses the posterior aspect of the lateral meniscus *(arrows)*.

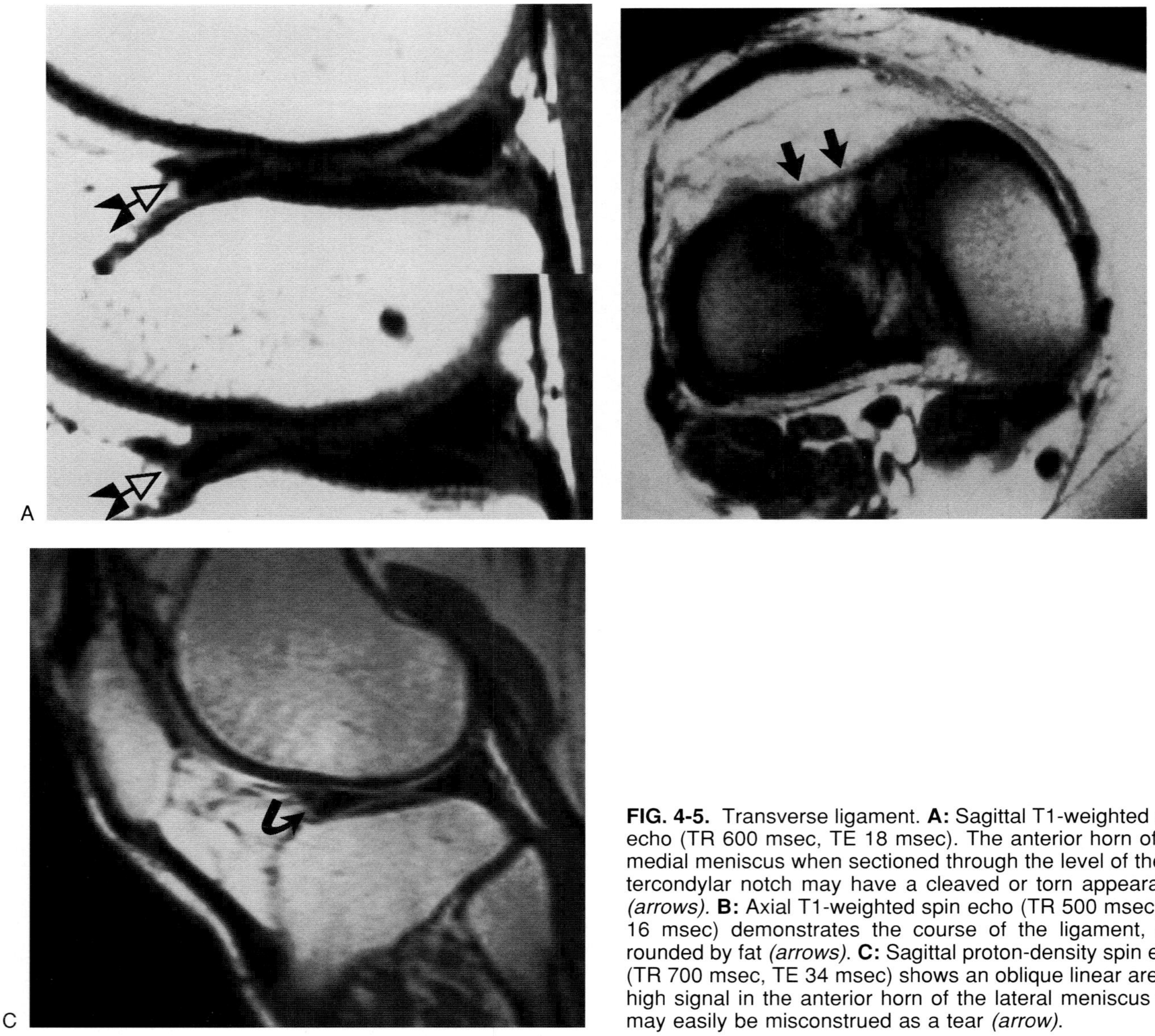

FIG. 4-5. Transverse ligament. **A:** Sagittal T1-weighted spin echo (TR 600 msec, TE 18 msec). The anterior horn of the medial meniscus when sectioned through the level of the intercondylar notch may have a cleaved or torn appearance *(arrows).* **B:** Axial T1-weighted spin echo (TR 500 msec, TE 16 msec) demonstrates the course of the ligament, surrounded by fat *(arrows).* **C:** Sagittal proton-density spin echo (TR 700 msec, TE 34 msec) shows an oblique linear area of high signal in the anterior horn of the lateral meniscus that may easily be misconstrued as a tear *(arrow).*

With meniscectomy the underlying articular cartilage is exposed to considerably more stresses, thereby accelerating degenerative changes (26,29,35,40–44). Compressive deformation of the articular cartilage and the subchondral bone following meniscectomy is approximately twice that seen in the normal joint. This deformation produces subchondral fracturing. Subsequent healing will produce increased subchondral bone density and decreased flexibility. The resultant decrease in the ability to attenuate applied forces allows these forces to be transmitted through the joint, causing articular cartilage destruction and further degenerative changes (45). The more extensive the removal of meniscus, the more rapidly degenerative changes are seen and the worse the long-term prognosis of the patient becomes (30). As might be expected, when the lateral meniscus is resected, the degenerative changes are more pronounced. If partial meniscectomy is done and meniscus regeneration occurs, the degenerative joint disease is considerably less severe. For reasons that are not entirely clear, these changes usually are more severe on the tibial side of the joint (43).

Other ancillary roles of the meniscus include prevention of impingement of the synovial membrane and increased efficacy of lubrication. It has been estimated that postmeniscectomy there is an approximately 20% increase in the coefficient of friction within the joint (29,46). Despite the many strong attachments of the menisci, they should not be thought of as static structures against which other things move. Knee motion is complex and requires simultaneous gliding, rolling, and rotary components. With maximum flexion the menisci undergo posterior displacement. Meniscal movement has been studied using cine-MRI in cadaveric knees, and mean meniscal motions of 5 mm medially and 11 mm lat-

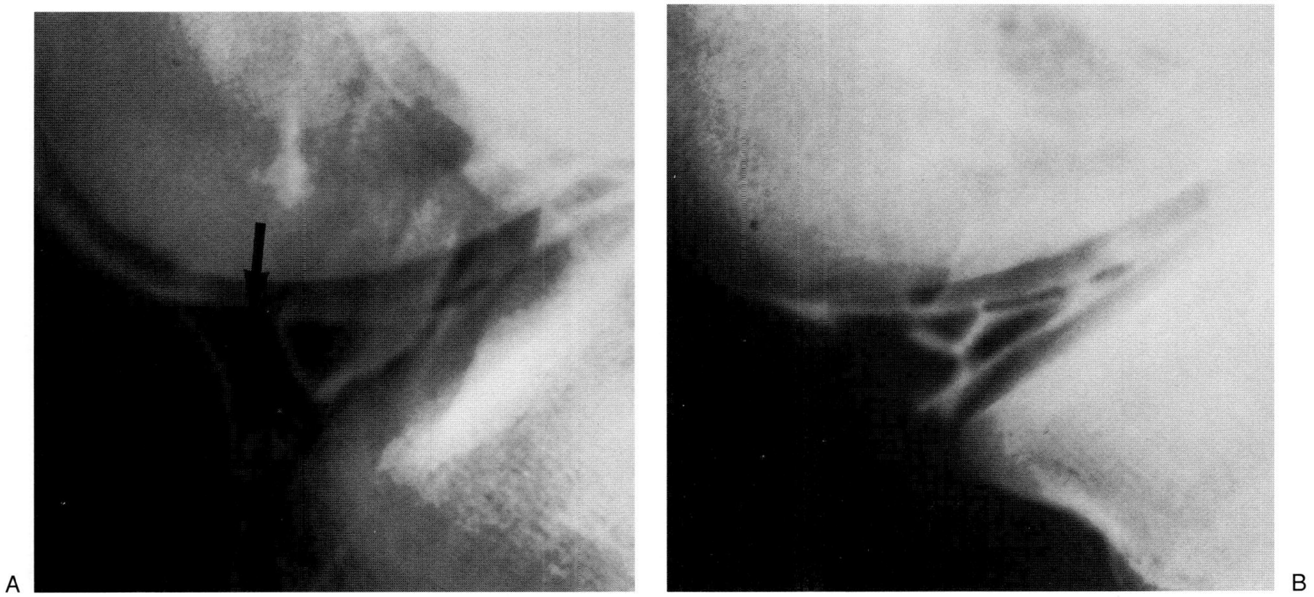

FIG. 4-6. Double-contrast knee arthrography. **A:** Torn and displaced posterior horn of the lateral meniscus. The *arrow* indicates gap in meniscus. **B:** Complex tear of the posterior horn of the medial meniscus.

erally have been demonstrated (47). This relatively lesser mobility of the medial meniscus is what accounts, in part, for the increased incidence of tears medially.

Because of the often ambiguous nature of clinical examination, a number of diagnostic techniques have been developed to evaluate the menisci for tears. Plain-film radiographic findings that reflect the presence of meniscal tears are unusual. Traditionally, arthrography has been widely used with the double-contrast technique, with both positive water-soluble contrast and air being the most favored (Fig. 4-6). Double-contrast arthrography is a demanding technique that requires considerable technical expertise and experience to achieve consistently reliable results (48–64). In experienced hands arthrography is approximately 95% accurate in the diagnosis of medial meniscal tears and 80% accurate in the diagnosis of lateral meniscal tears. Arthrography is a technique that to some degree depends on the operator. This may account for the wide range of reported accuracies, from 68% to in excess of 95%. The posterior horns have been an area of persistent difficulty, and tears of the lateral meniscus appear more difficult to diagnose than those of the medial meniscus. Arthrography appears to be the most accurate in the diagnosis of midbody and peripheral tears. Arthroscopy, on the other hand, is reputed to be more accurate in demonstrating anterior horn tears and tears involving the central edge of the meniscus. False-negative studies with arthrography have ranged from 2% to 13% compared with surgery (65). Besides the technical demands of this technique, arthrography has the disadvantage of entailing some discomfort and some risk (albeit minimal) because of contrast toxicity and possible inoculation of the joint with bacteria.

Diagnostic arthroscopy in the past 15 years has become increasingly prevalent, both as a diagnostic tool and as a treatment method in knee disorders. In skilled hands arthroscopy can be 95% accurate in the diagnosis of medial meniscal tears and 82% accurate in the diagnosis of lateral meniscal tears (49,59,66–69). These figures are highly variable because technical expertise varies markedly between different arthroscopists and is closely related both to experience and to the volume of examinations performed. The posterior horns of the menisci are often the sites of false-negative examinations. The undersurface of the menisci often require detailed probing to discover a small tear. To see the posterior horn of the medial meniscus adequately, it may be necessary for the surgeon to make an additional puncture of the knee joint so as to pass the arthroscope into an advantageous position for complete evaluation. Additional disadvantages of arthroscopy include its invasive nature, with its attendant low risks of infection, instrument breakage, thrombophlebitis, and vascular injury, as well as the attendant risks of regional or general anesthetic. Despite these drawbacks arthroscopy is highly accurate and must be considered the gold standard against which other methods are evaluated.

Computed tomography (CT) has also been used to evaluate meniscal lesions (Fig. 4-7). CT, however, has the disadvantage of being limited to the examination of the transaxial plane of the meniscus. This view does not advantageously demonstrate tears of the menisci. Although some investigators have reported good success with demonstration of meniscal abnormalities using CT, this technique has not found widespread favor and utilization. The examination may be performed with or without intra-articular contrast (52,70–75).

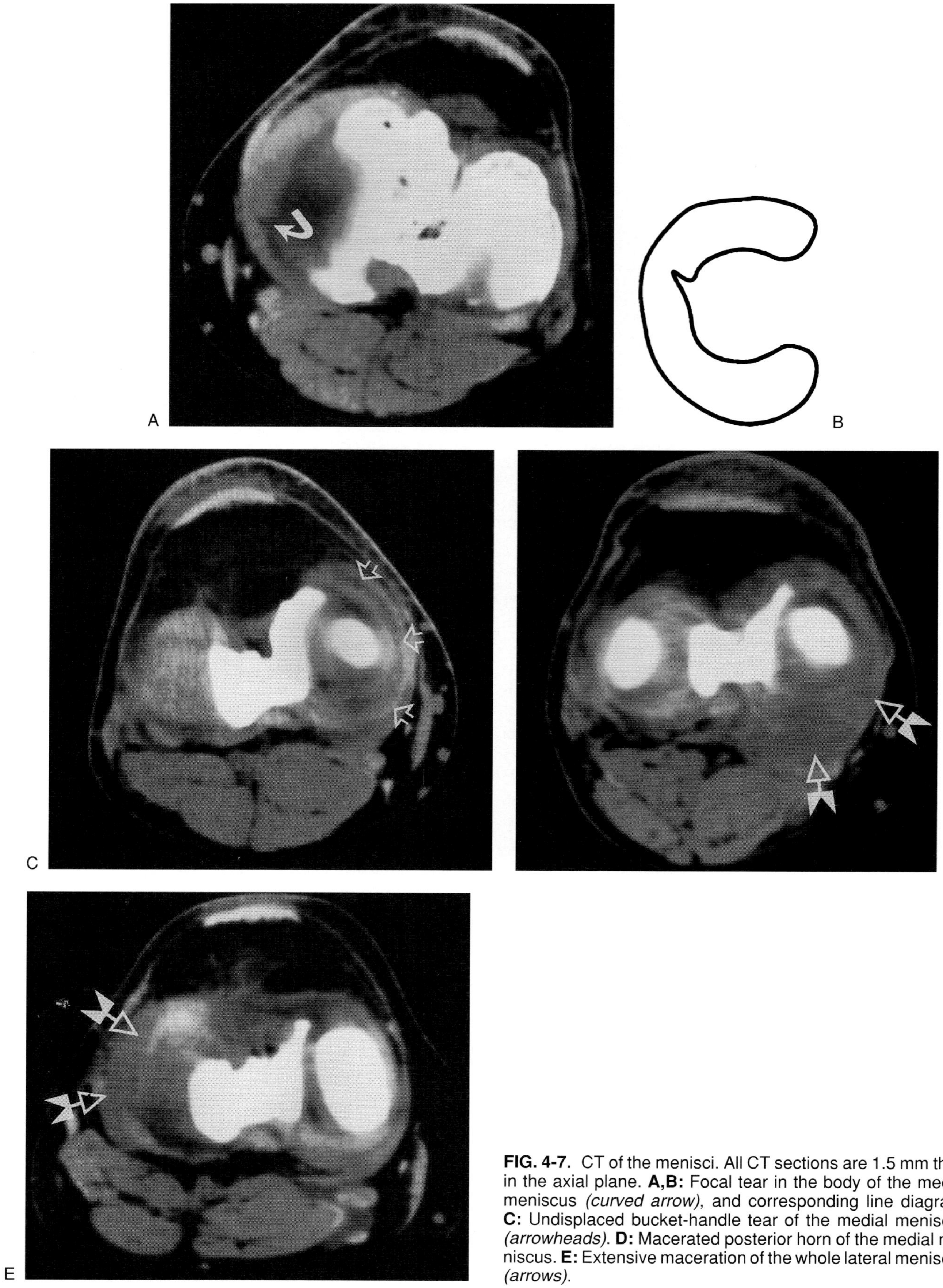

FIG. 4-7. CT of the menisci. All CT sections are 1.5 mm thick in the axial plane. **A,B:** Focal tear in the body of the medial meniscus *(curved arrow)*, and corresponding line diagram. **C:** Undisplaced bucket-handle tear of the medial meniscus *(arrowheads)*. **D:** Macerated posterior horn of the medial meniscus. **E:** Extensive maceration of the whole lateral meniscus *(arrows)*.

Ultrasound has been used with some success by a few investigators. Like CT, it has the advantage of not being invasive. Its use is highly operator dependent. At present, it is not widely used in the investigation of meniscal disorders. Intra-articular ultrasound with probes designed for endovascular work has been proposed for use during arthroscopy to aid in detection of difficult-to-find tears (76,77).

MRI APPEARANCE OF THE NORMAL MENISCUS AND MENISCAL DEGENERATION

Spin-echo imaging has been the most widely used sequence in the investigation of meniscal disorders. T1-weighted spin-echo sequences have been the most widely used because of their good spatial resolution with little noise, and relatively rapid acquisition time. In adults younger than 30 years the normal appearance of the meniscus is that of a uniformly dark structure with no evidence of any intrameniscal signal (Figs. 4-8A and 4-8B). In patients over the age of 30, even in asymptomatic patients with no evidence of meniscal tears, signal is often seen in the substance of the meniscus (78). It is normal to see high signal in the menisci of children. This is felt to be due to normal vascularity that diminishes with increasing age. The signal in this instance does not extend to the articulating surface of the meniscus (79–81). A grading system for intrameniscal signal consisting of three grades has been devised and is now widely used (Table 4-1) (82).

Grade 1 signal within the meniscus has a globular or ovoid configuration and does not communicate with the articulating surfaces of the meniscus (see Figs. 4-8C and 4-8D). With grade 2 signal the configuration is linear, but there is no evidence of communication with the surface (see Figs. 4-8E and 4-8F) (83). Grade 3 signal does communicate with the surface and may have a linear, globular, or complex configuration (see Figs. 4-8G and 4-8H). Grade 3 signal represents a meniscal tear; these patients are frequently symptomatic, unlike patients with grade 1 and grade 2 meniscal signals. The exact nature and significance of these areas of increased signal within the meniscus have been the subject of considerable interest and investigation over the past several years. If calcification is present (chondrocalcinosis of the meniscus), it may actually produce foci of increased signal, possibly because of scarring induced by the calcium deposits (84,85).

TABLE 4-1. *Meniscal signal*

Grade	Appearance on spin-echo images
0	No signal, uniformly dark
1	Globular or ovoid signal not communicating with meniscal articular surface
2	Linear signal not communicating with meniscal articular surface
3	Linear, complex, or diffuse signal communicating with meniscal articular surface

Grade 1 and 2 signal changes appear to remain relatively stable over short periods of time even in athletes. After strenuous exercise only minimal increases in signal are seen (no change in grade), this being especially rare among well-trained athletes (86,87).

Macroscopically, the normal meniscus is a supple structure with a semitranslucent white appearance on examination. With increasing age the meniscus becomes less supple and gradually changes color to a slightly yellowish appearance. The decreased suppleness and elasticity of the meniscus lead to an increased susceptibility to injury. This increased susceptibility may in part lead to the so-called degenerative changes often observed in the menisci of patients older than 30 years of age (88). The precise reason for these degenerative changes is somewhat speculative. However, it has been noted that the frictional forces of the superior and inferior surfaces of the meniscus differ, with the forces being greater on the tibial side. Because of this the central portion of the menisci, the middle perforating bundles, is subjected to shearing forces that may help promote these degenerative changes (89). The chronic trauma from asymmetric frictional forces may promote reactive secretion of mucopolysaccharides, resulting in abnormal accumulation of myxoid material in the substance of the meniscus. Microscopic examination of menisci with increased intrasubstance signal demonstrates numerous microscopic cysts and separation of collagen bundles as well as the presence of amorphous eosinophilic mucoid material. With time, increased collagenization and fragmentation of the collagen bundles occur and tears are found along collagen fibers.

Although not proven, the lesions noted in degenerating menisci probably represent a spectrum of stages, which may end in frank tears that communicate with the surface of the meniscus (90,91). Although grades 1 and 2 may stay stable for long periods, progression over time to grade 3 has been demonstrated (86,87,92–96). Interestingly, the prevalence of signal changes in the menisci does not greatly differ in those who are sedentary compared to well-trained athletes (97). Several investigators have also speculated that intrasubstance tears may exist that have the appearance of grade 2 lesions. This suggests that some patients with commonly asymptomatic grade 2 lesions may actually be symptomatic, because it is now known that the meniscus is innervated and that pain may be felt even though tears do not communicate with the articular surface of the meniscus (92).

With increasing use of higher-strength magnetic fields in the investigation of knee disorders, it is becoming apparent that an increasingly smaller proportion of menisci are totally free of signal. In addition, gradient-echo techniques and 3-D Fourier transform methods make it apparent that few, if any, menisci are entirely free of signal (Fig. 4-9). The precise significance of these findings is at present not entirely clear (90).

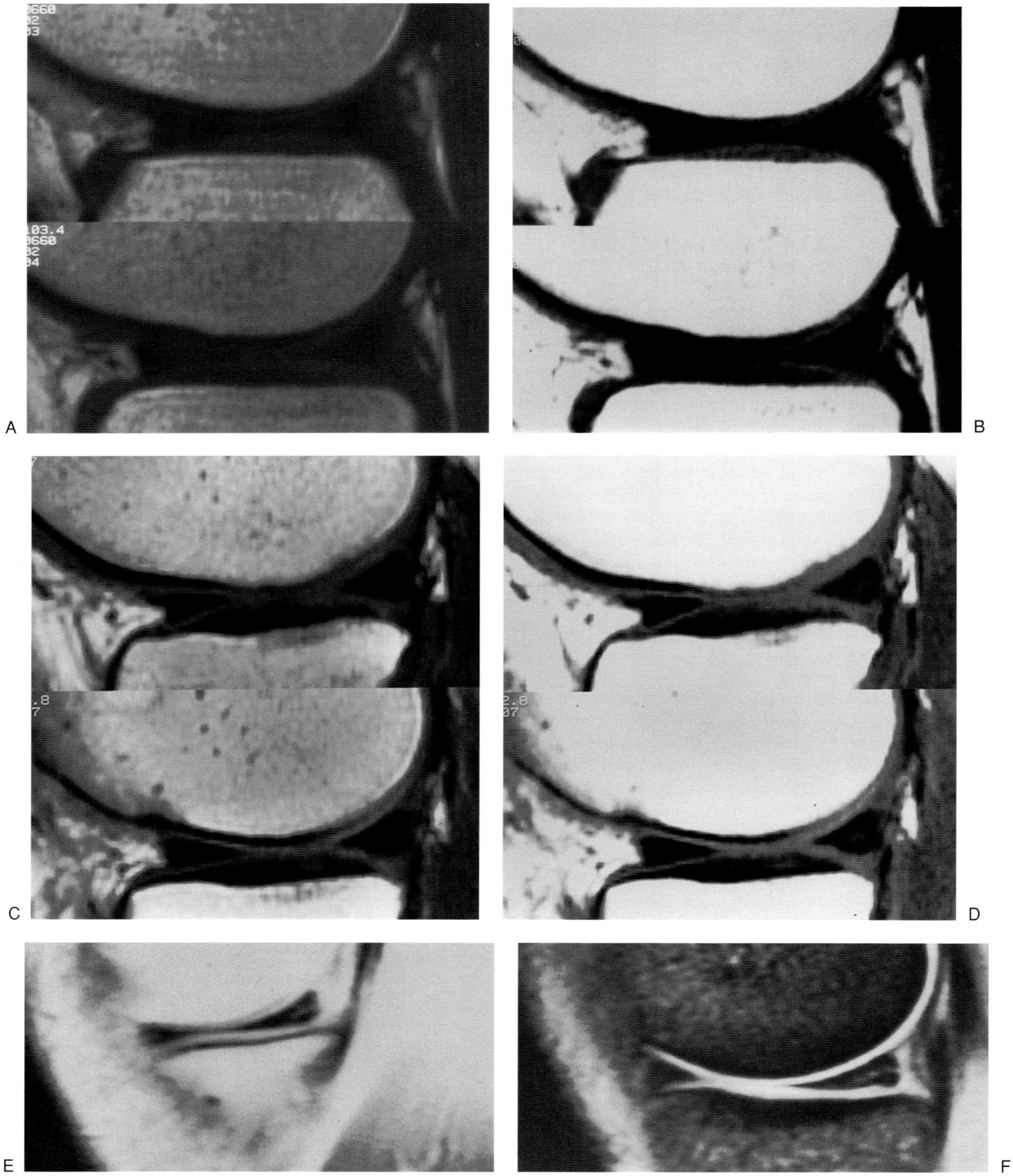

FIG. 4-8. Intrameniscal signal grading. **A,B:** Grade 0: regular and meniscal windows of a normal meniscus that is uniformly dark with no evidence of any mucoid degeneration whatever. **C,D:** Grade 1: regular and meniscal windows show an ovoid area of slightly increased signal within the substance of the meniscus. **E,F:** Grade 2: a linear area of increased signal is present on both T1- and T2*-weighted images of the posterior horn but does not extend to an articulating surface. **G,H:**

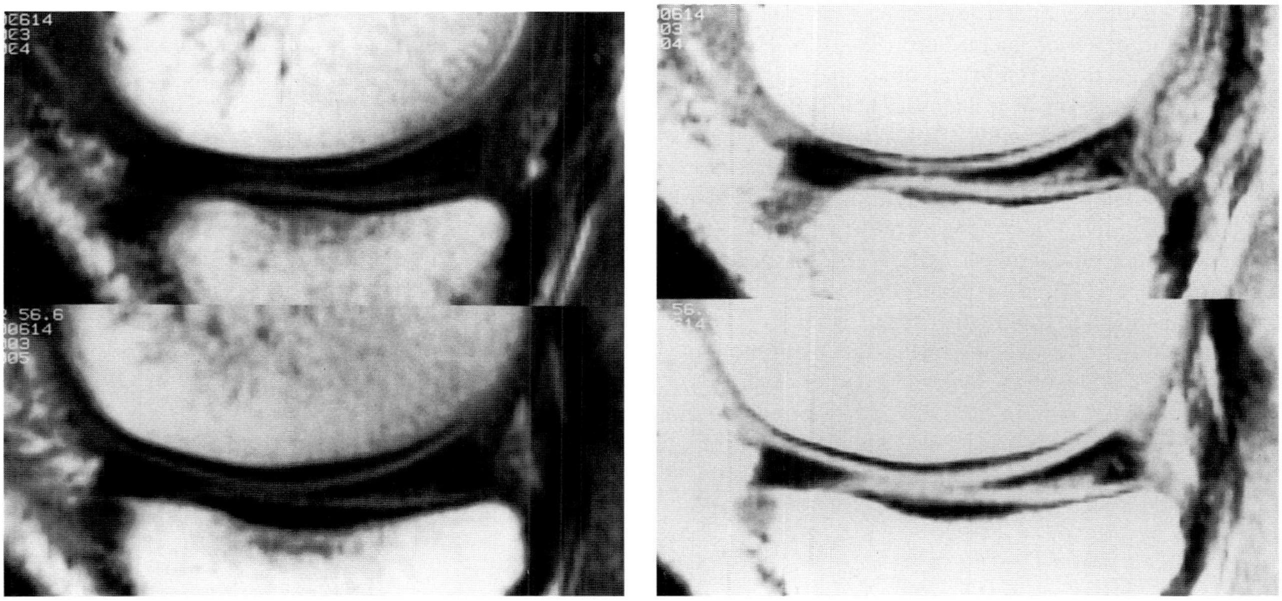

G H

FIG. 4-8. *(Continued).* Grade 3: regular and meniscal windows show a bandlike area of increased signal at the inferior aspect of the posterior horn that communicates with the articulating surface, consistent with a tear. **A** to **E** and **G and H:** Sagittal T1-weighted spin echo (TR 600 msec, TE 20 msec). **F:** Sagittal T2*-weighted gradient-echo MPGR (TR 400 msec, TE 20 msec, flip angle 20°).

PATHOLOGY

Meniscal Tears

Clinical Aspects

Meniscal tears (grade 3 signal) are commonly encountered in orthopedic practices that include a large number of young, active individuals. Medial meniscal tears are considerably more common than lateral meniscal tears, and although figures vary from one series to the next, medial tears are approximately five times as common. Furthermore, tears of the posterior horn are more frequently encountered than those of the anterior horn. Indeed, isolated anterior horn tears probably compose less than 1% of all meniscal tears (Fig. 4-10). The presence of a torn anterior cruciate often heralds the presence of meniscal tears which may be difficult to detect.

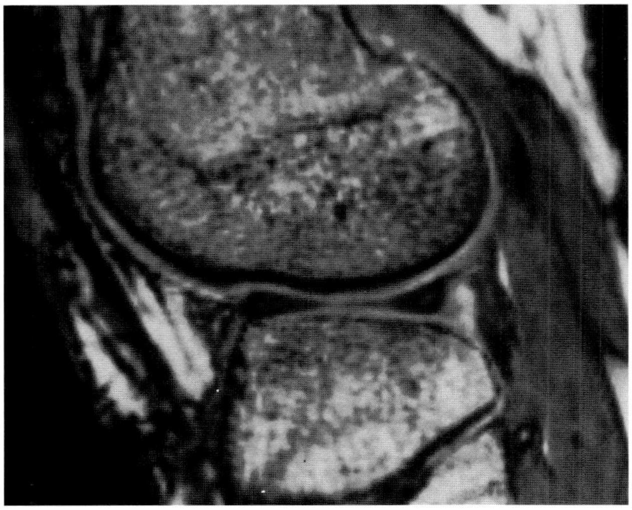

FIG. 4-9. Volumetric three-dimensional Fourier transform (3DFT) sagittal image. GRASS gradient echo (TR 55 msec, TE 15 msec, flip angle 30°) 1.7 mm thick. A small amount of globular signal is present within the substance of the meniscus, as is almost always the case with this technique.

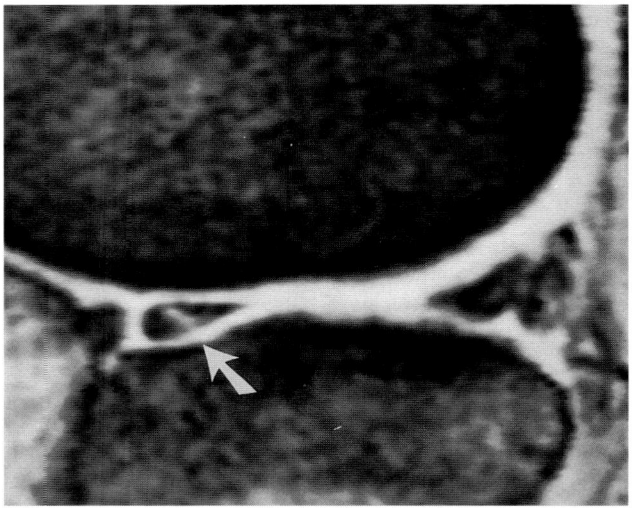

FIG. 4-10. Sagittal T2*-weighted gradient-echo MPGR (TR 400 msec, TE 20 msec, flip angle 20°). A small undisplaced anterior horn tear *(arrow)* is present in the medial meniscus.

In particular, subtle peripheral tears should be looked for, especially in the posterior lateral horn (98–100). If a long bone fracture (i.e., tibia, femur) or tibial plateau fracture is present, the likelihood of a meniscal tear being present increases considerably (101,102).

Menisci can be injured as a result of twisting, hyperflexion of the knee, and rotational instability resulting from ligamentous insufficiency. In addition, degenerative changes in the meniscus will predispose it to tearing. The clinical diagnosis of a meniscal tear is based on both physical examination and specific historical findings, such as the patient reporting an action resulting in the twisting of the knee with the foot firmly planted, or falling on the hyperflexed knee. Typically, the patient will report pain in the knee and swelling within hours to a day afterward. With rest the swelling often disappears but recurs rapidly following the resumption of activities. Often patients have a history of locking of the knee joint that occurs with the knee in a flexed position. Locking is a common feature of torn medial menisci and is less frequently seen with lateral meniscal tears.

On physical examination the knee will be seen to be tender and swollen. If a posterior tear is present, hyperflexion will reproduce the pain; if the tear is anterior, hyperextension will be painful. The clinical features of torn lateral menisci are often less clearly defined and the history may be vague. Although clinical accuracy in diagnosis of medial meniscal tears has been reported to be in excess of 90%, accuracy in diagnosis of lateral meniscal tears is often less than 60% (49).

Sequences and Findings

Meniscal tears are much more readily diagnosed with the use of MRI. In addition, injuries of the cruciate and collateral

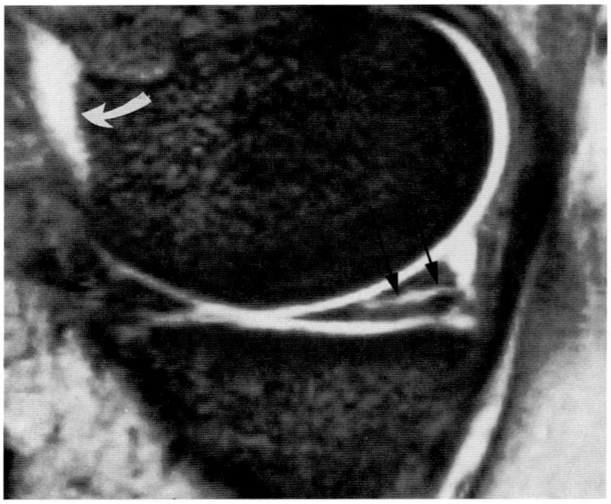

A

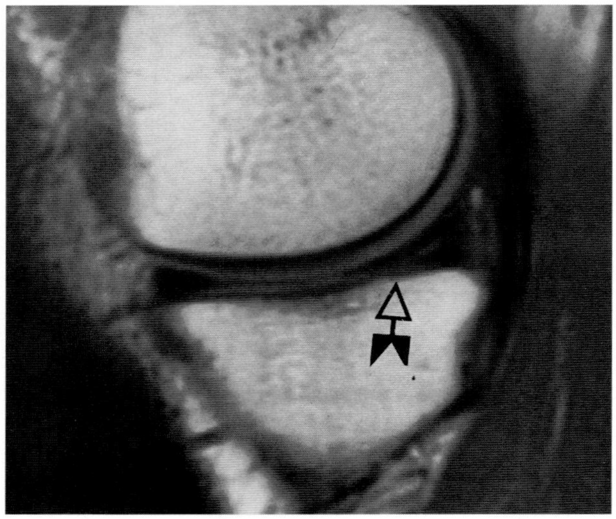

B

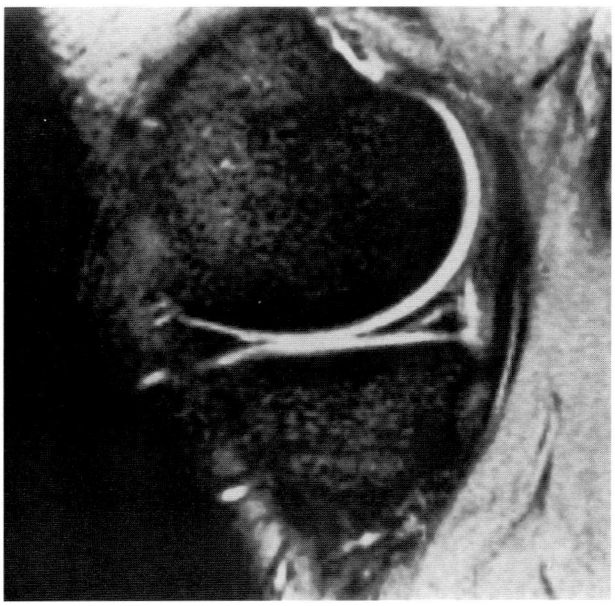

C

FIG. 4-11. Linear meniscal tears. **A:** Sagittal T2*-weighted gradient-echo MPGR (TR 400 msec, TE 20 msec, flip angle 20°). Linear tear of the posterior horn *(arrows)* extending to the superior surface of the meniscus. Incidental joint effusion *(curved arrow)*. (From Munk PL, *Canadian Association of Radiologists Journal* 1989;40:296–303. With permission.) **B:** Sagittal T1-weighted spin echo (TR 600 msec, TE 20 msec) with linear tear extending to inferior surface of the meniscus *(arrow)*. **C:** Sagittal T2*-weighted gradient echo MPGR (TR 400 msec, TE 20 msec, flip angle 20°). Same patient as in **B**. The tear is seen more vividly with T2* weighting in this instance.

ligaments, which often accompany meniscal tears, can be evaluated at the same time. When spin-echo sequences are utilized, meniscal tears are generally best seen with T1-weighted and proton-density images. With these sequences tears are visualized as areas of intermediate signal within the substance of the meniscus, extending to an articulating surface of the normally signal-free meniscus. The tears are seen as a result of the adsorption of water to the torn surface and of the mucopolysaccharides within degenerated menisci. Because the tears are visualized as a result of the presence of increased water (especially if an effusion is present), it might be expected that T2-weighted imaging would advantageously demonstrate tears; however, in general, most investigators have not found this to be the case. This is due to the diminished signal-to-noise ratio inherent in augmented T2 weighting as well as the coapting of the tear, which may decrease entry of high-signal water that would advantageously highlight it. This problem may be circumvented by using T1-weighted sequences following injection of gadolinium-chelate contrast agent into the joint (89,103).

Gradient-echo imaging techniques such as GRASS (gradient recall acquisition in the steady state) can also demonstrate tears. When flip angles of 40° or less are used, a T2-like image (T2*) is produced, which often advantageously demonstrates tears and may at times be superior to T1-weighted images (see Fig. 4-8F). These sequences also demonstrate mucoid degeneration very vividly to the point where virtually no menisci are ever entirely signal-free. In addition, gradient echo is sensitive to tiny amounts of gas within the joint—of the type present when vacuum phenomenon occurs. This can mimic meniscal surface irregularity (104).

Both gradient-echo sequences and spin-echo sequences may be utilized in volumetric imaging or 3-D Fourier transform images (see Fig. 4-9). This technique allows signal to be acquired from a volume of tissue and to be displayed as very thin slices of as little as 0.8 mm. In this way, even the smallest tears may be evaluated in great detail. Only a few studies have compared conventional spin-echo imaging with fast-scan 3-D Fourier transform using either axial or sagittal images (105). However, a few preliminary results have emerged; 3-D Fourier transform appears more sensitive for the diagnosis of meniscal tears, but the heightened sensitivity to intrameniscal signal may at times make it difficult to determine whether the abnormality communicates with the meniscal surface, hence diminishing the specificity of 3-D Fourier transform (106–113).

The longitudinal axis of the meniscus is the natural line along which meniscal tears occur, because the collagen fibers run in this direction. The tears may extend the whole length of the meniscus or affect only a portion of it and may emerge at either the superior or the inferior articulating surface (Fig. 4-11). The tears may extend to the free edge of the meniscus centrally, in which case a pedunculated tag may form (Fig. 4-12). If the tear extends along the length of the meniscus without communication with the free edge, the free edge may be displaced medially, producing a so-called bucket-handle fragment (Figs. 4-13 and 4-14) (50,114). This fragment may be seen on sagittal images as

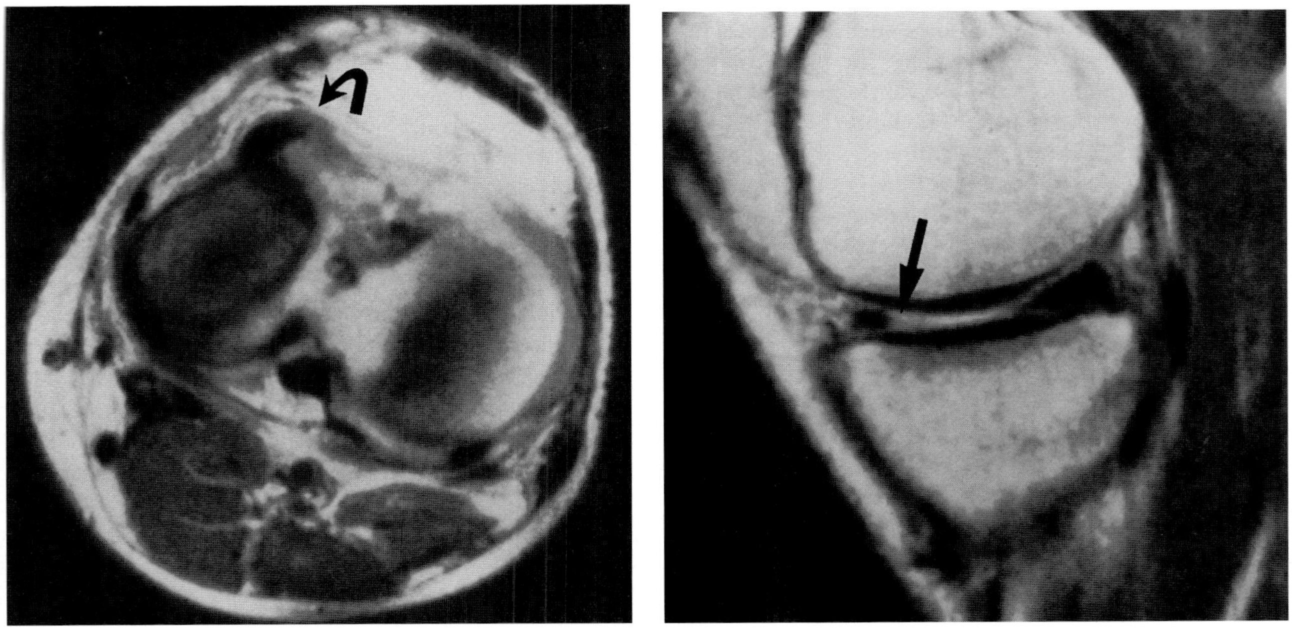

A B

FIG. 4-12. Pedunculated torn meniscus. **A:** Axial T1-weighted spin echo (TE 400 msec, TE 20 msec). Demonstrates a torn anterior horn of the medial meniscus, which has been rotated anteriorly and displaced into Hoffa's fat pad *(curved arrow)*. **B:** Sagittal T1-weighted spin echo (TR 600 msec, TE 20 msec). Anterior horn has a flattened, truncated apex *(arrow)* representing the donor site of the displaced meniscal fragment.

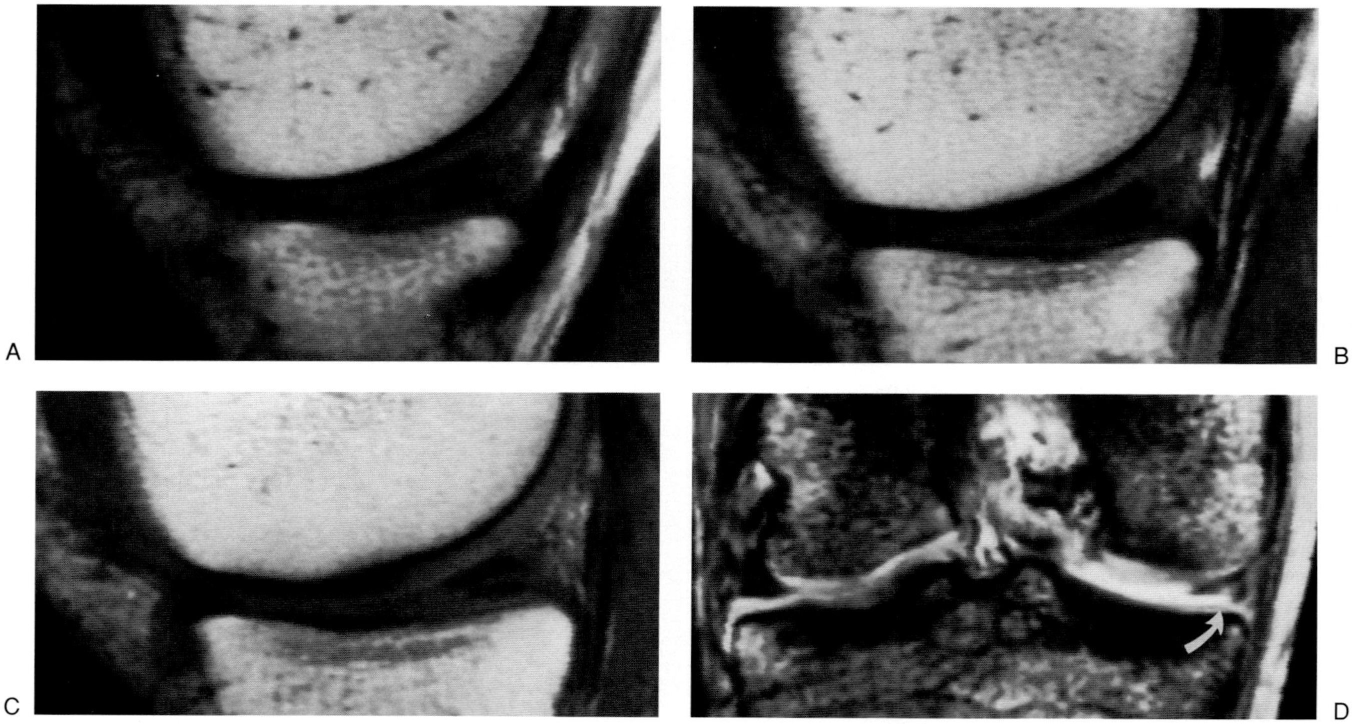

FIG. 4-13. Displaced bucket-handle meniscus tear **(A–C)**. Sagittal contiguous T1-weighted spin echo (TR 800 msec, TE 18 msec). None of these images through the medial meniscus show a normal body segment. Both anterior and posterior horns are truncated, and in addition, a horizontal tear is present through the posterior horn. **D:** Coronal T2*-weighted gradient-echo MPGR (TR 500 msec, TE 13 msec, flip angle 30°) from the same patient shows the torn meniscus, which has maintained a triangular cross-sectional configuration but is shortened *(arrow)*.

a dark band below the posterior cruciate ligament—the "double PCL" sign (this can also be seen on coronal images) (Figs. 4-15 and 4-16). The posterior horn of the meniscus may retain its triangular configuration but will be smaller than expected (the posterior horn should be larger than the anterior) (Fig. 4-17) (115,116). At times, a more complex pattern may exist, with multiple tears coexisting (Fig. 4-18) or the meniscus being macerated, with the abnormal portion being of diffusely increased signal with no discrete lines identified (Figs. 4-18 and 4-19). This is particularly common in the elderly. Although the majority of these will indeed be tears, some may represent the presence of calcium and associated scarring, which may mimic meniscal maceration (84). Although any type of tear may be seen at any location in the meniscus, longitudinal tears are especially common medially, and transverse or radial tears are often found laterally. Horizontal cleavage tears are said to be more common in the posterior horns (117). An abnormal meniscal contour is an obvious sign of a tear (118). Previous history of meniscal resection must first be excluded. On occasion the meniscus may appear buckled, when the free edge has a wavy, undulating appearance (meniscal flounce). This is a normal variant (119–121). Radial meniscal tears can also occur and have their plane of cleavage in the short axis of the meniscus (like radially oriented images) and can be quite subtle (122).

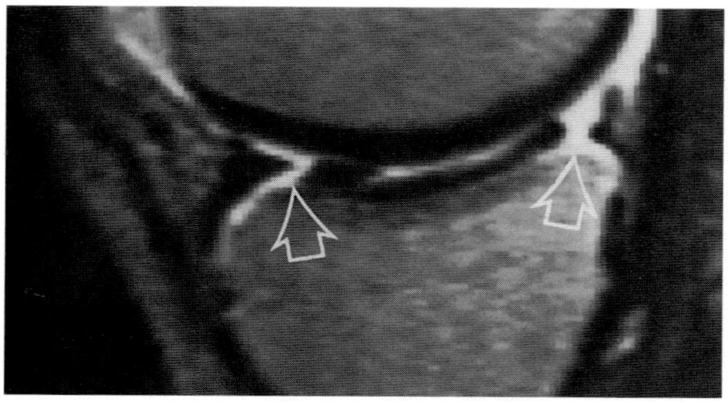

FIG. 4-14. Sagittal T2-weighted spin-echo (TR 2000 msec, TE 60 msec) image. Fluid within the joint outlines the meniscus. A bucket-handle tear is present with the long bucket-handle segment being between the two arrows. The posterior horn is noted to be truncated.

The problem of signal not clearly extending to an articular surface of the meniscus is a common one, frequently leading to equivocal calls. Recent work has suggested that when conventional spin-echo imaging is being done with 3–5-mm slices signal should be seen clearly extending to the surface of the meniscus on at least two slices. Addition of 3DFT images may help considerably in resolving difficult cases (105,106,110,111,113,123–125).

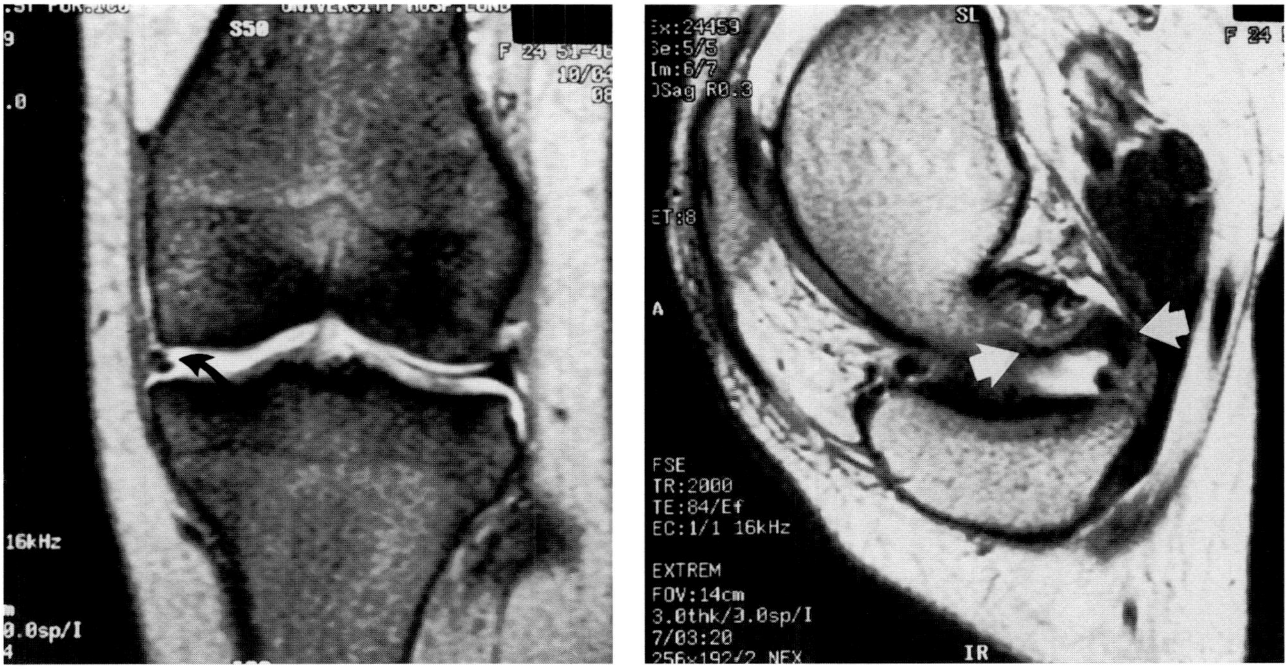

A B

FIG. 4-15. Bucket-handle tear with displacement centrally. **A:** Coronal T2*-weighted gradient echo MPGR (TR 500 msec, TE 20 msec, flip angle 20°). A tear of the medial meniscus is present with a truncated, cleft-appearing triangular outline *(arrow)*. **B:** Oblique Sagittal T2-weighted fast spin echo (TR 2000 msec, TEef 84 msec) shows an abnormally low signal structure in the center of the joint near the posterior cruciate *(arrows)* representing the displaced meniscal segment.

Regardless of the sequence, the single most useful plane for evaluating the meniscus is the sagittal plane, which also has the advantage of being satisfactory for examination of the cruciate ligaments. Some investigators have advocated radially oriented images to examine the meniscus, arguing that in this fashion it may be seen in cross section along its whole length (Fig. 4-20). Investigations to date have not shown any clear advantages of radial versus sagittal images (126).

Accuracy

MR, unlike arthroscopy and arthrography, is a noninvasive technique and, when standard imaging protocols are used, is not as operator dependent. It should also be remembered that arthroscopy is an imperfect gold standard. Many "missed" tears at MRI may be of little clinical significance (up to 47%) (96,127,128). Healed tears and prior meniscal surgery may also induce changes that can be misinterpreted as tears.

When the types of errors that do occur with MRI are analyzed, many are found to involve the free edge of the meniscus. These are often small tears that are easily hidden by volume-averaging artifacts, usually not requiring partial meniscectomy. In addition, most investigators have found that T1-weighted or proton-density images are more accurate than T2-weighted images, particularly for detection of these small abnormalities. This is presumably due to the poorer signal-to-noise ratio seen with T2-weighted images (129). Fast spin echo is reputedly less accurate than conventional spin echo, in part because of the inherent blurring with the technique, which is more pronounced if a long echo train is used (130). Gradient-echo images are also fairly accurate in the detection of meniscal tears, and in some instances, tear morphology may be better demonstrated. The sensitivity of gradient-echo images is enhanced further if 3-D Fourier transform volume acquisition techniques are utilized (125). This has the added advantage of diminishing the effect of volume-averaging artifacts. Meniscofemoral ligaments may also mimic tears (Fig. 4-21) (3,131,132).

Many studies have attempted to document the accuracy of MRI, usually compared with arthroscopy. Overall accuracy has been reported to be from 80% to 97%, with better results laterally than medially in some instances (133,134). A number of important pitfalls are recognized and are discussed fully in Chapter 6.

Treatment

The presence of a meniscal tear is not always an indication for resection or repair. Many meniscal tears are asymptomatic. A recent study of a large group of asymptomatic individuals demonstrated many clinically unsuspected, asymptomatic meniscal tears, especially in older individuals.

(text continues on page 101)

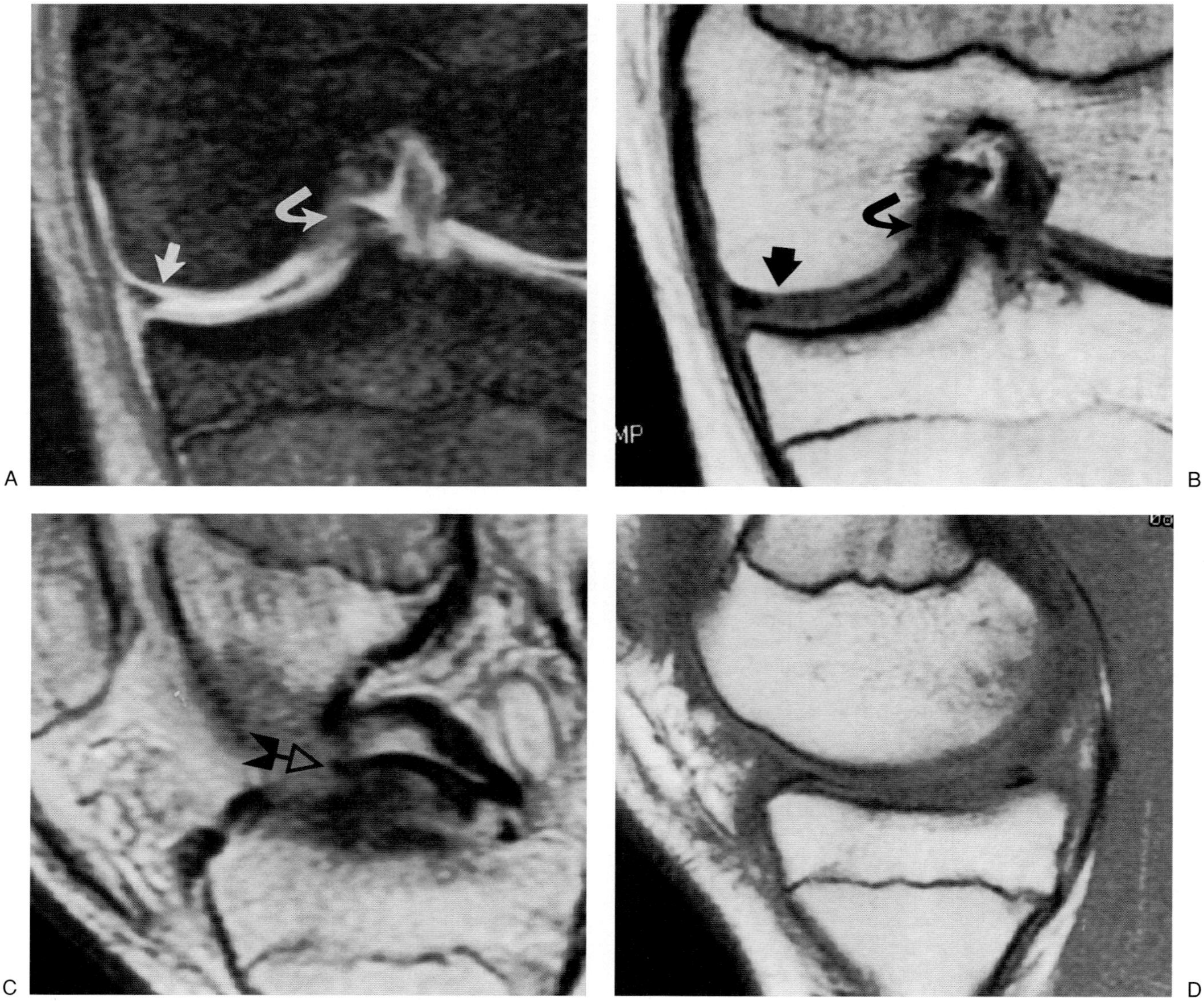

FIG. 4-16. Bucket-handle meniscal tear with double posterior cruciate sign. **Patient 1: A:** Coronal T2*-weighted MPGR (TR 400 msec, TE 20 msec, flip angle 20°). A truncated medial meniscus is seen *(arrow)*. The displaced bucket-handle fragment is seen in the intercondylar notch *(curved arrow)*. **B:** Coronal T1-weighted spin echo (TR 600 msec, TE 19 msec) shows similar findings; however, the displaced fragment is slightly more difficult to appreciate. **C:** Oblique sagittal T2-weighted spin echo (TR 2300 msec, TE 80 msec). Immediately below the curved posterior cruciate lies a similarly configured low signal band *(arrow)* representing the displaced medial meniscus bucket-handle fragment. **Patient 2: D:** Sagittal T1-weighted spin-echo (TR 500 msec, TE 15 msec) image shows a markedly truncated meniscus with virtually no posterior horn left *in situ*.

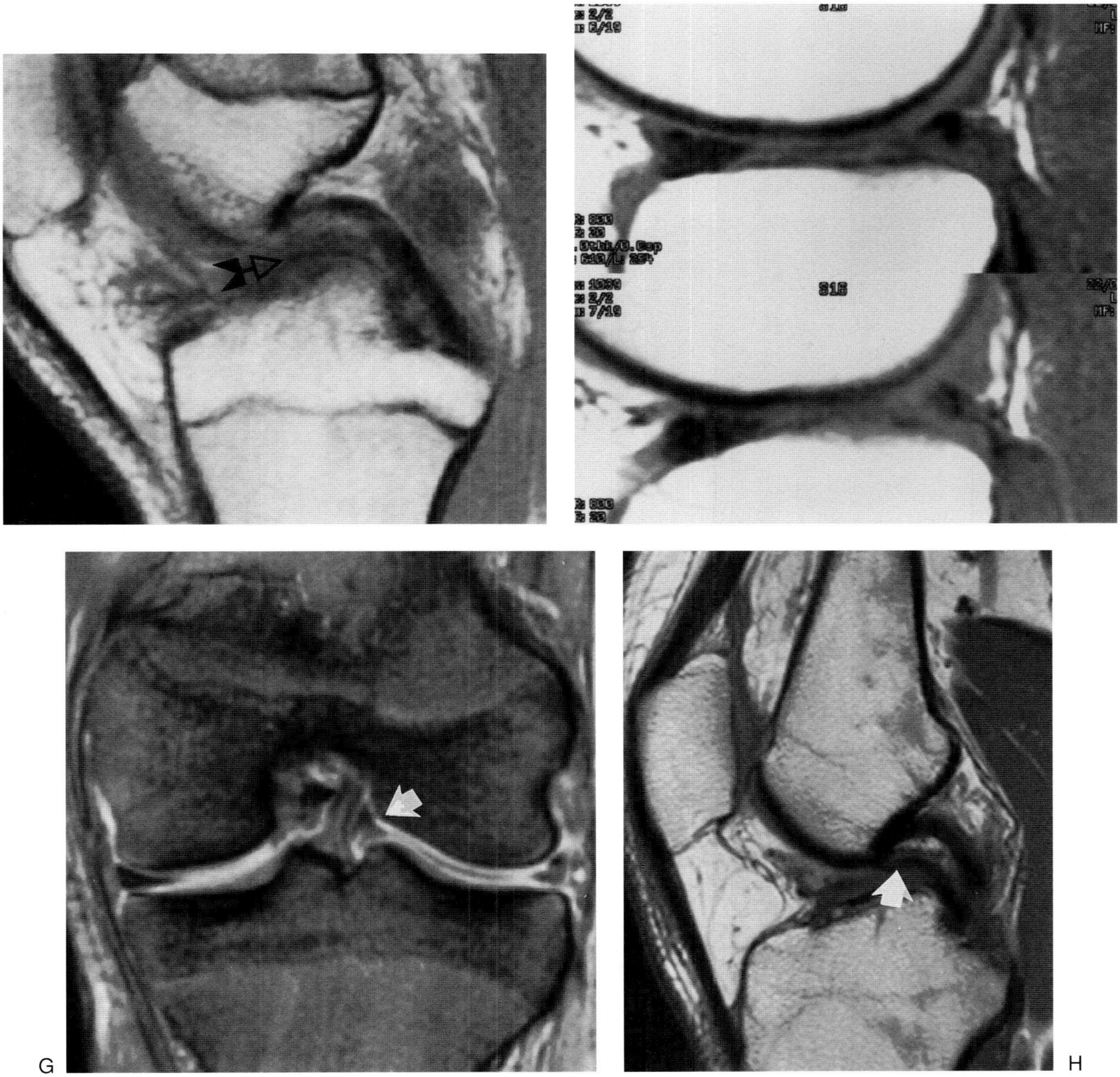

E F G H

FIG. 4-16. *(Continued).* **E:** From the same sequence the level of intercondylar notch, a thin band of decreased signal intensity representing the macerated medial meniscal bucket handle is seen *(arrow).* **Patient 3: F:** Contiguous sagittal T1-weighted spin-echo (TR 800 msec, TE 20 msec) image shows a complex tear of the medial meniscus with marked truncation of the posterior horn. **G:** Coronal T2*-weighted gradient echo MPGR (TR 400 msec, TE 20 msec, flip angle 20°) image shows a well-defined centrally displaced fragment tucked into the intercondylar notch immediately adjacent to the fibers of the anterior cruciate *(curved arrow).* **H:** Sagittal T1-weighted spin-echo (TR 800 msec, TE 20 msec) image at the level of the intercondylar notch once again demonstrates a bandlike structure mimicking the posterior cruciate—another displaced bucket-handle fragment.

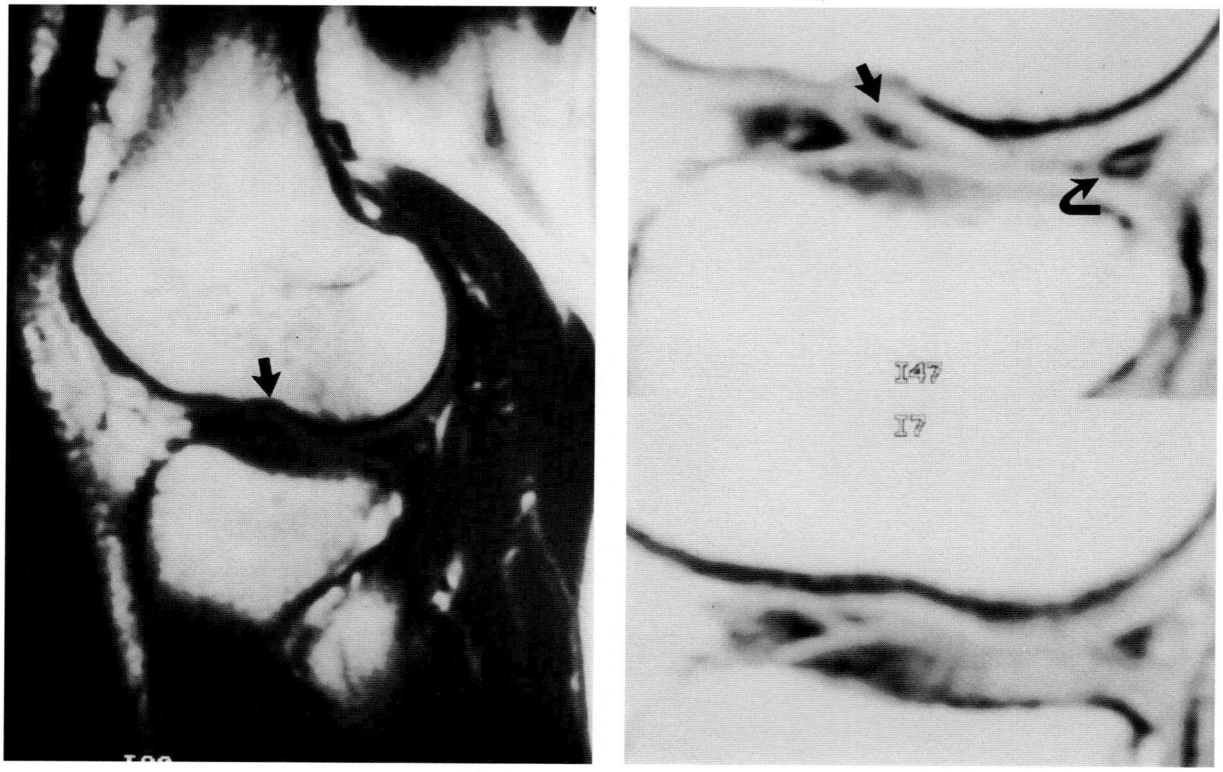

A B

FIG. 4-17. Bucket-handle tear lateral meniscus **(A)** and **(B)**. Sagittal T1-weighted spin-echo images (TR 600 msec, TE 18 msec) with meniscal windows in **B**. An anteriorly displaced fragment is noted to be located immediately posterior to the anterior horn *(arrows)*. A high-signal tear is visualized in the remaining portion of the posterior horn *(curved arrow)*.

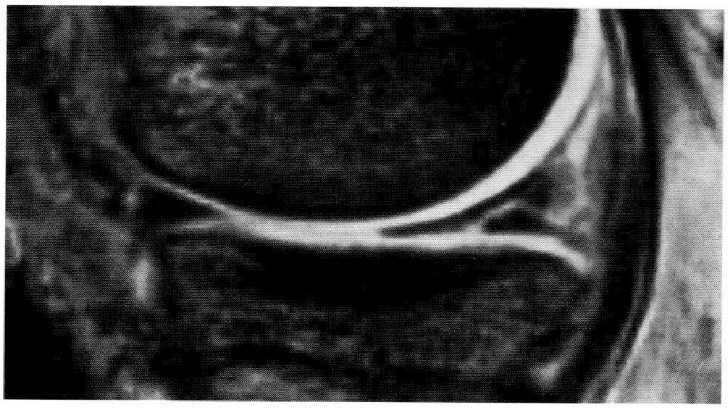

A

FIG. 4-18. Complex tear. **A:** Sagittal T2*-weighted gradient echo MPGR (TR 400 msec, TE 18 msec, flip angle 20°). A linear high-signal region with branching is present consistent with a complex tear. **B:** Sagittal T2*-weighted gradient-echo 3DFT GRASS images (TR 55 msec, TE 15 msec, flip angle 35°) from a different patient. An apical tear is present accompanied by diffuse high signal in the central portion of the meniscus. This appearance is referred to as maceration.

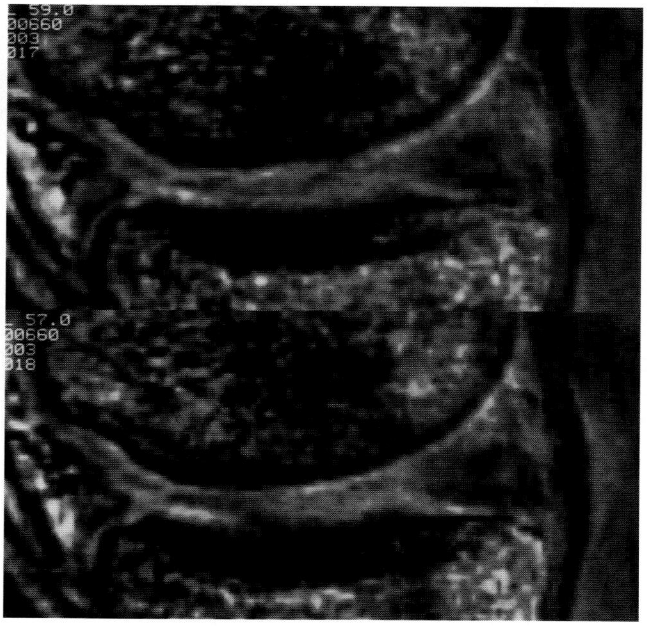

B

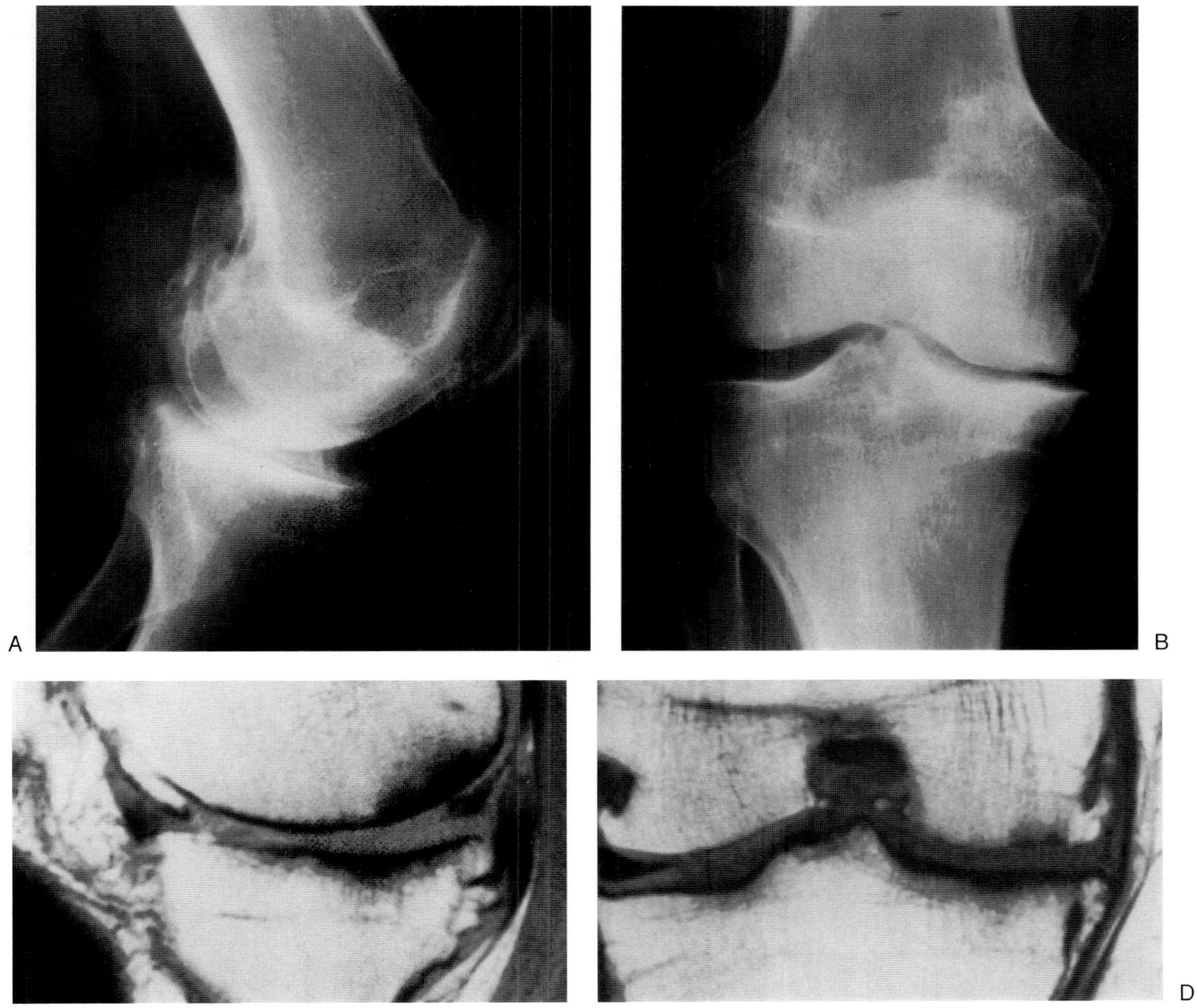

FIG. 4-19. Meniscal maceration. **A,B:** Lateral and anteroposterior radiographs demonstrate evidence of advanced osteoarthritis. **C,D:** Sagittal and coronal T1-weighted spin echo (TR 500 msec, TE 20 msec) show diffuse increased signal, especially through the apex of the medial meniscus, consistent with maceration.

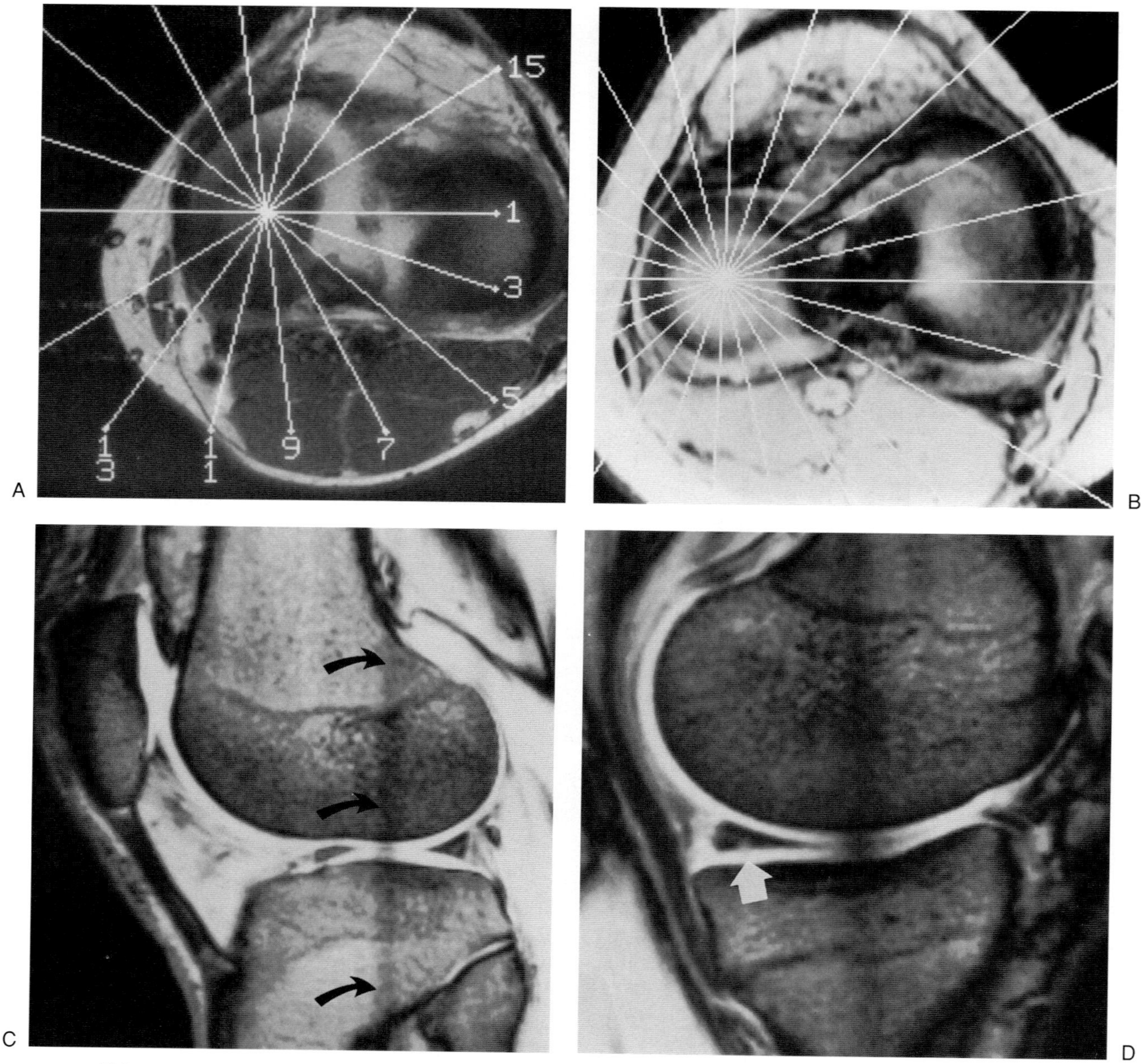

FIG. 4-20. Radial imaging of the meniscus T2*-weighted MPGR (TR 525 msec, TE 13 msec, flip angle 20°). Examples of medial meniscal **(A)** and lateral meniscal **(B)** prescriptions for radial imaging. **C:** Image from the lateral meniscus. (With gradient-echo imaging the menisci are seldom entirely free of signal, even when normal, as in this instance.) The axis of rotation is seen as a band of diminished signal down the length of the image *(curved arrows)*. **D:** In this section from the medial meniscus, a tear is seen in the posterior horn *(arrow)*.

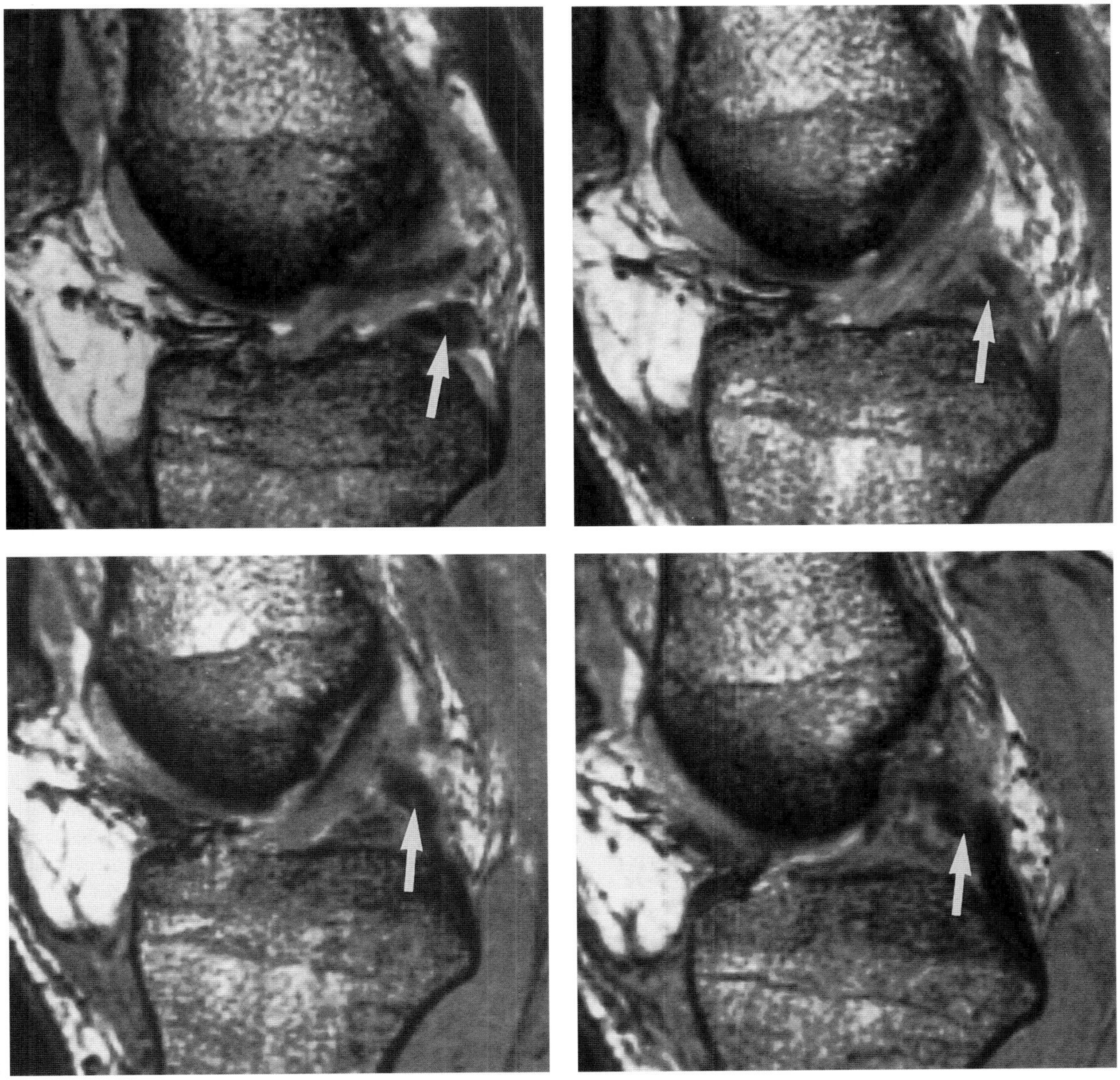

A B C D

FIG. 4-21. Meniscofemoral ligament mimicking a meniscal tear. Four 3DFT T2*-weighted gradient-echo MPGR images (TR 55 msec, TE 15 msec, flip angle 30°). Figures **A–D** show how a meniscofemoral ligament (in this case the ligament of Humphry) may mimic a posterior horn tear of the lateral meniscus *(arrows)*.

Asymptomatic tears are often seen in older or sedentary individuals (96). Even in active individuals, small flap tears or tiny tears of the free edge may not produce a clinical problem. With the greater appreciation in recent years of acceleration of degenerative changes in joints that have had menisci removed, there is an increasing tendency toward conservative procedures in the treatment of meniscal abnormalities (135). It has been remarked that, although an abnormal meniscus can be excised, once it is removed it cannot be replaced.

Certain meniscal tears can be left alone. These include partial-thickness tears that are split along the long axis of the meniscus and that are no more than 50% of the thickness of the meniscus at either the superior or the inferior surface. Such tears are seen especially in the lateral meniscus, often in association with anterior cruciate ligament tears. Similarly, full-thickness tears may occasionally be left alone if they are less than 5 mm long. Minor inner-margin tears along the free edge of the meniscus may also be safely left alone in most individuals, and minor flap tears at the meniscal surface are also frequently of little clinical significance (136).

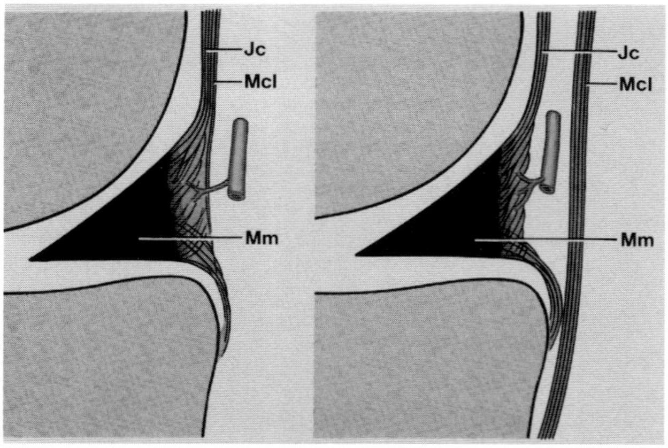

FIG. 4-22. Meniscal blood supply. The medial meniscus is illustrated here. On the left is the posterior portion of the meniscus; on the right a more anterior segment is shown. Only the periphery of the meniscus is well vascularized and amenable to repair. Jc, joint capsule; Mcl, medial collateral ligament; Mm, medial meniscus.

Certain tears are amenable to repair. This is particularly true of tears that are along the periphery of the meniscus, as this is the most vascularized portion (Fig. 4-22; see also color plate 6). Approximately 10–30% of the peripheral meniscus is vascularized and therefore may heal (16,137–139). Laser Doppler flowmetry has been used to evaluate the meniscus for suitability for repair. The anterior and posterior horns have a slightly larger area of vascularized meniscus, whereas the body of the meniscus generally has a slightly thinner zone. Approximately 20% of meniscal tears are suitable for repair. These usually are tears occurring in the posterior horns that have a vertical configuration. Patients who undergo meniscal repair often have longer recovery times than those with complete meniscectomy, but these patients usually have better long-term results. To maximize the success of repair, it is crucial that the surgeon be aware of any other accompanying derangements with the joint, especially damage to the anterior cruciate ligament. If the anterior cruciate ligament is not stabilized, the prognosis for a satisfactory outcome diminishes considerably and the retear rate is greatly increased (140,141).

Other lesions are more suitable for partial meniscectomy. Generally, the goal of partial meniscectomy is to remove torn, abnormally mobile segments of the meniscus, particularly if they are not in the peripheral portion of the meniscus. To do this it must be known that the peripheral rim of the meniscus is normal so as not to leave behind an unrepaired mobile segment that will break off following surgery. Long radial or bucket-handle tears of the lateral meniscus are particularly common lesions that are suitable for partial meniscectomy. Flap tears of the surface of the meniscus, especially if pedunculated, are also good candidates for resection and are usually found in the middle and anterior thirds of the menisci.

In patients who have extensive tearing or maceration of the meniscus, total meniscectomy is still appropriate and is likely to be the only treatment that will provide relief of symptoms. The more chronic a lesion, the less likely it is to respond adequately to conservative surgery. Approximately 50% of acute meniscal tears (those under 14 days old) are potentially repairable. After 14 days the figure falls to 20–25% or even less.

DISCOID MENISCI

The precise embryogenesis of the menisci is an issue of some debate. It is known that the menisci arise from primitive synovium, and in early development of the knee, a mass of mesenchyme exists between the cartilaginous precursors. This begins to break down at approximately 8 weeks of gestation. The menisci become recognizable at this time. One of the popular theories for the generation of discoid menisci is that incomplete resorption of the mesenchymal plate occurs, leaving a meniscus that extends farther centrally than normal (85,142,143). However, examination of fetal specimens has not verified this theory. A second theory postulates that the discoid meniscus is an acquired lesion that occurs because of altered knee mechanics, potentially related to a shortened meniscofemoral ligament attached to the posterior horn of the lateral meniscus (144,145).

Discoid menisci are seen much more frequently in the lateral meniscus than in the medial meniscus. Rarely, they have been reported bilaterally (146). The precise incidence of discoid meniscus is unknown; however, at least one series suggests that lateral discoid menisci can be seen in from 1.5% to 4.5% of individuals (147). Medial menisci are seen in, at most, 0.3% of individuals, and probably far fewer than that (142,143,148,149). Discoid menisci are clinically important because they are prone to tear, resulting in the typical symptoms of torn meniscus, including joint locking and knee pain. Occasionally, patients present with an untorn meniscus that produces a snapping sound on flexion or extension, the snapping knee syndrome. If the patient is symptomatic, meniscectomy (preferably partial) is the treatment of choice (150,151).

Several different classifications of discoid menisci exist (152). One popular classification divides discoid menisci into three groups. The first of these is the primitive discoid meniscus, which consists of a complete disc across the joint space. Over the years the stresses on the menisci cause the inferior surface of this complete disk to tear, which in turn causes sinking of the superior surface into the created cavity. Finally, a longitudinal tear usually appears through the full thickness of the discoid meniscus. The second category is the intermediate discoid meniscus, which consists of an incomplete or fenestrated membrane. The infantile discoid meniscus has a configuration that approaches normal; however, the apex of the meniscus protrudes more centrally within the joint than normal. This is probably the most commonly encountered type of discoid meniscus and is diagnosable

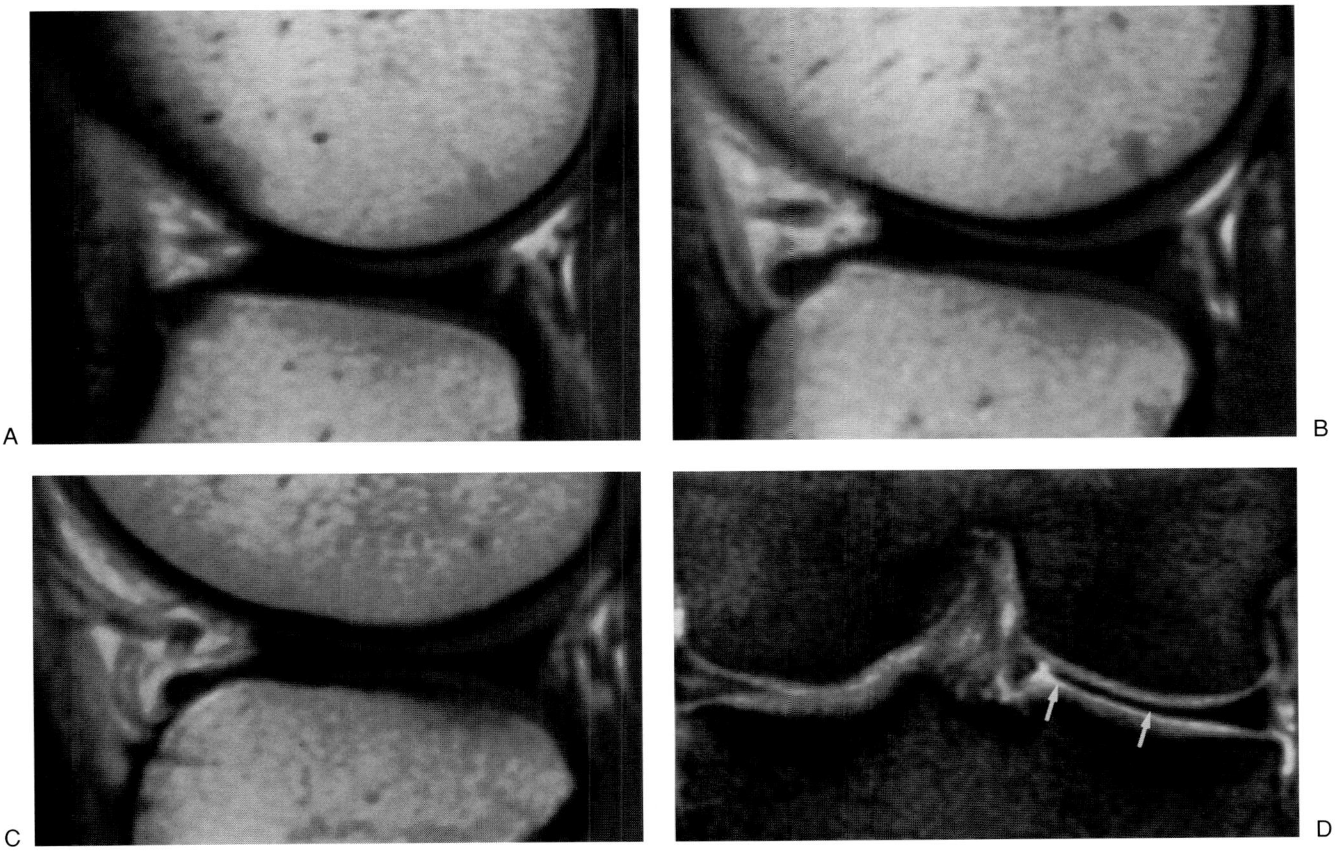

FIG. 4-23. Discoid lateral meniscus. **A–C:** Sagittal T1-weighted contiguous spin-echo images (TR 600 msec, TE 18 msec). These three 5-mm-thick sections show a bow-tie-shaped configuration extending centrally into the joint more than would normally be expected. **D:** Coronal T2*-weighted gradient-echo MPGR (TR 400 msec, TE 16 msec, flip angle 20°). The free edge of the meniscus is seen to extend almost to the intercondylar notch *(arrows)*.

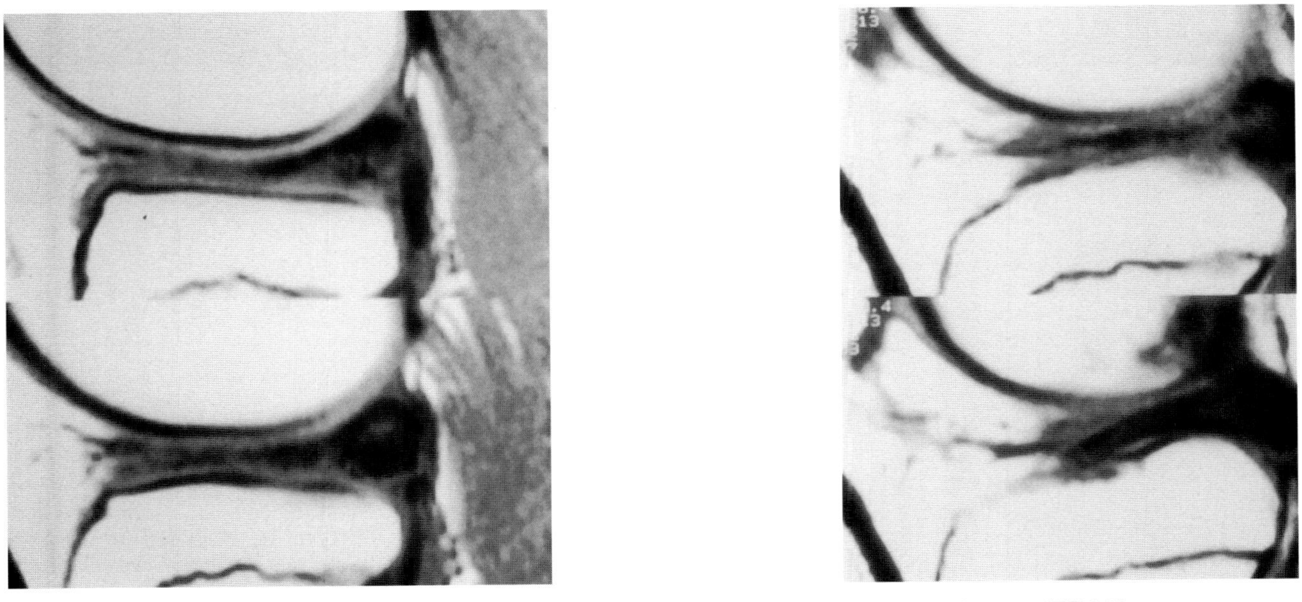

FIG. 4-24. Torn discoid meniscus. Series of four adjacent T1-weighted spin-echo images (TR 500 msec, TE 14 msec) shows a markedly thickened posterior horn of the lateral meniscus and protrusion of the central edge deep into the joint. The normal triangular configuration is not visible. Extensive signal is present within the meniscus substance, especially in the anterior horn and inferior surface, consistent with tears.

on arthrography because the apex of the meniscus is more centrally located than usual, sometimes so centrally displaced that it is not actually possible to demonstrate the apex of the meniscus clearly. Difficulty in diagnosing the presence of a discoid meniscus is particularly marked in instances of medial discoid menisci. Also, discoid menisci are more prone to develop meniscal cysts than other types of torn menisci (151,152).

Characteristic plain-film findings are associated with discoid menisci, particularly laterally located ones. Generally, there is hyperplasia of the lateral femoral condyle, and the fibular head is higher than normal. In addition, lateral joint space widening can be observed and there is decreased height of the lateral intercondylar tibial spine (153). No reliable plain-film findings with medial discoid menisci are known, although some authorities have postulated that the medial aspect of the joint may occasionally be widened. Arthrography and CT have been used to make the diagnosis (147,152,154).

Although some investigators accept a congenital origin for the development of discoid menisci, others have suggested that this is an acquired lesion. Discoid lateral menisci may evolve when the posterior horn of the meniscus is attached only to the meniscofemoral ligament, the so-called ligament of Wrisberg (144). When this is the situation, meniscal dislocation occurs when the joint is extended. With

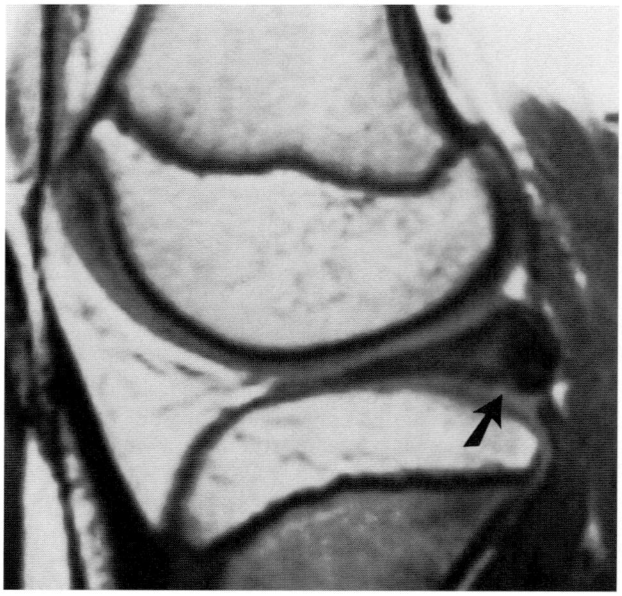

A

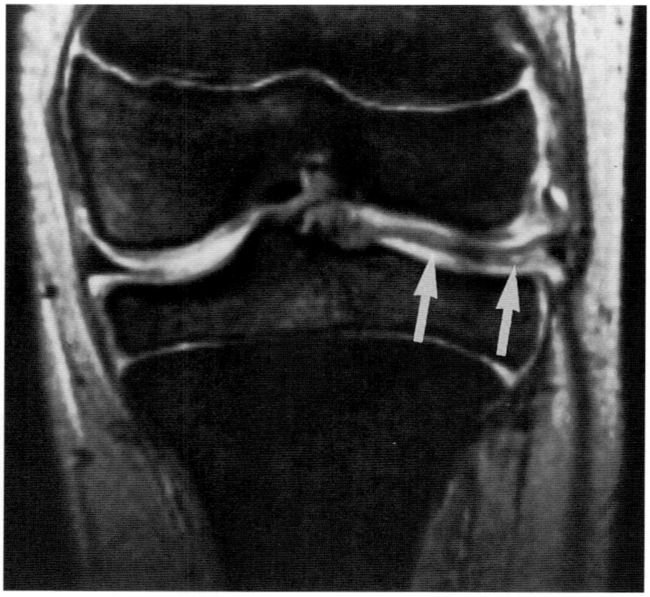

B

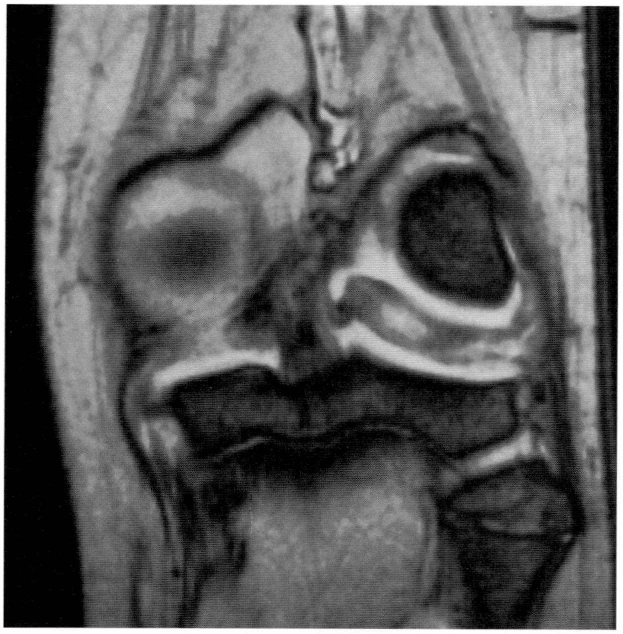

C

FIG. 4-25. Torn discoid menisci. **A:** Sagittal T1-weighted spin-echo image of a partially discoid (posterior horn) lateral meniscus *(arrow)*. **B:** Coronal $T2^*$-weighted gradient-echo image of a torn discoid medial meniscus *(arrows)*. Case courtesy of Royal North Shore Hospital, Sydney, Australia. **C:** Coronal $T2^*$-weighted gradient-echo image (TR 400 msec, TE 20 msec, flip angle 20°) shows a thick posterior horn of the lateral meniscus with areas of linear increased signal intensity within it. This represents a markedly macerated discoid meniscus.

flexion, meniscal dislocation is reduced. With time, stretching and hypertrophy of the meniscus occur until it acquires a discoid configuration (151).

On MRI the untorn discoid meniscus has signal characteristics similar to those of normal menisci. The discoid meniscus may be recognized by an unusually centrally located apex of the meniscus (Fig. 4-23). This is often elegantly demonstrated on coronal images but may also be recognized on sagittal images when an unusually large number of cuts is required to pass through the full extent of the meniscus (Fig. 4-24). If 5-mm-thick sagittal images are used, a discoid meniscus is considered to be present when three or more contiguous sections demonstrate a continuous band of meniscus from the front to the back of the tibial plateau. In addition, discoid menisci tend to be thicker than normal. If the height of the meniscus at the periphery of the midbody is 2 mm or more than the height of the opposite meniscus, it is likely to be discoid (146,155). Once the meniscus is torn, a displaced fragment can often be recognized. Arthroscopic treatment is more difficult than in normal menisci but is feasible (150). Frequently, discoid menisci have an extensively macerated appearance with diffuse high signal throughout the central portion of the meniscus (Fig. 4-25). As mentioned earlier, torn discoid menisci have a high incidence of lateral meniscal cysts (156).

MENISCAL CYSTS AND OTHER LESIONS

Cystic degeneration is commonly found in menisci, and several series that have examined resected menisci have placed the incidence at approximately 7%. Large, clinically obvious cysts are far less common. Meniscal cysts are usually clinically noted as an area of tenderness near the joint line often associated with a tense, hard lump and are only rarely fluctuant. Pain is typically dull and worsened by exercise. They at times reach large sizes, especially medially, with cysts being up to 6 cm in diameter. Meniscal cysts are associated with either horizontal or complex meniscal tears (Fig. 4-26) and probably have a degenerative rather than a traumatic etiology (91). Although debate persists on this point, in the case of discoid menisci, which are prone to develop cysts, a traumatic cause is more likely. The cysts form as synovial fluid is forced through the tear and then pushes its way through the meniscal capsular margin. Medial meniscal cysts are found posteriorly, in the weak areas immediately posterior to the medial collateral ligament. This weak zone allows the synovial fluid to penetrate the capsule more readily and to expand to form a clinically apparent cyst. Progressive posterior displacement may occur as a result of repeated knee flexion, and the cyst may be connected to the menisci by a long pedicle. These are often clinically mistaken for popliteal cysts. Lateral meniscal cysts are usually contained by the joint capsule. The weakest area is between the lateral collateral ligament and the iliotibial band, and most cysts seen in relation to the lateral meniscus are located in this area. Lateral meniscal cysts overall are more common than medial meniscal cysts, with a ratio of approximately five lateral cysts to one medial cyst. The cysts are often multiple (157).

The traditional method for demonstrating these cysts has been arthrography (156). The contrast medium, once introduced into the joint, passes through the meniscal tear and

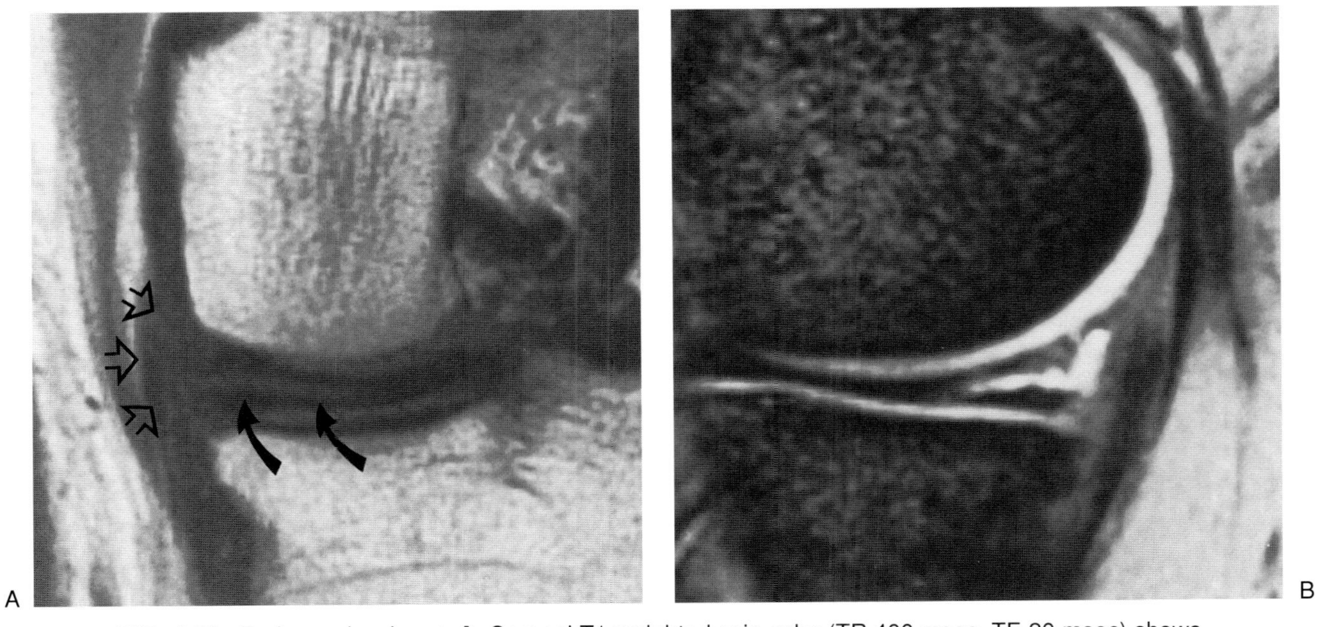

FIG. 4-26. Early meniscal cyst. **A**: Coronal T1-weighted spin echo (TR 400 msec, TE 20 msec) shows a horizontal menisca tear *(curved arrows)* communicating with a poorly defined zone of slightly increased signal intensity within the meniscal substance *(hollow arrows)*. **B:** Sagittal T2*-weighted gradient-echo MPGR (TR 400 msec, TE 18 msec, flip angle 20°) shows the meniscal tear to better advantage.

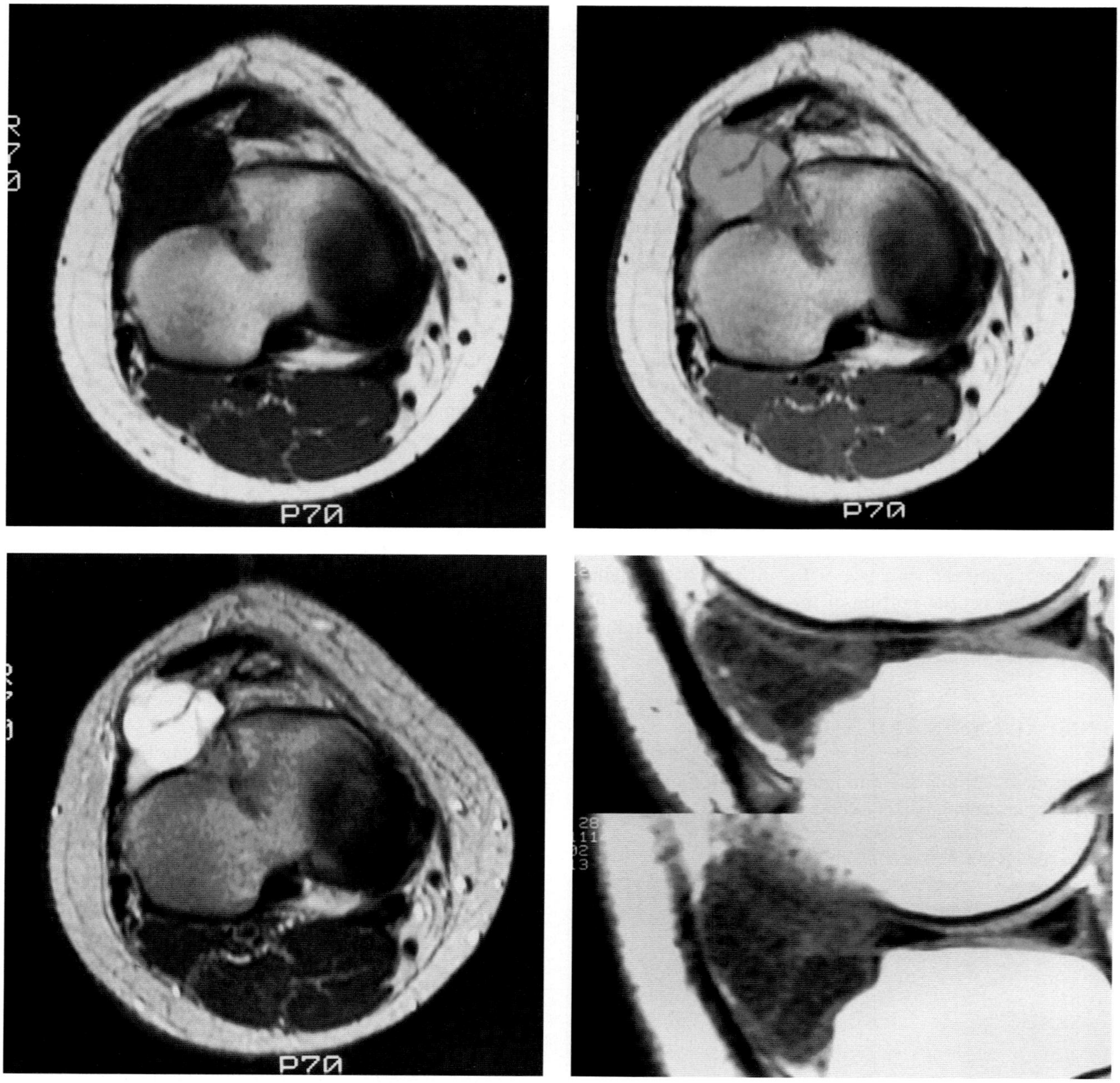

FIG. 4-27. Bulky meniscal cyst. **A:** Axial T1-weighted spin echo (TR 500 msec, TE 19 msec). **B,C:** Axial proton density and T2-weighted spin echo (TR 2000 msec, TE 30 and 70 msec). **D:** Sagittal T1-weighted spin echo (TR 500 msec, TE 20 msec). These images delineate a large, lobulated mass arising from the anterior horn of the lateral meniscus with several prominent septation. With augmented T2-weighting signal intensity increases. The mass is noted to extend into the Hoffa fat pad and to abut the patellar tendon.

into the cyst; however, because the cyst is often full of thick, viscous material, its size may be markedly underestimated and filling may only be seen on delayed films. CT will more accurately demonstrate the size of the cyst. Ultrasound may also demonstrate these lesions, but the viscous content may give them a solid appearance (158).

Generally, on MRI, meniscal cysts are noted to be smooth-walled structures. On T1-weighted images, the contents of the cysts are noted to be hypo- or isointense to adjacent muscles. As the degree of T2 weighting is augmented, the cyst becomes of increasingly higher signal and becomes readily apparent. The contents are almost always of uniform signal, and septation is common (Fig. 4-27). Although the cysts may be shown on axial, sagittal, or coronal scans, coronal scans usually demonstrate the cyst and the communicating meniscal tear best (Fig. 4-28 and 4-29) (159–161).

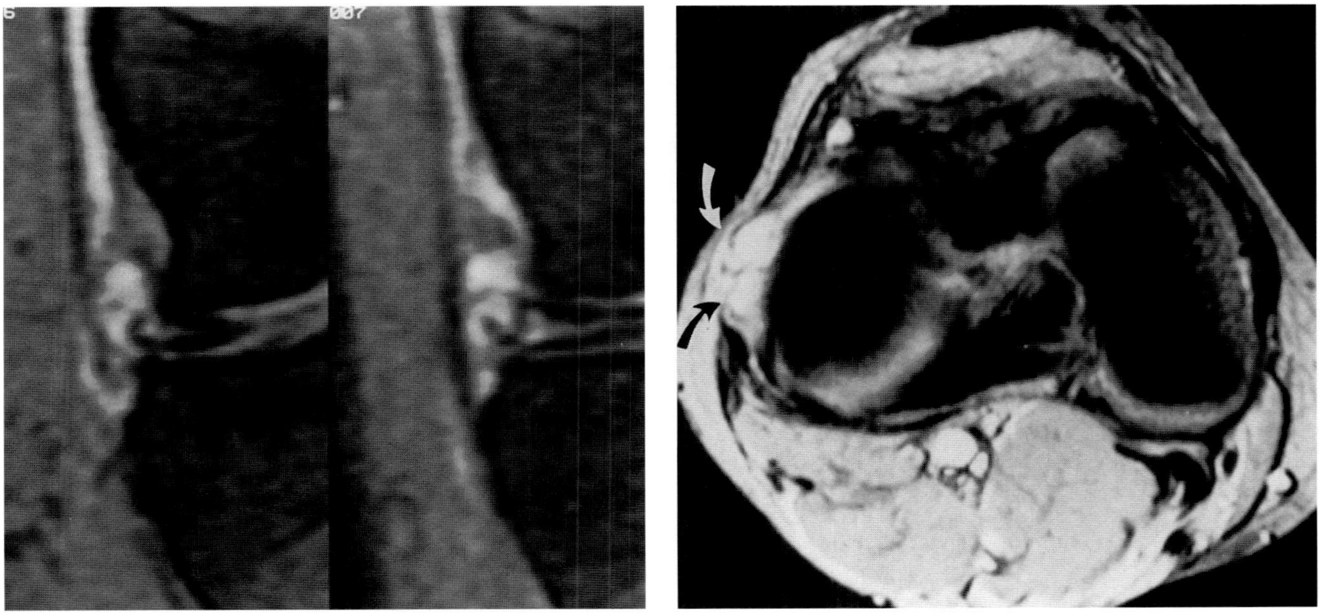

A B

FIG. 4-28. Small meniscal cyst with complex tear. **A:** Coronal T2*-weighted gradient-echo MPGR (TR 400 msec, TE 20 msec, flip angle 20°) shows the extensive tear involving the meniscus and containment of the cyst by the fascia. **B:** Axial T2*-weighted gradient-echo MPGR (TR 400 msec, TE 20 msec, flip angle 45°). The mensical cyst is seen to be septated *(arrows).*

Until recently it was accepted that a meniscal cyst could only be treated with meniscectomy, because otherwise the cyst would recur. A number of treatments have been devised that have been used with success in treatment of cysts consisting of cyst drainage and meniscal repair. At times removal of the meniscus is inevitable, especially if meniscal damage is diffuse or complex (162,163). On occasion meniscal cysts may be mistaken for pes anserine bursitis (159,164,165), although this usually is located more inferiorly, or for a rare synovial hemangioma (166).

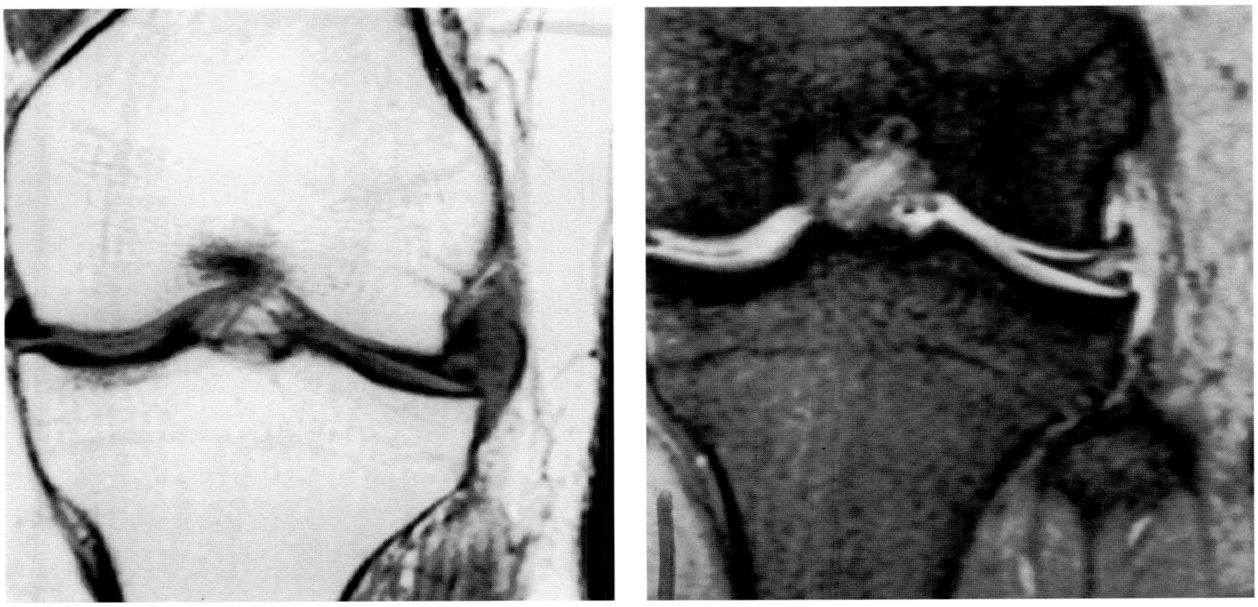

A B

FIG. 4-29. A: Coronal T1-weighted spin echo (TR 400 msec, TE 20 msec). **B:** Coronal T2*-weighted gradient-echo MPGR (TR 300 msec, TE 13 msec, flip angle 30°). Two examples of expanding meniscal cysts that are pushing aside the lateral retaining structures. Note the relatively intact-appearing menisci; triangular configuration has been retained.

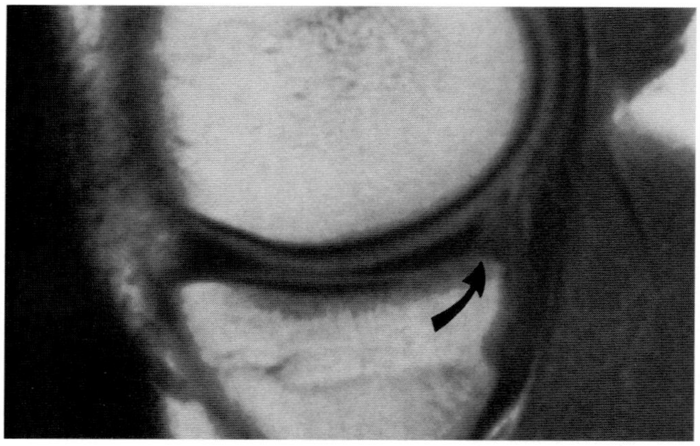

FIG. 4-30. Sagittal T1-weighted spin-echo image (TR 600 msec, TE 16 msec) showing meniscocapsular separation. A band of increased signal is seen immediately behind the posterior horn of the medial meniscus, representing a space separating the meniscus from the joint capsule *(arrow)*.

Meniscal ossicles are very rare. It is unclear if they are congenital or acquired. Both probably occur. At least some are symptomatic, probably because of the ossicle functioning as a stress riser in the meniscus, leading to a tear. On MRI the ossicle is of low signal intensity on all sequences and may have a high-signal center (167,168).

Chondrocalcinosis has been alluded to earlier. It is present commonly in older individuals and in those with certain metabolic disorders (e.g., calcium pyrophosphate deposition disease, renal failure, etc.). When calcification is very fine it may well go unnoticed on MRI. As it becomes more extensive, the meniscal signal may increase. This may be due to scarring around the deposits. High-signal calcium has also been encountered in the central nervous system, and there may be an analogous situation in the meniscus. When very heavy calcification is present, low signal is usually observed.

MENISCOCAPSULAR SEPARATION

At times when the injury to the knee occurs, the meniscus may actually separate from the joint capsule. This is more likely to occur at the posterior horns of the menisci, particularly medially. Once the meniscus is actually detached from the capsule it is less susceptible to becoming torn and is considered a stable injury by some authorities. Indeed, part of the reason the posterior horn of the medial meniscus is so frequently seen to be torn is its relative lack of mobility because of its firm adherence to the capsule (139).

To make the diagnosis, the presence of fluid interposed between the peripheral edge of the meniscus and capsule must be observed (Fig. 4-30). Hence, T2-weighted or T2* images are helpful in making this diagnosis. In addition, on sagittal MRI, the tibial plateau cartilage should be covered by the posterior horn of the medial meniscus; if this is not observed, the diagnosis of meniscocapsular separation should be entertained. This diagnosis is not easily made if the separation is narrow.

In this regard, arthrography may occasionally demonstrate a separation that is difficult to appreciate on MRI. MR arthrography either with saline or gadolinium may be helpful. The use of a tensor bandage to increase intra-articular pressure may further increase the chances of making the diagnosis by increasing the likelihood that fluid will find its way into the area of separation. Because meniscocapsular separations are often readily repaired, it is important to keep this diagnosis in mind when evaluating the posterior horn of the medial meniscus.

REFERENCES

1. Beltran J, Noto AM, Mosure JC, Weiss KL, Zuelzer W, Christoforidis AJ. The knee: surface-coil MR imaging at 1.5 T. *Radiology* 1986; 159:747–751.
2. Polly DW Jr, Callaghan JJ, Sikes RA, et al. The accuracy of selective magnetic resonance imaging compared with the findings of arthroscopy of the knee. *J Bone Joint Surg* 1988;70-A:192–198. Abstract.
3. Watanabe AT, Carter BC, Teitelbaum GP, Seeger LL, Bradley WG Jr. Normal Variations in MR imaging of the knee: appearance and frequency. *AJR* 1989;153:341–344.
4. Mink JH, Levy T, Crues JV, III. Tears of the anterior cruciate ligament and menisci of the knee: MR imaging evaluation. *Radiology* 1988; 167:769–774.
5. Reicher MA, Hartzman S, Bassett LW, Mandelbaum B, Duckwiler G, Gold RH. MR imaging of the knee. Part I. traumatic disorders. *Radiology* 1987;162:547–551.
6. Fischer SP, Fox JM, DelPizzo W, Friedman MJ, Snyder SJ, Ferkel RD. Accuracy of diagnoses from magnetic resonance imaging of the knee. *J Bone Joint Surg* 1991;73-A:2–10.
7. Mink JH, Deutsch AL. Magnetic resonance imaging of the knee. *Clin Orthop* 1989;244:29–47.
8. Mandelbaum BR, Finerman GAM, Reicher MA, et al. Magnetic resonance imaging as a tool for evaluation of traumatic knee injuries: anatomical and pathoanatomical correlations. *Am J Sports Med* 1986; 14:361–370.
9. Mesgarzadeh M, Schneck CD, Bonakdarpour A. Magnetic resonance imaging of the knee and correlation with normal anatomy. *Radiographics* 1988;8:707–733.
10. Bellon EM, Keith MW, Coleman PE, Shah ZR. Magnetic resonance imaging of internal derangements of the knee. *Radiographics* 1988; 8:95–118.
11. Jackson DW, Jennings LD, Maywood RM. Magnetic resonance imaging of the knee: arthroscopy confirms accuracy of MRI of the knee. *Am J Sports Med* 1988;16:29–38. Abstract.
12. Crues JV III, Ryu R, Morgan FW. Meniscal pathology: the expanding role of magnetic resonance imaging. *Clin Orthop* 1990;252:80–87.
13. Reicher MA, Hartzman S, Duckwiler GR, Bassett LW, Anderson LJ, Gold RH. Meniscal injuries: detection using MR imaging. *Radiology* 1986;159:753–757.
14. Crues JV, III, Mink JH, Levy TL, Lotysch M, Stoller DW. Meniscal tears of the knee: accuracy of MR imaging. *Radiology* 1987;164: 445–448.
15. Wojtys E, Wilson M, Buckwalter K, Braunstein E, Martel W. Magnetic resonance imaging of knee hyaline cartilage and intraarticular pathology. *Am J Sports Med* 1987;15:455–463.
16. Arnoczky SP, Warren RF. The microvasculature of the Meniscus and its response to injury: an experimental study in the dog. *Am J Sports Med* 1983;11:131–141.
17. Gray DJ, Gardner E. Prenatal development of the human knee and superior tibiofibular joint. *Am J Anat* 1950;86:235–286.
18. O'Rahilly R, Gardner E. The timing and sequence of events in the development of the limbs of the human embryo. *Anat Embryol* 1975; 148:1–23.
19. Kaplan EB. The embryology of the menisci of the knee joint. *Bull Hosp Joint Dis* 1955;16:111–124.

20. Gardner E, O'Rahilly R. The early development of the knee joint in staged human embryos. *J Anat* 1968;102:289–299.
21. Sledge CB, Zaleske DJ. Resnick D, Niwayama G, eds. *Diagnosis of bone and joint disorders,* 2nd ed. Philadelphia: WB Saunders, 1988; 18:604–624.
22. Ghosh P, Taylor TKF. The knee joint meniscus: a fibrocartilage of some distinction. *Clin Orthop* 1987;224:52–63.
23. Harley JD. An anatomic-arthrographic study of the relationships of the lateral meniscus and the popliteus tendon. *AJR* 1977;128:181–187.
24. Wickstrom KT, Spitzer RM, Olsson HE. Roentgen anatomy of the posterior horn of the lateral meniscus. *Radiology* 1975;116:617–619.
25. McIntyre JL. Arthrography of the lateral meniscus. *Radiology* 1972; 105:531–536.
26. DeHaven KE. Rationale for meniscus repair or excision. *Clin Sports Med* 1985;4:267–273.
27. Bray RC, Dandy DJ. Meniscal lesions and chronic anterior cruciate ligament deficiency: meniscal tears occurring before and after reconstruction. *J Bone Joint Surg* 1989;71B:128–130.
28. Henning CE, Lynch MA. Current concepts of meniscal function and pathology. *Clin Sports Med* 1985;4:259–265.
29. DiStefano VJ. Function, Post-traumatic sequelae and current concepts of management of knee meniscus injuries: a review article. *Clin Orthop* 1980;151:143–146.
30. Hazel WA, Rand JA, Morrey BF. Results of meniscectomy in the knee with anterior cruciate ligament deficiency. *Clin Orthop* 1993; 292:232–238.
31. Warren RF, Levy IM. Meniscal lesions associated with anterior cruciate ligament injury. *Clin Orthop* 1983;172:32–37.
32. Warren RF. Meniscectomy and repair in the anterior cruciate ligament-deficient patient. *Clin Orthop* 1990;252:55–63.
33. Levy IM, Torzilli PA, Gould JD, Warren RF. The effect of lateral meniscectomy on motion of the knee. *J Bone Joint Surg* 1989;71A: 401–406.
34. Sturup J, Iversen BF, Lauersen N. Abnormal knee mobility and meniscal injury. *Acta Orthop Scand* 1987;58:655–657.
35. Burr DB, Radin EL. Meniscal function and the importance of meniscal regeneration on preventing late medial compartment osteoarthrosis. *Clin Orthop Rel Res* 1982;171:121–126.
36. Fithian DC, Kelly MA, Mow VC. Material properties and structure-function relationships in the menisci. *Clin Orthop* 1990;252:19–31.
37. McDevitt CA, Webber RJ. The ultrastructure and biochemistry of meniscal cartilage. *Clin Orthop* 1990;252:8–18.
38. Jelaso DV. The fascicles of the lateral meniscus: an anatomic-arthrographic correlation. *Radiology* 1975;114:335–339.
39. Baratz ME, Fu FH, Mengato R. Meniscal tears: the effect of meniscectomy and of repair on intraarticular contact areas and stress in the human knee. *Am J Sports Med* 1986;14:270–360.
40. Krause WR, Pope MH, Johnson RJ, Wilder DG. Mechanical changes in the knee after meniscectomy. *J Bone Joint Surg* 1976;58-A: 599–604.
41. Lanzer WL, Komenda G. Changes in articular cartilage after meniscectomy. *Clin Orthop* 1990;252:41–48.
42. DeHaven KE. Meniscus repair in the athlete. *Clin Orthop* 1985;198: 31–35.
43. Abdon P, Turner MS, Pettersson H, Lindstrand A, Stenstrom A, Swanson JG. A long-term follow-up study of total meniscectomy in children. *Clin Orthop* 1990;257:166–170.
44. Ringertz HG. Arthrography of the Knee. II. Isolated and combined lesions. *Acta Radiol Diagn* 1976;17:235–248.
45. Ghosh P, Sutherland J, Bellenger C, Read R, Darvodelsky A. The influence of weight-bearing exercise on articular cartilage of meniscectomized joints: an experimental study in sheep. *Clin Orthop* 1990; 252:101–113.
46. Dowson SD, Wright V. Functions of the menisci: a preliminary study. *Ann Rheum Dis* 1974;33:111
47. Niitsu M, Anno I, Fukubayashi T, Shimojo H, Kuno S, Akisada M. Tears of cruciate ligaments and menisci: evaluation with cine MR imaging. *Radiology* 1991;178:859–864.
48. Tegtmeyer CJ, McCue FC, Higgins SM, Ball DW. Arthrography of the knee: a comparative study of the accuracy of single and double contrast techniques. *Radiology* 1979;132:37–41.
49. Gillies H, Seligson D. Precision in the diagnosis of meniscal lesions: a comparison of clinical evaluation, arthrography, and arthroscopy. *J Bone Joint Surg* 1979;61A:343–346.
50. Shakespear DT, Rigby HS. The bucket-handle tear of the meniscus: a clinical and arthrographic study. *J Bone Joint Surg* 1983;65B: 383–387.
51. DeSmet AA. Meniscal tears on knee arthrography: patterns of arthrographic abnormalities. *Skeletal Radiol* 1985;14:280–285.
52. Manco LG, Berlow ME. Meniscal tears-comparison of arthrography, CT, and MRI. *Crit Rev Diagn Imaging* 1989;29:151–179.
53. Turner AF, Budin E. Arthrography of the knee: a simplified technique. *Radiology* 1970;97:505–508.
54. Angell FL. Fluoroscopic technique of double contrast arthrography of the knee. *Radiol Clin North Am* 1971;9:85–98.
55. Leven H. Evaluation of a modified method for arthrography of the knee. *Acta Radiol Diagn* 1977;18:351–356.
56. Butt WP, McIntyre JL. Double-contrast arthrography. *Radiology* 1969;92:487–499.
57. Dalinka MK, Coren GS, Wershba M. Knee arthrography. *CRC Crit Rev Radiol Sci* 1973;September:1–59.
58. Hall FM. Further pitfalls in knee arthrography. *J Can Assoc Radiol* 1978;29:179–184.
59. Dumas J, Edde DJ. Meniscal abnormalities: prospective correlation of double-contrast arthrography and arthroscopy. *Radiology* 1986;1986: 453–456.
60. Freiberger RH, Pavlov H. Knee arthrography. *Radiology* 1988;166: 489–492.
61. Kaye JJ. Knee arthrography today. *Radiology* 1985;157:265–266.
62. O'Malley BP. Value of delayed films in knee arthrography. *J Can Assoc Radiol* 1974;25:144–146.
63. Kiss J, Moir JD. Experience with arthrographic examination of the knee joint. *J Can Assoc Radiol* 1968;19:187–191.
64. Olson RW. Knee arthrography. *AJR* 1967;101:897–914.
65. Hall FM. Pitfalls in knee arthrography. *Radiology* 1976;118:55–62.
66. Bonamo JJ, Shulman G. Double contrast arthrography of the knee: a comparison to clinical diagnosis and arthroscopic findings. *Orthopedics* 1988;11:1041–1046.
67. Thijn CJP. Accuracy of double-contrast arthrography and arthroscopy of the knee joint. *Skeletal Radiol* 1982;8:187–192.
68. Levinsohn EM, Baker BE. Prearthrotomy diagnostic evaluation of the knee: review of 100 cases diagnosed by arthrography and arthroscopy. *AJR* 1980;134:107–111.
69. Selesnick FH, Noble HB, Bachman DC, Steinberg FL. Internal derangement of the knee: diagnosis by arthrography, arthroscopy, and arthrotomy. *Clin Orthop* 1985;198:26–30.
70. Manco LG, Kavanaugh JH, Lozman J, Colman ND, Bilfield BS, Fay JJ. Diagnosis of meniscal tears using high-resolution computed tomography: correlation with arthroscopy. *J Bone Joint Surg* 1987;69A: 498–502.
71. Manco LG, Lozman J, Coleman ND, Kavanaugh JH, Bilfield BS, Dougherty J. Noninvasive evaluation of knee meniscal tears: preliminary comparison of MR imaging and CT. *Radiology* 1987;163: 727–730.
72. Manco LG, Berlow ME, Czajka J, Alfred R. Bucket-handle tears of the meniscus: appearance at CT. *Radiology* 1988;168:709–712.
73. Buttner-Janz K, Schellnack K, Rieder T. Noninvasive diagnosis of cruciate ligament damage with particular reference to computed tomography with arthrography. *Am J Sports Med* 1989;17:501–504.
74. Passariello R, Trecco F, De Paulis F, Masciocchi C, Bonanni G, Beomonte Zobel B. Meniscal lesions of the knee joint: CT diagnosis. *Radiology* 1985;157:29–34.
75. Ghelman B. Meniscal tears of the knee: evaluation by high-resolution CT combined with arthrography. *Radiology* 1985;157:23–27.
76. McDonnell CH, Jeffrey RB, Bjorkengren AG, Li KCP. Intraarticular sonography for imaging the knee menisci: evaluation in cadaveric specimens. *AJR* 1992;159:573–574.
77. Selby B, Richardson ML, Nelson BD, Graney DO, Mack LA. Sonography in the detection of meniscal injuries of the knee: evaluation in cadavers. *AJR* 1987;149:549–553.
78. Li KC, Henkelman M, Poon PY, Rubenstein J. MR imaging of the normal knee. *J Comput Assist Tomogr* 1984;8:1147–1154.
79. Juhl M, Boe S. Arthroscopy in children, with special emphasis on meniscal lesions. *Injury* 1986;17:171–173.
80. Munk PL. Magnetic resonance imaging of the knee: an overview. *J Can Assoc Radiol* 1989;40:296–303.
81. Munk PL, Vellet AD, Levin MF. MRI evaluation of the knee meniscus. *Australas Radiol* 1993;37:40–46.

82. Stoller DW, Martin C, Crues JV, III, Kaplan L, Mink JH. Meniscal tears: pathologic correlation with MR imaging. *Radiology* 1987;163: 731–735.
83. Dillon EH, Pope CF, Jokl P, Lynch K. The clinical significance of stage 2 meniscal abnormalities on magnetic resonance knee images. *Magn Reson Imaging* 1990;8:411–415.
84. Hodler J, Haghighi P, Pathria MN, Trudell D, Resnick D. Meniscal changes in the elderly: correlation of MR imaging and histologic findings. *Radiology* 1992;184:221–225.
85. Hough AJ Jr, Webber RJ. Pathology of the meniscus. *Clin Orthop* 1990;252:32–40.
86. Kursunoglu-Brahme S, Schwaighofer B, Gundry C, Ho C, Resnick D. Jogging causes acute changes in the knee joint: an MR study in normal volunteers. *AJR* 1990;154:1233–1235.
87. Shellock FG, Mink JH. Knees of trained long-distance runners: MR imaging before and after competition. *Radiology* 1991;179:635–637.
88. Ferrer-Roca O, Vilalta C. Lesions of the meniscus. Part I: Macroscopic and histologic findings. *Clin Orthop* 1980;146:289–300.
89. Hajek PC, Gylys-Morin VM, Baker L, Sartoris DJ, Haghighi P, Resnick D. The high signal intensity meniscus of the knee: magnetic resonance evaluation and in vivo correlation. *Invest Radiol* 1987;22: 883–890.
90. Kornick J, Trefelner E, McCarthy S, Lange R, Lynch K, Jokl P. Meniscal abnormalities in the asymptomatic population at MR imaging. *Radiology* 1990;177:463–465.
91. Ferrer-Roca O, Vilalta C. Lesions of the meniscus. Part II: horizontal cleavages and lateral cysts. *Clin Orthop* 1980;146:301–307.
92. Dillon EH, Pope CF, Jokl P, Lynch JK. Follow-up of grade 2 meniscal abnormalities in the stable knee. *Radiology* 1991;181:849–852.
93. Reing JW, McDevitt ER, Ove PN. Progression of meniscal degenerative changes in college football players: evaluation with MR imaging. *Radiology* 1991;181:255–257.
94. Brunner MC, Flower SP, Evancho AM, Allman FL, Apple DF, Fajman WA. MRI of the athletic knee: findings in asymptomatic professional basketball and collegiate football players. *Invest Radiol* 1989; 24:72–75.
95. Tersegno MM. Meniscal tears in marathon runners (Letter). *AJR* 1992; 159:434
96. Boden SD, Davis DO, Dina TS, Stoller DW, Brown SD, Vailas JC, Labropoulos PA. A prospective and blided investigation of magnetic resonance of the knee: abnormal findings in asymptomatic subjects. *Clin Orthop* 1992;282:177–185.
97. Shellock FG, Deutsch AL, Mink JH, Kerr R. Do asymptomatic marathon runners have an increased prevalence of meniscal abnormalities? An MR study of the knee in 23 volunteers. *AJR* 1991;157:1239–1241.
98. DeSmet AA, Graf BK. Meniscal tears missed on MR imaging: relationship to meniscal tear patterns and anterior cruciate ligament tears. *AJR* 1994;162:905–911.
99. Binfield PM, Maffulli N, King JB. Patterns of Meniscal tears associated with anterior cruciate ligament lesions in athletes. *Injury* 1993; 24:557–561.
100. Zarins B, Adams M. Knee injuries in sports. *New Engl J Med* 1988; 318:950–961.
101. Vangsness CT, DeCampos J, Merritt PO, Wiss DA. Meniscal injury associated with femoral shaft fractures. *J Bone Joint Surg* 1993;75-B:207–209.
102. Vangsness CT, Ghaderi B, Hohl M, Moore T. Arthroscopy of meniscal injuries with tibial plateau fractures. *J Bone Joint Surg* 1994;76-B: 488–490.
103. Beltran J, Noto AM, Mosure JC, Bools JC, Zuelzer W, Christoforidis AJ. Meniscal tears: MR demonstration of experimentally produced injuries. *Radiology* 1986;158:691–693.
104. Shogry MEC, Pope TL. Vacuum phenomenon simulating meniscal of cartilaginous injury of the knee at MR imaging. *Radiology* 191; 180:513–515.
105. Araki Y, Ootani F, Tsukaguchi I, Ootani M, Furukawa T, Yamamoto T, Tomoda K, Mitomo M. MR diagnosis of meniscal tears of the knee: value of axial three-dimensional Fourier transformation GRASS images. *AJR* 1992;158:587–590.
106. Tyrrell RL, Gluckert K, Pathria MN, Modic MT. Fast three-dimensional MR imaging of the knee: comparison with arthroscopy. *Radiology* 1988;166:865–872.
107. Soloman SL, Totty WG, Lee JKT. MR imaging of the knee: comparison of three-dimensional FISP and two-dimensional spin-echo pulse sequences. *Radiology* 1989;173:739–742.
108. Harms SE, Flamig DP, Fisher CF, Fulmer JM. New method for fast MR imaging of the knee. *Radiology* 1989;173:743–750.
109. Spritzer CE, Vogler JB, Martinez S, et al. MR imaging of the knee: preliminary results with a 3DFT GRASS pulse sequence. *AJR* 1988; 150:597–603.
110. Reeder JD, Matz SO, Becker L, Andelman SM. MR Imaging of the knee in the sagittal projection: comparison of three-dimensional gradient-echo and spin-echo sequences. *AJR* 1989;153:537–540.
111. Adam G, Bohndorf K, Drobnitzky M, Guenther RW. MR imaging of the knee: three-dimensional volume imaging combined with fast processing. *J Comput Assist Tomogr* 1989;13:983–988.
112. Harms SE, Muschler G. Three-dimensional MR imaging of the knee using surface coils. *J Comput Assist Tomogr* 1986;10:773–777.
113. Haggar AM, Froelich JW, Hearshen DO, Sadasivan K. Meniscal abnormalities of the knee: 3DFT fast-scan GRASS MR imaging. *AJR* 1988;150:1341–1344.
114. Haramati N, Staron RB, Rubin S, Shreck EH, Feldman F, Kierman H. The flipped meniscus sign. *Skeletal Radiol* 1993;22:273–277.
115. Singson RD, Feldman F, Staron R, Kiernan H. MR imaging of displaced bucket-handle tear of the medial meniscus. *AJR* 1991;156: 121–124.
116. Weiss KL, Morehouse HT, Levy IM. Sagittal MR images of the knee: a low-signal band parallel to the posterior cruciate ligament caused by a displaced bucket-handle tear. *AJR* 1991;156:117–119.
117. Mesgarzadeh M, Moyer R, Leder DS, et al. MR imaging of the knee: expanded classification and pitfalls to interpretation of meniscal tears. *Radiographics* 1993;13:489–500.
118. Davis SJ, Teresi LM, Bradley WG, Burke JW. The "notch" sign: meniscal contour deformities as indicators of tear in MR imaging of the knee. *J Comput Assist Tomogr* 1990;14:975–980.
119. Hall FM. Buckled meniscus revisited (letter). *AJR* 1991;156:200
120. Chew FS. Medial meniscal flounce: demonstration on MR imaging of the knee. *AJR* 1990;155:199
121. Hall FM. Buckled meniscus. *Radiology* 1978;126:89–90.
122. Tuckman GA, Miller WJ, Remo JW, Fritts HM, Rozansky MI. Radial tears of the menisci: MR findings. *AJR* 1994;163:395–400.
123. Kaplan PA, Nelson NL, Garvin KL, Brown DE. MR of the knee: the significance of high signal in the meniscus that does not clearly extend to the surface. *AJR* 1991;156:333–336.
124. DeSmet AA, Norris MA, Yandow DR, Quintana FA, Graf BK, Keene JS. MR Diagnosis of meniscal tears of the knee: importance of high signal in the meniscus that extends to the surface. *AJR* 1993;161: 101–107.
125. Disler DG, Kattapuram SV, Chew FS, Rosenthal DI, Patel D. Meniscal tears of the knee: preliminary comparison of three-dimensional MR reconstruction with two-dimensional MR imaging and arthroscopy. *AJR* 1993;160:343–345.
126. Quinn SF, Brown TR, Szumowski J. Menisci of the knee: radial MR imaging correlated with arthroscopy in 259 patients. *Radiology* 1992; 185:577–580.
127. Quinn SF, Brown TF. Meniscal Tears Diagnosed with MR imaging versus arthroscopy: how reliable a standard is arthroscopy? *Radiology* 1991;181:843–847.
128. DeSmet AA, Tuite MJ, Norris MA, Swan JS. MR diagnosis of meniscal tears: analysis of causes of errors. *AJR* 1995;163:1419–1423.
129. Evancho AM, Fajman WA, Stiles RG, Brunner MC, Peterson J, Fleming L. Magnetic resonance imaging of knee menisci: comparison of spin echo pulse sequences. *Invest Radiol* 1990;25:1224–1227.
130. Rubin DA, Kneeland JB, Listerud J, Underberg-Davis SJ, Dalinka MK. MR diagnosis of meniscal tears of the knee: value of fast spin-echo vs conventional spin-echo pulse sequences. *AJR* 1994;162: 1131–1135.
131. Watanabe AT, Carter BC, Teitelbaum GP, Bradley WG Jr. Common pitfalls in magnetic resonance imaging of the knee. *J Bone Joint Surg* 1989;71-A:857–862.
132. Herman L, Beltran J. Pitfalls in MR imaging of the knee. *Radiology* 1988;167:775–781.
133. DeSmet AA, Norris MA, Yandrow DR, Graf BK, Keene JS. Diagnosis of meniscal tears of the knee with MR imaging: effect of observer variation and sample size on sensitivity and specificity. *AJR* 1993; 160:555–559.
134. Raunest J, Oberle K, Loehnert J, Hoetzinger H. The clinical value of

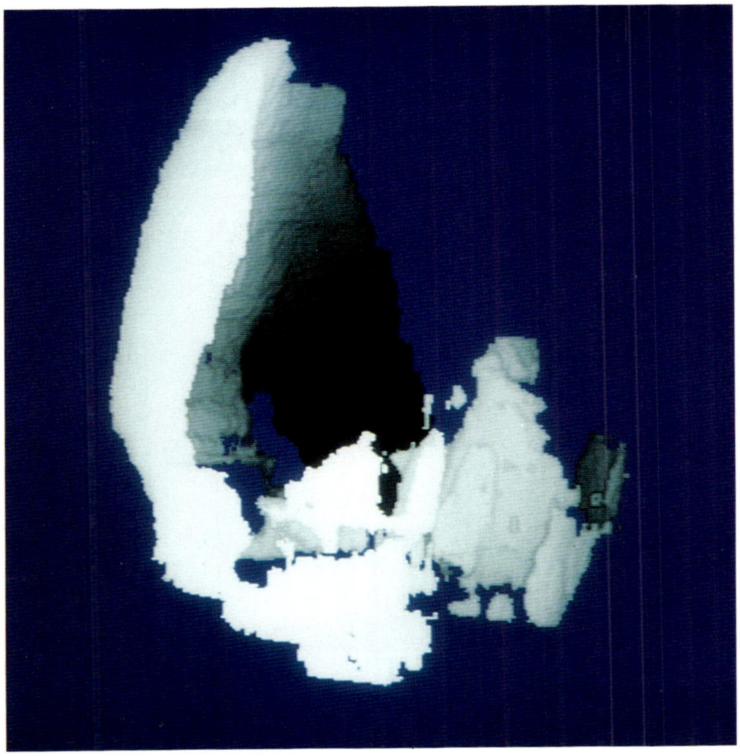

Color plate 1. Three-dimensional display. A large joint effusion is displayed as viewed from the posterolateral aspect. (Courtesy of A. Heuck and P. Lang, Berlin, Federal Republic of Germany, and H. Genant, San Francisco, California.)

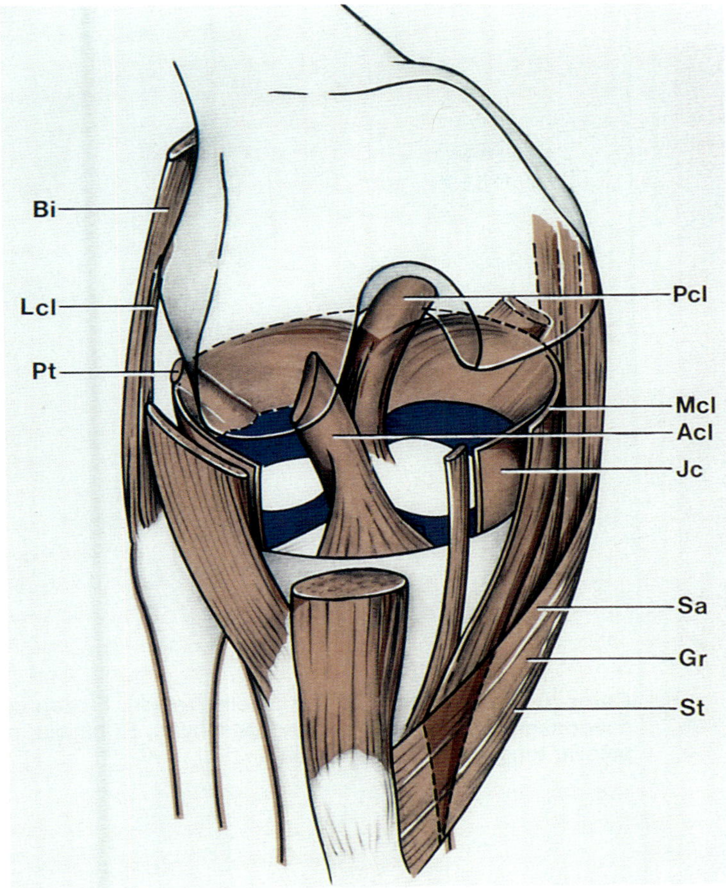

Color plate 2. Diagram of the cruciate ligaments. View of the knee from anterior perspective with the joint partially flexed. Bi, biceps femoris; Lcl, lateral collateral ligament; Pt, popliteus tendon; Pcl, posterior cruciate ligament; Mcl, medial collateral ligament; Acl, anterior cruciate ligament; Sa, sartorius; Gr, gracilis; St, semitendinosus; Jc, joint capsule.

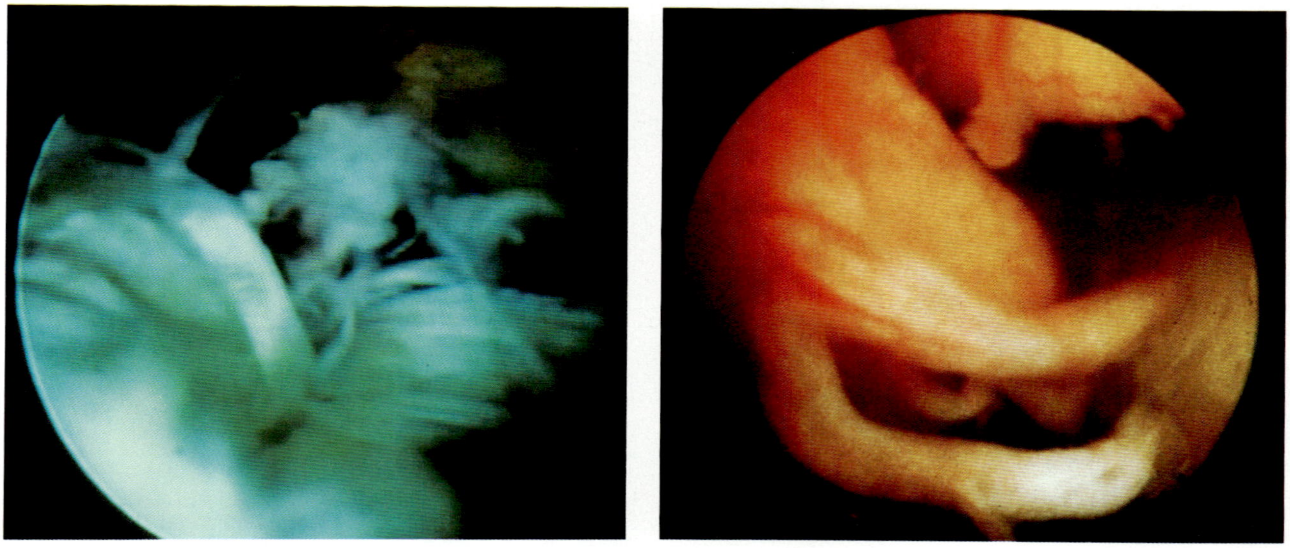

A B

Color plate 3. Arthroscopic evaluation of anterior cruciate **(A,B).** Two arthroscopic images of disrupted anterior cruciate ligaments. In **(A)** the torn end is more frayed than in **(B).**

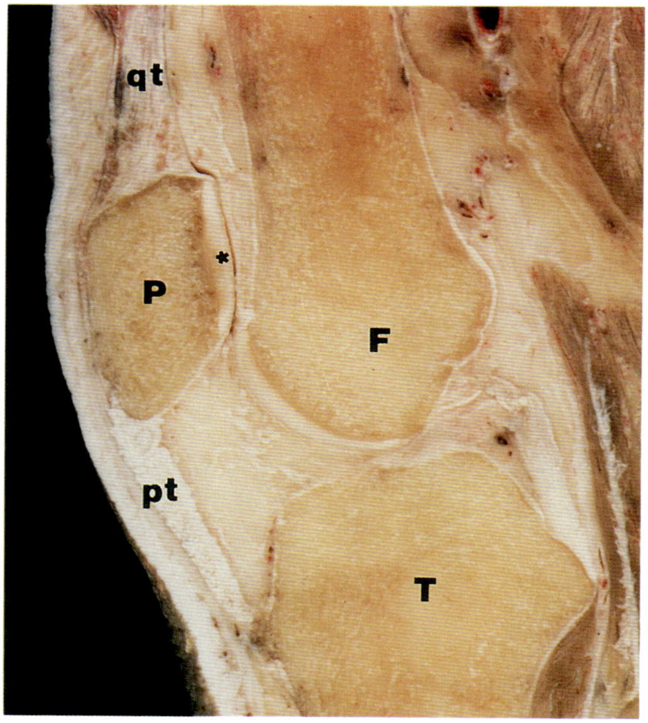

Color plate 4. Anatomy of the patellar region. Frozen cadaver sagittal section. qt, quadriceps tendon; P, patella; pt, patellar tendon; F, femur; T, tibia.

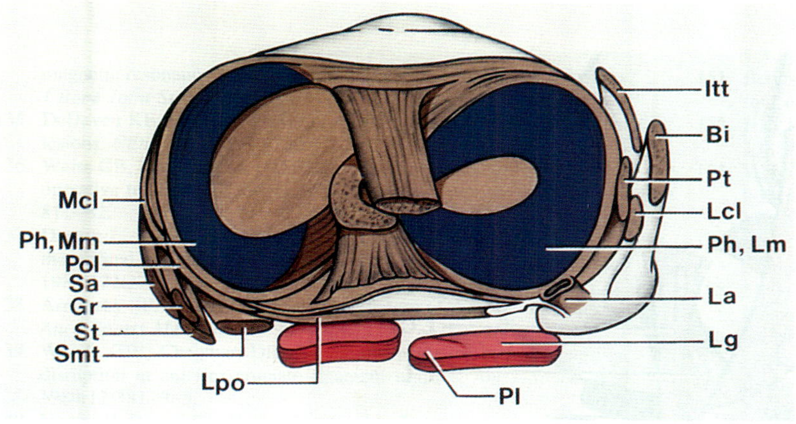

Color plate 5. Schematic diagram of the menisci. Mcl, medial collateral ligament; Ph, Mm, posterior horn medial meniscus; Pol, popliteal oblique ligament; Sa, sartorius; Gr, gracilis; St, semitendinosus; Smt, semimembranosus; Lpo, posterior oblique ligament; Pl, popliteus ligament; Lg, lateral head gastrocnemius; La, arcuate ligament; Ph, Lm, posterior horn lateral meniscus; Lcl, lateral collateral ligament; Pt, popliteus tendon; Bi, biceps femoris; Itt, iliotibial tract.

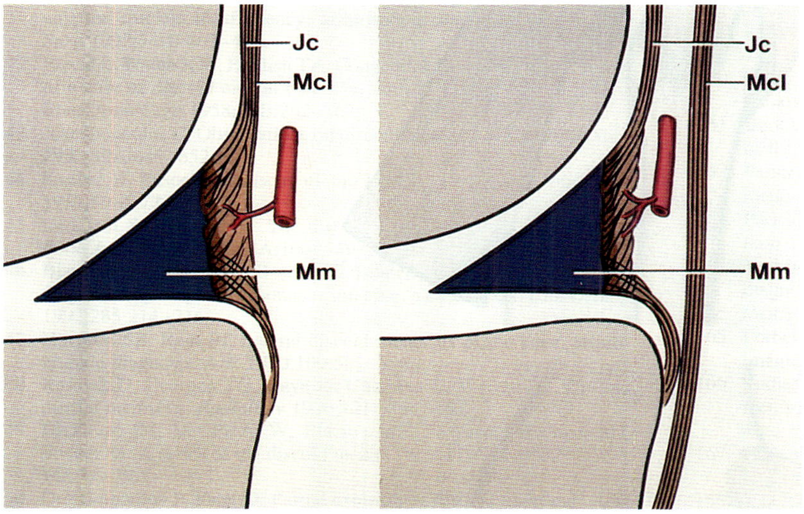

Color plate 6. Meniscal blood supply. The medial meniscus is illustrated here. On the left is the posterior portion of the meniscus; on the right a more anterior segment is shown. Only the periphery of the meniscus is well vascularized and amenable to repair. Jc, joint capsule; Mcl, medial collateral ligament; Mm, medial meniscus.

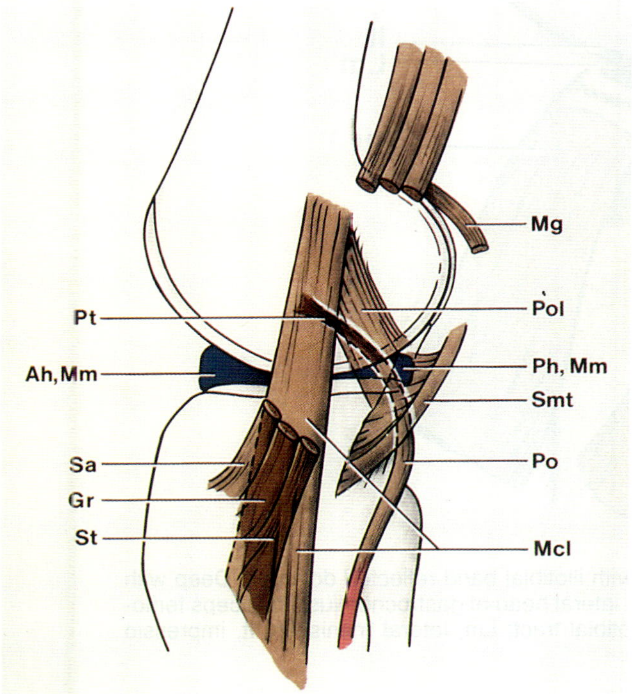

Color plate 7. Medial aspect of the knee. Sa, sartorius; Ah, Mm, anterior horn, medial meniscus; Gr, gracilis; St, semitendinosus; Mcl, medial collateral ligament; Ph, Mm, posterior horn, medial meniscus; Smt, semimembranosus; Mg, medial head of gastrocnemius.

MRI of the Knee, Second Edition,
edited by P. L. Munk and C. A. Helms.
Lippincott-Raven Publishers, Philadelphia © 1996.

CHAPTER 5

Collateral Ligaments and Related Structures

Peter L. Munk, A. Dale Vellet, and Dennis L. Janzen

The knee is a complex joint in terms both of kinematics and function and of anatomy. Instability in particular has been an important problem, from the point of view of orthopedic practice, and a vast amount of literature has appeared in the orthopedic journals addressing this topic. At present, considerable debate persists as to the role of the different structures of the knee joint in providing stability. Even the anatomy of the collateral ligaments and their associated structures is not fully agreed upon. In this chapter we review the anatomy and function of the collateral ligaments and other supporting structures of the knee.

ANATOMY AND FUNCTION

The knee joint depends on many different structures to maintain stability as it goes through its complex range of motion. It is generally accepted that the cruciate ligaments play an important role in maintaining stability (1,2). Considerable debate exists as to the precise contribution of the posterior cruciate to joint stability, with some feeling that the anterior cruciate is the most important structure contributing to stability and that the posterior cruciate plays only a relatively minor role (3,4). On the other hand, some authorities, such as Hughston and others, advocate an absolutely crucial role for the posterior cruciate ligament and feel that knee stability is fundamentally dependent on this structure (5–8). In addition, the menisci play an important role in stabilizing the knee, particularly when cruciate ligament insufficiency exists. Finally, the so-called supporting structures of the knee also contribute to knee stability, although again their precise contribution is a matter of considerable debate (9,10).

P. L. Munk: Department of Diagnostic Imaging, British Columbia Cancer Agency, and Department of Radiology, University of British Columbia, Vancouver, British Columbia, Canada V5Z 4E6.

A. D. Vellet: Department of Diagnostic Imaging, University of Calgary, Foothills Hospital, Alberta, Canada T2N 2T9.

D. L. Janzen: Department of Radiology, Vancouver Hospital and Health Sciences Center, Vancouver, British Columbia, Canada V5Z 1M9.

The supporting structures of the knee can best be divided into two major groups. The first of these has been referred to as the static stabilizers, which consist essentially of ligaments that can be divided into capsular and noncapsular groups (11–13). The second category is made up of the dynamic stabilizers, which consist of musculotendinous units and their aponeuroses. The structures of the medial and lateral aspects of the knee have many similarities, but they also have differences, especially posteriorly. The supporting structures of the medial compartment are considered to extend medially from the patellar tendon to the posterior cruciate ligament, and those of the lateral compartment are defined in a similar fashion at the opposite side of the knee. The anterior and middle thirds of the supporting structures of the two compartments are similar, with marked differences residing in the posterior third.

At the medial side of the knee (Fig. 5-1; see also color plate 7), the anterior third of the supporting structures consists of the anterior capsule of the joint with reinforcement from the vastus medialis retinaculum. The ligaments are thin and loose and obtain much of their strength from the overlying dynamic stabilizing aponeurosis of the vastus medialis component of the quadriceps mechanism. This portion of the quadriceps is important in maintaining stability, particularly when the knee is flexed. In the middle third the capsular ligaments are very strong. The deep portions of these supporting structures are often called the deep layer of the medial ligament, which is composed of a strong upper meniscofemoral portion, with a weaker lower meniscotibial portion. The upper part is attached to the medial femoral condyle more anteriorly than the more superficial tibial collateral ligament (14). It has a strong attachment to the middle third of the medial meniscus and functions in part to hold the meniscus to the femur for stabilization during flexion and extension. The lower portion of the deep layer of the medial collateral ligament continues downward as the so-called coronary ligament and is attached to the tibia immediately below the articular surface of the joint (15). The laxity inher-

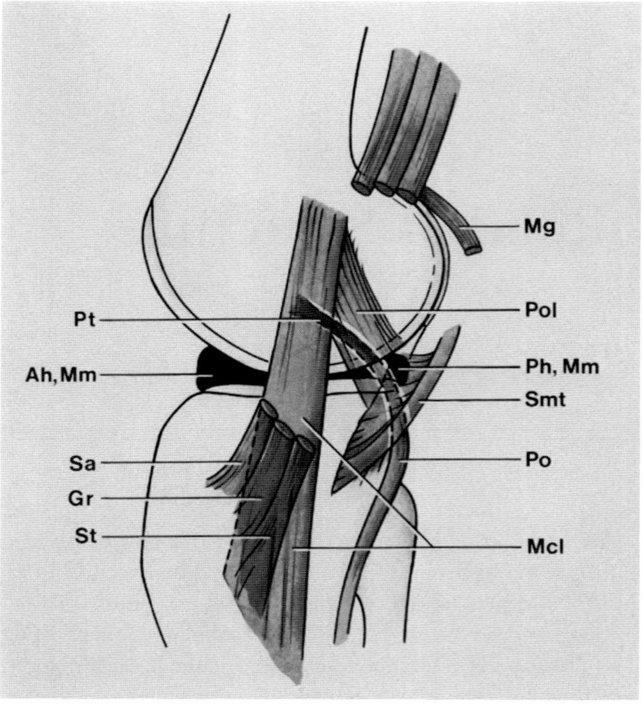

FIG. 5-1. Medial aspect of the knee. Sa, sartorius; Ah, Mm, anterior horn, medial meniscus; Gr, gracilis; St, semitendinosus; Mcl, medial collateral ligament; Ph, Mm, posterior horn, medial meniscus; Smt, semimembranosus; Mg, medial head of gastrocnemius.

ent in this structure permits the meniscus to move to some degree on the tibia as the knee joint flexes, extends, and rotates.

More superficially, the tibial collateral ligament (sometimes called the superficial portion of the medial ligament) lies over the middle third of the medial portion of the knee joint (12,14). It arises from the medial femoral epicondyle and passes inferiorly to insert into the medial surface of the tibia, some 7–8 cm below the joint line. It is separated from the underlying capsule by a bursa that facilitates free movement between these structures. On extension this ligament moves forward and tightens. A portion of its fibers swing obliquely posteriorly to reinforce the posterior portion of the medial compartment. The superficial and deep components are more integral posteriorly and difficult to separate. The bursa is no longer present in this region.

At the posterior third of the medial compartment, the joint capsule is supported by the posterior extension of the medial capsular ligament, which is termed the *posterior oblique ligament*. The more superficial portion of the oblique ligament consists of fibers made up from contributions of the vastus medialis, adductor magnus, and semimembranosus muscles. These muscles also constitute important dynamic stabilizers of the medial aspect of the joint.

The lateral compartment, especially in its anterior two-thirds, demonstrates many similarities to the medial compartment (Fig. 5-2; see also color plate 8) (16). At the anterior third, the deepest layer is formed by the joint capsule, which is reinforced by the patellar retinaculum, a component of the quadriceps mechanism. In the middle third, these structures are reinforced by the overlying iliotibial tract, which forms an important dynamic stabilizer. The iliotibial tract is seen to be a central condensation of fascia along the lateral thigh receiving part of the insertion of the tensor fascia lata and gluteus maximus, directly joining the intermuscular septum to insert along the distal border of the linea aspera and continuing inferior to insert onto Gerdy's tubercle at the anterolateral aspect of the tibia. Its strong structure permits it to function as both a dynamic and static stabilizer. It stabilizes when varus stress is exerted and limits anteroposterior motion during flexion and extension (17). Deep to the iliotibial tract is found the posterior extension of the patellar retinaculum. Deep to the retinaculum are found the capsular structures that are attached to the joint margins at the tibia and femur at the outer edge of the lateral meniscus (12).

At the posterior third of the lateral compartment, the anatomy of the supporting structures becomes extremely complex (Fig. 5-3) (18,19). A collection of structures forms the so-called arcuate complex. This consists of the fibular collateral ligament, the popliteal muscle tendon, the arcuate ligament, and the lateral head of the gastrocnemius muscle. The elements of this complex blend together, and it is extremely difficult to dissect one from the other (16,18,20,21). In addition, the biceps femoris is an important dynamic stabilizer in this region.

The deepest of these structures is the popliteus tendon, which passes through the posterolateral aspect of the lateral meniscus through its tunnel. It plays an important role in restraining varus instability and unlocking the joint in flexion (9). The tendon has fibers interwoven with the arcuate complex in some patients, although most individuals have little or no insertion of the popliteus onto the lateral meniscus. This makes the once postulated role of the popliteus in retracting and protecting the meniscus less likely (9,22). The joint capsule overlies the lateral meniscus slightly more superficially. The next layer encountered is the lateral collateral ligament, which is shorter than its counterpart medially. It courses from the lateral aspect of the lateral femoral condyle distally and slightly posteriorly to insert onto the styloid process of the fibular head. Immediately posterior to its insertion lies the insertion of the biceps femoris muscle, and when these structures are viewed from the lateral perspective, they form a V-like arrangement opening superiorly. The arcuate ligament, which also lies roughly at this depth, is more posteriorly located and blends into the popliteus muscle. The next layer, inconstantly found, is the fabellofibular ligament, which is often absent in patients with hypoplastic or absent fabellas. More superficial yet and located slightly posteriorly is the biceps femoris tendon.

The importance and interrelationship of these structures have been closely investigated, with particular attention to

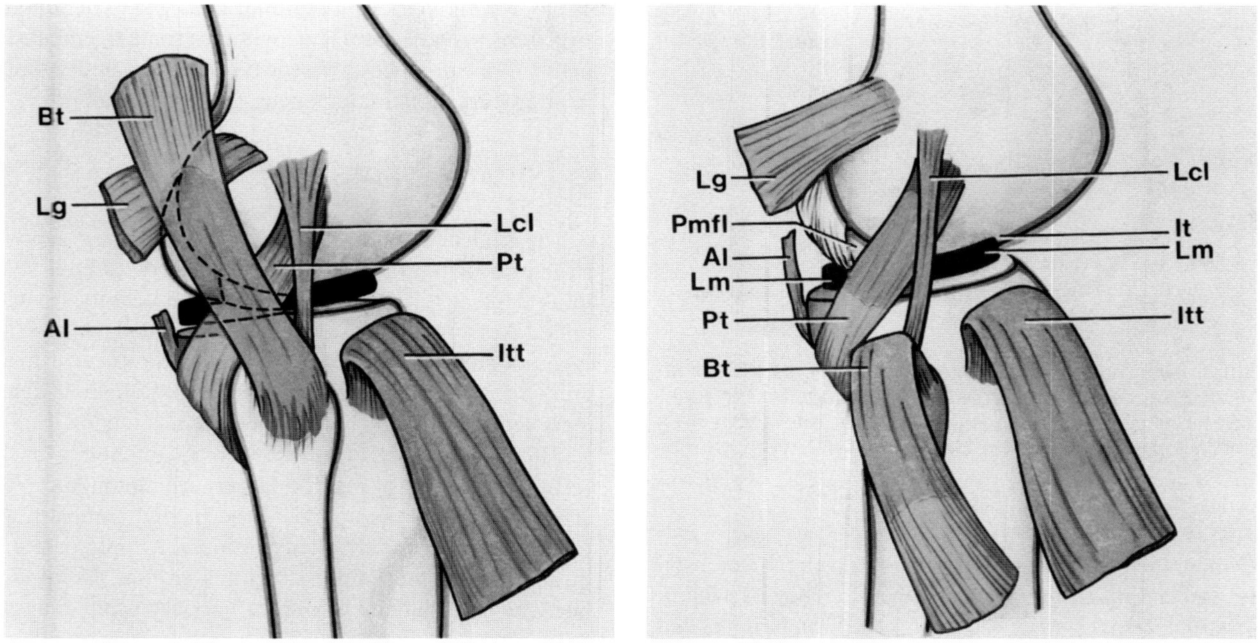

A B

FIG. 5-2. Lateral aspect of knee. **A:** superficial with iliotibial band reflected down. **B:** Deep with biceps femoris reflected down. Al, arcuate ligament; Lg, lateral head of gastrocnemius; Bt, biceps femoris; Lcl, lateral collateral ligament; Pt, popliteus; Itt, iliotibial tract; Lm, lateral meniscus; It, impressio terminalis; Pmfl, posterior meniscofemoral ligament.

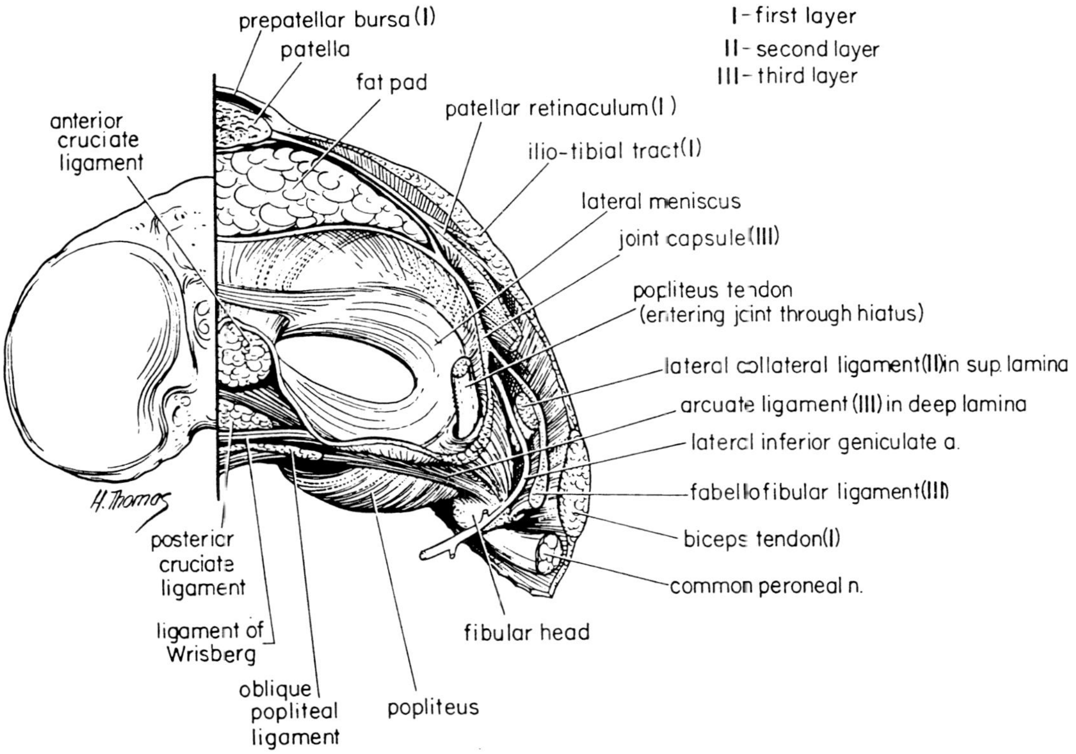

FIG. 5-3. Cross-sectional diagram of the lateral aspect of the knee. (From Seebacher JR et al. The structure of the posterolateral aspect of the knee. *J Bone Joint Surg* 1982;64A:536–541. With permission.)

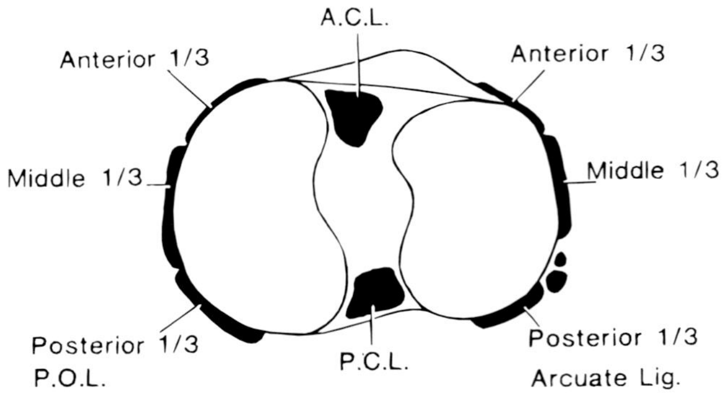

FIG. 5-4. Diagram of the ligaments of the knee. The ligaments of the knee have been divided into categories by Hughston in his classification of knee instability (see Table 5-1). (From *Orthop Clin North Am* 1985;16:69–82. With permission.)

their importance in the classification of knee ligament instability. Depending on the degree of insufficiency of each of these structures, different types of knee instability occur. Probably the most easily understood classification is that produced by Hughston (Fig. 5-4). He classified knee instabilities into eight different categories (Table 5-1). The instabilities have been classified into straight instabilities and rotary instabilities, with the latter occurring most frequently (21,23,24). Although most clinically significant instability is the result of trauma, it can also be seen with degenerative disease (25).

Straight instabilities fall into four main types—medial, lateral, anterior, and posterior—and are classified according to the motion of the tibia in relationship to a stabilized femur. By this very definition these instabilities consist of motion of the tibia without associated rotational components. Joints afflicted in such a fashion demonstrate opening of the joint comparable to the opening of a book. As can be seen from Table 5-1, the deficiency of a specific group of supporting structures (usually associated with a cruciate ligament abnormality) will produce different types of instability that will include a rotational component (26).

TABLE 5-1. *Classification of knee instability*

Knee instability type	Structures frequently torn (see Fig. 5-4)
Straight medial	Anterior cruciate Posterior cruciate Middle and posterior medial thirds
Straight lateral	Anterior cruciate Posterior cruciate Middle and posterior lateral thirds
Straight anterior	Anterior cruciate Posterior cruciate Middle medial and lateral thirds
Straight posterior	Posterior cruciate Posterior medial and lateral thirds
Anteromedial	Anterior cruciate Middle and posterior medial thirds
Anterolateral	Anterior cruciate Middle lateral third ± iliotibial band
Posterolateral	Posterior lateral third
Combined	Variable

CLINICAL ASPECTS

The clinical manifestations of disruption of the supporting structures of the knee joint are extremely variable. Symptoms depend to a large degree on the activities a patient undertakes. Certain histories are associated with different types of injuries; for example, traumatic knee dislocation are associated with a high incidence of collateral ligament tears accompanied by biceps and popliteal tendon tears (27). Sedentary individuals or those who do not engage in sports (especially running) may be largely asymptomatic. For instance, complete disruption of the medial compartment of the knee can occur with only minimal symptomatology or disability, provided other structures are not damaged. Isolated medial collateral ligament injury can occur and is often encountered in sports (14). These often respond well to conservative treatment (28). Acutely localized edema and tenderness may be found and are often helpful in determining the site of disruption of the supporting structures, particularly the tibial collateral ligament. Careful clinical examination is essential to determine which components of the supporting structures in addition to the cruciate ligaments are disrupted; in an acute setting this can often be a very challenging undertaking. Muscle spasm and guarding may make assessment particularly difficult.

Lateral instability of the knee occurs considerably less frequently than medial instability; however, it is much more disabling. Unfortunately, the clinical diagnosis of lateral instabilities is more subtle and they are more frequently misinterpreted. In the acute setting, symptoms are often minimal, with no more than mild to moderate pain over the lateral joint line. With time, instability often progresses and evidence of meniscal and cruciate pathology becomes more evident. In these individuals symptoms are often not apparent until they engage in athletics, particularly those involving running, with rapid change in direction of motion. The greater the number of supporting structures that are torn, the worse the symptoms usually are. In particular, if the posterolateral supporting structures are torn, symptoms may be severe even during normal walking (19,29). As the symptoms become more chronic, sudden pain and instability are seen more frequently (30).

IMAGING

Assessment of the supporting structures of the knee has been largely dependent on clinical examination and acumen. The role of various imaging procedures was very limited until the advent of MRI.

On plain films very few specific findings are available suggesting the presence of supporting structure abnormalities. One of the best known is the so-called Segond fracture, which is manifested as a small vertical avulsion injury of the lateral aspect of the proximal tibia immediately distal to the plateau (31,32). Typically, the bone fragment is less than 10 mm long, and its site of origin may be difficult to see. An accompanying avulsion fracture at the proximal aspect of the fibular head may be present. Investigation has demonstrated that this finding is specific for the diagnosis of detachment of the capsular portion of the lateral collateral ligament. Its significance lies in the high association of concomitant anterior cruciate ligament tears and meniscal injury. Rarely, avulsion of the iliotibial tract may be diagnosed by observing the presence of a small chip of bone arising from Gerdy's tubercle. Most other plain-film findings are nonspecific and consist merely of soft-tissue swelling, an inaccurate indicator of ligamentous disruption.

A number of findings have been reported with arthrography that relate to tears of the ligamentous structures of the knee. When the ligamentous structures and underlying joint capsule are torn, contrast material will leak to form an amorphous, ill-defined area of contrast in the soft tissues. This is only seen under two conditions, however. The examination must usually be performed within the first 48 hours following the injury; otherwise the synovial membrane tends to seal over the area of disruption. Also, the deep portion of the medial collateral ligament or the middle portion of the lateral capsule ligament must be disrupted. Disruption at other sites is usually not demonstrated with arthrography. Because of these problems the accuracy of arthrography is low. A delay in obtaining films for the diagnosis of collateral ligament disruption is not critical because the fine detail needed to assess anterior cruciate and meniscal lesions is not required.

Computed tomography has been widely used in assessing meniscal and cruciate ligament lesions. However, often collateral ligament abnormalities can also be detected. The medial collateral ligament can almost invariably be identified on transaxial computed tomography; it has a thin, bandlike, homogeneous appearance with low attenuation. The lateral collateral ligament is found more posteriorly with a density similar to that of its medial counterpart; however, its morphology is more cordlike. The biceps femoris tendon is found slightly posterior to the lateral collateral ligament and has a similar appearance and size. With tears of the collateral ligaments in the acute stage, thickening indistinct borders, increased attenuation, and lack of homogeneity are observed. When healing occurs, the ligaments thicken markedly and are once again of low attenuation in the chronic state. If a complete tear has occurred, the ligament may not be identifiable in its usual site. The accuracy of computed tomography has not been well investigated.

MAGNETIC RESONANCE IMAGING

Assessment of the collateral ligaments has been a subject that has been very sparsely addressed in the radiologic litera-

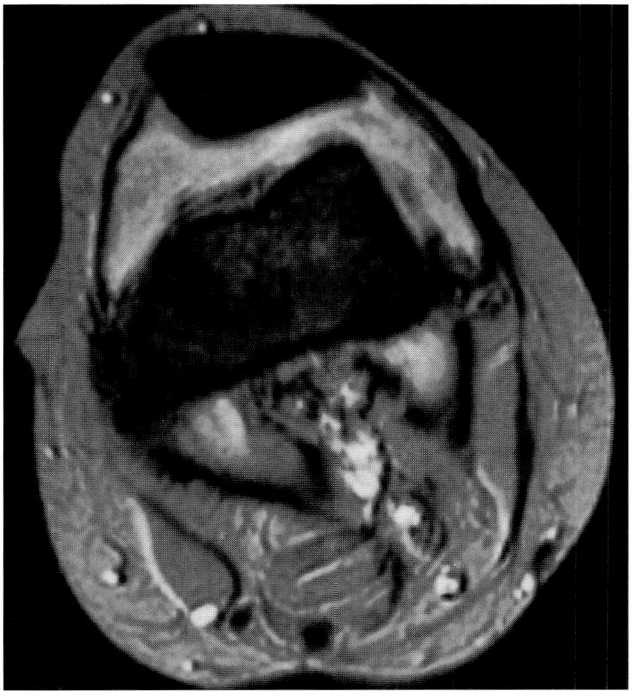

A

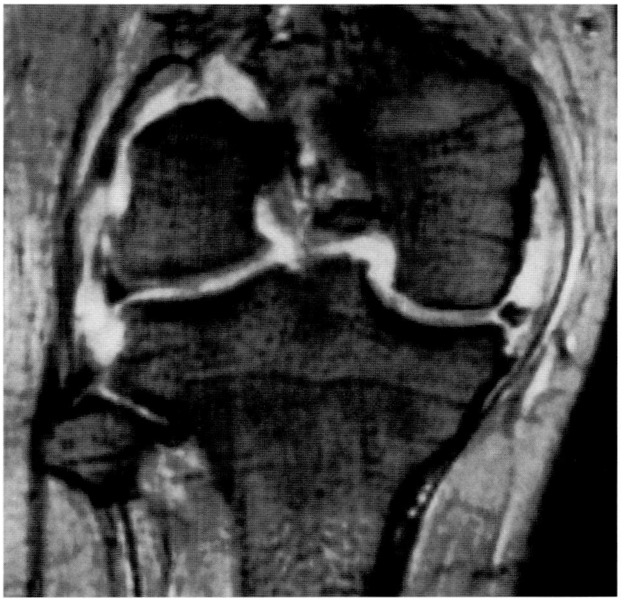

B

FIG. 5-5. Joint effusion. **(A)** Axial and **(B)** coronal T2*-weighted gradient-echo MPGR (TR 400 msec, TE 13 msec, flip angle 20°). Marked joint distension is present allowing the joint capsule, collateral ligaments and other structures to be seen to advantage. Note how the meniscus medially is drawn outward from the joint line due to its extensive adherence to the joint capsule.

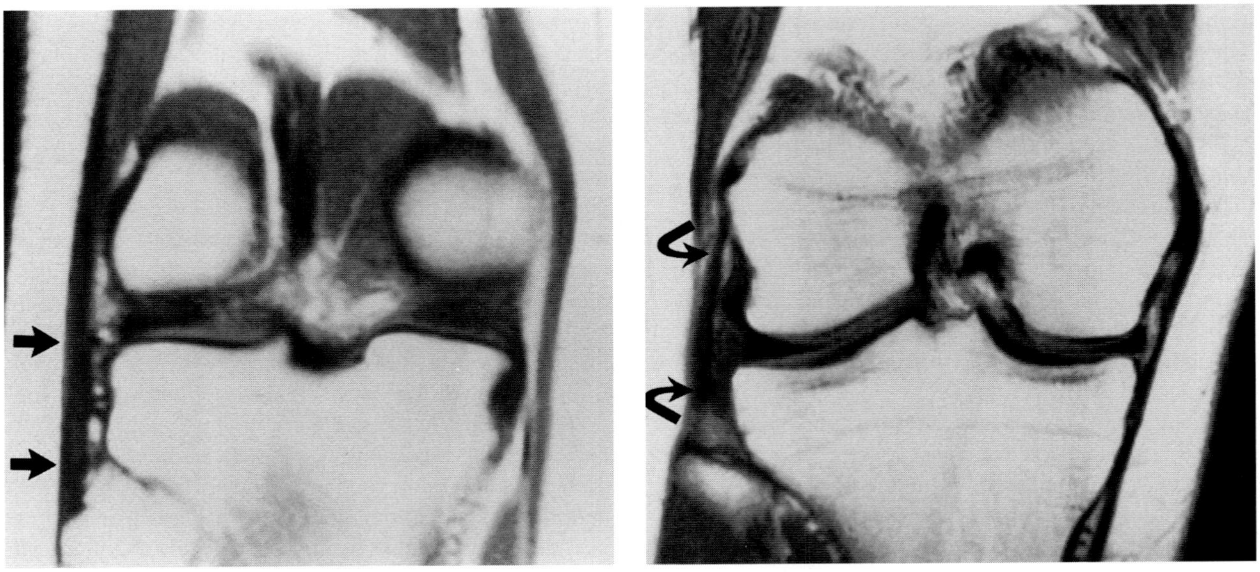

A B

FIG. 5-6. Posterolateral aspect of the knee. Coronal images T1-weighted spin echo (TR 400 msec, TE 15 msec). **A:** Insertion of the biceps tendon onto the fibular head *(arrows)*. **B:** Slightly more anteriorly, the lateral collateral ligament is seen *(curved arrows)*.

ture. Consequently, detailed evaluation of normal anatomy has not been completely elucidated and evaluation of traumatic and other disorders has been treated only in a cursory fashion.

The ideal plane for MRI evaluation of the collateral ligaments is the coronal plane. The details of the collateral ligaments and their associated structures are particularly well seen when fast scan techniques are used. Regardless of the sequence employed, the collateral ligaments will invariably be seen as bands of low-signal tissue outlined by adjacent high-signal fat and bursa. Although certain portions of the collateral ligaments and other associated supporting structures can be defined on both axial and sagittal images, these are often more difficult to interpret than coronal plane images (Fig. 5-5).

The fibular collateral ligament, as noted previously, courses obliquely posteroinferiorly to attach on the fibular head (Fig. 5-6). Because of this it is infrequently seen in its

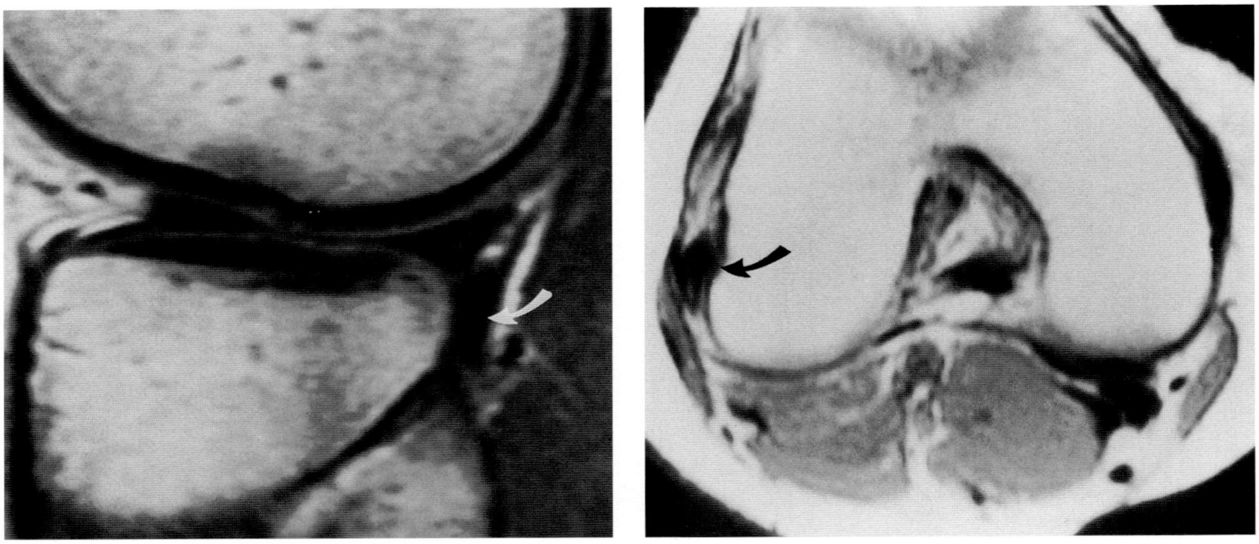

A B

FIG. 5-7. Popliteal tendon. **A:** Sagittal T1-weighted spin echo (TR 600 msec, TE 18 msec). The tendon is seen as a flat, often oval structure behind the posterior tibial margin *(curved arrow)*. **B:** Slightly tilted axial image T1-weighted spin echo (TR 400 msec, TE 20 msec). Low-signal tendon is shown by *curved arrow*.

A 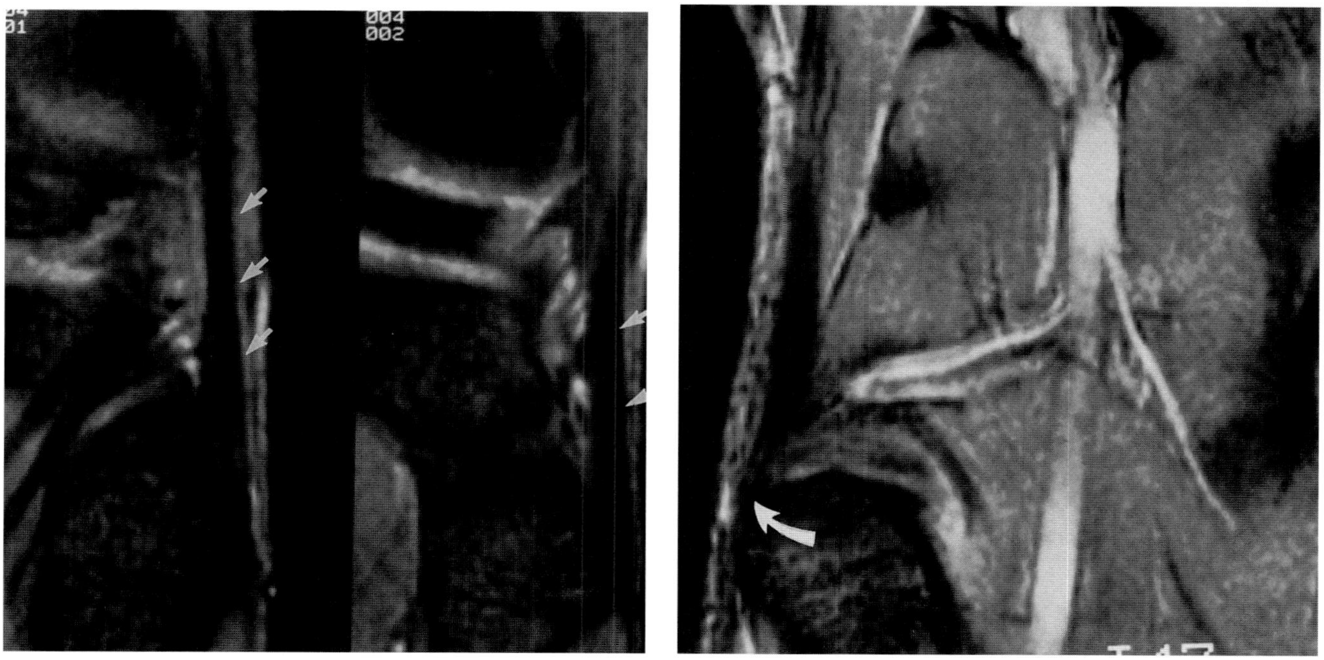 B

FIG. 5-8. Biceps femoris tendon. **A:** Adjacent coronal $T2^*$-weighted gradient-echo MPGR images (TR 400 msec, TE 12 msec, flip angle 20°). The dark tendon *(small arrows)* is seen to insert onto the lateral aspect of the fibular head. Because of its oblique orientation it is not usually seen on a single image. **B:** Coronal $T2^*$-weighted gradient-echo MPGR (TR 400 msec, TE 14 msec, flip angle 22°). The biceps tendon is seen as a dark band inserting on the femoral head. Frequently its distal insertion may appear slightly attenuated *(arrow)*. Note the high signal intensity from the popliteal artery and its geniculate branches.

entirety on a single coronal image. Frequently, the popliteus tendon, which separates the fibular collateral ligament from the posterior segment of the lateral meniscus, can be distinguished separately (Fig. 5-7). These two structures, as well as the biceps femoris, are often separated from one another by small amounts of fat (Figs. 5-8 and 5-9).

The tibial collateral ligament is usually seen in a more anteriorly placed slice and is overlaid by the sartorius and gracilis tendons, which blend together at this point to form the pes anserinus (Fig. 5-10). The more distal part of the tibial collateral ligament near its insertion is overlaid by the third component of the pes anserinus, which is the complex tendinous extension of the semimembranous muscle. The tibial collateral ligament may be separated from the pes anserinus by either small quantities of fat or a bursa that may at times be distended with fluid (Figs. 5-11 and 5-12). This collection of structures has sometimes been misinterpreted as representing layers of the medial collateral ligament. More anteriorly, at the lateral aspect of the knee, the iliotibial tract and band may be identified as a straight, low-signal region that inserts in the proximal portion of the tibial metaphysis (Fig. 5-13). It is frequently separated from the lateral meniscus by a layer of high-signal fat (33,34).

Numerous structures may be identified on the transaxial images that, not unexpectedly, have an appearance similar to that observed on CT. The margins of the joint capsule

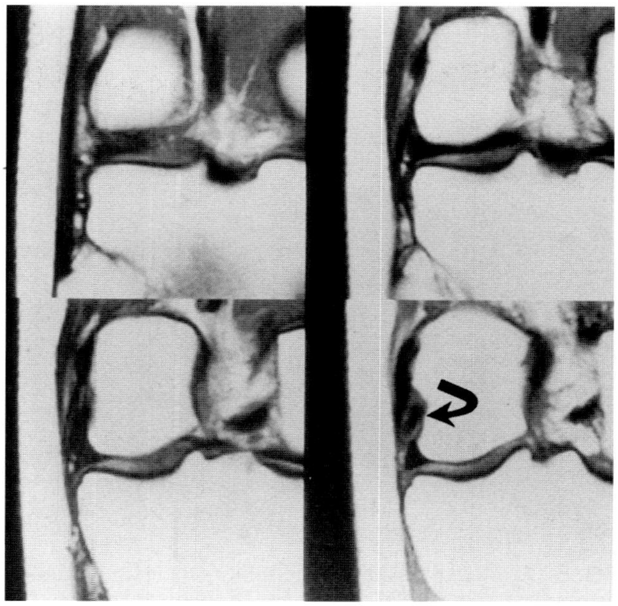

FIG. 5-9. Arcuate complex. Coronal T1-weighted spin echo (TR 400 msec, TE 16 msec) contiguous images through the posterolateral aspect of the knee (*curved arrow* indicates popliteus tendon).

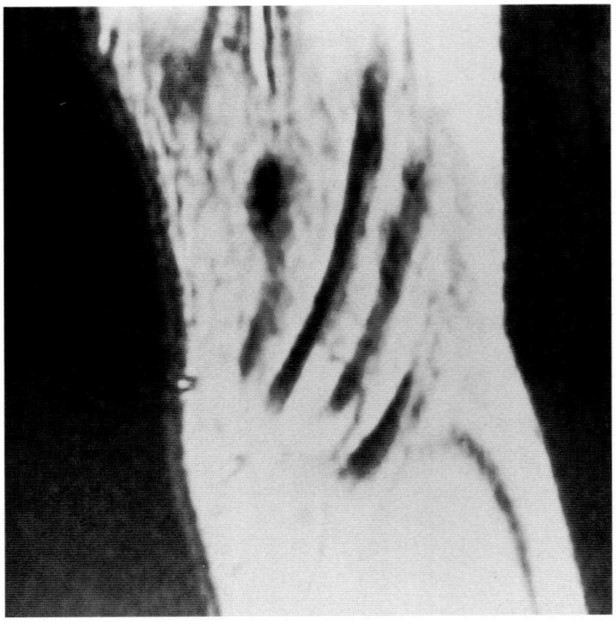

FIG. 5-10. Pes anserinus. Sagittal T1-weighted spin echo (TR 800 msec, TE 20 msec) demonstrates the tendons of the pes anserinus ("goose foot") outlined by fat.

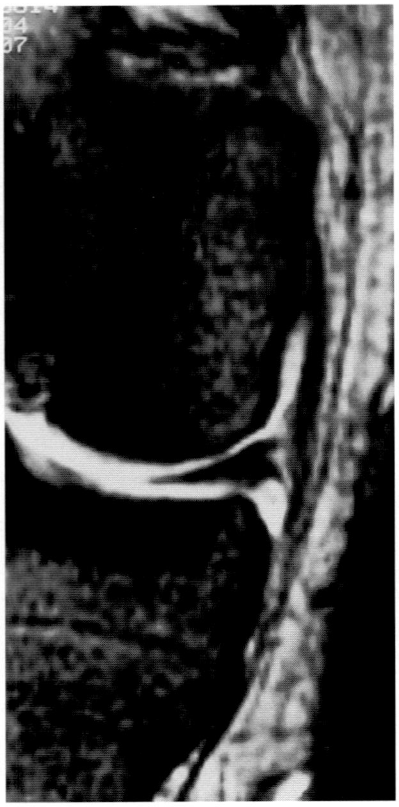

FIG. 5-12. Coronal T2*-weighted gradient-echo MPGR (TR 400 msec, TE 18 msec, flip angle 20°) of a normal medial collateral ligament shows the zone of separation between them.

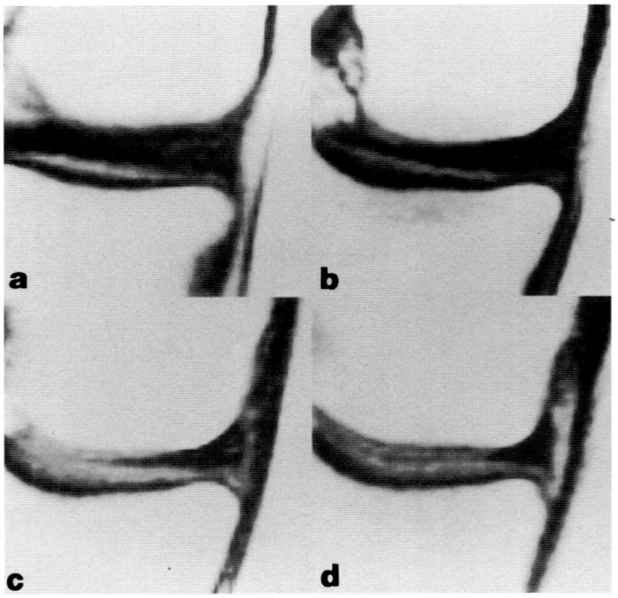

FIG. 5-11. Medial collateral ligament complex. Coronal T1-weighted spin-echo (TR 400 msec, TE 20 msec) images from posterior **(A)** to anterior **(B)**. The ligament is tightly applied to the underlying medial meniscus at its posterior aspect. Separation from the overlying fibers of the pes anserinus can be impossible to appreciate.

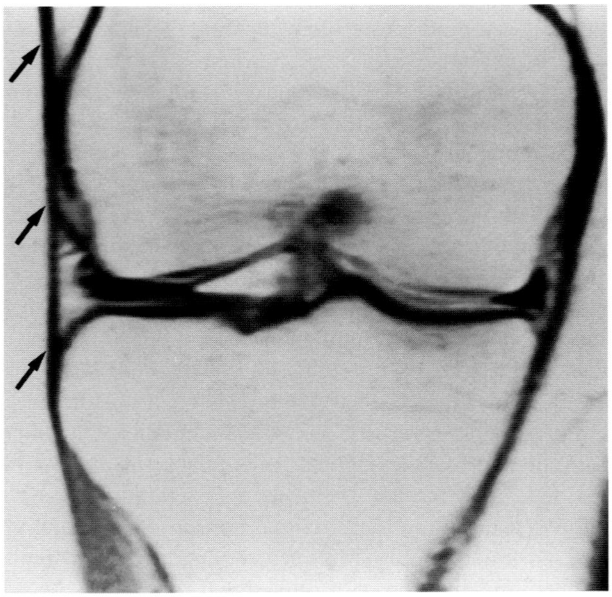

FIG. 5-13. Coronal T1-weighted spin echo (TR 400 msec, TE 20 msec). The iliotibial tract is seen as a narrow, low-signal line that inserts inferiorly on the tibia *(arrows)*.

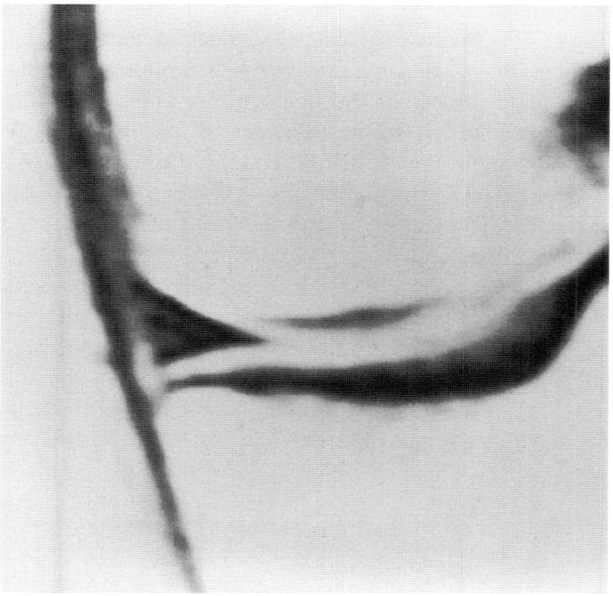
A

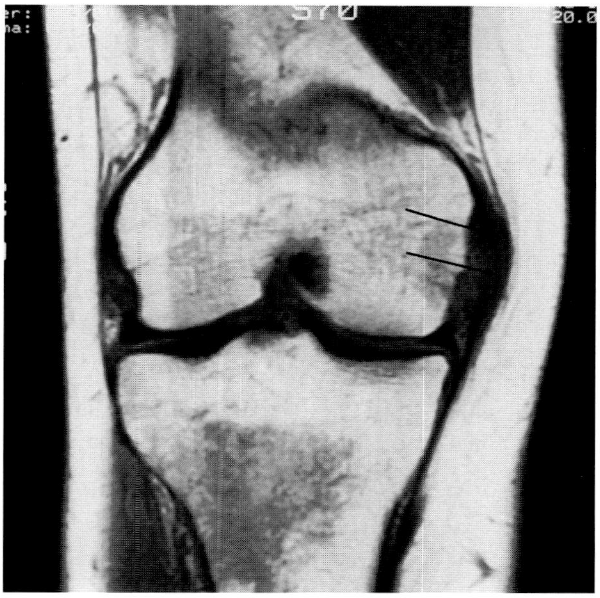
B

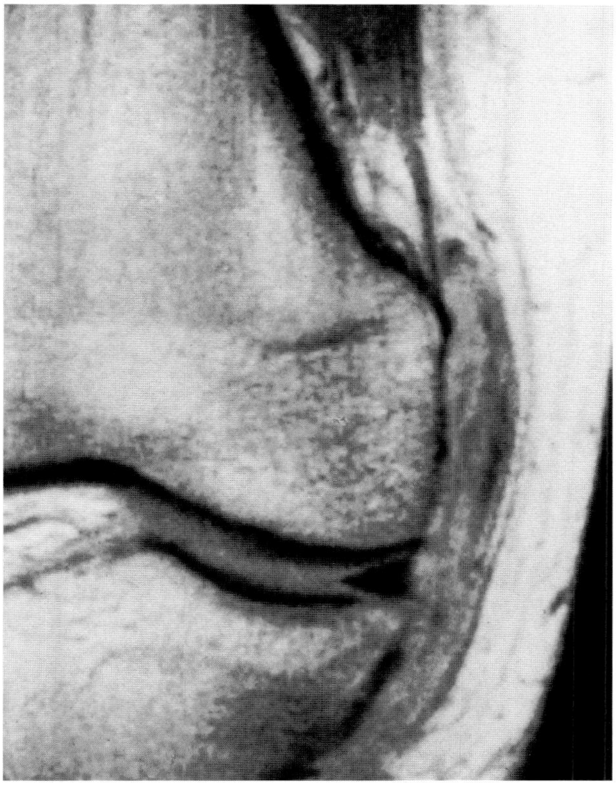
C

FIG. 5-14. Medial collateral ligament tears. **A:** Coronal T1-weighted spin echo (TR 400 msec, TE 20 msec). Mild tear showing only minimal ligament broadening and increased signal. **B:** Coronal T1-weighted spin echo (TR 500 msec, TE 13 msec). Moderate tear affecting cranial portion ligament, which is surrounded by slightly higher-signal edema/blood. Low-signal fibers of the ligament are just barely seen as a low signal line *(arrows)*. Incidentally seen are patches of diminished signal intensity within the normally bright bone marrow—red marrow islands. **C:** Coronal proton-density spin echo (TR 1000 msec, TE 40 msec). The ligament is grossly thickened with marked increase in signal intensity consistent with a severe tear. Low-signal fibers are not readily identifiable. (From Munk PL. *Can Assoc Radiol J* 1989;40:296–303. With permission.)

itself are occasionally well defined and seen as a thin, low-signal band. This is particularly well appreciated posteriorly when a joint effusion is present.

The most frequently injured structure among the supporting structures is the medial collateral ligament (Fig. 5-14). Attempts have been made to correlate the clinical grades of injury with MRI findings. Grade 0 is a normal ligament consisting of a thin, low-intensity band that extends from the medial femoral epicondyle to the proximal medial tibial metaphysis. In grade 1 injury the ligament is either of normal thickness or slightly thickened, with slight contour irregularity at its medial aspect. A halo of edema is often seen. The substance of the ligament itself does not show evidence of increased signal with T2- or T2*-weighted images. The ligament is also not displaced by edema; however, edema and hemorrhage may be apparent in the subcutaneous tissues (Fig. 5-15). In grade 2 lesions, evidence of hemorrhage and edema is more extensive, and partial disruption and displacement of the fibers of the ligament are apparent, with increased signal within the substance of the ligament. With grade 3 tears, complete disruption occurs and gross edema is evident (35–37). In children epiphyseal avulsion may occur before the ligament gives way. In adults the strength of the ligament is greater than in children, but fusion of the epiphysis makes bone avulsion less frequent. Avulsion is more likely to occur laterally than medially (38,39). With tears of the collateral ligaments, anterior cruciate ligament tears are often present and contralateral bone contusions are found representing associated trabecular bone fractures and hemorrhage within the bone marrow (40–42). These bony changes

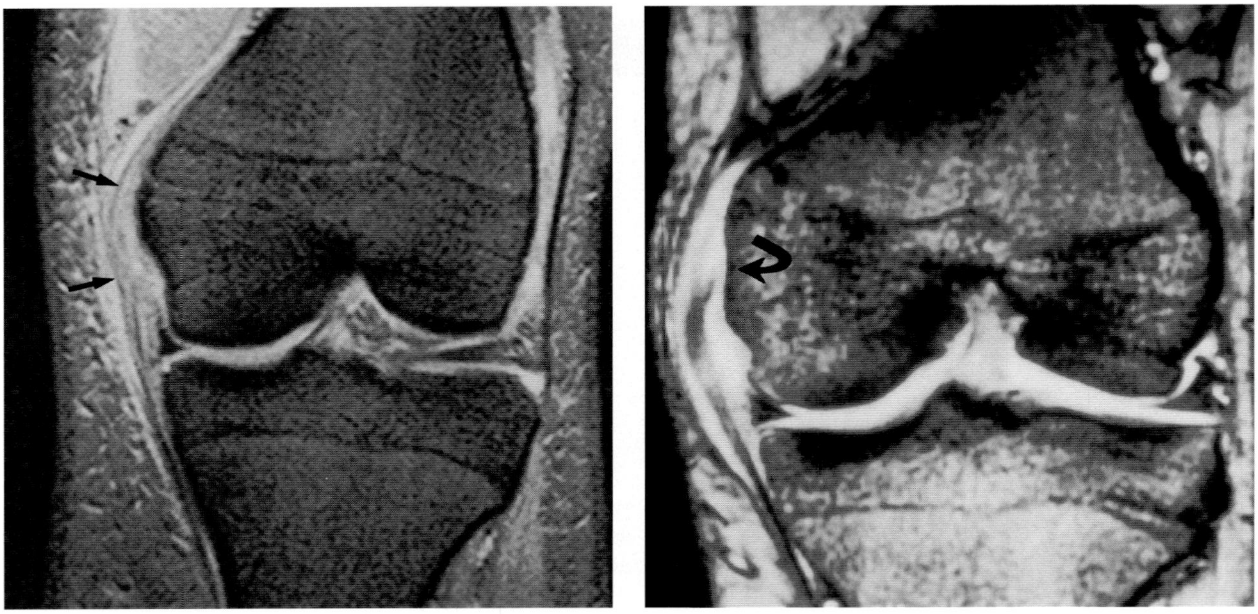

A B

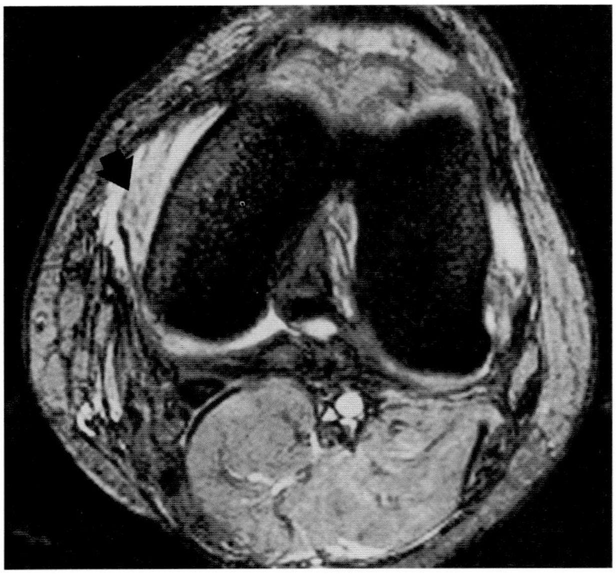

C

FIG. 5-15. Medial collateral ligament tears seen with gradient echo. **A:** Coronal T2*-weighted gradient-echo MPGR (TR 700 msec, TE 13 Msec, flip angle 20°). Partial tear of the cranial medial collateral is outlined by surrounding high-signal-intensity edema/blood. Low-signal-intensity fibers *(arrows)* can still be seen and are in continuity. **B:** Coronal T2*-weighted gradient-echo MPGR (TR 500 msec, TE 18 msec, flip angle 30°) shows a more severe tear. The cranial aspect of the ligament is completely detached *(arrow)*. **C:** Axial T2*-weighted gradient-echo MPGR (TR 650 msec, TE 27 msec, flip angle 30°). The torn medial collateral ligament has a wavy contour *(arrow)* and is surrounded by high signal intensity.

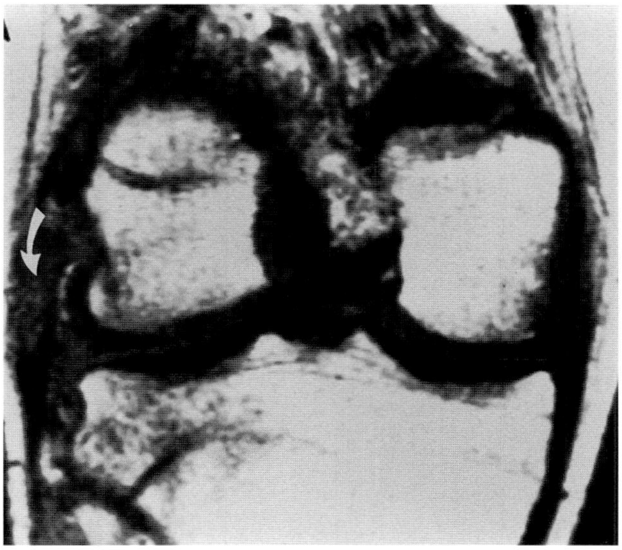

FIG. 5-16. Coronal T1-weighted spin echo (TR 500 msec, TE 17 msec). The proximal portion of the lateral collateral ligament cannot be defined and is replaced by hematoma *(curved arrow)*. Note the linear low signal in the lateral medullary region of the lateral tibia. This represents a fracture, with poorly defined, low-signal blood/edema around it replacing the normal high-signal bone marrow.

may occur in the tibia, femur, or both. Changes in the lateral collateral ligament, although less frequently seen, are similar in terms of their MRI appearance (Fig. 5-16). Discontinuity, widening of the ligament, ligamentous displacement, increased signal within the ligament, and serpentine contours are all signs consistent with disruptions both laterally and medially. All these changes are well noted on T1-weighted images (40). Edema is more marked and easily appreciated with T2- or T2*-weighted sequences or with fat suppression (37,41,43,44) (Figs. 5-17–5-20).

OTHER LESIONS OF THE SUPPORTING STRUCTURES

Although many other lesions of the supporting structures other than collateral ligament tears are known to occur, most have not been investigated with MRI. Among those that have been demonstrated are lesions of the dynamic stabilizers, particularly muscular hematomas and avulsion injuries at the site of musculotendinous insertions.

Muscular hematomas may occur as a result of abnormal

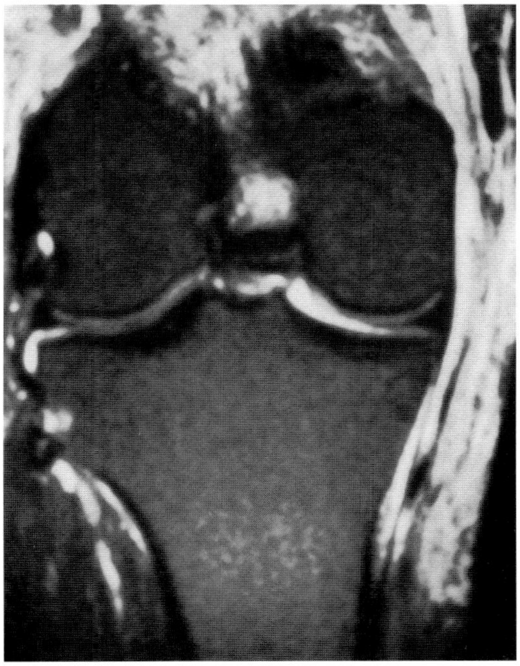

FIG. 5-17. Coronal T2-weighted fast spin echo (TR 3500 msec, TEef 102 msec) with fat saturation. The completely disrupted medial collateral ligament is replaced by high-signal-intensity blood/edema that has been accentuated by suppressing the fat signal.

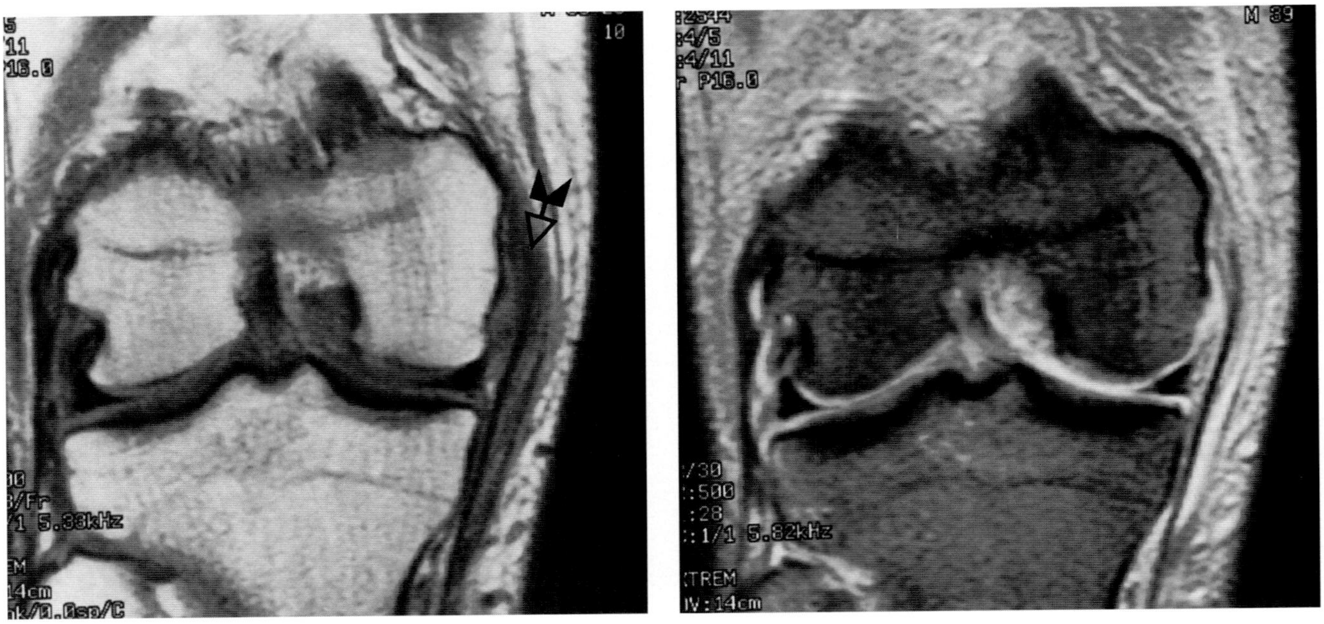

A B

FIG. 5-18. Subacute medial collateral ligament tear. **A:** Coronal T1-weighted spin echo (TR 500 msec, TE 18 msec) from a patient who had been injured more than 2 months previously. Slight irregularity and prominence in soft tissues is present at the cranial aspect of the medial collateral ligament *(arrow)*. **B:** Coronal $T2^*$-weighted gradient-echo MPGR (TR 500 msec, TE 28 msec, flip angle 30°) shows only slight increase in signal, signifying that relatively little edema/fluid is present at the site of injury.

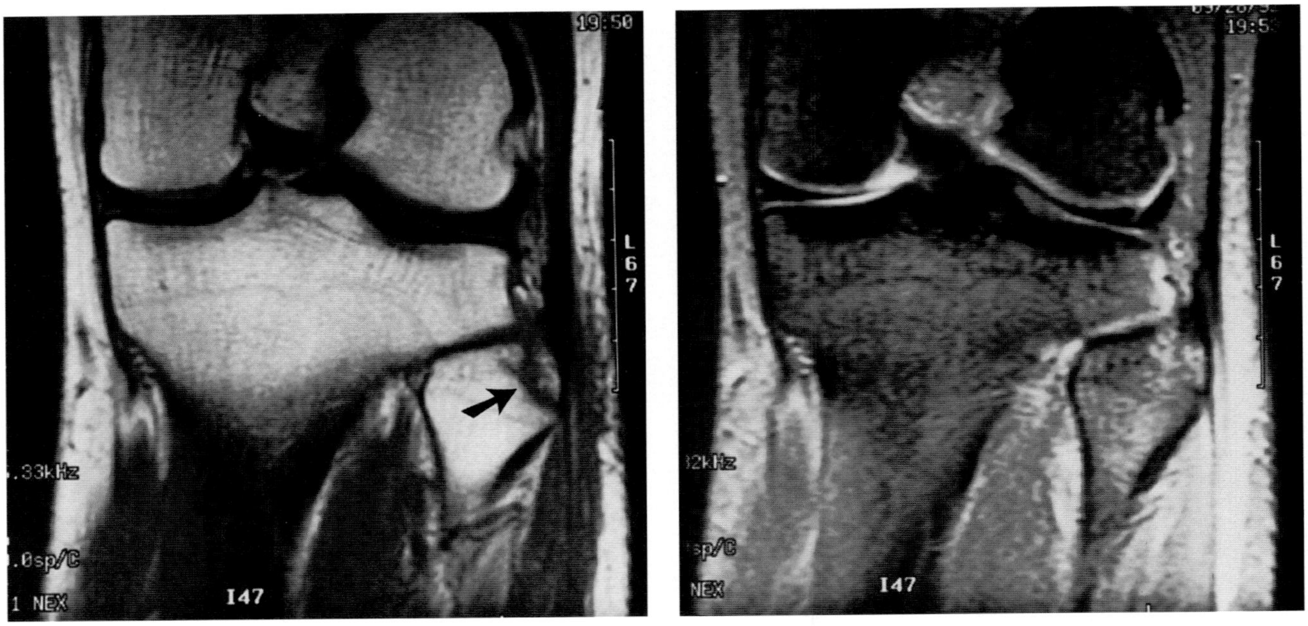

A B

FIG. 5-19. Partial avulsion fibular collateral ligament. **A:** Coronal T1-weighted spin echo (TR 500 msec, TE 18 msec) shows only slight irregularity at the lateral, superior aspect of the fibular head *(arrow)*. **B:** Coronal $T2^*$-weighted gradient-echo MPGR (TR 500 msec, TE 28 msec, flip angle 30°) demonstrates increased signal at the site of the avulsion, as well as fluid in the adjacent proximal tibiofibular joint.

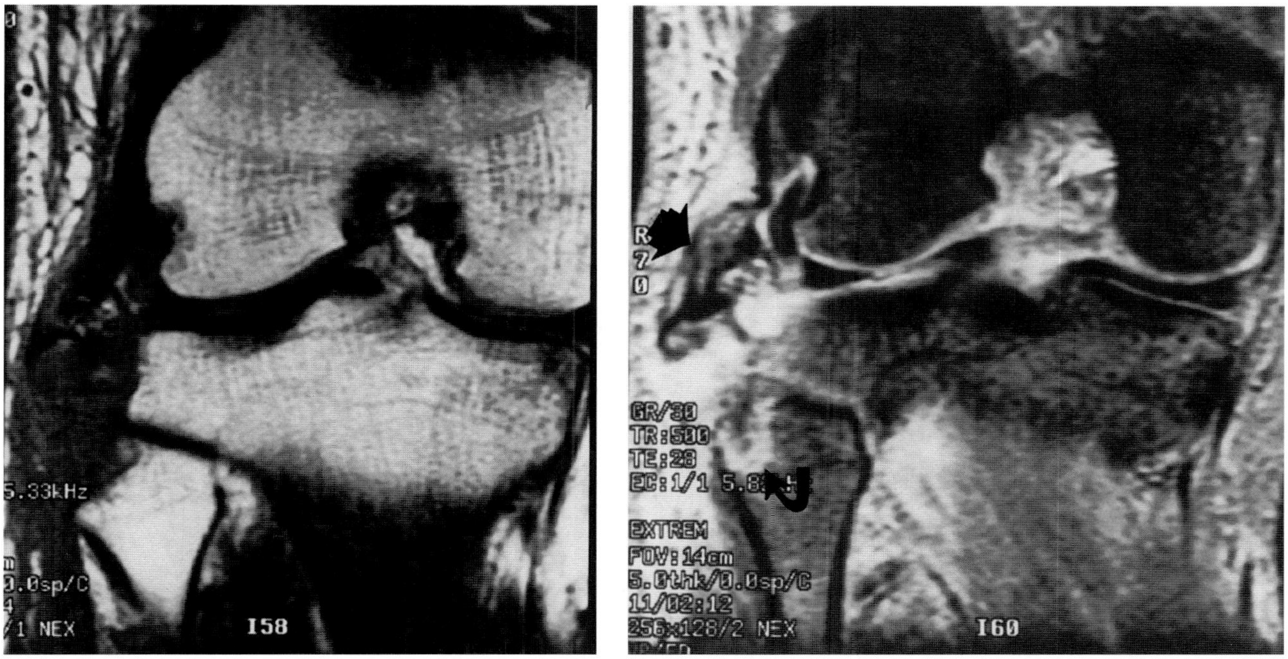

A B

FIG. 5-20. Displaced avulsion fragment from fibular head. **A:** Coronal T1-weighted spin echo (TR 500 msec, TE 18 msec) shows an area of low signal intensity, but greater than that of bone cortex or ligament at the inferior aspect of the lateral joint margin. **B:** Coronal T2*-weighted gradient-echo (TR 500 msec, TE 28 msec, flip angle 30°) displays these abnormalities more vividly. The avulsed and retracted fibular collateral ligament is surrounded by high-signal edema/blood *(arrow)* lifting a segment of low signal cortex from the donor site *(curved arrow).*

stresses that result in muscle tears. These hematomas are well delineated on T2-weighted images as areas of high signal, often extending along the long axis of the muscle and possessing at times indistinct or serrated margins. As the hematoma matures, low-signal areas gradually become apparent as hemosiderin is deposited. This is appreciated to greater advantage with gradient-echo sequences. In addition, at the insertion of tendons, avulsion of small segments of bone or of the tendon itself may occur. An example of this is the avulsion of the posteromedial tibial plateau by the semimembranosus tendon that has been diagnosed by MRI in a number of instances.

Often, plain films demonstrate displacement of a small fleck of bone. Although high-signal-intensity material is present on T2-weighted images at the site of the avulsion, the tendon itself usually maintains its low-signal appearance (31). Rarely, a similar appearance may be identified related to the popliteus tendon on the lateral side of the knee, which is very firmly attached to the femoral condyle. When of sufficient size the fragment may be surgically reattached (Fig. 5-21). Complete dislocation of the knee will often be accompanied by disruption of medial and lateral collateral ligaments and by tears of the popliteus and biceps tendons (27).

Abnormalities of the fabella have been seen on plain films and computed tomography. To our knowledge, dislocation of the fabella and tear of the associated fibulofabellar ligament have not been reported using MRI, but presumably they could be detected. Abnormalities of the quadriceps mechanism and retinacula are common and are addressed in Chapter 3.

A bursa is often seen at the insertion of the pes anserinus in the proximal tibia. This bursa may become inflamed and sometimes reaches great size. Occasionally, if the bursitis is chronic, erosion of the underlying cortical bone may be seen and the distended bursa can be detected easily by ultrasonography or CT. Bony spurs may also be seen at this site and be misinterpreted as osteochondromas. Their etiology is unclear but probably relates to abnormal stresses on the bone due to tension from the pes anserinus and/or chronic bursitis. On MRI the bursa is seen as a brightly demonstrated region on T2-weighted images displacing the overlying interdigitated segments of the pes anserinus muscle tendons (Fig. 5-22). Immediately deep to the pes anserinus bursa lies the tibial insertion of the medial collateral ligament, which is seen as a low-signal structure. Interestingly, most patients with this lesion are obese females.

Disruptions of the iliotibial tract may occur and are seen as discontinuity of the thin, straight black line representing the distal portion of the tract. Rarely, avulsion of the distal insertion may carry off a small segment of bony cortex. In either event, edema and hemorrhage will be manifested on T2-weighted images as areas of increased signal.

MR findings in the iliotibial band friction syndrome have

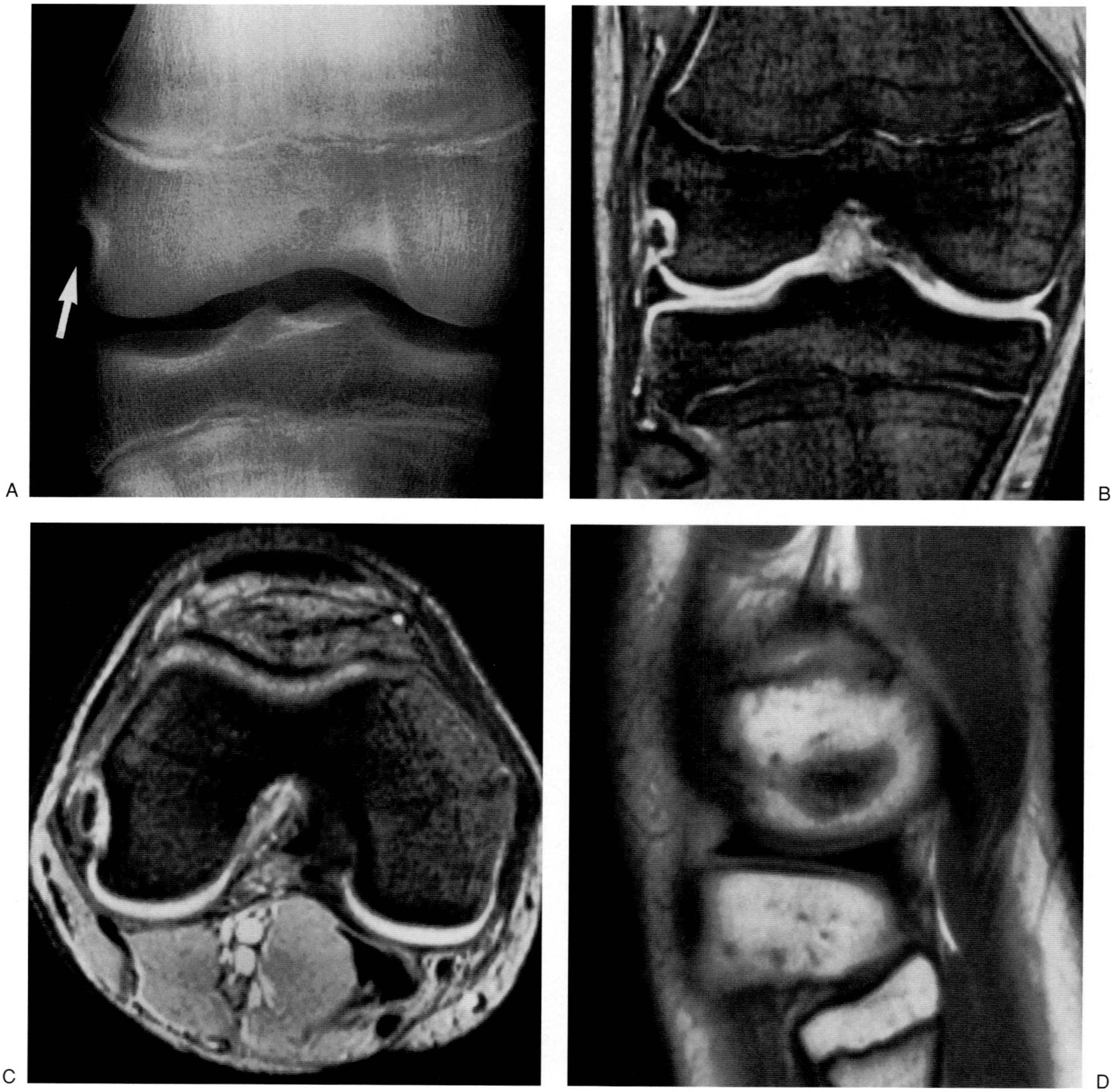

FIG. 5-21. Popliteus avulsion. **A:** Anteroposterior radiograph shows a tiny fleck of bone just barely seen *(arrow)*. **B,C:** Coronal and axial T2*-weighted gradient-echo MPGR (TR 400 msec, TE 20 msec, flip angle 20°) readily demonstrate the small, low-signal bone fragment outlined by bright fluid. **D:** Sagittal T1-weighted spin echo (TR 600 msec, TE 18 msec) shows the low-signal donor site at the lateral aspect of the femoral condyle.

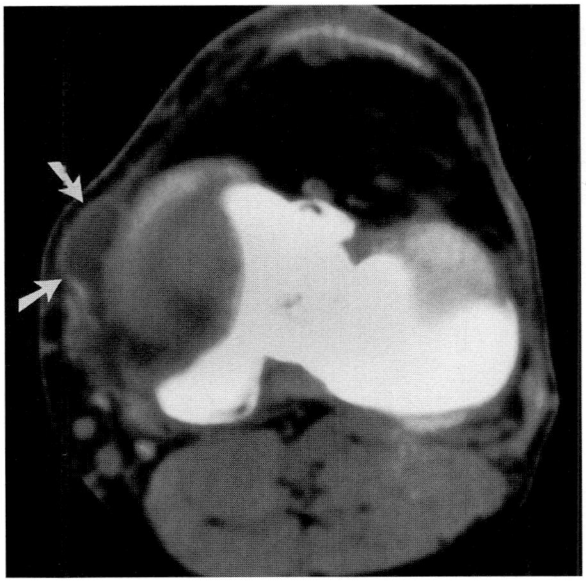
A

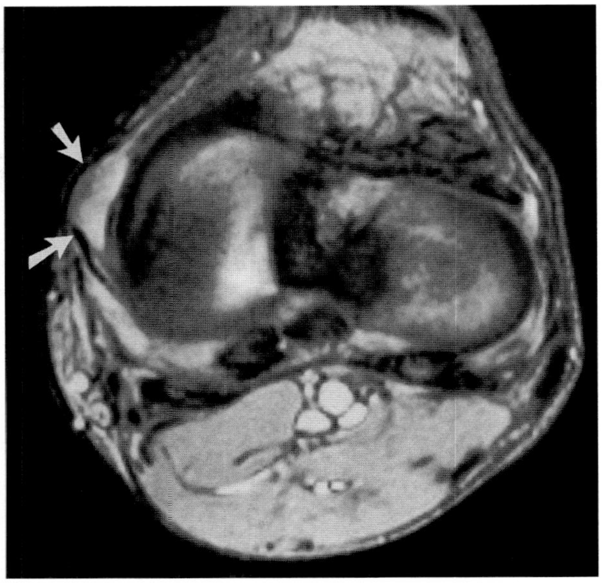
B

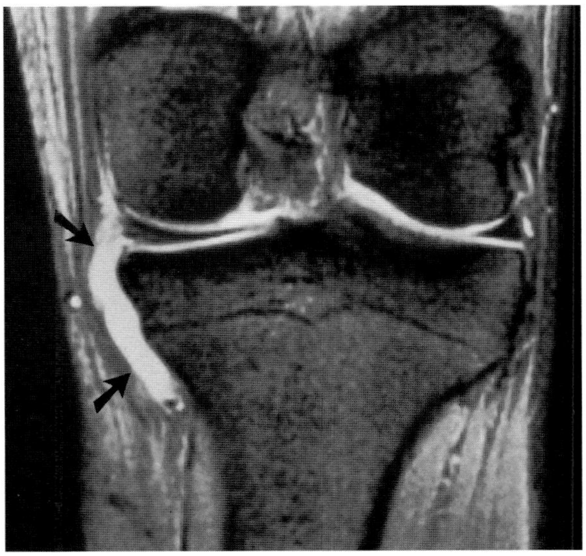
C

FIG. 5-22. Pes anserine bursitis. **A:** Axial CT scan shows a small cystic structure *(arrows)* originally thought to be a meniscal cyst. **B:** Axial T2*-weighted gradient-echo MPGR (TR 500 msec, TE 23 msec, flip angle 40°) shows the bursa to be of high signal. **C:** Coronal T2*-weighted gradient-echo MPGR (TR 400 msec, TE 20 msec, flip angle 20°) shows the relationship of the bursa to the joint. No meniscal tear was demonstrated and at surgery the bursa was readily peeled off.

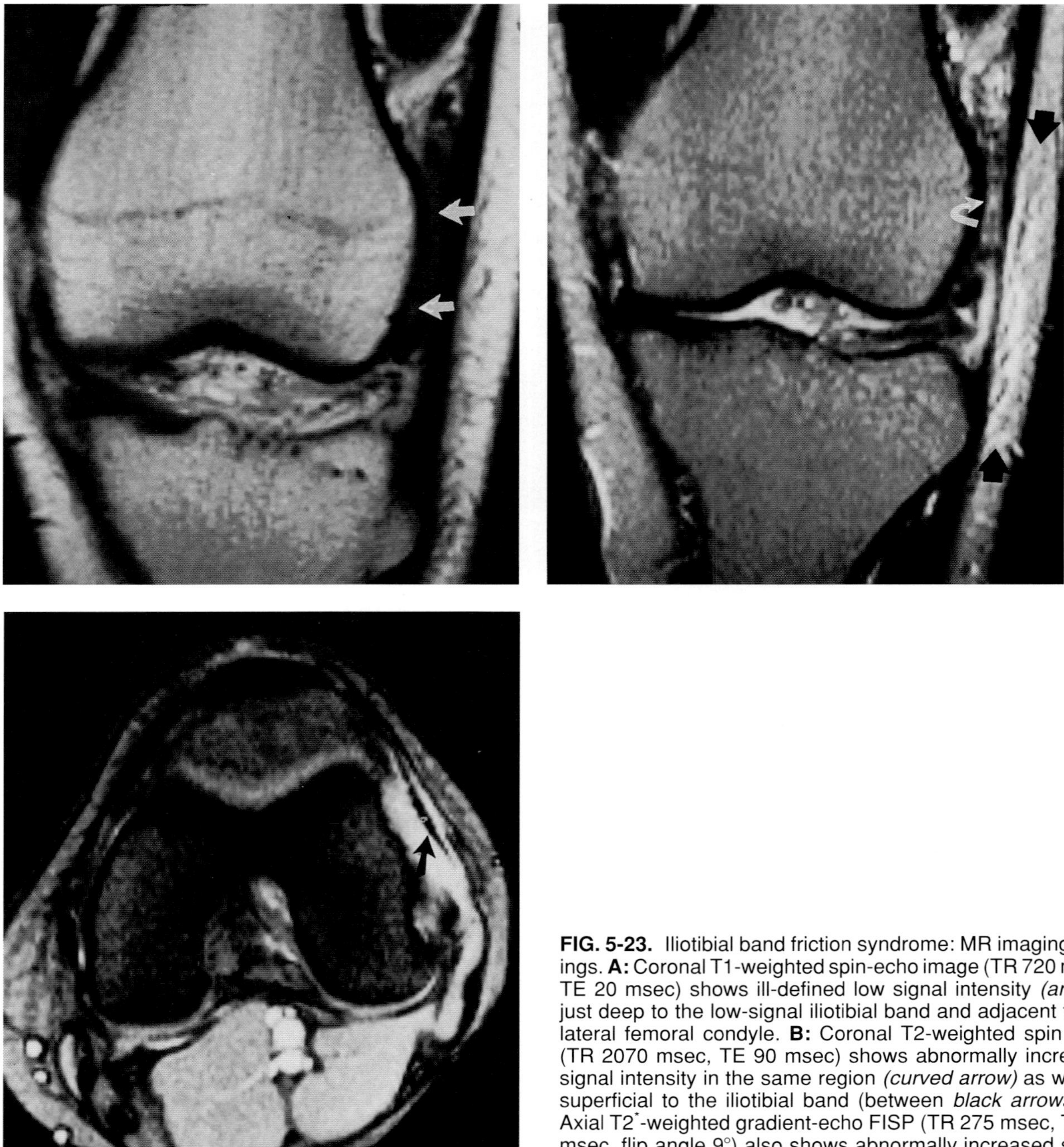

A B C

FIG. 5-23. Iliotibial band friction syndrome: MR imaging findings. **A:** Coronal T1-weighted spin-echo image (TR 720 msec, TE 20 msec) shows ill-defined low signal intensity *(arrows)* just deep to the low-signal iliotibial band and adjacent to the lateral femoral condyle. **B:** Coronal T2-weighted spin echo (TR 2070 msec, TE 90 msec) shows abnormally increased signal intensity in the same region *(curved arrow)* as well as superficial to the iliotibial band (between *black arrows*). **C:** Axial T2*-weighted gradient-echo FISP (TR 275 msec, TE 12 msec, flip angle 9°) also shows abnormally increased signal intensity both superficial and deep to the iliotibial band *(arrow)*. (From Murphy BJ, et al. *Radiology* 1992; 185:569–571. With permission.)

also been reported. This is an overuse injury most often found in long-distance runners (45–47). It is characterized by poorly localized pain over the outer aspect of the knee in relation to the lateral femoral epicondyle. Treatment is with rest and anti-inflammatory agents, although surgical release of the posterior fibers of the iliotibial band may be performed (48). On MRI ill-defined decrease in signal on T1-weighted images in the tissues deep to the iliotibial band can be encountered. On T2 weighting this becomes of increased signal (49) (Fig. 5-23).

REFERENCES

1. Rong G, Wang Y. The role of cruciate ligaments in maintaining knee joint stability. *Clin Orthop Rel Res* 1987;215:65–71.
2. Girgis FG, Marshall JL, Al Monajem ARS. The cruciate ligament of

the knee joint: anatomical, functional and experimental analysis. *Clin Orthop Rel Res* 1975;106:216–231.
3. Van Dommelen BA, Fowler PJ. Anatomy of the posterior cruciate ligament: a review. *Am J Sports Med* 1989;17:24–29.
4. Parolie JM, Bergfeld JA. Long-term results of nonoperative treatment of isolated posterior cruciate ligament injuries in the athlete. *Am J Sports Med* 1986;14:35–38.
5. Kennedy JC, Grainger RW. The posterior cruciate ligament. *J Trauma* 1967;7:367–377.
6. Covey DC, Sapega AA. Injuries of the posterior cruciate ligament. *J Bone Joint Surg* 1993;75-A:1376–1386.
7. Hughston JC, Bowden JA, Andrews JR, Norwood LA. Acute tears of the posterior cruciate ligament: results of operative treatment. *J Bone Joint Surg* 1980;62-A:438–450.
8. Barton TM, Torg JS, Das M. Posterior cruciate ligament insufficiency: a review of the literature. *Sports Med* 1984;1:419–430.
9. Nielson S, Helmig P. The static stabilizing function of the popliteal tendon in the knee: an experimental study. *Arch Orthop Trauma Surg* 1986;104:357–362.
10. McLeod WD. The biomechanics and function of the secondary restraints to the anterior cruciate ligament. *Orthop Clin North Am* 1985; 16:165–170.
11. Butler DL, Noyes FR, Grood ES. Ligamentous restraints to anterior-posterior drawer in the human knee. *J Bone Joint Surg* 1980;62A: 259–270.
12. Hughston JC, Andrews JR, Cross MJ, Moschi A. Classification of knee ligament instabilities. Part I: the medial compartment and cruciate ligaments. *J Bone Joint Surg* 1976;58A:159–172.
13. Warren LF, Marshall JL, Girgis F. The prime static stabilizer of the medial side of the knee. *J Bone Joint Surg* 1974;56A:665–674.
14. Indelicato PA. Nonoperative management of complete tears of the medial collateral ligament. *Orthop Rev* 1989;18:947–952.
15. El-Khoury GY, Usta HY, Berger RA. Meniscotibial (coronary) ligament tears. *Skeletal Radiol* 1984;11:191–196.
16. Andrews JR, Axe MJ. The classification of knee ligament instability. *Orthop Clin North Am* 1985;16:69–82.
17. McNicol K, Taunton JE, Clement DB. Iliotibial tract friction syndrome in athletes. *Can J Appl Sports Sci* 1981;6:76–80.
18. Seebacher JR, Inglis AE, Marshall JL, Warren RF. The structure of the posterolateral aspect of the knee. *J Bone Joint Surg* 1982;64A: 536–541.
19. Veltri DM, Warren RF. Posterolateral instability of the knee. *J Bone Joint Surg* 1994;76-A:460–472.
20. Kennedy JC, Hawkins RJ, Willis RB, Danylchuk KD. Tension studies of human knee ligaments. *J Bone Joint Surg* 1976;58A:350–355.
21. Hughston JC, Andrews JR, Cross MJ, Moschi A. Classification of knee ligament instabilities. Part II: the lateral compartment. *J Bone Joint Surg* 1976;58A:173–179.
22. Tria AJ, Johnson CD, Zawadsky JP. The popliteus tendon. *J Bone Joint Surg* 1989;71-A:714–716.
23. Slocum DB, Larson RL. Rotatory instability of the knee: its pathogenesis and a clinical test to demonstrate its presence. *J Bone Joint Surg* 1968;50A:211–225.
24. Norwood LA, Andrews JR, Meisterling RC, Glancy GL. Acute anterolateral rotatory instability of the knee. *J Bone Joint Surg* 1979;61A: 704–709.
25. Msika CC, Sedlin ED. Postero-lateral rotatory instability in osteoarthritis of the knee. *Int Orthop* 1990;14:25–28.
26. Fleming RE, Blatz DJ, McCarroll JR. Lateral reconstruction for anterolateral rotatory instability of the knee. *Am J Sports Med* 1983;11: 303–307.
27. Yu JS, Goodwin D, Salonen D, et al. Complete dislocation of the knee: spectrum of associated soft-tissue injuries depicted by MR imaging. *AJR* 1995;164:135–139.
28. Indelicato PA, Hermansdorfer J, Huegel M. Nonoperative management of complete tears of the medial collateral ligament of the knee in intercollegiate football players. *Clin Orthop Rel Res* 1990;256:174–177.
29. Baker CL Jr, Norwood LA, Hughston JC. Acute combined posterior cruciate and posterolateral instability of the knee. *Am J Sports Med* 1984;12:204–208.
30. Terry GC, Hughston JC. Associated joint pathology in the anterior cruciate ligament-deficient knee with emphasis on a classification system and injuries to the meniscocapsular ligament-musculotendinous unit complex. *Orthop Clin North Am* 1985;16:29–39.
31. Dietz GW, Wilcox DM, Montgomery JB. Segond tibial condyle fracture: lateral capsular ligament avulsion. *Radiology* 1986;159:467–469.
32. Woods GW, Stanley RF Jr, Tullos HS. Lateral capsular sign: x-ray clue to a significant knee instability. *Am J Sports Med* 1979;7:27–33.
33. Mink JH, Deutsch AL. Magnetic resonance imaging of the knee. *Clin Orthop Rel Res* 1989;244:29–47.
34. Munk PL. Magnetic resonance imaging of the knee: an overview. *J Can Assoc Radiol* 1989;40:296–303.
35. Turner DA, Prodromos CC, Petasnick JP, Clark JW. Acute injury of the ligaments of the knee: magnetic resonance evaluation. *Radiology* 1985;154:717–722.
36. Pope TL. MRI of knee ligaments. *Semin Ultrasound CT MR* 1994;15: 366–382.
37. Staron RB, Haramati N, Feldman F, et al. O'Donoghue's triad: magnetic resonance imaging evidence. *Skeletal Radiol* 1994;23:633–636.
38. Woo SL, Orlando CA, Gomez MA, Frank CB, Akeson WH. Tensile properties of the medial collateral ligament as a function of age. *J Orthop Res* 1986;4:133–141.
39. Sullivan JA. Ligamentous injuries of the knee in children. *Clin Orthop Rel Res* 1994;255:44–50.
40. Garvin GJ, Munk PL, Vellet AD. Tears of the medial collateral ligament: magnetic resonance imaging findings and associated injuries. *Can Assoc Radiol J* 1993;44:199–204.
41. Yao L, Dungan D, Seeger LL. MR imaging of tibial collateral ligament injury: comparison with clinical examination. *Skeletal Radiol* 1994;23: 521–524.
42. Newberg AH, Wetzner SM. Bone bruises: their patterns and significance. *Semin Ultrasound CT MR* 1994;15:396–409.
43. Forster BB, Helms CA. Importance of routine T2-weighted or T2*-weighted coronal images in magnetic resonance imaging of the knee. *Can Assoc Radiol J* 1993;44:396–398.
44. Mirowitz SA, Shu HH. MR imaging evaluation of knee ligaments and related injuries: comparison of T1-weighted, T2-weighted and fat-saturated T2-weighted sequences-correlation with clinical findings. *J Magn Reson Imaging* 1994;4:725–732.
45. Noble CA. Iliotibial band friction syndrome in runners. *Am J Sports Med* 1980;8:232–234.
46. Noble CA. The treatment of iliotibial band friction syndrome. *Br J Sports Med* 1979;13:51–54.
47. Orava S. Iliotibial tract friction syndrome in athletes: an uncommon exertion syndrome on the lateral side of the knee. *Br J Sports Med* 1978;12:69–73.
48. Martens M, Libbrecht P, Burssens A. Surgical treatment of the iliotibial band friction syndrome. *Am J Sports Med* 1989;17:651–654.
49. Murphy BJ, Hechtman KS, Uribe JW, Selesnick H, Smith RL, Zlatkin MB. Iliotibial band friction syndrome: MR imaging findings. *Radiology* 1992;185:569–571.

MRI of the Knee, Second Edition,
edited by P. L. Munk and C. A. Helms.
Lippincott-Raven Publishers, Philadelphia © 1996.

CHAPTER 6

Pitfalls in Magnetic Resonance Imaging of the Knee

Clyde A. Helms

Multiple pitfalls have emerged in imaging the knee with MR that can cause confusion and misdiagnosis and result in inappropriate or unnecessary surgery (1–4). Because of the high diagnostic accuracy achieved with knee MR, surgeons are prone to operate solely on the MR diagnosis; therefore, even uncommon pitfalls should be recognized. This chapter divides the various pitfalls into anatomic categories: menisci, ligaments, bones, and some additional pitfalls.

MENISCI

Several pitfalls that can simulate meniscal tears exist that, once learned, are easy to differentiate from real tears. One of the most common is caused by the transverse ligament. The transverse ligament is a horizontally oriented structure that attaches to the anterior horns of the medial and lateral menisci (Fig. 6-1). It often mimics a tear of the anterior horn of the lateral meniscus at its insertion into the meniscus (Fig. 6-2). Its presence is variable, ranging from 22–38% in several series (1,2) to 43% in our own series of 67 arthroscopically proven cases at the University of California at San Francisco.

A pseudotear secondary to the insertion of the transverse ligament to the anterior horn of the medial meniscus is seen less frequently (only 13% in our series) (Fig. 6-3). The transverse ligament was erroneously referred to as the superior lateral geniculate artery in early publications; however, this structure is clearly not an artery because of its constant nonvascular appearance on flow-sensitive imaging sequences.

Occasionally, a tear of the anterior horn of the lateral meniscus is misinterpreted as a normal transverse ligament (Fig. 6-4). If a presumed transverse ligament can be followed into the body of the meniscus, a tear is likely to be present. More important, a transverse ligament should be followed across the knee in Hoffa's fat pad.

It has been shown that the accuracy of MR imaging for meniscal tears suffers when an anterior cruciate ligament (ACL) tear is present (5). DeSmet showed in a series of 400 patients that the sensitivity for a torn medial meniscus dropped from 97% to 88%, and in the lateral meniscus the sensitivity dropped from 94% to 69%. The predominant pattern of tears that were missed were subtle peripheral tears, especially those involving the posterior horn of the lateral meniscus. Therefore, when a torn ACL is noted, careful attention to this area is recommended. Several pitfalls can make the posterior horn of the lateral meniscus difficult to assess. These include pulsation artifact from the popliteal artery, magic-angle phenomenon, the popliteus tendon interface, and insertion of the meniscofemoral ligaments. These are discussed in detail in this chapter.

An entity very similar to the insertion of the transverse ligament on the anterior horn of the lateral meniscus occurs on the posterior horn of the lateral meniscus from the insertion of the anterior meniscofemoral ligament of Humphry and the posterior meniscofemoral ligament of Wrisberg (6). These ligaments attach on the superior aspect of the posterior horn of the lateral meniscus in its most medial portion and course obliquely superiorly and medially to the medial femoral condyle (Fig. 6-5). A meniscal tear can be simulated at the insertion of the ligaments on the posterior horn of the lateral meniscus (Fig. 6-6). This was seen in 27% of our series of 67 cases, 12% from the ligament of Humphry and 15% from the ligament of Wrisberg. These ligaments can usually be identified on contiguous sagittal images and followed to their usual recognizable positions anterior or posterior to the posterior cruciate ligament.

Another process that can mimic a tear on the posterior horn of the lateral meniscus is the popliteus recess. The pop-

C. A. Helms: Department of Radiology, Duke University Medical Center, Durham, North Carolina 27710.

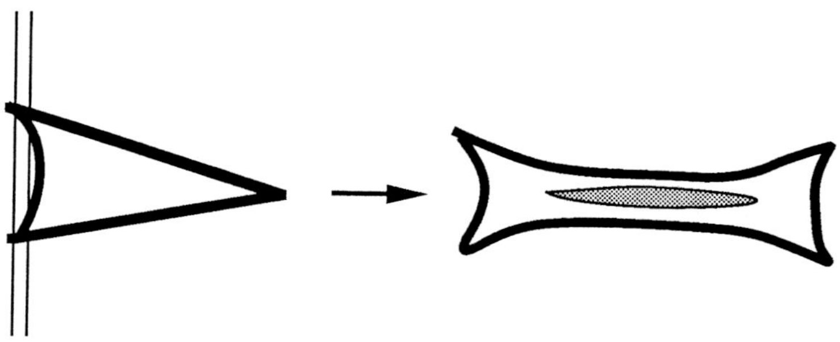

A

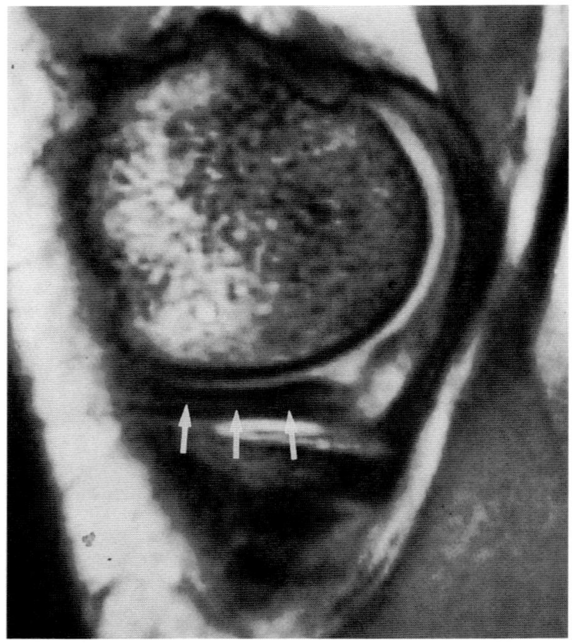

B

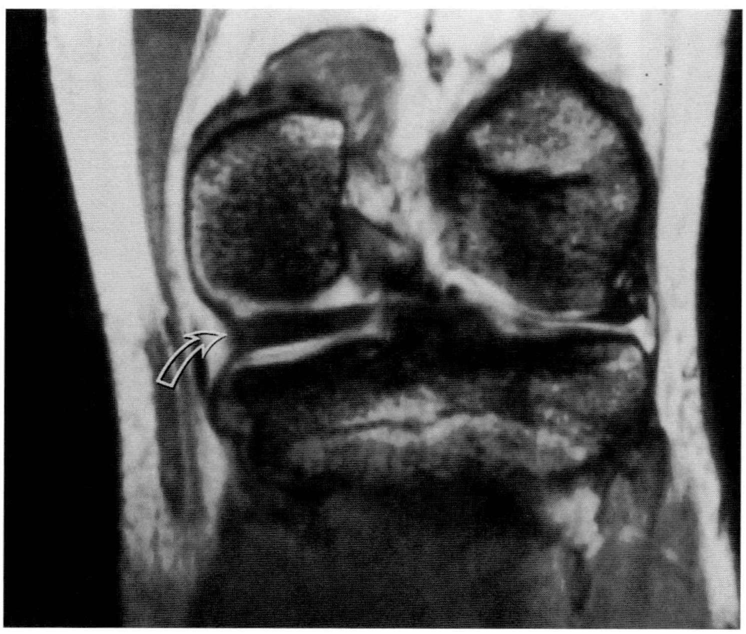

C

FIG. 6-11. Partial volume averaging of meniscus edge. **A:** This diagram shows how the edge of the meniscus can appear to have linear grade 2 degeneration in the sagittal plane secondary to partial volume averaging of the concave meniscus edge. **B:** Sagittal image through the most medial aspect of the body of the medial aspect of the body of the medial meniscus shows apparent grade 2 meniscus degeneration *(arrows).* **C:** This coronal image reveals that the medial meniscus has a concave edge *(arrow)* that allows partial volume averaging to show a linear high signal mimicking grade 2 degeneration in the sagittal plane as shown in **B**.

images. On the sagittal images only two cuts should be of the body (if the cuts are 5 mm thick) because the body of the meniscus averages 12 mm in width (9).

If a coronal image has the fibula or condyles of the femur visible, be wary of suggesting the diagnosis of a discoid meniscus. If the meniscus is discoid only in its anterior or posterior horns, one can occasionally rely on the increased height of the affected portion as compared to the opposite meniscus. If a meniscus is 2 mm thicker than the opposite meniscus as measured in its periphery, it should be considered abnormal (Fig. 6-14). This is not an extremely reliable sign, but it is helpful when present.

As with the previously mentioned pitfall of the posterior coronal images mimicking a discoid meniscus, the posterior coronal images can mimic a bucket-handle tear (Fig. 6-15). The more posterior cuts can go through the body and then through the posterior horn as it makes its C configuration. This gives the appearance of meniscal tissue that is removed from the body and displaced into the more central part of the joint. Again, beware of calling a bucket-handle tear with a displaced fragment using only the far posterior coronal slices (when the fibula is visualized). This can also be seen on the far anterior cuts, but not as commonly. Unfortunately, a true bucket-handle tear often has the displaced central frag-

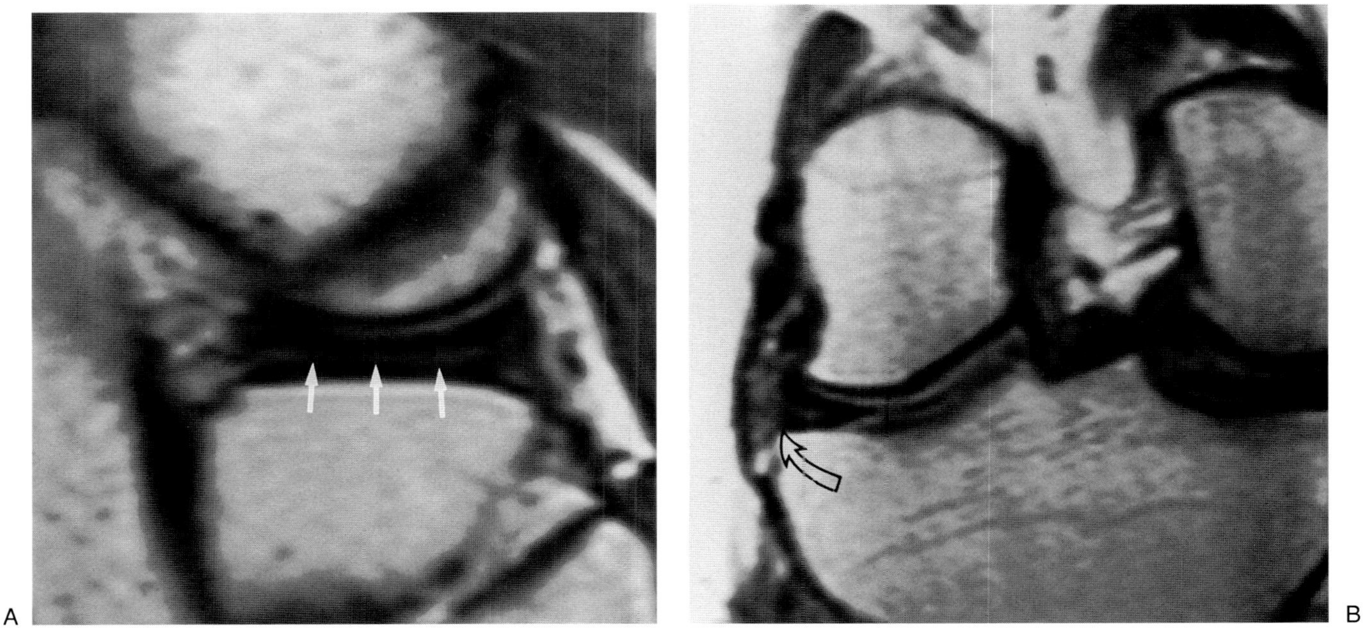

FIG. 6-12. Meniscal cyst mimicking partial volume artifact. **A:** Sagittal image through the lateral-most aspect of the lateral meniscus in this patient shows a linear high-signal region in the body of the meniscus *(arrows)* that resembles the partial volume artifact illustrated in Fig. 6-11. **B:** Coronal image in this patient shows that the high signal seen in the meniscus on the sagittal image is caused by a large meniscal cyst *(arrow)* that extends from the meniscus into the adjacent soft tissues.

ment seen only on the far anterior or posterior cuts. Therefore, other criteria must be present to diagnose a bucket-handle tear.

A bucket-handle tear can be difficult to diagnose when it is not large. There are several ways to improve detection of a bucket-handle tear. First, it is necessary to understand exactly what a bucket-handle tear is. This type of tear is a vertically oriented tear through the body of the meniscus that may or may not involve the anterior or posterior horns. If the central portion of the meniscus is displaced, it forms the "handle" of the bucket and the remaining rim of meniscus appears smaller (Fig. 6-16). The remaining meniscus may have a truncated appearance or a normal configuration, but smaller. If its configuration appears normal except for its size, it can be very difficult to detect. It is important, therefore, to count how many sagittal images show the "bowtie" shape of the meniscus body. The average width of the body of the meniscus is 9–12 mm; thus, with 5-mm-thick slices, at least two images should be through the meniscus body. If the body can only be visualized on one image, or on none at all, a bucket-handle tear should be considered (Fig. 6-17). An inspection of the intercondylar notch and the Hoffa's fat pad region anteriorly will often reveal the remainder of the meniscus as a free fragment or as the displaced "handle" of the bucket.

In a similar fashion, a parrot-beak tear can be diagnosed by noting a small gap in the second bowtie image. A parrot-beak tear is a radial or free-edge tear (Fig. 6-18), which is uncommon; usually, symptoms are not severe enough to warrant surgery. However, most surgeons will debride the torn free edge if it is encountered. A parrot-beak tear should be suspected if the second bowtie segment is not complete (Fig. 6-19). If there is blunting or rounding of the separated portions, the diagnosis can be made with assurance.

A meniscocapsular separation of the medial meniscus is one of the more commonly missed diagnoses in the knee. This is a crucial diagnosis to make with MR because it can be difficult to diagnose clinically and the treatment afforded the patient is dependent on the diagnosis. These tears can be treated with immobilization, allowing the vascular meniscal periphery to rejoin with the capsule. Alternatively, some orthopedists prefer to suture the meniscus to the capsule. Failure to make the diagnosis with continuing weight bearing and stress to the area can result in nonunion of this tear and further meniscal degeneration.

Meniscocapsular separation can be diagnosed by seeing high-signal-intensity joint fluid extending between the normally adherent medial meniscus and the medial capsule on T2-weighted images. If only T1-weighted images are obtained, a separation of the medial meniscus from the capsule can be very difficult to appreciate (Fig. 6-20). T2-weighted images should be obtained in the coronal plane so that a meniscocapsular separation is not overlooked. If no joint effusion is present, it can be very difficult to diagnose this type of tear. Fast spin-echo T2 coronal images can be employed; however, fat saturation should be utilized. On fast spin-echo T2 images fat and fluid can have similar signal; a small fat pad, often present between

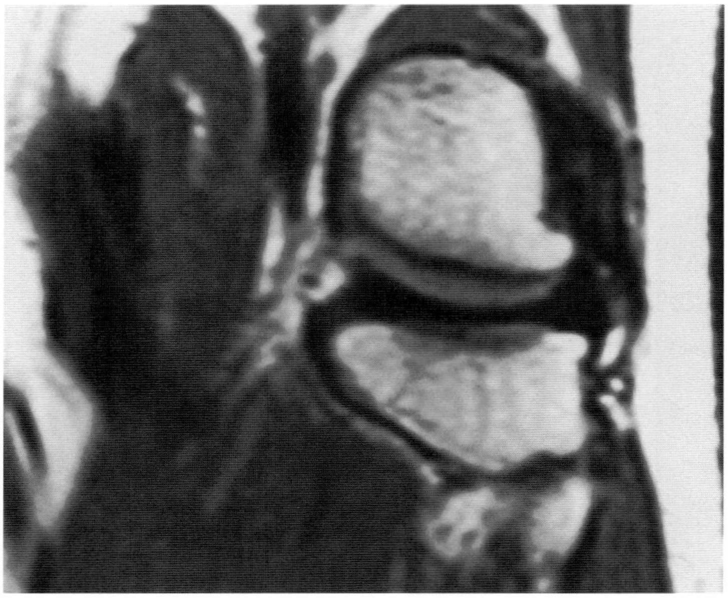

A

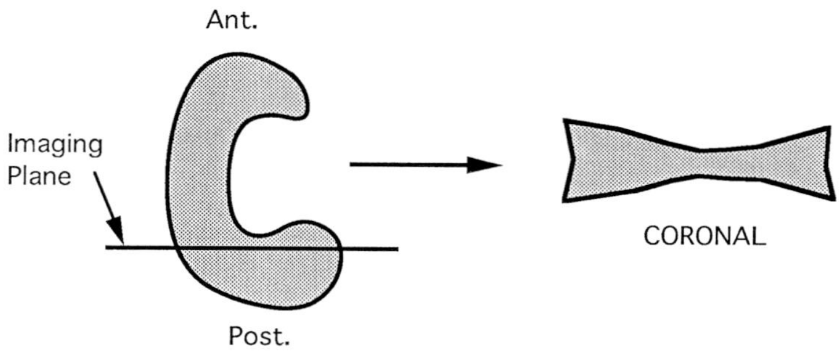

B

FIG. 6-13. Pseudodiscoid meniscus. **A:** The medial meniscus in this T1-weighted coronal image through the posterior horn of the menisci has a discoid appearance, with the meniscus extending almost into the intercondylar notch. This is the usual appearance of a normal meniscus on the posterior coronal cuts. Note that the fibular head is present, which is a tip-off that the image is through the posterior horns. **B:** This drawing illustrates how a coronal image through the posterior horn of the meniscus can mimic a discoid meniscus.

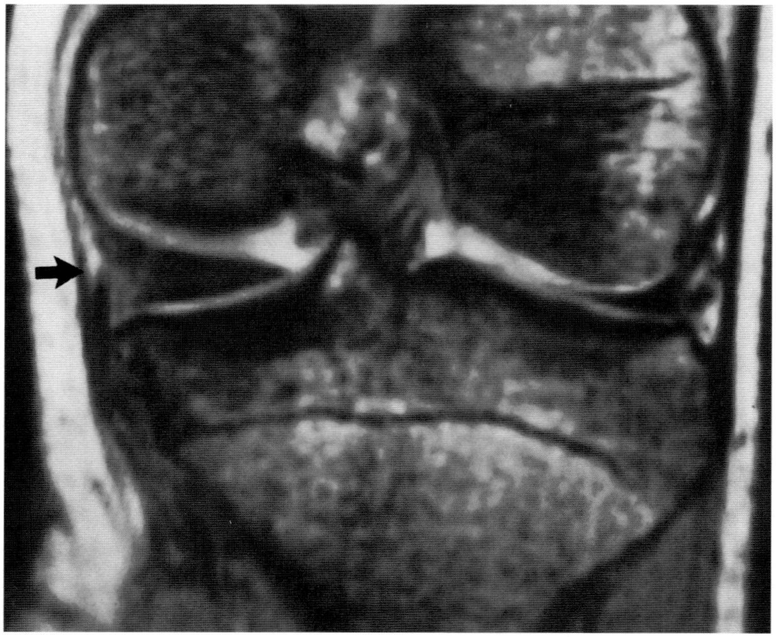

FIG. 6-14. Discoid meniscus with increased height. This coronal image demonstrates a medial meniscus with an abnormally large height as measured at the meniscocapsular junction *(arrow)*. This is a discoid medial meniscus.

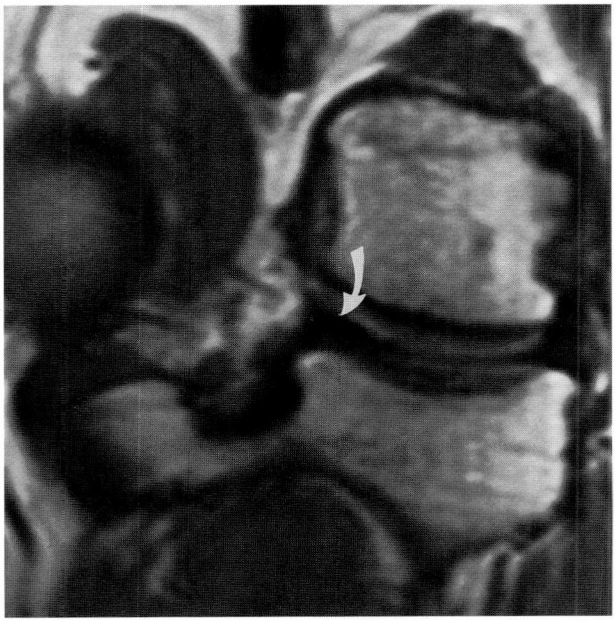

A

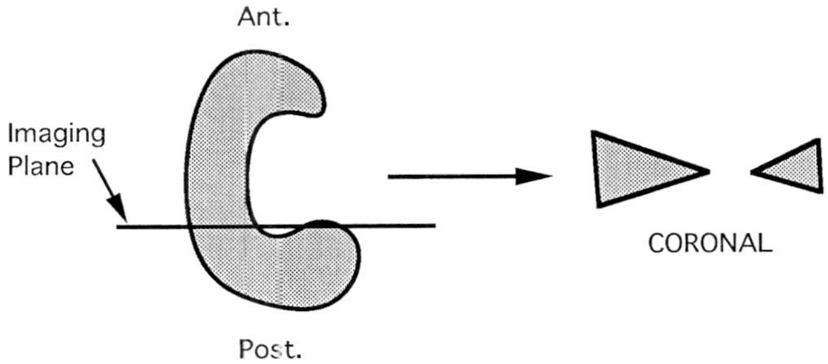

B

FIG. 6-15. Pseudo-bucket-handle tear. **A:** This coronal image shows a normal triangle of medial meniscus with a second triangular piece of meniscus *(arrow)* seen near the intercondylar notch that mimics a free fragment as seen with a bucket-handle tear. This image is a far posterior cut, however, which can produce this appearance normally and mimic a bucket-handle tear. **B:** This drawing illustrates how a far posterior coronal image can give the appearance of a free fragment and mimic a bucket-handle tear.

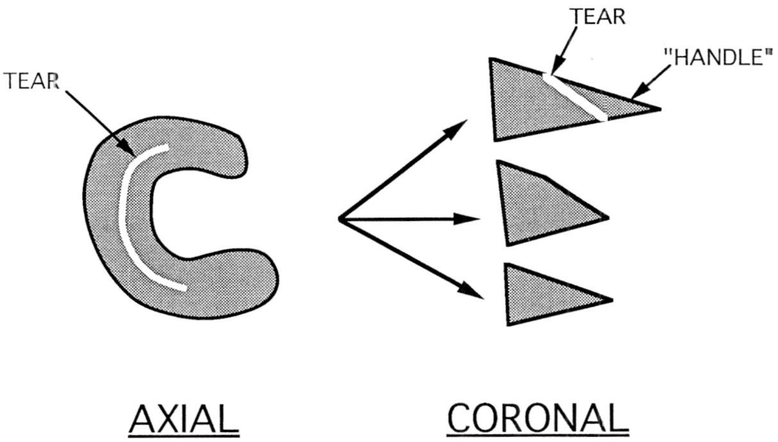

A

FIG. 6-16. Drawing of a bucket-handle tear. **A:** This drawing shows the configuration of a bucket-handle tear and how the residual meniscus can appear in coronal images before and after the "handle" has become displaced. **B:** This drawing shows a meniscus with a bucket-handle tear in which the "handle" separates from the body and extends into the intercondylar notch. **C:** This drawing shows how the "handle" in a bucket-handle tear can flip into the notch.

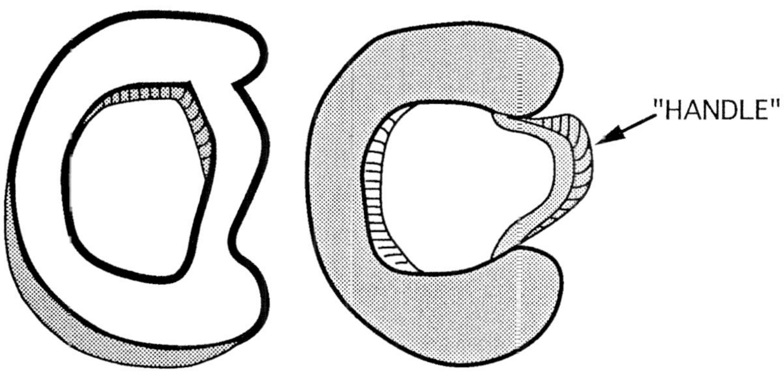

B

C

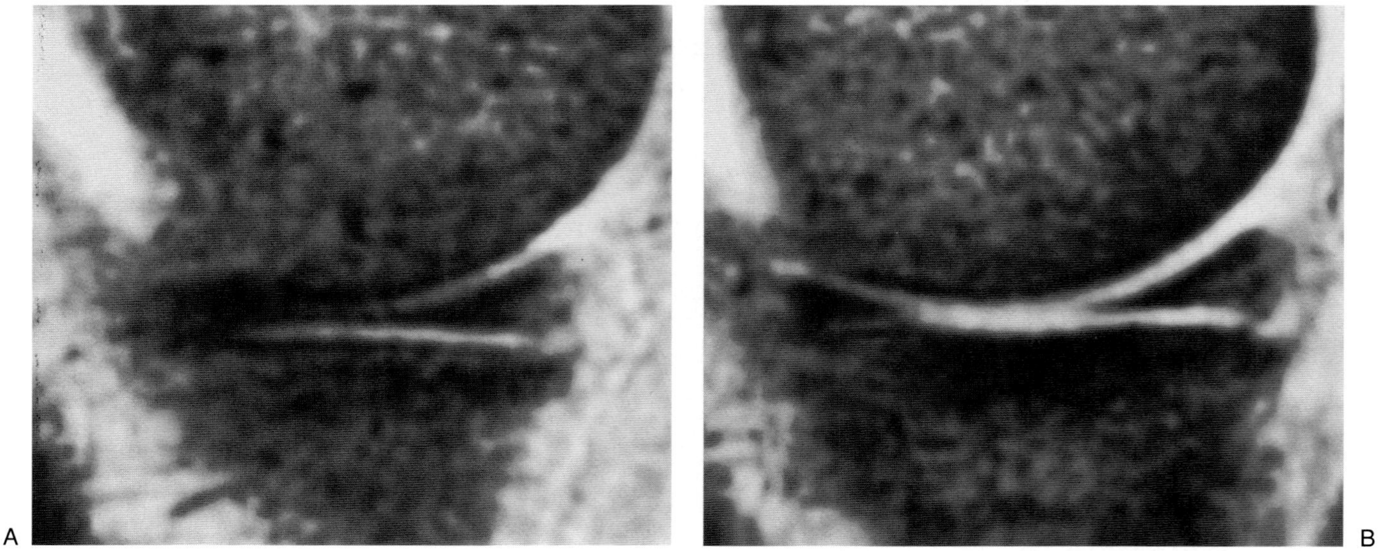

FIG. 6-17. Bucket-handle tear with one "bowtie" image. **A:** The lateral-most sagittal image in this patient reveals a normal-appearing body segment of the lateral meniscus. It typically has a "bowtie" shape that should be present on two consecutive images. The adjacent image **(B)** has what appears to be a normal anterior and posterior horn; however, since this image should have a "bowtie" configuration, a bucket-handle tear should be considered. This was a large bucket-handle tear.

the medial collateral ligament and the medial meniscus, can be mistaken for fluid, allowing a false diagnosis of meniscocapsular separation. Also, a tibial collateral ligament bursa has been described (10) that can present as fluid between the medial meniscus and the capsule at the tibial collateral ligament (Fig. 6-21). It can usually be easily differentiated from a meniscocapsular separation if it is present on only one coronal image and the fluid is contained in a sac rather than being free.

If the meniscus is separated from the capsule it occasionally displaces into the joint, leaving a gap at the meniscocapsular junction. Unfortunately, the normal distance that the meniscus maintains with the capsule varies widely, reflecting the normal mobility of the meniscus. On the far anterior or posterior cuts the normal meniscus can appear to be displaced into the joint somewhat, mimicking a meniscocapsular separation with displacement.

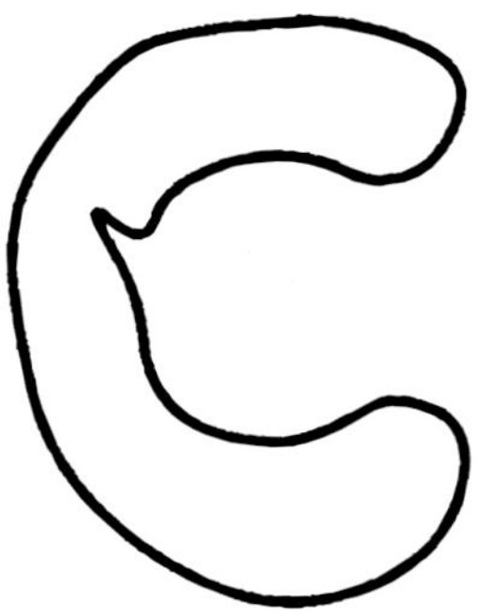

FIG. 6-18. Parrot-beak tear. This schematic illustrates the appearance of a radial or free-edge tear that is called a parrot-beak tear.

If a 256 × 128 matrix is employed a Gibbs truncation artifact can occur and mimic a meniscal tear (11,12). These artifacts characteristically occur at sharp, high-contrast interfaces and result in a series of regularly spaced bands of high signal that are mismapped in the phase-encoding direction. In the knee this is exhibited as a curvilinear stripe of high signal that parallels the femoral condyle and is mismapped onto the meniscus (Fig. 6-22). It can usually be appreciated as an artifact if it extends off of the meniscus, but often this is not appreciated and a torn meniscus is mistakenly diagnosed. Gross motion artifacts can have an identical appearance. If a pseudo-tear that resembles a Gibbs truncation artifact is present and the imaging matrix is not 256 × 128, it is probably a motion artifact.

In general, grades 1 and 2 meniscus degeneration are not important findings, but it is important that they not be mistaken for complete meniscal tears. Occasionally, however, the signal in some areas of presumed degeneration is of such magnitude that an intrasubstance tear should be considered. This is a true meniscal tear that does not extend to the articular surface of the meniscus. It has been reported to be capable of causing symptoms (13) but cannot be seen at arthrography or with surface inspection of the meniscus at arthroscopy. It is a somewhat controversial entity and is very uncommon. It may, in fact, be nothing more than a meniscal cyst that has collapsed. When this occurs it is usually associated with a parameniscal fluid collection or cyst that has been extruded from the meniscus.

Following meniscectomy, an intermediate-signal "ghost

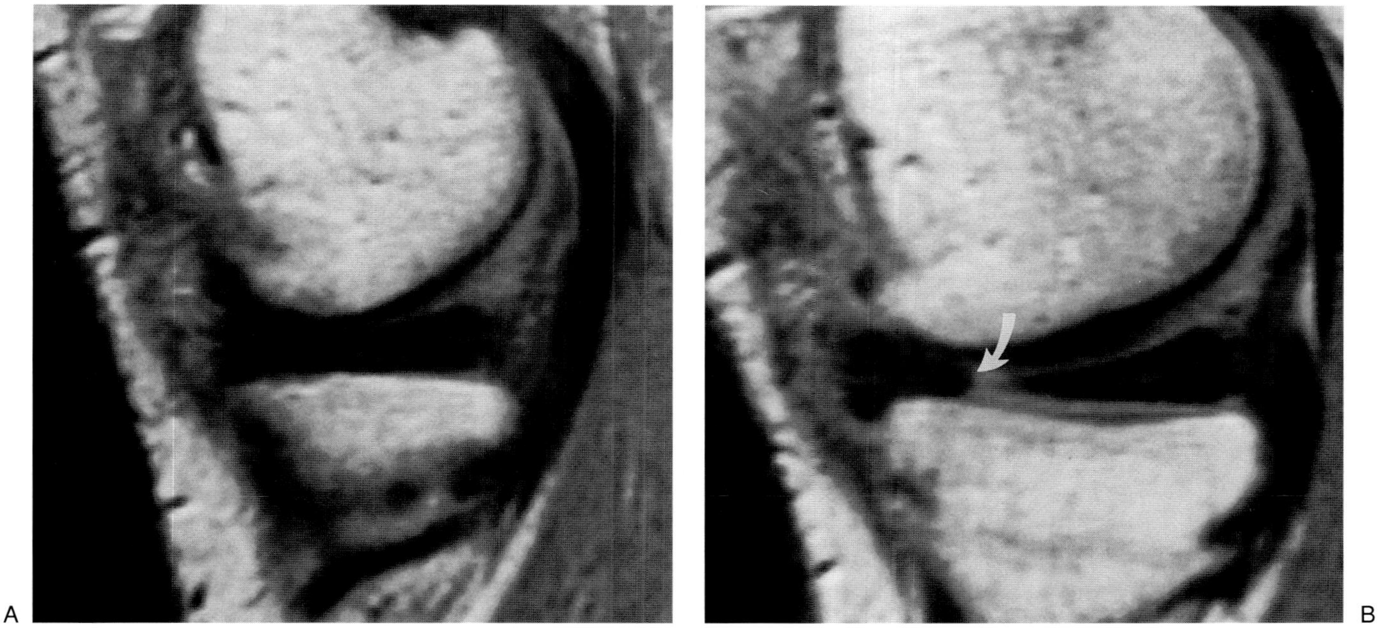

FIG. 6-19. Parrot-beak tear. A: A sagittal proton-density image through the far medial aspect of the medial meniscus shows the normal bowtie appearance of the body segment. The next adjacent sagittal image (B) should be another bowtie segment, but instead reveals a small gap that represents a tear in the free edge of the meniscus. Note the rounded anterior portion *(arrow)* that makes the diagnosis of a parrot-beak tear even easier.

meniscus'' can be seen filling the space of the former meniscus (Fig. 6-23). Initially, the space is filled with fluid, but with time it takes on a more intermediate signal. This may represent fibrous tissue that has filled in the space. A ''ghost meniscus'' can also be seen following a peripheral tear with complete displacement of the meniscus or of the anterior or posterior horn. Sometimes diminished signal throughout the anterior or posterior horn in the form of a ''ghost meniscus'' is all that is present to tell that the meniscus is completely torn loose and displaced.

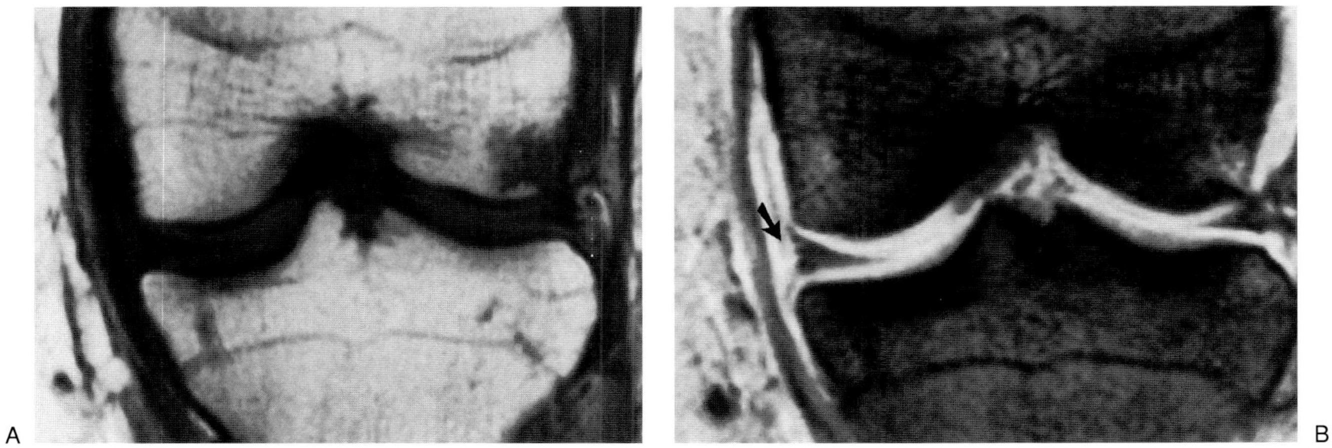

FIG. 6-20. Meniscocapsular separation. A: T1-weighted coronal image shows no definite abnormalities. It is difficult to ascertain whether joint fluid is separating the medial collateral ligament/capsule complex from the medial meniscus on a T1-weighted image. B: This T2-weighted image reveals fluid between the medial meniscus and the capsule *(arrow)* that could not be appreciated on the T1-weighted image. This is a meniscocapsular separation. On the lateral side, this can be very difficult to diagnose with MRI because the attachment to the capsule is very loose and the popliteus tendon and bursa can contain fluid that mimics a separation. On the medial side, however, fluid between the meniscus and the capsule should generally be considered abnormal.

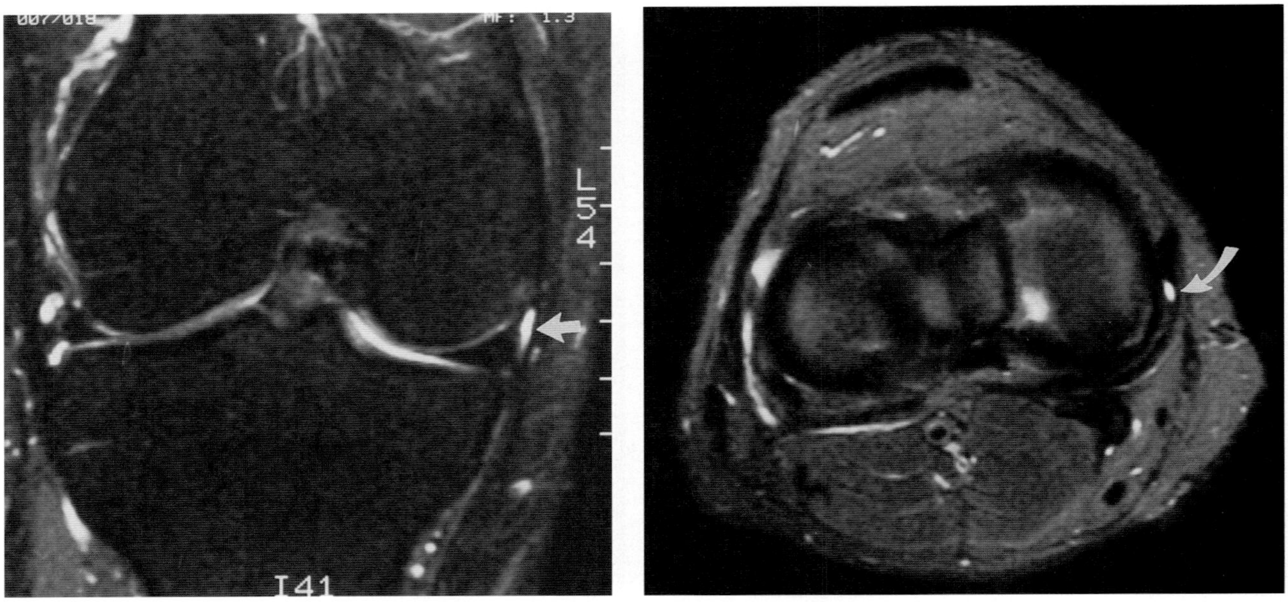

A B

FIG. 6-21. Tibial collateral ligament bursa. **A:** A coronal gradient-echo image shows fluid between the medial meniscus and the medial or tibial collateral ligament *(arrow)*. This should indicate a meniscocapsular separation; however, the adjacent images anterior and posterior to this one appeared normal. Also, the fluid seems very well defined, rather than diffuse throughout the soft tissues. The axial gradient-echo image **(B)** showed the fluid to be a rounded collection *(arrow)* characteristic for a tibial collateral ligament bursa.

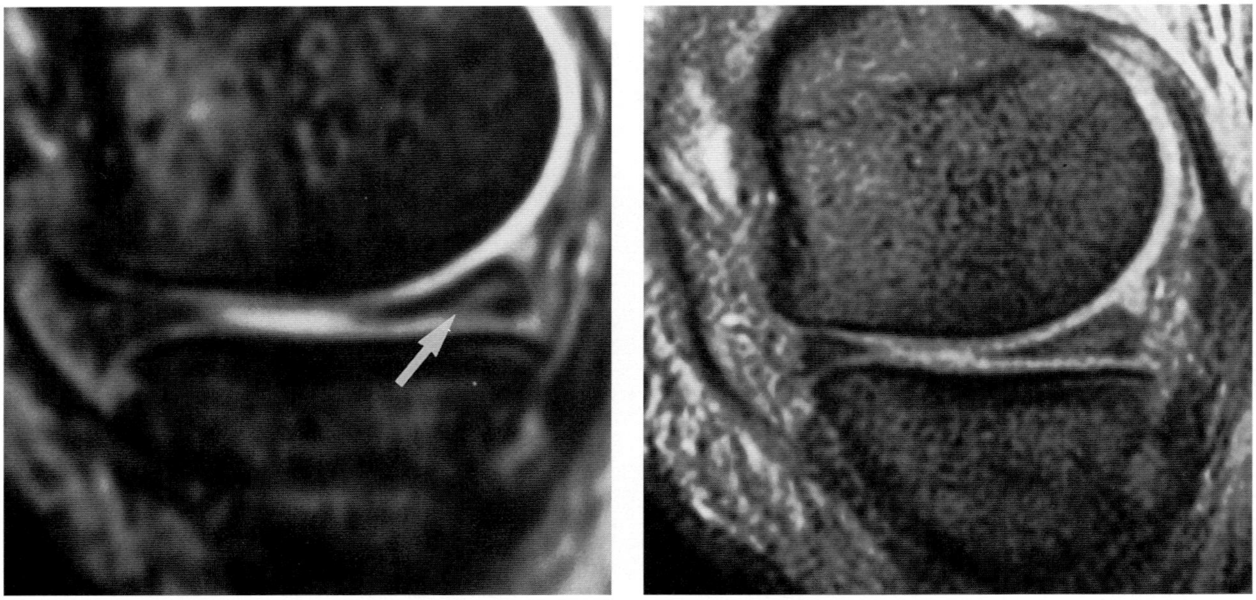

A B

FIG. 6-22. Gibbs truncation artifact. **A:** The high signal in the meniscus *(arrow)* in this patient is suspicious for an artifact because of its curvilinear appearance and because it was not found in other images through the same area taken with other parameters **(B).** This is characteristic for a Gibbs truncation artifact. Patient motion can cause a similar appearance.

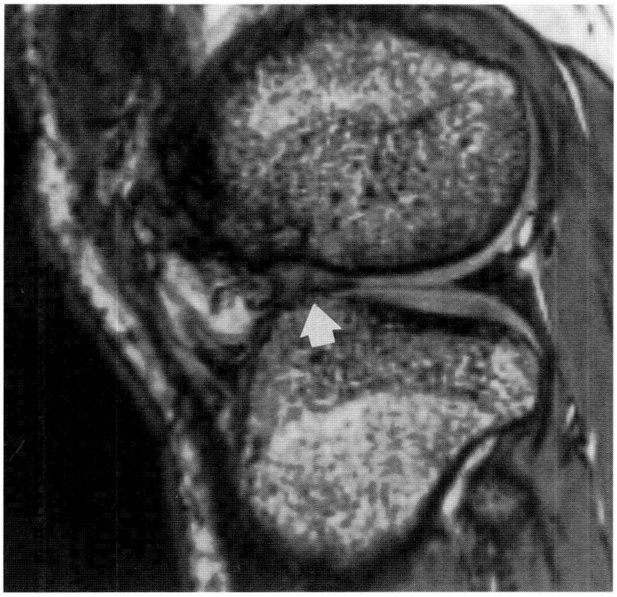

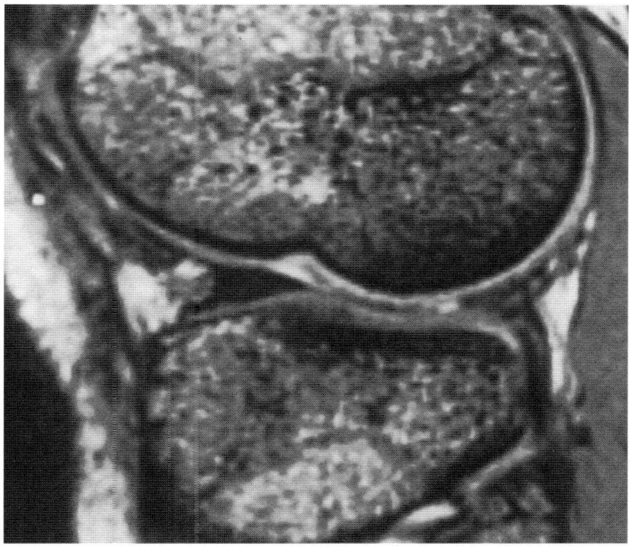

A B

FIG. 6-23. "Ghost meniscus." **A:** The anterior horn of the medial meniscus *(arrow)* has a uniformly higher signal than the posterior horn. The anterior horn has been torn and is displaced, leaving a ghost meniscus appearance. Often this uniformly higher signal is all that will be present to denote an absent section of meniscus. This is frequently seen following meniscectomy. **B:** This three-dimensional image shows the posterior horn of the lateral meniscus to be considerably higher in signal than the anterior horn. The posterior horn has been surgically removed, and now there is the appearance of a ghost meniscus.

The body of the medial meniscus sometimes will be found to have a wavy or folded appearance (Fig. 6-24). This is a normal variant called a meniscal flounce (14).

LIGAMENTS

The meniscofemoral ligaments of Humphry and Wrisberg course obliquely across the posterior aspect of the knee from the posterior horn of the lateral meniscus superiorly to the medial femoral condyle. The ligament of Humphry courses anteriorly to the posterior cruciate ligament (Fig. 6-25), and the ligament of Wrisberg passes just posterior to the posterior cruciate ligament (Fig. 6-26). The ligament of Humphry has been reported in 24–33% of patients (2,4) (42% in our own series), whereas the ligament of Wrisberg has been reported in 23–33% (2,4) (27% in our series). They are visualized simultaneously in only 3–12% of cases (2,4) (7% in our series). They have been confused for partial tears of the posterior cruciate ligament with fibers "balled up" around the tear. They are also occasionally confused for free fragments of meniscal tissue or cortical bone (Fig. 6-27). Since meniscal fragments often migrate anteriorly or posteriorly to the cruciate ligaments in the intercondylar notch, it is important to recognize the normal meniscofemoral ligaments and not to confuse them for free fragments.

The anterior cruciate ligament is considered to be torn if its fibers are not seen intact and taut on the sagittal images. Occasionally, however, the fibers of the anterior cruciate

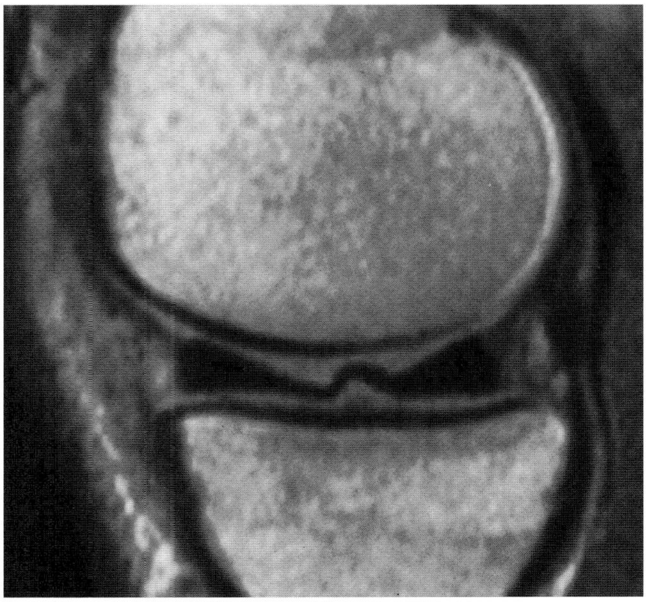

FIG. 6-24. Meniscal flounce. A sagittal T1-weighted image through the medial meniscus shows the meniscus to have a wavy or buckled appearance. This is a normal finding termed a meniscal flounce.

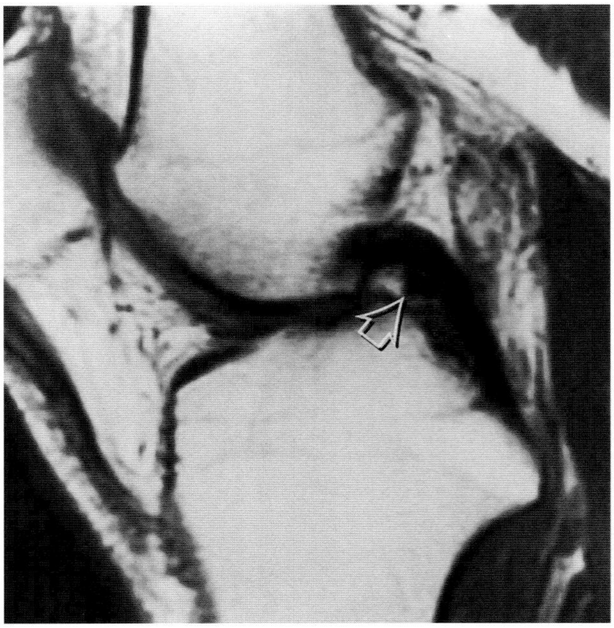

FIG. 6-25. Ligament of Humphry. This T1-weighted image through the posterior cruciate ligament shows the ligament of Humphry *(arrow)* just anterior to the posterior cruciate.

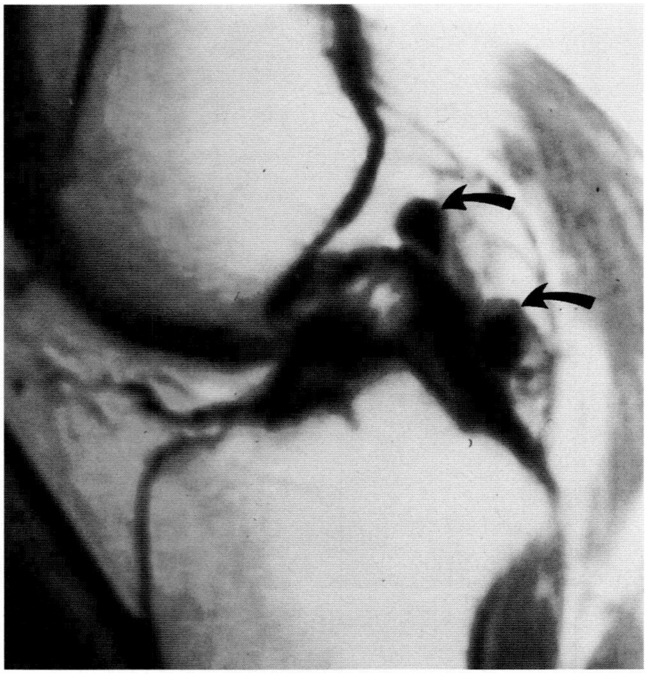

FIG. 6-27. Free fragments mimicking ligament of Wrisberg. Sagittal T1-weighted image through the posterior cruciate ligament shows two low-signal round structures *(arrows)*, either of which could be confused for the ligament of Wrisberg. These are free fragments of a torn meniscus, one of which could be followed to the medial side of the knee.

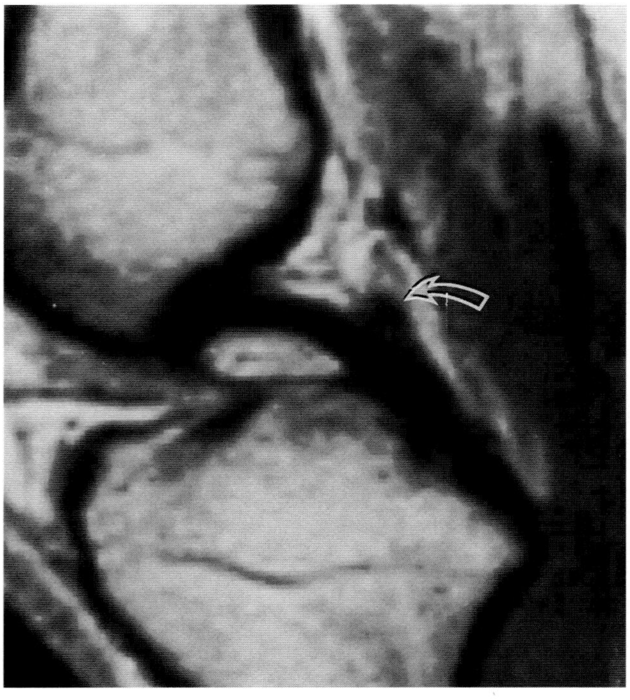

FIG. 6-26. Ligament of Wrisberg. This T1-weighted sagittal image through the posterior cruciate ligament demonstrates the ligament of Wrisberg *(arrow)* just dorsal to the posterior cruciate.

ligament and the bony margin of the intercondylar notch are partially volume averaged and the anterior cruciate appears to be disrupted proximally (Fig. 6-28). It is rare for this to occur on both the T1- and the T2-weighted images in the same patient. Hence, if the anterior cruciate appears torn in one set of images and not in the other, it is likely to be from partial volume averaging of the femur.

The medial collateral ligament is best identified on T2-weighted coronal images. If T1-weighted coronal images are acquired to examine the collateral ligaments, a joint effusion can obscure visualization of the medial collateral ligament (Fig. 6-29). With T2-weighted images the medial collateral ligament and the joint effusion can be differentiated, resulting in increased conspicuity of ligamentous rupture. Also, partial tears and strains of the ligament can be diagnosed by the presence of increased signal in an intact ligament. As mentioned earlier, T2-weighted coronals are necessary for diagnosing meniscocapsular separations. For these reasons we acquire our coronal images with T2 weighting. As mentioned previously, if fast spin-echo T2 is used for the coronal images, we employ fat saturation.

Axial images are obtained primarily to examine the patellar cartilage. If an effusion is present the cartilage cannot be seen with T1-weighted images; therefore, as in the coronal images, T2 weighting should be used on the axial images (Fig. 6-30). With gradient-echo T2* weighting, the hyaline

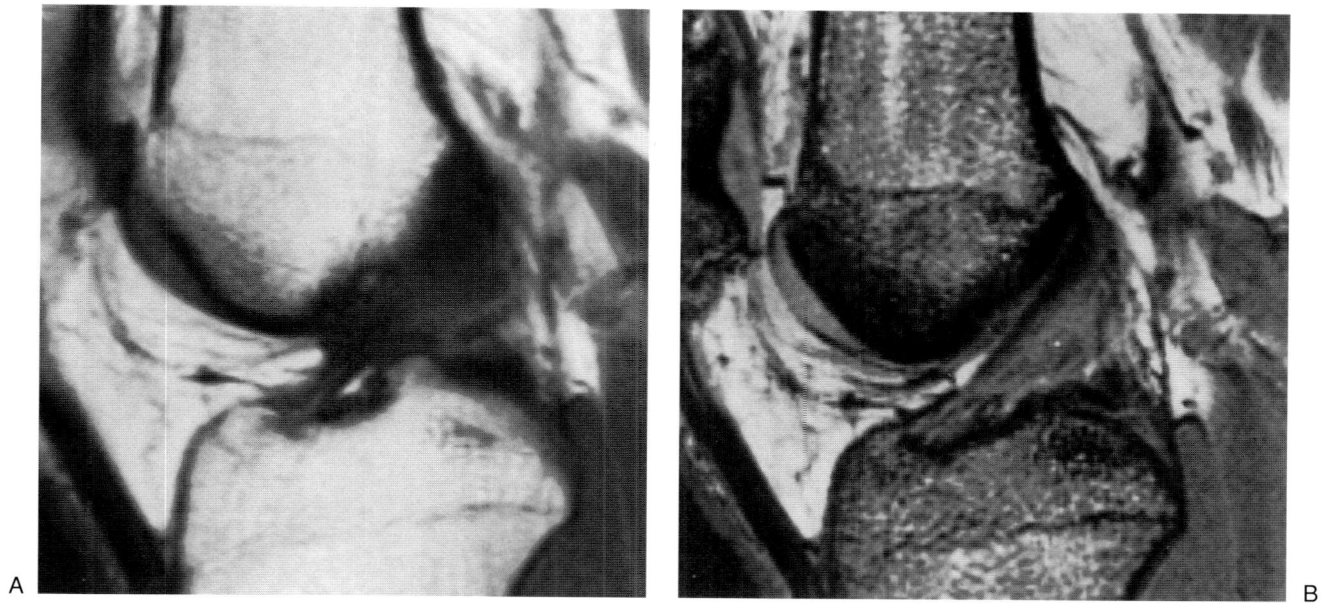

FIG. 6-28. Anterior cruciate ligament pseudotear. **A:** T1-weighted sagittal image (5 mm thick) through the intercondylar notch in this patient shows the anterior cruciate ligament to be poorly delineated from its origin on the femur to its midportion. **B:** A three-dimensional sagittal image (3 mm thick) shows the same anterior cruciate ligament to be intact throughout. The appearance in **A** is due to partial volume averaging of the ligament with the bony portion of the notch. This is seen more frequently in thicker section slices and decreases with thinner sections.

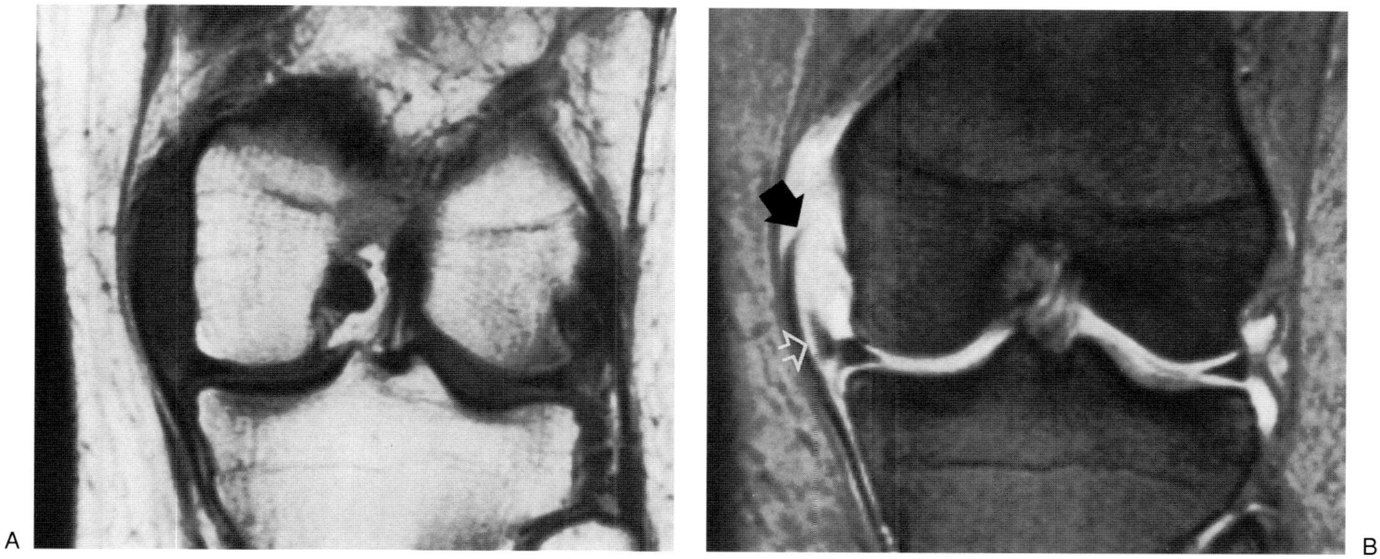

FIG. 6-29. Medial collateral ligament on T1- and T2-weighted images. **A**: *This T1-weighted coronal image demonstrates the difficulty of examining the medial collateral ligament when an effusion is present. The ligament cannot be differentiated from the joint fluid with T1 weighting. Also, a meniscocapsular separation cannot be diagnosed because joint fluid cannot be identified extending between the medial meniscus and the capsule.* **B:** The same knee with a T2* image shows that the medial collateral ligament is disrupted proximally *(large arrow)* and that the medial meniscus is separated from the capsule *(small arrow)*, as evidenced by the high-signal joint fluid extending between the meniscus and the capsule.

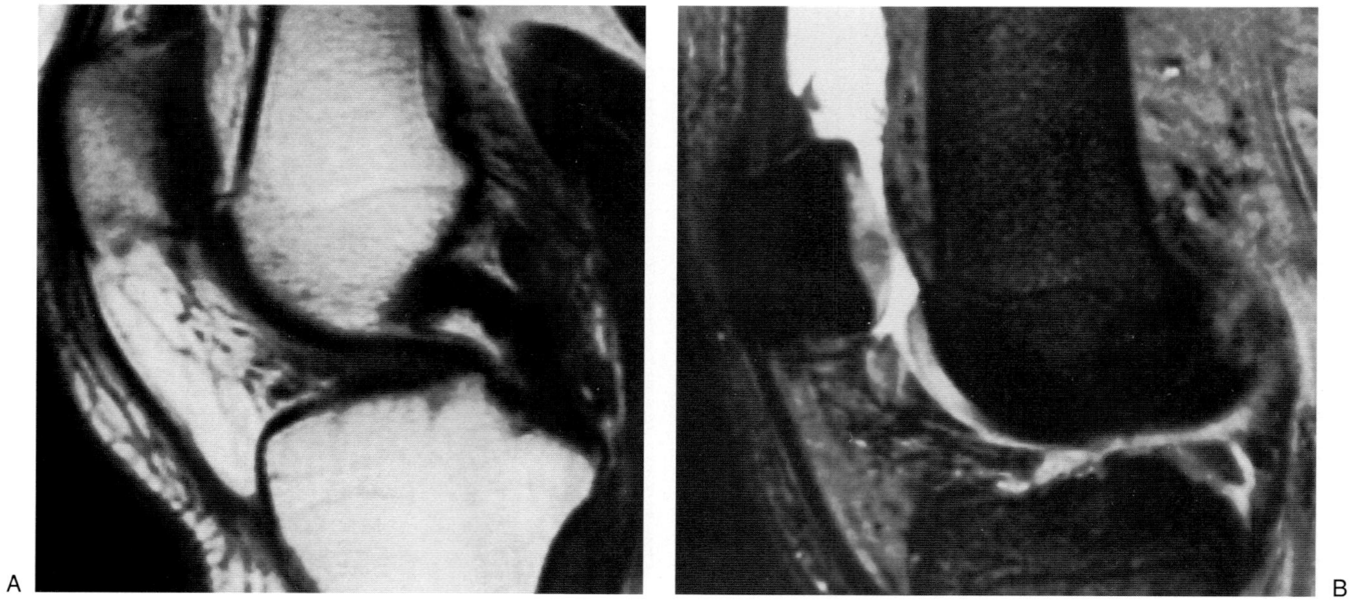

FIG. 6-30. Patellar articular cartilage on T1- and T2-weighted axial images. **A:** This T1-weighted sagittal image fails to show the hyaline articular cartilage due to the isointense joint fluid. **B:** With T2* weighting, the fluid and the patellar cartilage can be differentiated, allowing examination of the cartilage.

articular cartilage cannot be differentiated from joint fluid in every case unless a long TE is used. Hence, a dual echo should be considered for the axial images if gradient-echo sequences are used. The joint fluid will be clearly differentiated from the cartilage on either the first or the second echo image in every case. STIR and fast spin-echo T2-weighted axial images are also satisfactory for examining the patellar cartilage.

The T2-weighted axial images are also useful for identifying the medial patellar plica, which is present in up to 70% of all knees but only rarely causes symptomatology, the so-called plica syndrome (15). If T1-weighted axial images are obtained the plica cannot be differentiated from joint fluid. On T2-weighted images the plica is easily seen extending from the medial joint capsule toward the medial patella facet, but only if the joint is distended with fluid.

The normal medial patellar plica is a thin, fibrous band of tissue that varies in extent from a few millimeters to several centimeters as seen on axial images (Fig. 6-31). A thickened plica should be mentioned when it is noted to be more than a millimeter or two thick (Fig. 6-32); however, no measurements have been published to reliably determine an abnormal plica. A thick plica can cause signs and symptoms indistinguishable from a torn meniscus—clicking, locking, and a feeling of instability. Hence, it should be preoperatively noted so the surgeon will be forewarned of the correct pathology. A plica can be easily removed at arthroscopy.

Rarely, an infrapatellar plica will be identified. The infrapatellar plica, also called the ligamentum mucosum, extends from Hoffa's fat pad to the anterior cruciate ligament in a

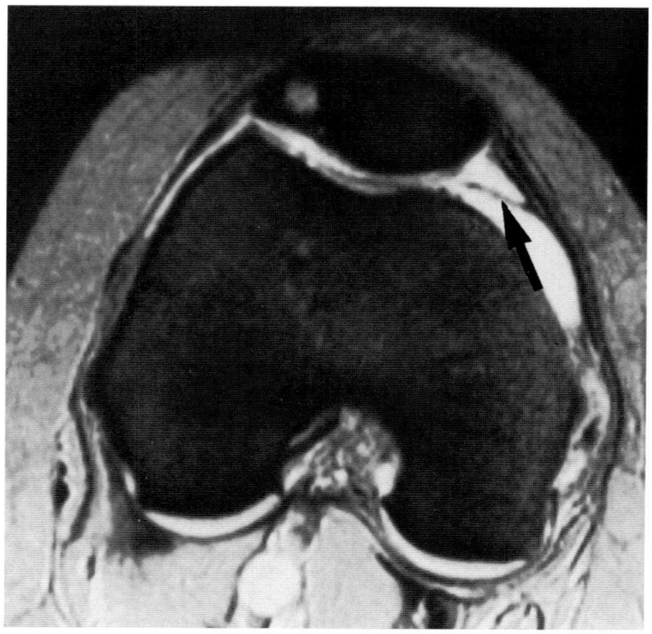

FIG. 6-31. Medial patellar plica. This axial T2-weighted image shows a thin, low-signal linear structure *(arrow)* with joint fluid on either side. It extends into the medial facet of the patella. This is a medial patellar plica.

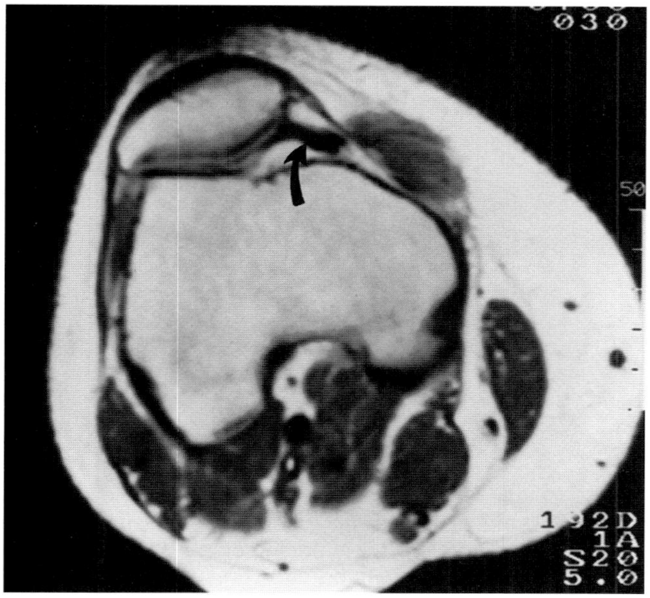

FIG. 6-32. Abnormal plica. This axial T1-weighted image shows a thick band of low signal in the expected location of a medial patellar plica *(arrow)*. Since this is a T1-weighted image, it is possible this may be merely joint fluid. The sagittal T2-weighted images showed no joint fluid to be present, however. This is an extremely thickened plica that clinically mimicked a torn medial meniscus.

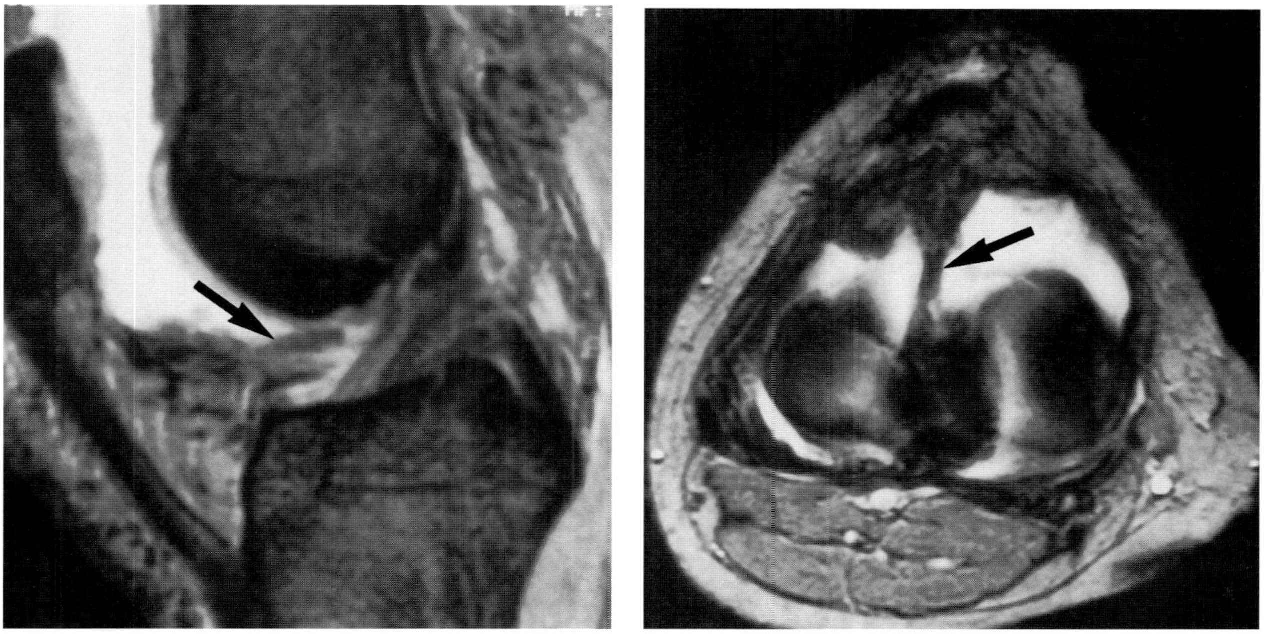

A B

FIG. 6-33. Infrapatellar plica. **A:** A sagittal T2-weighted image through the intercondylar notch shows a band of low-signal-intensity tissue extending from Hoffa's fat pad toward the anterior cruciate ligament *(arrow)*. **B:** The axial image shows this midline band of tissue again *(arrow)*. This is an infrapatellar plica.

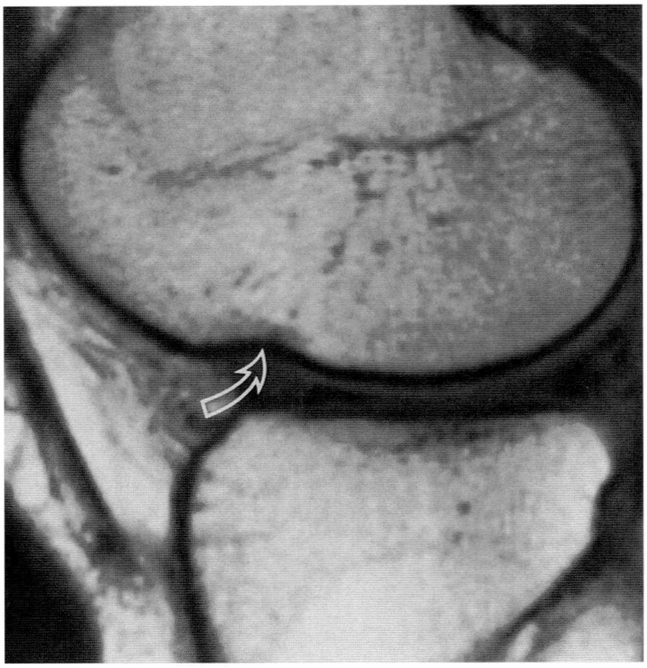

FIG. 6-34. Depression on anterolateral femoral condyle. This depression on the anterolateral portion of the femoral condyle *(arrow)* is a normal variant that is often present and should not be confused with an osteochondral defect secondary to trauma or avascular necrosis unless it is greater than 1.5 mm in depth. It then seems to correlate with a torn anterior cruciate ligament.

A

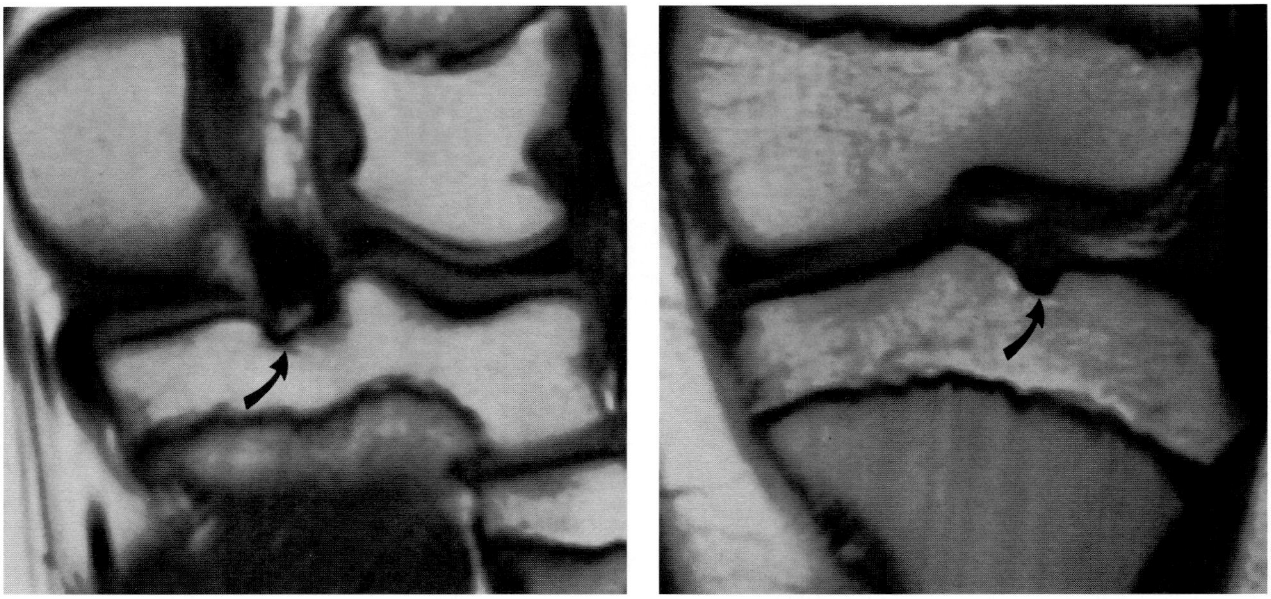

B

FIG. 6-35. Posteromedial and anterolateral tibial pits. **A:** T1-weighted coronal image through the posterior knee demonstrates a large bony depression or defect on the medial tibial plateau *(arrow)* that mimics an osteochondral fracture. This is the insertion of the posterior cruciate ligament, found in 100% of knees. **B:** This T1-weighted coronal image through the anterior knee shows a bony depression on the lateral tibial plateau *(arrow)* that is found in up to 95% of all knees. It represents the insertion of the anterior cruciate ligament.

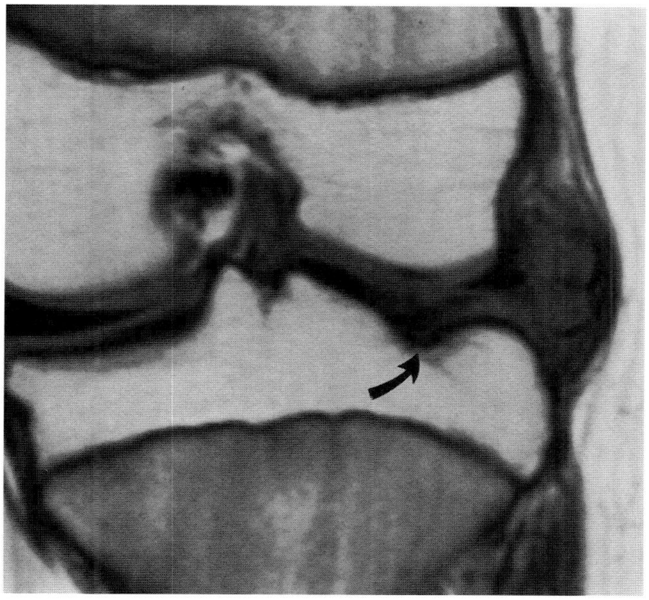

FIG. 6-36. Osteochondral defect. This T1-weighted coronal image shows a defect on the posterior lateral tibial plateau *(arrow)* that is similar to the normal depressions illustrated in Fig. 35; however, this is a true osteochondral fracture. This depression is located on the posterior *lateral* part of the tibial plateau rather than on the posterior *medial* side.

sagittal band and divides the joint into medial and lateral compartments when complete. It can be seen as a band of tissue anterior to the anterior cruciate ligament on sagittal images, and as a linear strand of tissue in the anterior joint space on axial images (Fig. 6-33). It has not been described as causing symptoms.

BONES

A smooth depression on the anterior portion of the lateral femoral condyle is a commonly seen normal variant that, if shallow, should not be confused for an impaction fracture or an osteochondral defect. Its characteristic location, smooth margins, and lack of underlying bony contusion or sclerosis all help in recognizing this depression as normal (Fig. 6-34). The normal depression should be around 0.5 mm. If it is greater than 1.5 mm deep it has been reported to have an association with a torn anterior cruciate ligament (16). It is then presumed to be an impaction defect from the pivot-shift phenomenon in which the lateral femoral condyle impacts the posterior lateral tibial plateau.

Two additional bony irregularities that often are confused

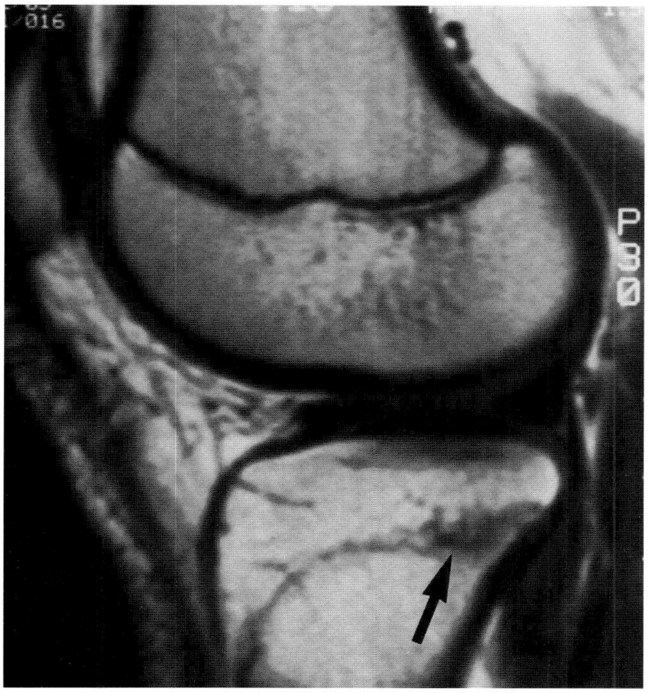

FIG. 6-37. Physeal line mimicking a fracture. This T1-weighted image in a child who suffered trauma to the knee demonstrates the appearance of the normal physeal plate *(arrow)*, which can mimic a fracture line.

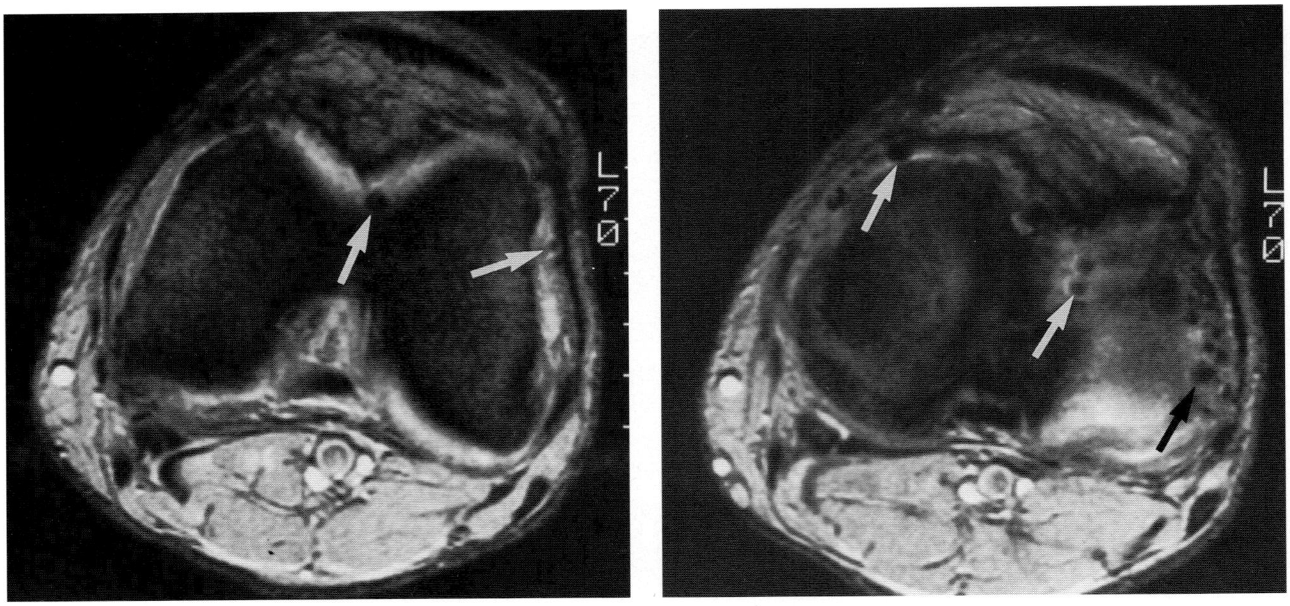

A B

FIG. 6-38. Susceptibility artifacts mimicking loose bodies. **A,B:** Multiple low-signal round structures *(arrows)* that mimic loose bodies in the joint are identified on these axial T2* images. These are susceptibility artifacts from tiny bits of metallic debris left during a prior arthroscopic procedure. Note that several display a high-signal "halo" that is characteristically seen with susceptibility artifacts.

for osteochondral fractures occur on the posteromedial and anterolateral tibial plateau. These are best seen on coronal images and are the insertion points of the anterior and posterior cruciate ligaments (Fig. 6-35). In a series of 100 knee MR studies we found these tibial pits in 100% of those taken posteromedially and in 95% of those done anterolaterally. They ranged in size from 4 to 10 mm on the posteromedial tibia and from 1 to 6 mm on the anterolateral tibia. True osteochondral fractures or defects can be differentiated from these normal variants primarily by their location (Fig. 6-36).

The normal epiphysis or old physeal line scar can mimic a bony fracture (Fig. 6-37). Ordinarily, the differentiation is no problem, but on occasion it is difficult to be certain if the linear low signal is a physeal scar or a fracture. Observing the adjacent bones for physeal scars will often help make the distinction.

Following joint surgery, one will often see multiple small low-signal artifacts that resemble loose bodies (Fig. 6-38). These represent susceptibility artifacts from microscopic pieces of metal left behind by the metallic surgical instru-

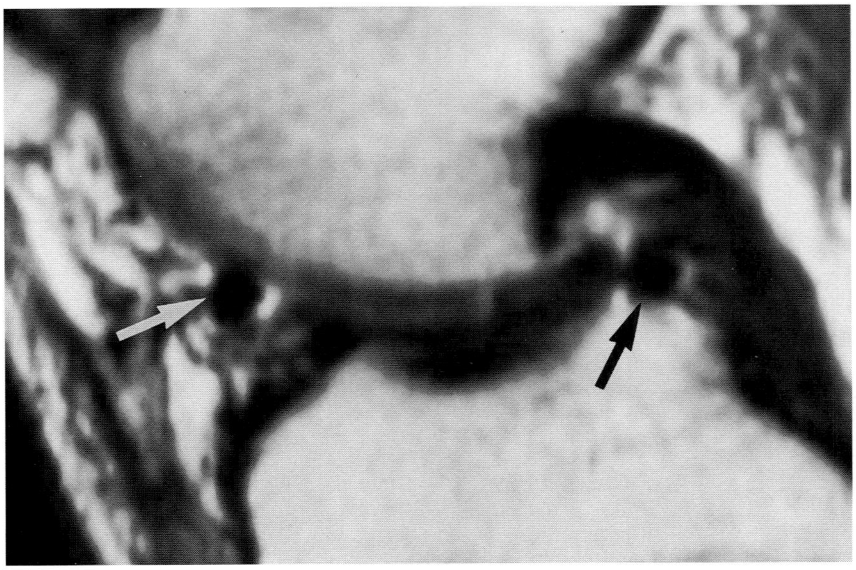

FIG. 6-39. Metallic artifact mimicking loose body. A loosebody *(black arrow)* is seen just anterior to the posterior cruciate ligament in this patient with a bucket-handle tear of the meniscus. What appears to be another loose body is seen in the anterior region of the knee *(white arrow)* but is actually a metallic artifact from prior surgery. Note the high-signal halo around the anterior artifact.

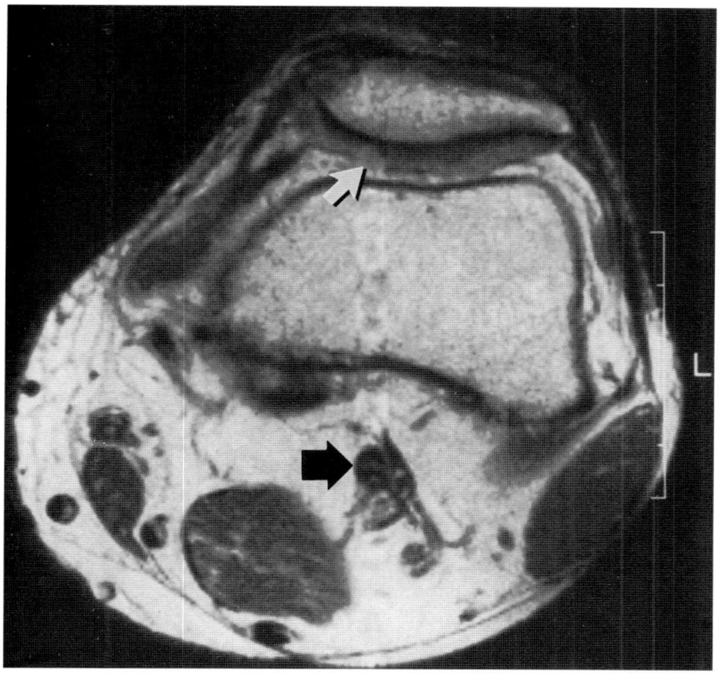

FIG. 6-40. Pulsation artifact on patellar cartilage. An apparent defect in the hyaline articular cartilage of the patella *(small arrow)* is caused by a pulsation artifact from the popliteal artery *(large arrow)*.

ments. They are almost never visible on plain films or CT, but they can be quite pronounced on MR. They should be more prominent on gradient-echo sequences and often have a halo of high signal, which should alert the examiner to their true nature (Fig. 6-39).

The same pulsation artifact from the popliteal artery that was discussed earlier in this chapter can cause an apparent irregularity of the patellar hyaline articular cartilage and subchondral bone that can be confused with chondromalacia patellae (Fig. 6-40). As mentioned, changing the phase-encoding direction from anteroposterior will eliminate this artifact.

A dorsal defect of the patella (DDP) is a round, lytic defect as seen on plain films that occurs solely in the upper outer quadrant of the patella and is thought to be an incidental normal variant (17). Said to occur in 1–2% of the population, it has a nonspecific appearance on MR of low signal on T1-weighted sequences with high signal on T2 (Fig. 6-41); however, its characteristic location should allow the diagnosis to be made.

Residual red marrow may occasionally be seen in the distal femur of healthy adults. Complete signal loss may be seen in these regions of red marrow on gradient-echo sequences because of magnetic susceptibility and out-of-phase chemical shift effects (Fig. 6-42). Care must be taken to recognize this process as a variation of normal rather than as an infiltrative marrow process. Red marrow may also be diffusely hyperplastic and resemble an infiltrative marrow disorder on T1-weighted images (Fig. 6-43) leading to an unnecessary biopsy (18). Normal red marrow characteristically spares the epiphyses and the patella and does not brighten significantly on T2-weighted images.

ADDITIONAL PITFALLS

Pes anserinus bursitis can mimic a torn meniscus or plica syndrome and therefore can result in unnecessary surgery if it goes unrecognized (19). The pes anerinus (''goose's foot'') is so named because of the webbed-foot appearance to its insertion on the anterior medial aspect of the tibia. The pes anserinus is made up of the tendons of the sartorius, gracilis, and semitendinosus muscles. The bursa lies deep to the tendons and can become inflamed as a result of chronic overuse such as that which occurs in jogging. The patients present with medial pain near the joint line (mimicking a meniscus tear on exam) or anteromedially on the tibia, near the patella (mimicking a plica syndrome). MR imaging shows a cystic fluid collection associated with the pes anserinus (Fig. 6-44). Treatment consists of rest and anti-inflammatory medication, but in refractory cases surgery has proved efficacious.

A recently described bursa, the semimembranosus-tibial collateral ligament bursa (20), lies just superior to the pes anserinus bursa, adjacent to the semimembranosus at the level of the joint (Fig. 6-45). It can mimic a pes anserinus bursa clinically, but because on physical exam it lies more proximal and is situated more laterally and posteriorly, it often confuses the clinician into disregarding a bursitis and mistakenly thinking the meniscus or a plica is responsible for the symptoms.

Injury of the plantaris muscle is occasionally encountered and has two distinctly different appearances on MR imaging that should be recognized (21). The plantaris muscle arises on the lateral femoral condyle and runs inferiorly just deep to the lateral head of the gastrocnemius and superficial to

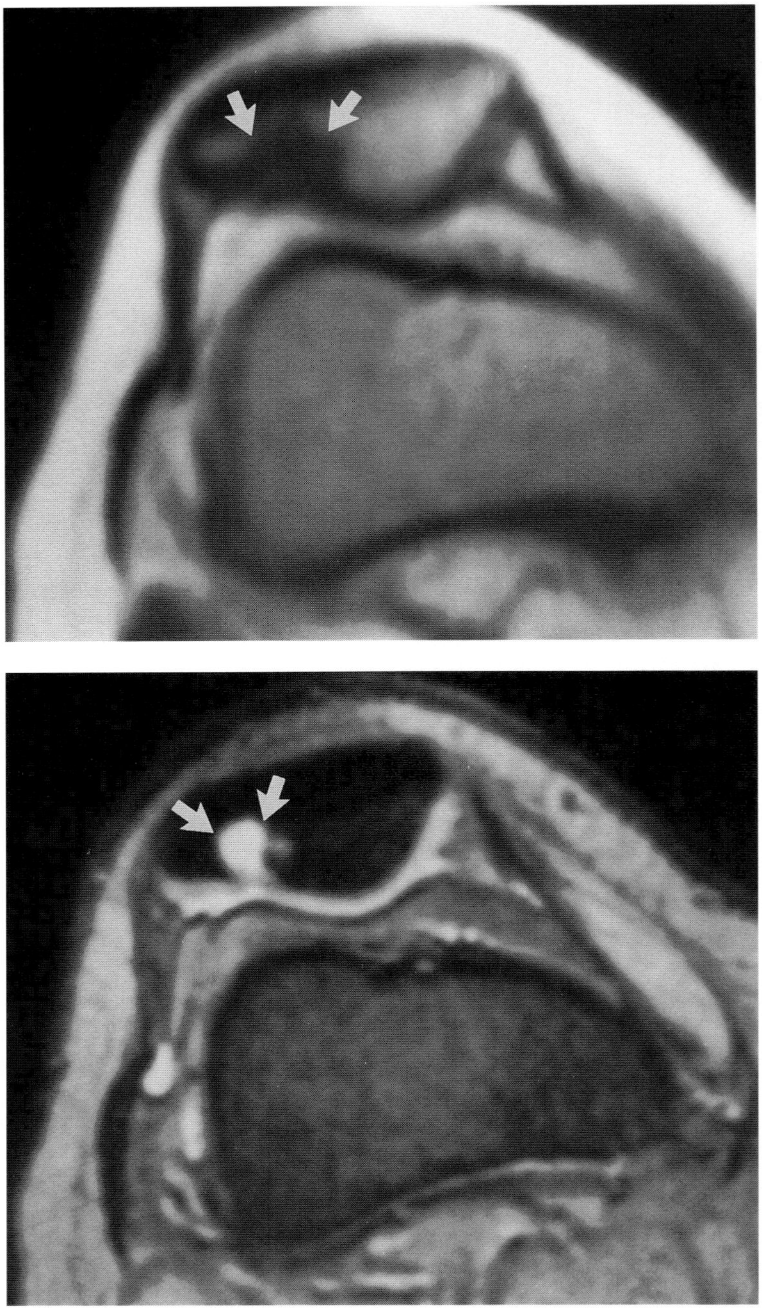

A

B

FIG. 6-41. Dorsal defect of the patella. A bony depression or defect *(arrows)* is seen in the superior lateral portion of the patella on T1-weighted **(A)** and $T2^*$ **(B)** images that represents a dorsal defect of the patella. This is a normal variant that should not be confused with a lytic lesion.

the soleus muscle. Its tendon begins in the upper part of the lower leg and courses medially deep to the medial head of the gastrocnemius and continues adjacent to the achilles tendon to the calcaneus (Fig. 6-46). Tears of the plantaris tendon have been termed "tennis leg" because of its frequent association with that activity. The patient presents with acute calf pain and occasionally displays swelling. These symptoms can clinically resemble a torn medial head of the gastrocnemius, which requires different treatment than a torn plantaris tendon, or they can resemble those of deep venous thrombosis. MR imaging through the calf will show fluid between the soleus and the medial head of the gastrocnemius (Fig. 6-47). A torn, retracted tendon may be visualized. The fluid collection is often very tubular in configuration (Fig. 6-48). If the plantaris muscle itself is injured, MR images through the knee will show the plantaris muscle to have increased signal on T2-weighted sequences because of the edema and hemorrhage. The muscle may be retracted proximally, giving it a "balled-up" appearance (Fig. 6-49). An association between an injured plantaris muscle and a torn anterior cruciate ligament has been noted.

A coronal or axial T2-weighted image occasionally

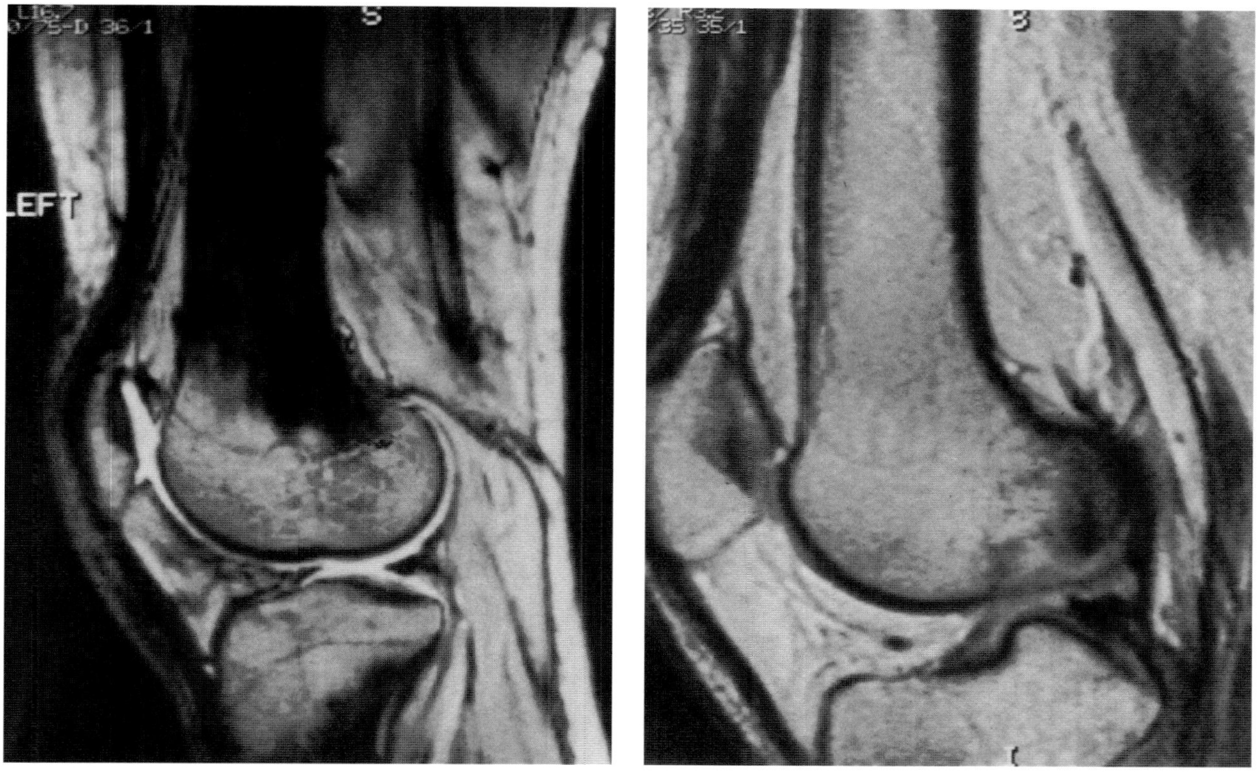

A B

FIG. 6-42. Red marrow on out-of-phase gradient-echo images. **A:** Residual red marrow can occasionally manifest dramatic signal loss on gradient-echo images when the TE is such that fat and water are out of phase. This image was obtained with a 0.35-T unit with TR = 1000 ms, TE = 30 ms, f = 75°. **B:** The marrow appears completely normal on this proton-density spin-echo sagittal image (TR = 2500 ms, TE = 35 ms).

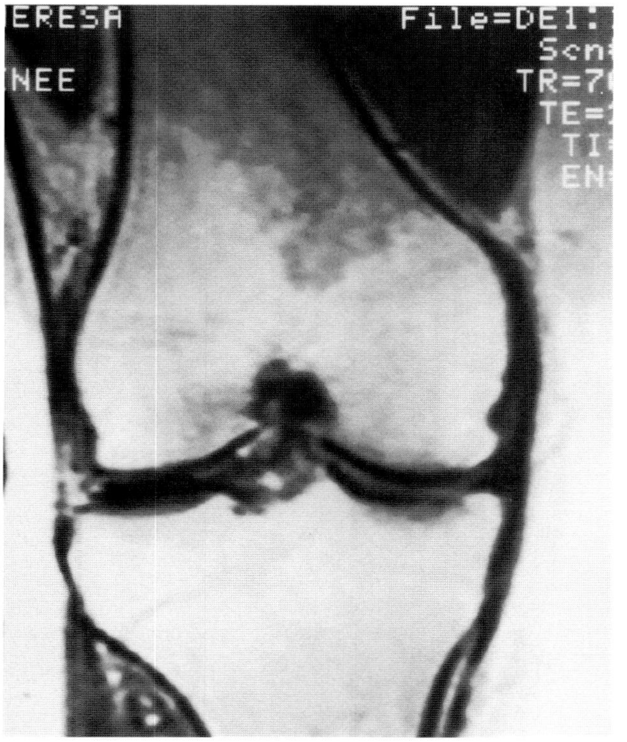

FIG. 6-43. Red marrow hyperplasia. This T1-weighted image demonstrates low-signal red marrow that may mimic tumor infiltration. Characteristic epiphyseal sparing is noted. Although tumor involvement of the marrow can have this identical appearance, biopsy is not recommended unless other findings suggesting a tumor are present.

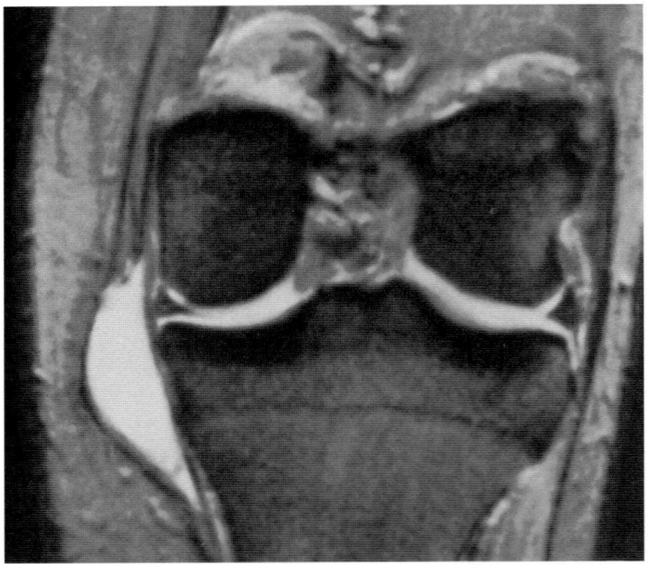

FIG. 6-44. Pes anserinus bursitus. A coronal T2-weighted image shows a large fluid collection on the medial side of the knee which is just beneath the pes anserinus tendons. This is pes anserinus bursitus.

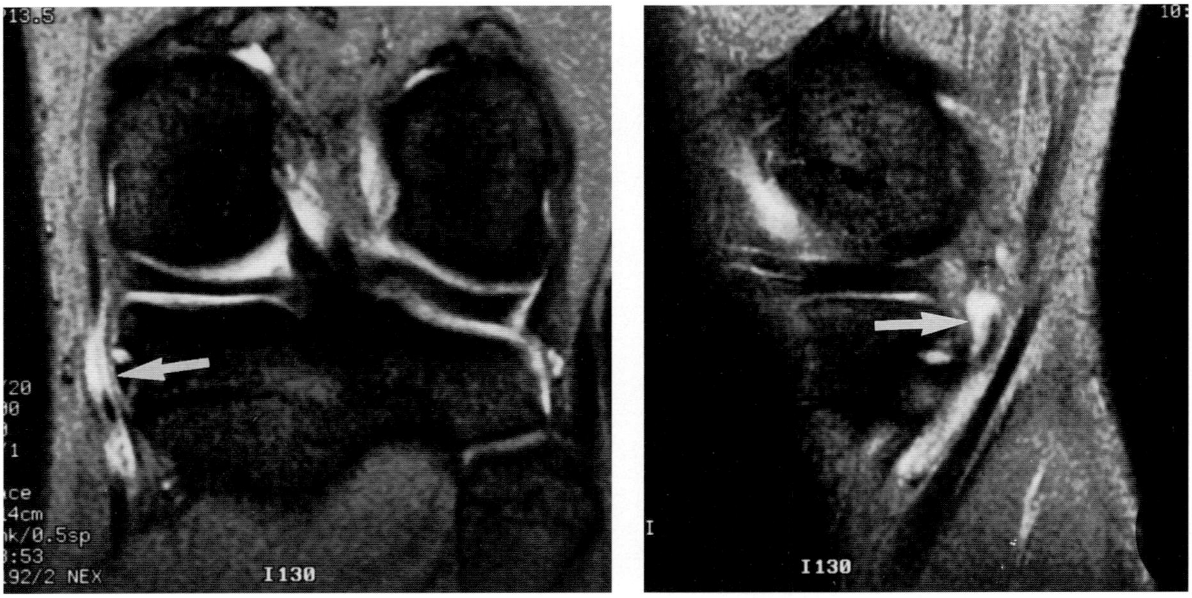

A B

FIG. 6-45. Semimembranosus-tibial collateral ligament bursa. **A:** A coronal T2-weighted image reveals a fluid collection *(arrow)* adjacent to the medial meniscus that is intimately associated with the semimembranosus tendon. **B:** A sagittal T2-weighted image shows this fluid collection draped over the semimembranosus tendon *(arrow)* that is characteristic for the semimembranosus-tibial collateral ligament bursa. It is usually somewhat more proximal than the aforementioned pes anserinus bursa.

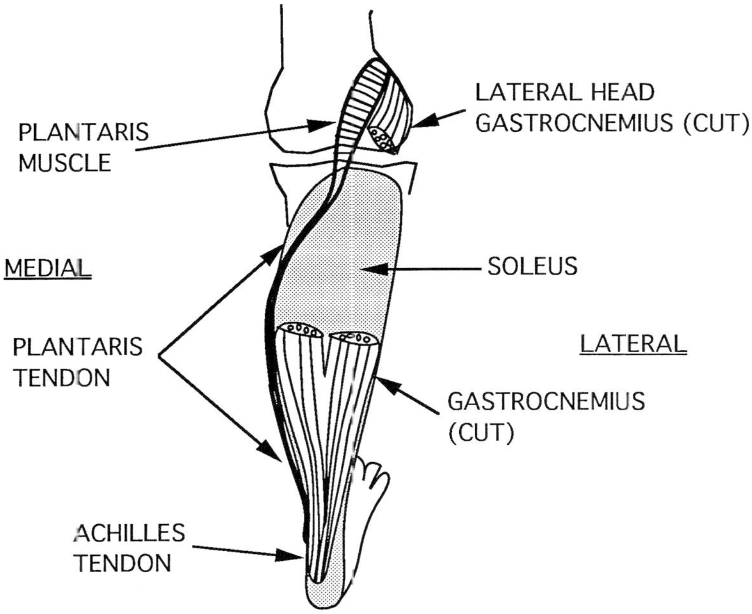

FIG. 6-46. Anatomy of plantaris muscle and tendon. This schematic shows the normal anatomy of the plantaris muscle as it arises from the lateral femoral condyle and courses medially with the tendon adjacent to the achilles tendon.

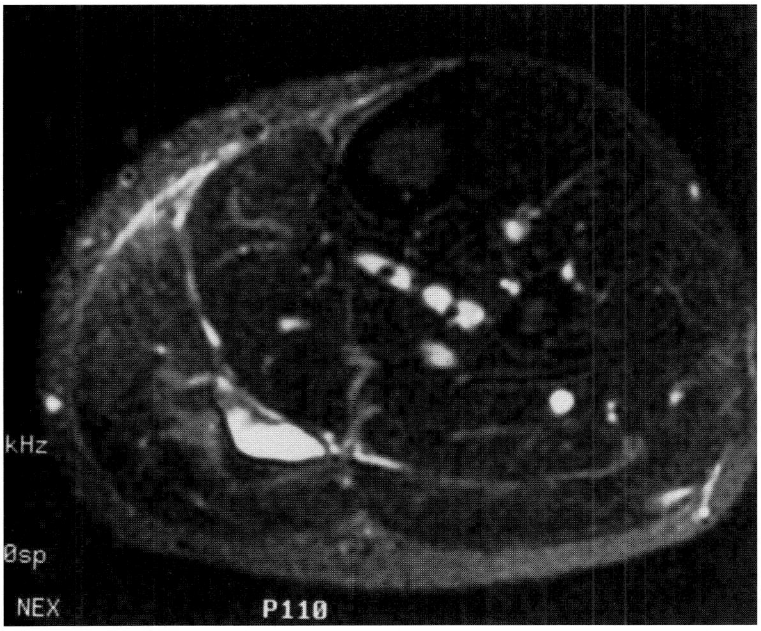

FIG. 6-47. Torn plantaris tendon. An axial T2-weighted image through the calf in this patient with pain following exercise shows a fluid collection between the soleus muscle and the medial head of the gastrocnemius. This is characteristic for a torn plantaris tendon.

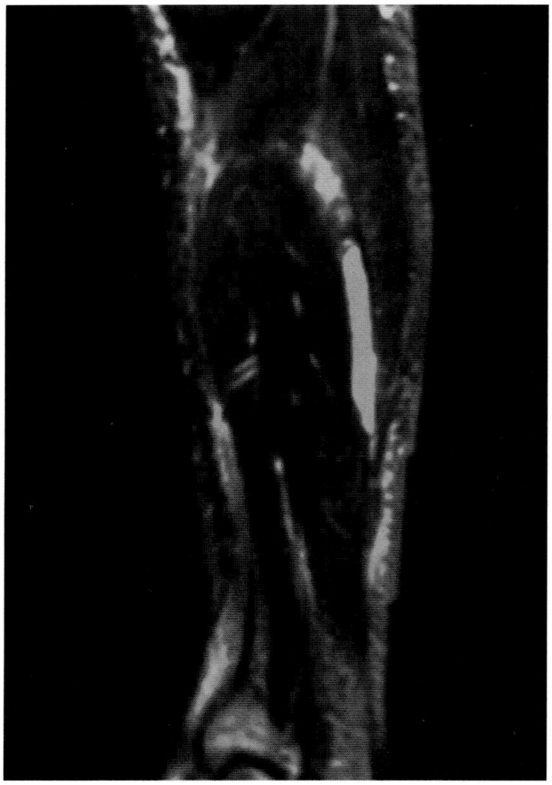

FIG. 6-48. Torn plantaris tendon. This sagittal T2-weighted image through the calf in a patient with a torn plantaris tendon shows how a tubular fluid collection can form between the soleus and the medial head of the gastrocnemius.

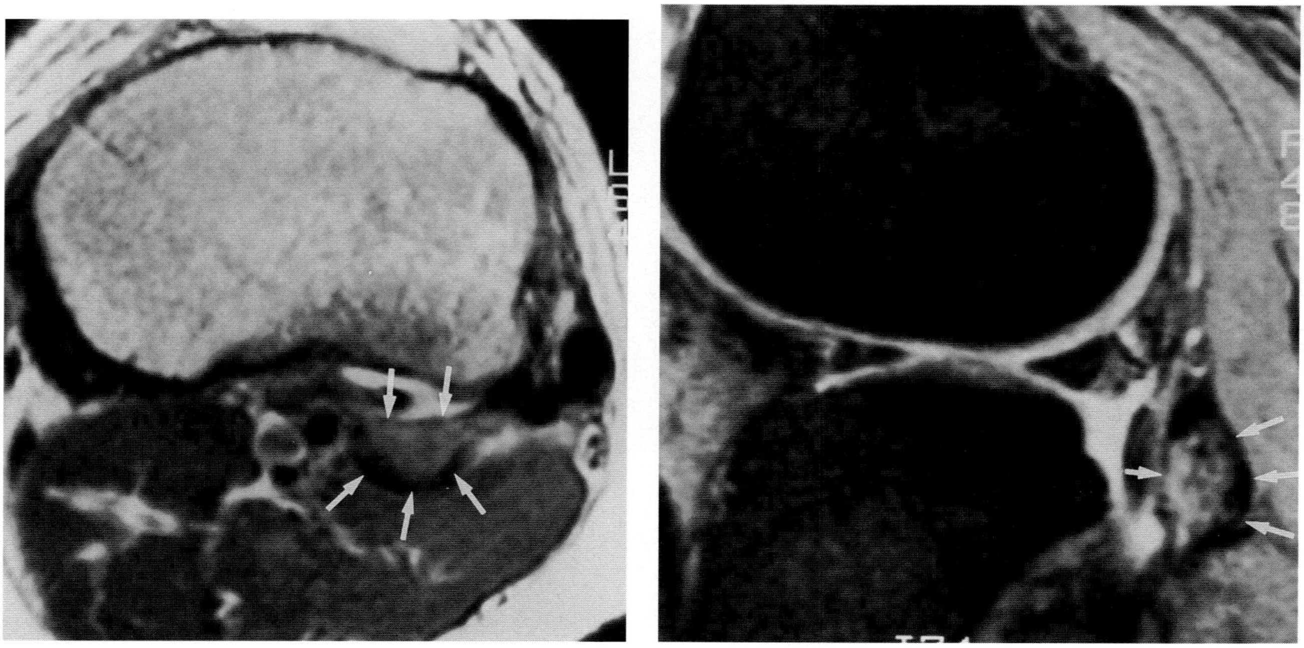

A B

FIG. 6-49. Torn plantaris tendon. **A:** An axial proton density image through the proximal lower leg, near the knee joint, in a patient with a torn plantaris tendon shows the plantaris muscle to be retracted and balled up *(arrows)*. **B:** A sagittal T2-weighted image in the same patient shows the plantaris *(arrows)* to be balled up and retracted proximally. It has high signal within it as a result of edema and hemorrhage.

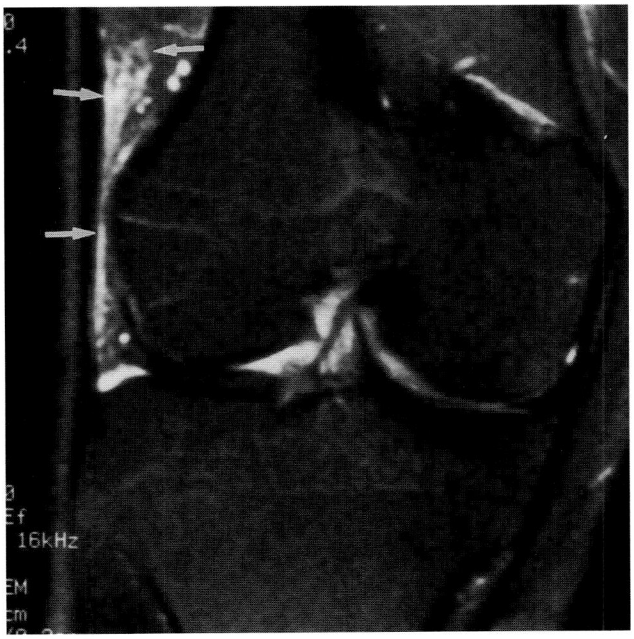

FIG. 6-50. Iliotibial band syndrome. This coronal T2-weighted image reveals high signal around the iliotibial band *(arrows)* laterally. This patient was a runner with pain in this area from overuse.

shows fluid around the lateral aspect of the knee associated with the iliotibial band (Fig. 6-50). This is seen frequently in overuse situations, as is the case when runners develop pain and irritation from the iliotibial band rubbing or snapping on the lateral femoral condyle. A simple joint effusion can give this appearance, so it is necessary to rely on increased signal outside of the joint (22). This is called iliotibial band friction syndrome and is usually treated conservatively.

REFERENCES

1. Herman LJ, Beltran J. Pitfalls in MR imaging of the knee. *Radiology* 1988;167:775–781.
2. Watanabe AT, Carter BC, Teitelbaum GP, Bradley WG Jr. Common pitfalls in magnetic resonance imaging of the knee. *J Bone Joint Surg* 1989;71-A:857–862.
3. Watanabe AT, Carter BC, Teitelbaum GP, Seeger LL, Bradley WG Jr. Normal variations in MR imaging of the knee: appearance and frequency. *AJR* 1989;153:341–344.
4. Grover JS, Bassett LW, Gross ML, Seeger LL, Finerman GAM. Posterior cruciate ligament: MR imaging. *Radiology* 1990;174:527–530.
5. DeSmet A, Graf B. Meniscal tears missed on MR imaging: relationship to meniscal tear patterns and anterior cruciate ligament tears. *AJR* 1994;162:905–911.
6. Vahey T, Bennett H, Arrington L, Shelbourne K, Ng J. MR imaging of the knee: pseudotear of the lateral meniscus caused by the meniscofemoral ligament. *AJR* 1990;154:1237–1240.
7. Peterfy C, Janzen D, Tirman P, van Dijke C, Pollack M, Genant H. "Magic-angle" phenomenon: a cause of increased signal in the normal lateral meniscus on short-TE MR images of the knee. *Radiology* 1994;163:149–154.
8. Erickson S, Prost R, Timins M. The "magic angle" effect: background physics and clinical relevance. *Radiology* 1993;188:23–26.
9. Silverman JM, Mink JH, Deutsch AL. Discoid menisci of the knee: MR imaging appearance. *Radiology* 1989;173:351–354.
10. Lee J, Yao L. Tibial collateral ligament bursa: MR imaging. *Radiology* 1991;178:855–859.
11. Czervionke LF, Cervionke JM, Daniels DL, Haughton VM. Characteristic features of MR truncation artifacts. *AJR* 1988;151:1219–1228.
12. Turner D, Rapoport M, Erwin W, McGould M, Silvers R. Truncation artifact: a potential pitfall in MR imaging of the menisci of the knee. *Radiology* 1991;179:629–633.
13. Crues JV, Ryu R, Morgan FW. Meniscal pathology. *Clin Orthop Rel Res* 1990;252:80–87.
14. Chew F. Medial meniscal flounce: demonstration on MR imaging of the knee. *AJR* 1990;155:199.
15. Patel D. Plica as a cause of anterior knee pain. *Orthop Clin North Am* 1986;17:273–277.
16. Cobby M, Schweitzer M, Resnick D. The deep lateral femoral notch: an indirect sign of a torn anterior cruciate ligament. *Radiology* 1992;184:855–858.
17. Ho VB, Kransdorf MJ, Jelinek JS, Kim CK. Dorsal defect of the patella: MR features. *JCAT* 1991;15:474–476.
18. Deutsch A, Mink J, Rosenfelt F, Waxman A. Incidental detection of hematopoietic hyperplasia on routine knee MR imaging. *AJR* 1989;152:333–336.
19. Forbes JR, Helms CA, Janzen DL. Acute pes anserinus bursitis: MR imaging. *Radiology* 1995;194:525–527.
20. Hennigan S, Schneck C, Mesgarzadeh M, Clancy M. The semimembranosus-tibial collateral ligament bursa: anatomical study and MR imaging. *J Bone Joint Surg* 1994;76-A:1322–1327.
21. Helms CA, Fritz RC, Garvin G. Plantaris muscle injury: evaluation with MR imaging. *Radiology* 1995;195:201–203.
22. Murphy B, Hechtman K, Uribe J, Selenesnick H, Smith R, Zlatkin M. Iliotibial band friction syndrome: MR imaging findings. *Radiology* 1992;185:569–571.

MRI of the Knee, Second Edition,
edited by P. L. Munk and C. A. Helms.
Lippincott-Raven Publishers, Philadelphia © 1996.

CHAPTER 7

Traumatic Osteochondral Disease of the Knee Joint and Related Disorders

A. Dale Vellet and Peter L. Munk

An increasingly important application of magnetic resonance imaging (MRI) is in the evaluation of the posttraumatic osteochondral diseases of joints and their short, intermediate, and long-term sequelae. With the increasing application of MRI in traumatic disorders of the musculoskeletal system, new light is being cast on the pathophysiology of acute and chronic posttraumatic joint disorders. This chapter addresses the MRI characteristics and role of MRI in the evaluation of known and presumed traumatic disorders of the knee joint.

EMBRYOLOGY

Much of our understanding of the morphogenesis and histogenesis of the human appendicular skeleton and its respective joints comes from animal embryologic studies (1–5).

The embryogenesis of the bones and joints of the limbs occurs between 25 and 50 days (4–7 weeks) of intrauterine gestation, with upper limb development preceding that of the lower limb by approximately 24 hours. The first discernible vestige of the arm bud (of cellular blastema) occurs at approximately 26 days of age. The primitive chondrogenic and myogenic precursors within the mesenchymal blastema undergo differentiation in two mature osseous and muscular components of the mature skeleton.

Joint development occurs in the following sequential, interdependent stages: segmentation, formation of articular surfaces, joint cavitation, and development of intra-articular meniscoligamentous structures and synovial lining. At approximately 44 days of age, chondrification of the mesenchymal blastema has progressed to the point at which the rudimentary analage of the tibia and femur exist. The approximating end of each analage is organized into arcades of flattened chondrocytes, separated by intervening zone of mesenchymal cells distinct from the chondrocytes (the precursors of the epiphysis) and termed the *interzone*. Although initially loosely organized, there is progressive peripheral cellular condensation with collagenization peripherally and eventually cavitation centrally. The peripheral zones give rise to the articular cartilage and joint capsule with further differentiation. The central region of cavitation occurs simultaneously with vascularization of the interzone. Residual islands of vascularized persistent mesenchyme within the interzone eventually give rise to the meniscoligamentous complex and the synovial lining of the joint.

OSTEOCHONDRAL ANATOMY

Joints are classified as fibrous, cartilaginous, or synovial. The knee joint represents a synovial diarthrodial hinged joint. The fundamental constituents of synovial joints, such as the knee, are an investing articular fibrous capsule with its superficial tendinous and ligamentous reinforcements lined by synovial membrane consisting of an intimal and subintimal layer, apposed articular surfaces consisting of a subchondral bony plate surfaced by articular hyaline cartilage, and in the knee, intra-articular fibrocartilaginous menisci (6). The structures defining a synovial diarthrodial joint are contained by the fibrous capsule and bathed by synovial fluids created by the intimal component of the synovial membrane. The MRI anatomic and signal intensity characteristic of the knee joint are illustrated in other chapters of this text.

Articular Capsule

The knee joint is enveloped by a fibrous capsule of variable thickness consisting of dense bundles of fibrous tissue.

A. D. Vellet: Department of Diagnostic Imaging, University of Calgary, Foothills Hospital, Alberta, Canada T2N 2T9.

P. L. Munk: Department of Radiology, University of British Columbia, Department of Diagnostic Imaging, British Columbia Cancer Agency, Vancouver, British Columbia, Canada V5Z 4E6.

The fibrous capsule is adherent to the periosteum of both the tibia and femur at the site of its insertion. The periosteal attachment to the tibia, with the exception of the tibial tubercle, closely approximates the articular margin of the tibia. In the instance of the femur, the fibrous capsule merges with the periosteum of the epicondyles, resulting in an intraarticular location of the distal femoral metaphysis, physis, and epiphysis.

The fibrous capsule merges imperceptibly with patellar retinaculum expansion, the patellar periosteum, and the patellar tendon. The joint capsule is reinforced medially by the medial collateral ligament and is thickened medially in the regions of the meniscofemoral and posterior oblique ligaments. The capsule is relatively deficient posteriorly within the popliteal fossa.

The fibrous capsule demonstrates evidence of variable compactness and in regions such as the meniscal femoral ligament may adopt histological features suggestive of tendon. The fibrous capsule is relatively vascular, in part reflecting the rich vascular supply of the loosely adherent subintima of the subjacent synovial membrane.

Synovial Membrane

The subintimal layer of the synovial membrane is loosely adherent throughout the fibrous capsule through its deep subintimal layer. The synovial membrane is deficient over the articular surface of the joint. The synovium extends from the fibrous capsule to adjacent periosteal bone surfaces to the level of the osteochondral junction. These regions demonstrate the greatest degree of capsular and subintimal vascularity.

The synovial membrane is described in more detail in the chapter on inflammatory disorders of the knee.

Articular Cartilage

Articular cartilage consists of a 1.0–3.0-mm-thick layer of hyaline cartilage lining the articular surface of the joint. The articular cartilage in conjunction with the lubricating synovial fluid allows for motion with a relatively low coefficient of friction. The deep layers of the cartilage are also involved in enchondral ossification.

Histologically, articular cartilage consists of four discrete microscopic zones. The most superficial layer is referred to as the superficial tangential zone of cartilage. This consists of densely packed collagen fibers, the majority of which parallel the articular surface. The chondrocytes in this region are relatively loosely packed, smaller in size than chondrocytes within the remainder of the cartilage, flattened, and relatively parallel to the articular surface. The next zone of cartilage is referred to as the tangential zone. This consists of a region of less densely packed and randomly oriented collagen fibers, which are larger than those within the superficial zone. The chondrocytes in this region are larger and less parallel than those within the superficial layer. Cells in this region tend to cluster. The next deepest layer of cartilage is referred to as the radial zone. This is characterized by a degraded degree of cellularity, with further increase in size of individual chondrocytes. The chondrocytes tend to be arranged in columns and are interspersed within a collagen matrix similar to that seen in the transitional zone. The radial zone consists of the largest layer of the cartilage. Radial zone cartilage is bound to the subchondral endplate by a calcified zone of articular cartilage termed the *tidemark*. The tidemark zone appears to serve an anchoring function between the deepest layer of the radial zone and the subchondral endplate. The latter structure consists of trabecular bone, which merges imperceptibly with subchondral cortex. The subchondral endplate serves as a conduit for small blood vessels, which perforate the subchondral bone plate and the calcified zone of articular cartilage to supply the deepest portions of the radial zone of the cartilage.

Hyaline cartilage has relatively poor regenerative capacity and, except for its deepest layers, heals by fibrocartilaginous repair. The importance of the basal vascular supply is becoming more widely recognized in the evolution of posttraumatic osteochondral defects and osteonecrosis.

Despite the relatively high concentration of water by weight in cartilage (approximately 70%) the water is bound to macromolecular collagen, chondroid, and sulfate, the latter being in turn bound to protein. Consequently, there is T1 and T2 relaxation enhancement of hydrogen ions in cartilage. This translates to intermediate to high signal intensity of cartilage on T1-weighted images and intermediate to high signal intensity on T2-weighted images. The individual layers of cartilage can be identifiable, although inconsistently, on high-resolution MRI, particularly inversion recovery pulse sequences (Fig. 7-1). The cartilage surface within the knee varies in thickness, depending on its location. The articular cartilage lining the tibial plateau is of relatively uniform thickness (1.0–2.0 mm), although the cartilage surface may be more substantive toward the non-weight-bearing surface relative to the slope of the tibial spines. The articular cartilage of the femoral condyles is thicker anteriorly and posteriorly, measuring between 4.0 and 7.0 mm. Although global thinning of the articular cartilage occurs with age, it is always thinnest relative to the inferior articular surfaces of the condyles.

Subchondral Bone

Subchondral bone plate merges indiscernibly with the lamellar cortical bone surface of the femur and tibia. The subchondral bone is uniformly thick throughout the tibia and femur, measuring approximately 1.0–3.0 mm. Cortical bone is free of signal on T1, T2, and GE sequences and can be differentiated because of high SI differences versus the surrounding structures (bone marrow, cartilage, fat). The subchondral epiphyseal marrow cavity consists of cancellous

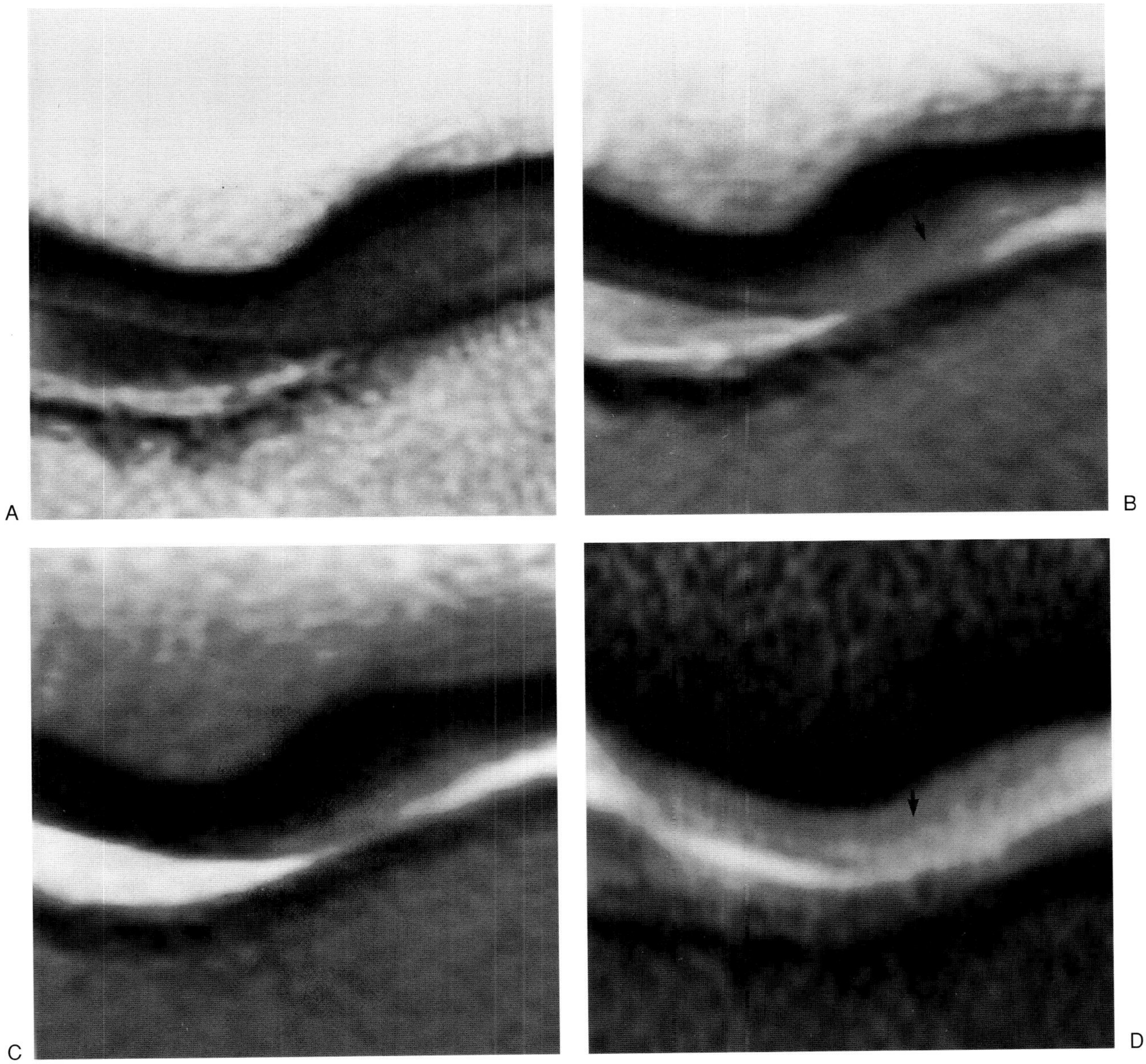

FIG. 7-1. High resolution articular cartilage (*arrows*). **A:** T1-weighted (SE 600/20). **B:** Proton density weighted (SE 2000/30). **C:** T2-weighted (SE 2000/70). **D:** T1-weighted inversion recovery image (STIR 2500/150/20).

trabecular bone that usually demonstrates fatty marrow at all ages. Trabecular bone is not normally visualized on spin-echo sequences except in areas of normal stress-bearing trabecular condensations that form low-signal bands. With GE sequences the magnetic susceptibility effect of the trabeculae on the surrounding fat is responsible for the low signal of bone marrow in the epiphyseal region.

OSTEONECROSIS

Osteonecrosis involving the knee can be divided into four broad categories: idiopathic or primary osteonecrosis of the femur, idiopathic or primary osteonecrosis of the tibia, posttraumatic osteonecrosis, and secondary osteonecrosis.

Idiopathic or Primary Osteonecrosis of the Femoral Condyle

The entity of idiopathic osteonecrosis of the femoral condyle was originally described in 1968 by Ahlbach and colleagues (7). Since this description, many articles have addressed its etiology, pathogenesis, radiographic and scintigraphic appearances, and progression (7–30).

Idiopathic osteonecrosis presents as chronic, persistent,

unilateral knee pain of relatively acute onset, involving the medial joint compartment of the knee. Most patients (approximately 65%) are elderly, postmenopausal women, with the remainder of the patients being elderly men. Although this characteristically is a unilateral process confined to the articular, weight-bearing surface of the medial femoral condyle, reports of involvement of the lateral femoral condyles bilaterally are cited (13,14,30).

In contradistinction to secondary forms of osteonecrosis, a history of systemic etiological factors associated with this disorder is conspicuously absent (see later). In many instances, a history of unusual mechanical stress often precedes the onset of symptoms, suggesting that subliminal stress in a relatively osteoporotic skeleton represents an inciting event in the etiology of osteonecrosis.

The clinical course of osteonecrosis is varied, with management decisions based on clinical history and radiographic manifestations (12,25,28,30–33). A few patients will have symptoms compatible with idiopathic osteonecrosis, but at no time will they demonstrate radiographic abnormalities consistent with osteonecrosis. This stage can be regarded as stage 0. Such patients are treated conservatively, with protected weight bearing, anti-inflammatory agents, and analgesia. Although subsidence of symptoms over a course of months is not invariable, recovery is usual. Stage I–IV lesions show a progressive spectrum of radiographic manifestations proportionate to the magnitude of osteonecrosis and complicating osteoarthritis (28). In patients with relatively early stage I (radiographic flattening of the articular surface with or without regional osteopenia) and stage II (linear subchondral radiolucency) lesions at presentation, conservative, non-weight-bearing management may result in spontaneous resolution (11–25).

Initially favorable prognostic estimates of conservative management have been revised, acknowledging the high incidence of progression of such lesions to osteoarthritis within the medial compartment of the knee. Lesions other than stage I that are symptomatic should be treated surgically (11,25,28). Surgical options include drilling, tibial osteotomy, allograft repair, hemarthroplasty, and total knee arthroplasty (30–33).

The MR features of osteonecrosis are similar regardless of the location of the lesion and are best understood if they are correlated with its pathogenic evolution (34–38). Table 7-1 represents a proposed correlation of the pathologic, radiographic, and MRI stages of idiopathic osteonecrosis.

Preinfarction (Stage A)

Although not strictly applicable to idiopathic osteonecrosis, preinfarction will be discussed at this point because it is relevant to other forms of osteonecrosis and may be pertinent to future MRI applications. Although the etiology of osteonecrosis is complex and undoubtedly multifactorial, an underlying theme is a relative vascular insufficiency to the medullary bone at risk. A distinction between vascular occlusions (either arterial insufficiency or intravascular sinusoidal) and extravascular sinusoidal occlusions can be made (29). It is postulated that in preinfarction there is disruption of sinusoidal blood flow, as a consequence of either diminished vascular inflow to medullary sinusoidal spaces or extrinsic pressure on the spaces. MRI is not yet able to evaluate microvascular circulation quantitatively. It is theoretically possible to obtain an indexed quantification of medullary fat composition utilizing a variety of pulse sequences to evaluate alterations in its composition and abundance. Consequently, a MRI may prove valuable in patients receiving steroid therapy in identifying those at risk for the development of osteonecrosis.

TABLE 7-1. *Proposed correlation of pathologic radiographic, and MR stages of idiopathic osteonecrosis of the femur*

Pathologic stage	Radiographic stage	MR stage
Preinfarction	—	Stage A
Cell Death	Stage 0	Stage B
Early Reparative	Stage I	Stage C
Late Reparative	Stage II	Stage D
Collapse	Stage III	Stage E
Osteoarthritis	Stage IV	Stage F

Phase of Initial Cell Death (Stage B)

The marrow cavity consists of hemopoietic cells, osteocytes, and lipocytes. Within 48 hours following an infarctive insult, both hemopoietic cells and osteocytes will have undergone cell death (39,40). If the infarctive territory is sufficiently large, the necrobiosis of hemopoietic elements, in particular the erythrocytic mass, will result in a focal region of diminished signal intensity within the medullary fat on both T1- and T2-weighted images, which reflects the presence of intracellular deoxyhemoglobin. Within 2–7 days, the signal intensity on both T1- and T2-weighted images of this region will increase because of the conversion of intracellular deoxyhemoglobin to intracellular and extracellular methemoglobin. This would occur peripherally in the first instance, possibly resulting in a complex focus of low central and high peripheral signal intensity on T1-weighted images. In isolation this could be difficult to perceive because of the lack of differentiation between methemoglobin and marrow fat. However, with ensuing lipocyte cell death (occurring at 5 days), there is passive transudation of fluid in relation to the infarcted focus, which in isolation would present as diminished signal intensity on T1-weighted images and as increasing intensity on T2-weighted images. In most instances the signal characteristics will be dominated by liquified fat. Small areas of infarction consequently may not be perceived as such at this stage. Osteoblastic cell death is not perceptible at our present level of resolution.

Early Reparative Phase (Stage C)

The early reparative phase consists of a circumferential zone of reactive hyperemia surrounding successive zones of cellular infarction and ischemia. The hyperemia is primarily a response to the products of cell death and results in a progressive transudation of fluid, serum protein, and inflammatory cells. This is an exaggeration of the early transudation and presents with an exaggeration of findings cited earlier on spin-echo and inversion recovery pulsed sequences.

Late Reparative Phase (Stage D)

The late reparative phase is characterized by the progressive intrusion into the zone of infarction of a peripheral fibrovascular interface between adjacent normal bone and infarction. In its wake peripheral new bone is formed, presenting as a serpiginous region of low signal intensity on both T1- and T2-weighted images. Immediately subjacent to this zone is a region of immediate signal intensity on T2-weighted images, corresponding to the fibrovascular interface. The irregular central infarction zone is of increased signal intensity on T1- and T2-weighted images, reflecting the predominance of liquified fat on signal intensity.

Established Chronic Infarct

Established infarcts contained within the metaphyseal or epiphyseal medullary fat present as serpiginous regions of diminished signal intensity on both T1- and T2-weighted images surrounding a somewhat geographic central core of high signal intensity on pulsed sequences (Fig. 7-2).

Primary Osteonecrosis

Infarcts that abut the subchondral cortical bone as seen in idiopathic osteonecrosis appear distinct in that remodeling of the infarction weakens cortical bone and with repeated impactive loading results in subsequent collapse of the overlying osteochondral complex.

Reports in the radiological literature reflect features that are generic to osteonecrosis and those that are unique to femoral osteonecrosis (34–38). Most instances cited concern the features noted in advanced lesions with no reports available describing the MRI features of early femoral osteonecrosis.

Early lesions present as regions of focal, discrete, subcortical low signal intensity on T1-weighted images (Fig. 7-3). These regions are of variable signal intensity on T2-weighted images, depending on their age. The mature lesions present as regions of intermediate to increasing intensity on T2-weighted images with an apparently intact overlying osteochondral complex (Fig. 7-4). This increased signal intensity is a reflection of edema, intruded synovial fluid, and/or hemorrhage. The latter possibility is suggested by potential high signal intensity noted on T1-weighted images in lesions of this age. With time, lesions become marginated by a fibro-

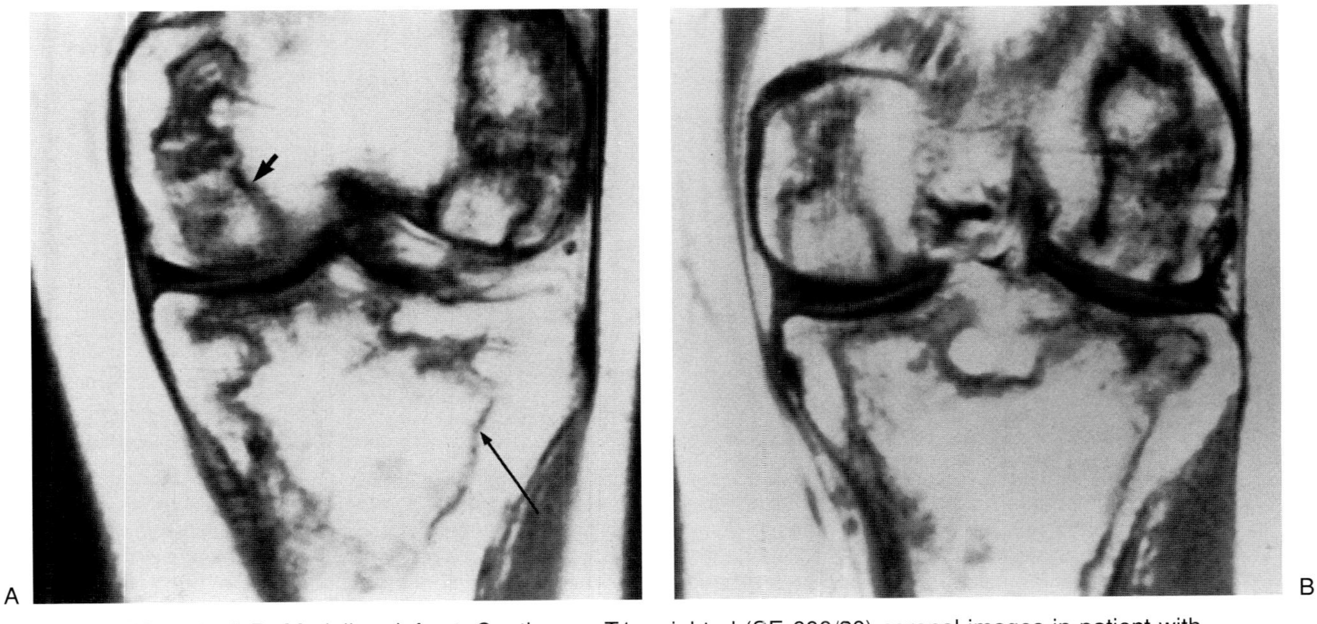

FIG. 7-2. A,B: Medullary infarct. Contiguous T1-weighted (SE 600/20) coronal images in patient with SLE demonstrates extensive medullary infarction within both the femoral and tibial epiphyseal and metaphyseal regions. The central, nonviable regions of the infarcts are isointense with noninfarcted marrow fat. The margins of the infarcts demonstrate variable-signal characteristics dependent upon the age of the infarction. More mature regions demonstrate discrete marginal T2 shortening consistent with reactive new bone formation with little intervening intermediate-signal-intensity reactive interface *(long arrows)*. Less mature regions of infarction demonstrate less discrete, wider marginal zones of T2 shortening with demonstrable zones of intervening reactive interface *(short arrows)*.

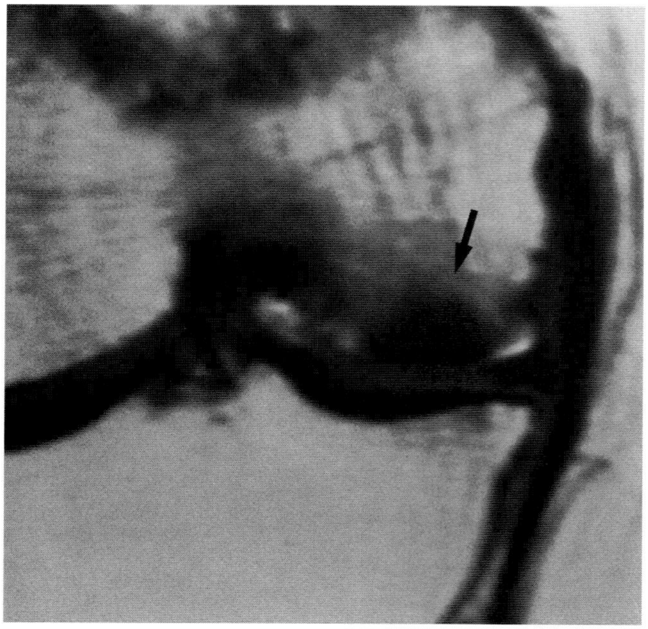

FIG. 7-3. Spontaneous femoral osteonecrosis (SON). T1-weighted (SE 600/20) coronal image demonstrates a focal low-signal-intensity subcortical, subarticular region within the medial femoral condyle. The low-signal-intensity region fades gradually into the epiphyseal fat, the periphery of the lesion representing marrow edema *(arrow)*. The cortical surface is intact.

vascular interface as described earlier (Fig. 7-5). Progressive reactive medullary osteosclerosis separates the fibrovascular interface from normal medullary marrow fat. Ensuing collapse of the osteochondral complex results in a multitude of imaging permutations on spin-echo and gradient-echo sequences. Lesions of diminished signal intensity remain on T1-weighted images, although they become increasingly marginated by T2 shortening coordinating with osteosclerosis seen in the late reparative phase (Fig. 7-5). Internal and intra-articular regions of T2 shortening correspond to free cortical or osteochondral fragments. Once breach of the articular osteochondral complex is evident, free intra-articular communication allows intrusion of synovial fluid into the core of the lesion, thus resulting in increased signal intensity on T2-weighted images surrounded by and containing regions of T2 shortening corresponding to bone on T1-weighted images.

Conditions that may mimic primary osteonecrosis differ, depending on the evolutionary phase of the lesion at the time of MRI examination.

Early Lesions

During the earliest phase of such lesions, when discrete reactive demarcation is not evident, acute posttraumatic subcortical occult fractures and subarticular synovial cysts have similar appearances on T1-weighted images (Figs. 7-6 and 7-7). On T2-weighted and inversion recovery images occult

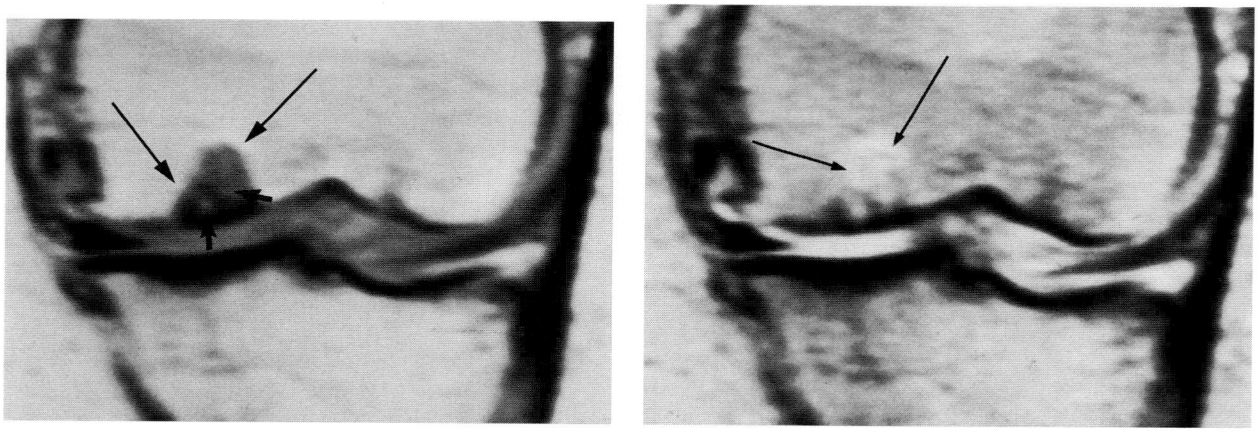

A

B

FIG. 7-4. A: Spontaneous femoral osteonecrosis (SON). T1-weighted (SE 600/20) coronal image of SON of the medial femoral condyle demonstrates a pyramidal region of predominantly low signal intensity with a subtle halo of high signal intensity *(long arrows)* and patchy central high signal intensity *(short arrows)* consistent with hemorrhage. The degree to which the central high signal intensity reflects composite signal intensity from fat and hemorrhage is uncertain. A small focus of subcortical, subarticular low signal intensity is noted subjacent to the lateral femoral condyle. Although not documented, this may represent a resolving SON lesion in its late phase. **B:** Spontaneous femoral osteonecrosis (SON). Corresponding T2-weighted (SE 2000/70) coronal image of same SON lesion of the medial femoral condyle demonstrates complex signal characteristics. The peripheral boundary and bulk of the lesion are of increased signal intensity *(long arrows)*. There are multiple, discrete crescents of consecutive T2 shortening consistent with regions of sequential deoxyhemoglobin or reactive new bone, most likely the latter. These regions demarcate regions of ischemic bone. These appearances support the thesis of posttraumatic hemorrhage occurring intercurrently during the early stages of SON. The more mature subcortical lesion within the lateral femoral condyle remains of diminished signal intensity.

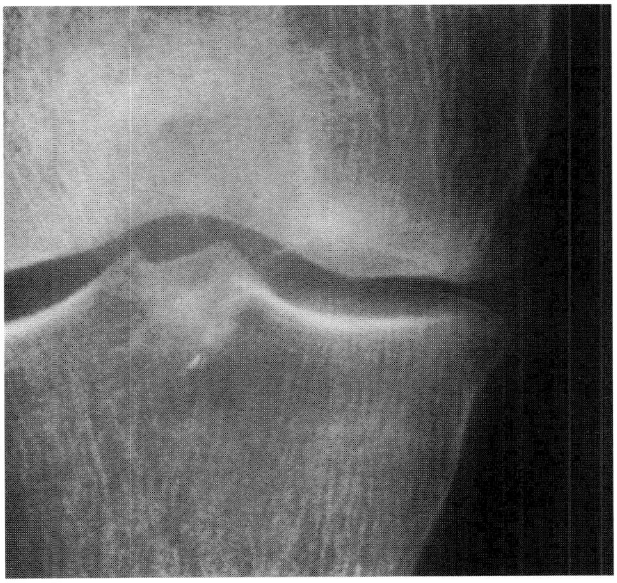

A

FIG. 7-5. A: Spontaneous femoral osteonecrosis (SON). AP plain film of resolving SON. There is mild collapse of the articular surface of the medial femoral condyle with subcortical osteosclerosis above this location. **B,C:** Spontaneous femoral osteonecrosis (SON). Corresponding T1-weighted (SE 600/20) coronal (B) and sagittal (C) images of medial femoral SON. The lesion is more extensive than appreciated on the plain film. The periphery of the lesion is of low signal intensity and poorly defined, with subtle high signal intensity within its center *(arrows)*. **D,E:** Spontaneous femoral osteonecrosis (SON). Corresponding T2-weighted (SE 2000/70) coronal (D) and sagittal (E) images of medial femoral SON. There is subtle high signal intensity along the spiculated boundary corresponding to the poorly defined margin on the T1-weighted images *(long arrows)*. Subjacent to this there is a crescentic halo of T2 shortening corresponding to reactive new bone formation *(short arrows)*. Subjacent to this region are locular high signal intensity regions corresponding to methemoglobin, which in turn surround subcortical regions of T2 shortening *(white arrowheads)*. It is impossible both to define a definite reactive interface and to differentiate deoxyhemoglobin from endosteal sclerosis.

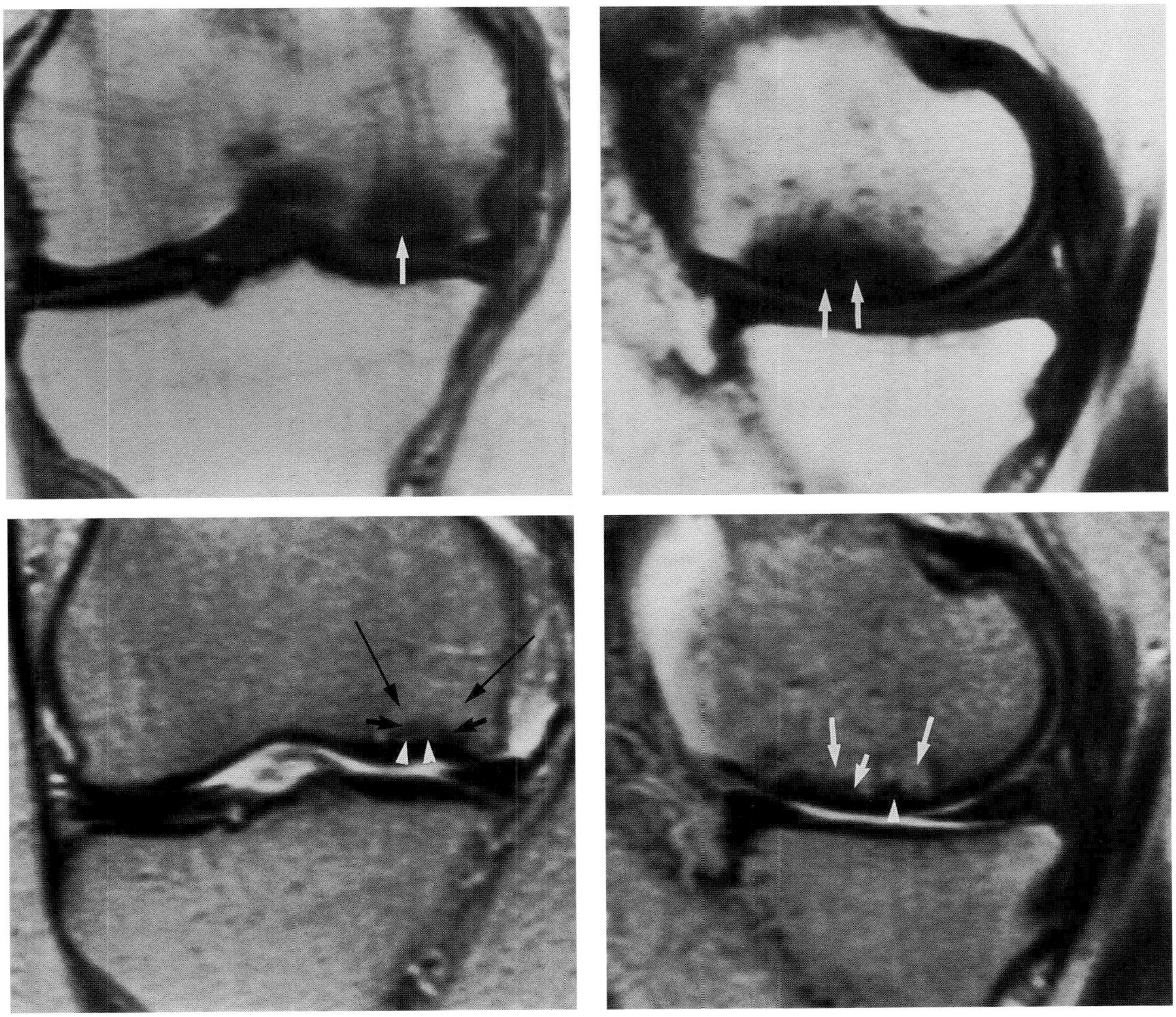

B C D E

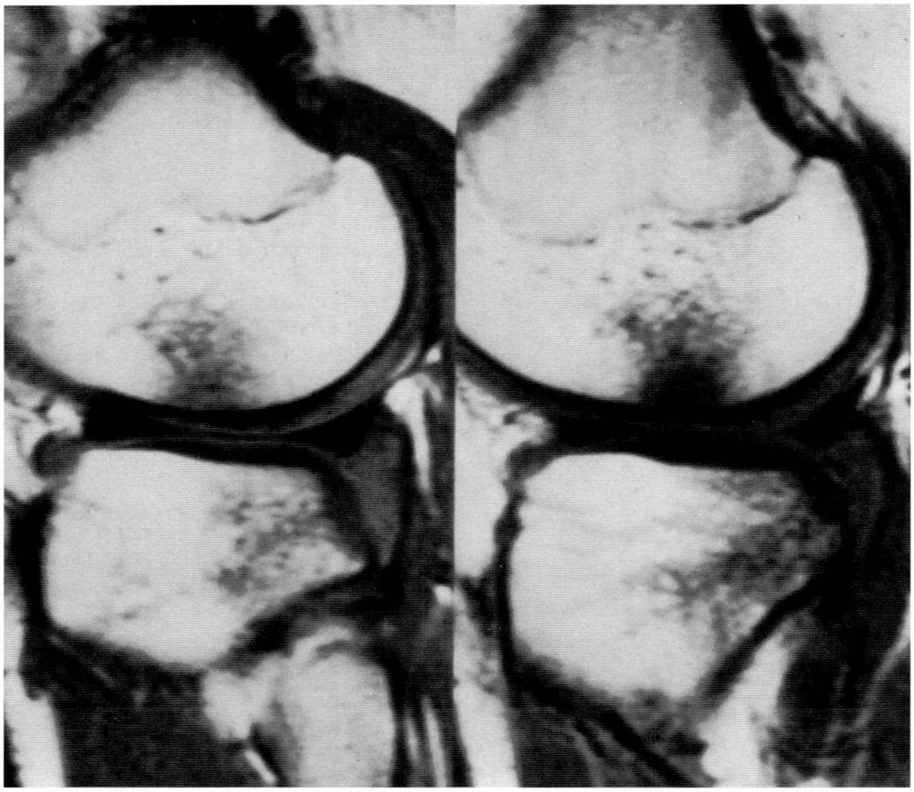

FIG. 7-6. A: Occult subcortical fracture. T1-weighted (SE 600/20) sagittal image of focal low signal intensity occult subcortical fracture within lateral femoral condyle. The lesion is similar in appearance to femoral SON on T1-weighted images.

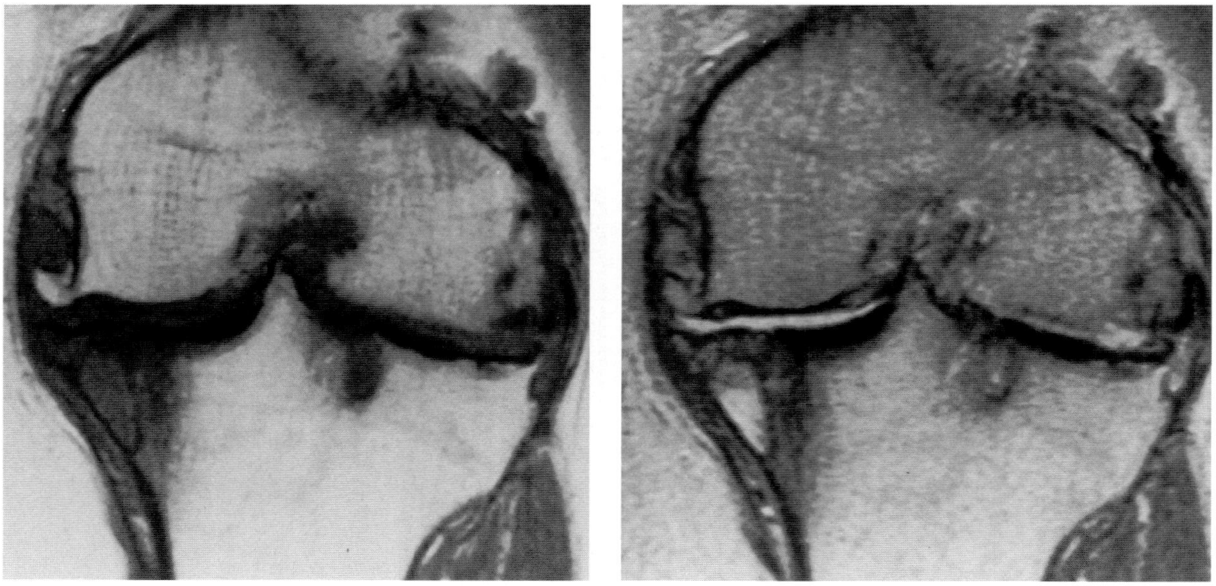

A B

FIG. 7-7. A: Subarticular synovial cyst. T1-weighted (SE 600/20) coronal image of discrete circular subarticular synovial cyst demonstrating similar signal characteristics to SON on T1-weighted images but more discretely defined. **B:** Subarticular synovial cyst. T2-weighted (SE 2000/70) sagittal image of the same subarticular synovial cyst. The cyst is of high signal intensity and demarcated by a discrete zone of T2 shortening consistent with reactive trabecular new bone.

fractures demonstrated patchy increased signal intensity (see Fig. 7-7) although experience with early osteonecrosis lesions is limited, similar appearances may theoretically be evident. In the final analysis, reliance on clinical history may be necessary. In contradistinction, although of even greater signal intensity on T2-weighted images, synovial cysts are relatively homogeneous and usually demarcated from medullary fat by a discrete, thin rim of T2 shortening consistent with reactive osteosclerosis (see Fig. 7-7). Although theoretically such an appearance may overlap that seen in osteonecrosis in evolution, the degree of marginating osteosclerosis would be expected to be greater, and invariably, the majority of synovial cysts are associated with evidence of osteoarthritis.

Late Lesions

During the late phase of primary osteonecrosis, its distinction from posttraumatic osteonecrosis (see later) and the potential osteochondral sequelae of occult, subcortical fractures may be impossible (Fig. 7-8) (41). Conservative management of primary osteonecrosis that is asymptomatic at presentation may be successful. However, the majority of patients require surgical intervention. Initial enthusiasm concerning allograft repair of primary osteonecrosis has waned because of high failure rates in this condition (21). However, allografts are utilized in posttraumatic osteonecrosis. In this latter instance, MRI may be of value in the assessment of allograft incorporation. Allografts consist of a fashioned, crescentic fragment of osteochondral bone and medullary fat. The granulation interface between the allograft and the recipient site appears to be as a low signal intensity rim on T1-weighted images and a high signal intensity focus on T2-weighted images. With progressive incorporation of the allograft, the granulation reaction is replaced by a bridging bone interface that is seen as a region of diminished signal intensity on T1- and T2-weighted images. Failure of the allograft incorporation is indicated when there is increasing width and signal intensity on the granulation interface on T2-weighted images, with eventual disruption, disintegration, and dislodgement of the allograft.

Idiopathic or Primary Osteonecrosis of the Tibia

Originally described as an osteonecrosis-like syndrome, osteonecrosis of the tibial plateau has a clinical history very similar to that seen in idiopathic femoral osteonecrosis (42). The condition usually involves the medial tibial plateau and has a relatively benign course with a high incidence of spontaneous recovery with conservative medical management. There is a relatively high incidence of concomitant osteoarthritic change within the medial joint compartment. It is hypothesized that the pathogenesis of this condition relates to shear stress-induced microinfraction of attenuated tibial cortical bone through preexisting osteoarthritic cartilaginous defects (30,31). Consequent intrusion of synovial fluid within the subcortical medullary space may result in symptoms but not necessarily in osteonecrosis. This may account

A 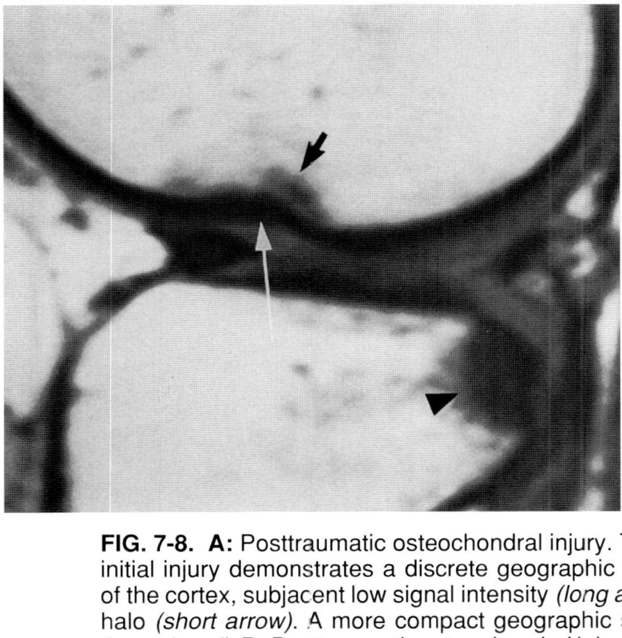 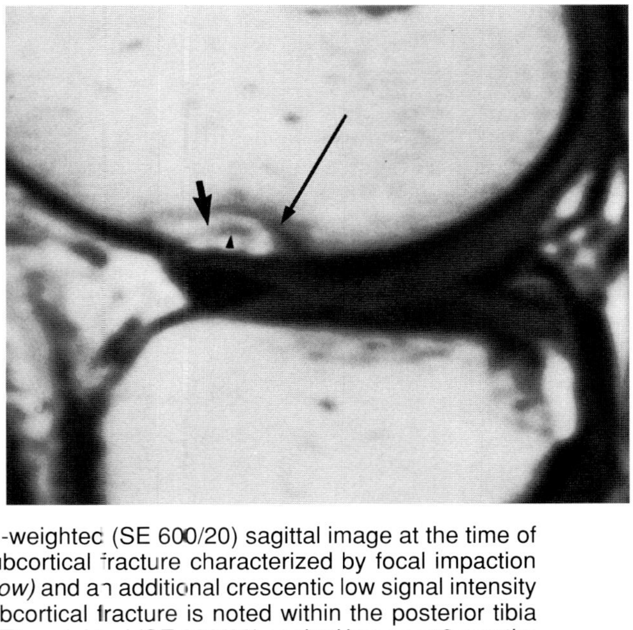 B

FIG. 7-8. A: Posttraumatic osteochondral injury. T1-weighted (SE 600/20) sagittal image at the time of initial injury demonstrates a discrete geographic subcortical fracture characterized by focal impaction of the cortex, subjacent low signal intensity *(long arrow)* and an additional crescentic low signal intensity halo *(short arrow)*. A more compact geographic subcortical fracture is noted within the posterior tibia *(arrowhead)*. **B:** Posttraumatic osteochondral injury. T1-weighted (SE 600/20) sagittal image at 8 months follow-up demonstrates thinning of the cortex at the site of the original injury in (A), with evidence of a subjacent subcortical hematoma [central T2 shortening of deoxyhemoglobin *(arrowhead)* and peripheral high-signal-intensity methemoglobin *(short arrow)*], demarcated by a halo of T2 shortening *(long arrow)*.

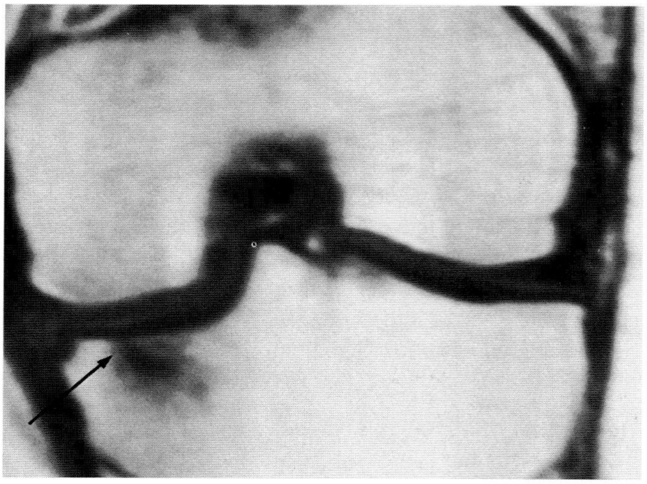

FIG. 7-9. Spontaneous tibial osteonecrosis. T1-weighted (SE 600/20) coronal image demonstrates an irregular epiphyseal low-signal-intensity subarticular focus within the medial tibial plateau. A discrete extension to the cortical surface *(arrow)* is evident.

for the low incidence of radiographic detectability and relatively high incidence of spontaneous recovery. The development of true osteonecrosis may reflect the type of cortical microinfraction and the architecture of the intruding fluid. There is no MRI experience in the evaluation of early examples of tibial osteonecrosis. Published reports cite examples of relatively advanced lesions (Fig. 7-9) (43). Theoretically, MRI would be able to differentiate isolated intruded synovial fluid from overt loss of cortical integrity and sequestration of osteochondral fragments from parent bone.

Posttraumatic Osteonecrosis

The histologic characteristics and MRI appearances of posttraumatic osteonecrosis are similar to those of idiopathic osteonecrosis. However, posttraumatic osteonecrosis can occur at any age, and a definite history of significant trauma is available.

The response of posttraumatic osteonecrosis to allograft therapy is more rewarding than that of primary osteonecrosis (27,28). With advances in cryopreservation techniques, the likelihood of allograft therapeutic success for osteonecrosis will increase.

Secondary Osteonecrosis

Medullary avascular necrosis (AVN) may occur within the metaphysis and/or epiphysis of the tibia, femur, or fibula in a number of systemic disorders (44). The majority of such disorders (e.g., systemic lupus erythematosus) are associated with a microvascular vasculopathy, although the production of osteonecrosis may be multifactorial in most cases.

The MRI appearances of such lesions are characteristic and similar in most respects to primary osteonecrosis of both the femur and tibia and to osteonecrosis of the femoral capital epiphysis (45–50). On all pulse sequences, lesions are defined by a serpiginous low signal intensity halo, defining medullary new bone adjacent to the fibrovascular reactive interface that is of low to intermediate signal intensity on T1-weighted and intermediate to high signal intensity on T2-weighted images. This interface may be exaggerated by chemical shift artifact when the peripheral reactive new bone is poorly established during the earlier stages of evolution (48–50). The center of such lesions consists of necrotic marrow fat, hemopoietic contents, and bone surrounded by a region of ischemic marrow and bone. The central necrotic zone is of intermediate to increased signal intensity on T1-weighted images and increased signal intensity on T2-weighted images. Medullary fat peripheral to the serpiginous halo is of increased intensity on T2-weighted and fat-suppressed images and is compatible with edema. The magnitude of such edema is a reflection of disease activity and acuity. With progressive evolution, the medullary core diminishes in size secondary to remodeling (Fig. 7-10). There is also no longer a distinct intermediate to high signal intensity fibrovascular interface. The majority of such medullary infarcts eventually become mature, asymptomatic, and

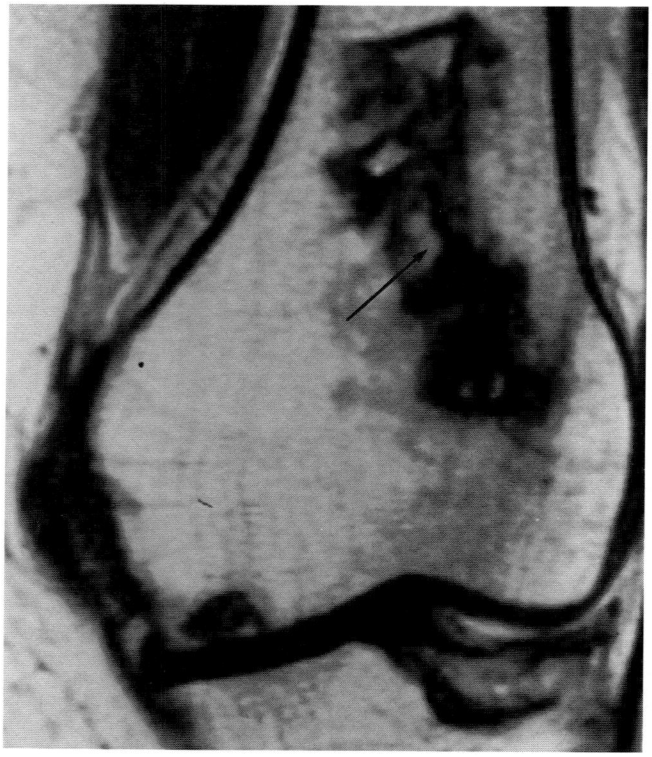

FIG. 7-10. Chronic medullary infarct. T1-weighted (SE 600/20) coronal image of mature medullary infarct. The infarct consists of extensive serpiginous low signal intensity, reactive new bone with a small residual island of necrotic marrow (*arrow*).

quiescent; however, a small percentage of such lesions are associated with malignant transformation (51,52). This most commonly represents the development of a fibrosarcoma, malignant fibrohistiocytoma, chondrosarcoma, or osteogenic sarcoma upon the antecedent region of osteonecrosis. The MRI appearance of such lesions will be the combination of the features of mature medullary osteonecrosis and the supervening tumor. However, when identified late in its stage of development, the tumor may obliterate the preexistent region of medullary osteonecrosis.

OSTEOCHONDROSES

Although many disorders demonstrating similar clinical radiographic manifestations are collectively termed *osteonecroses*, they are often very dissimilar in their pathogenesis. Although the radiographic features of fragmentation, collapse, sclerosis, and reossification are similar in all disorders and characteristic of osteonecrosis, it is now recognized that histologically many of these disorders do not represent aseptic necrosis or osteonecrosis of the involved epiphysis or apophysis. Osgood-Schlatter's disease, Blount's disease, and Sinding-Larsen-Johansson disease are the three osteochondroses that involve the immature skeleton about the knee, and they will be described. These disorders represent a true osteonecrosis.

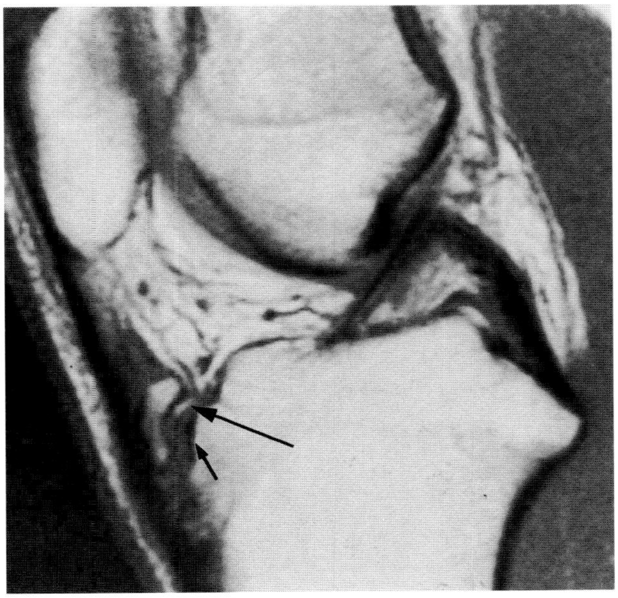

FIG. 7-11. Osgood-Schlatter's disease. T1-weighted (SE 600/20) sagittal image through the midpatellar tendon demonstrates distraction of the nonfragmented tibial tuberosity ossification center that is separated from the irregular tibial epiphysis *(arrow)* by an intervening intermediate-signal-intensity cleft. There is also some intervening fat extending from the infrapatellar fat pad *(long arrow)*. The patellar tendon insertion is irregular, with some prepatellar tendon edema.

Osgood-Schlatter's Disease

Osgood-Schlatter's disease represents a disorder of abnormal patellar traction upon the secondary ossification center of the tibial chondroepiphysis (53–56). The disease occurs predominantly in boys between the ages of 11 and 15 years. The disease is usually unilateral, although it may be bilateral in approximately 25% of cases. However, it is generally asymmetric in its distribution.

Scattered reports concerning Osgood-Schlatter's disease are found in the MRI literature (43,57,58). The changes noted on MRI depend on the age of the patient at the time of initial presentation and the stage of the disease. Secondary ossification of the tibial tuberosity may develop from multiple discrete osseous centers (56). Consequently, the relationship of the patellar tendon insertion to the respective osseous centers of ossification of the tibial tuberosity is highly variable. Such ossification centers will be noted as focal regions of increased signal intensity on T1-weighted images marginated by cortical T2 shortening. With increased age these ossification centers coalesce with their parent hyaline cartilage. The latter cartilage demonstrates evidence of intermediate signal intensity on T1- and T2-weighted images.

Osgood-Schlatter's disease represents an avulsive injury of the patellar tendon relative to the tibial tuberosity. Major changes are noted at the interface between the tendon and the tuberosity. In the acute phase, there is evidence of perifocal edema in relation to both the anterior and the posterior surfaces of the patellar tendon. This is reflected in the presence of intermediate signal intensity on T1-weighted images marginating the patellar tendon, which is of increased signal intensity on T2-weighted images (Fig. 7-11). Depending on the magnitude of injury, there may be evidence of interstitial edema within the patellar tendon that may be noted best on gradient-echo or T2-weighted images as linear regions of increasing signal intensity within the tendon. The inflammatory process deep to the patellar tendon results in secondary blunting of the normal sharp inferior angle of the infrapatellar fat pad (Fig. 7-12). Edema may be noted extending to involve the physis and extending between the proximal tibia and the tuberosity (see Figs. 7-11 and 7-12). The anterior margin of the tibial epiphyseal ossification center may normally be irregular, and it is unlikely that traction abnormalities of the patellar tendon would result in altered signal characteristics within the epiphysis. Redundancy of the patellar tendon may also be evident. During the later stages the peritendinous edema is less evident, and features consistent with healing of an avulsive or traction abnormality may be evident within the osseous centers of the tuberosity. These will be demonstrated as low signal intensity cortical irregularity of the ossification centers or center. At the region of such traction abnormalities there may be evidence of increasing intensity on T2-weighted images consistent with a focal region of edema. With eventual resolution, the ossification centers of the tuberosity coalesce and eventually fuse with the tibial epiphysis.

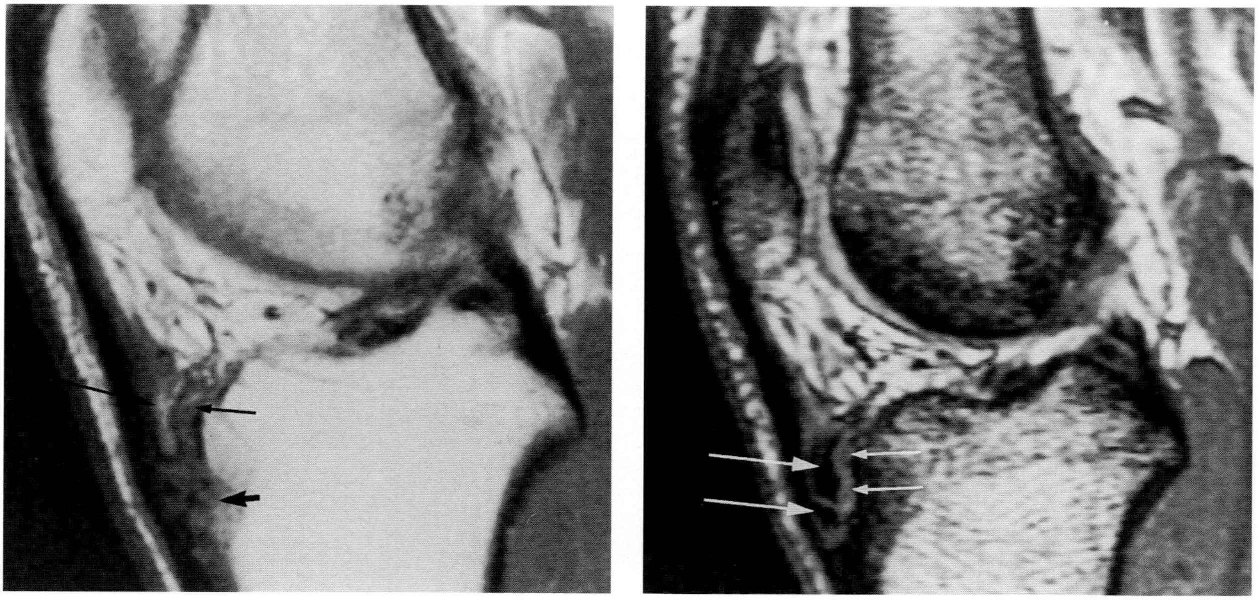

A B

FIG. 7-12. A,B: Osgood-Schlatter's disease. T1-weighted (SE 600/20) (A) and corresponding gradient-echo (55/13) (B) sagittal images demonstrate fragmentation of the ossification center of the tibial tuberosity *(long arrow)*, irregularity of the tibial epiphysis *(short arrow)*, subacute intermediate signal intensity inflammatory changes intervening between the distracted tuberosity ossification center and the epiphysis *(arrows)*, irregularity and blunting of the inferior angle of the infrapatellar fat pad, anterior bulging of the tuberosity ossification center, and thinning of the overlying patellar tendon.

Blount's Disease

Blount's disease or tibia vara is most likely the result of abnormal stress on the medial aspect of the proximal tibia, although its etiology may be multifactorial (59,60). The disease is classified into two forms, infantile tibia vara and adolescent tibia vara. The appearances depend on the age at the presentation.

Infantile Tibia Vara

Infantile tibia vara occurs in children between the ages of 1 and 3 years. It is bilateral in approximately 60% of patients. There is a high incidence of associated obesity, limb shortening, tibial torsion, and pronation of the feet. With increased age there is progressive varus deformity of the involved knee.

The MRI description of Blount's disease is limited (43). In the early stages of the disease (1, 2, and 3 years of age), although there may be depression of the medial tibial metaphysis and corresponding physis, the axial alignment of the joint is preserved, with no significant evidence of varus deformity about the knee secondary to hypertrophic change within the medial epiphyseal cartilage. At this stage the epiphyseal cartilage is unossified, demonstrating an intermediate signal intensity on T1- and T2-weighted images. Although histologically at this stage there is evidence of alteration in the composition of the physis, narrowing has not yet occurred and the physis signal in MRI is of intermediate signal intensity on T1-weighted images and of increasing intensity on T2-weighted images.

As the child becomes older, there is evidence of progressive depression of the medial tibial epiphysis and metaphysis. Although the medial epiphysis remains unossified, depression is not evident despite the hypertrophic change. There is now evidence of medial narrowing of the physis, with an irregular endosteal margin. This is reflected in the irregularity of both the physeal and osteal margins of the cortical signal void of the medial metaphysis. With increasing age (4–6 years), there is progressive deepening of the metaphyseal depression, with progressive wedging of the medial ossified epiphysis. The epiphysis within the metaphyseal depression undergoes enchondral ossification, which is identified as focal punctate regions of T2 shortening within the depressed intermediate signal intensity epiphysis adjacent to the physis. There is progressive narrowing of the physis. With progression there is further depression of the medial tibial metaphysis, narrowing and bridging of the physis, and depression of the medial epiphysis. The epiphyseal ossification center continues to be dysplastic, and a bipartite ossification center eventually forms within the medial aspect of the depressed epiphysis. This remains until eventual incorporation of the united, disorganized, and deformed medial epiphysis with the tibia, resulting in premature closure of the physis.

Adolescent Tibia Vara

Adolescent tibia vara occurs as an isolated, progressive, idiopathic varus deformity of the knee secondary to premature fusion of the medial physis in children between 8 and 15 years of age (61). Approximately 90% of cases are unilateral, with pain and progressive varus deformity of the knee. In the majority of cases, the etiology is not clear, although a few have a defined history of trauma. There are no radiologic reports of MR appearances of adolescent tibia vara. Adolescent tibia vara may be difficult to differentiate from advanced infantile tibia vara on MRI characteristics alone. Consequently, the MR features described for the latter condition are applicable. However, the medial tibial physis in adolescent tibia vara tends to remain intact, although medial wedging and relative hypoplasia occur. Consequently, low-signal-intensity fibrous bands partitioning the epiphysis would not be evident. Rather, bridging T2 shortening across the narrowed medial physis would be the dominant feature, with pronounced diminished signal intensity marginating the wedged medial epiphysis consistent with reactive new bone.

Sinding-Larsen-Johansson Disease

Sinding-Larsen-Johansson disease represents a postavulsive fragmentation of the inferior pole of the patella, similar in many respects to Osgood-Schlatter's disease (61,62). It occurs in the same population with the same distribution and displays similar clinical features.

The MR features depend on the acuity of presentation. In acute cases, there is partial avulsive distraction of the inferior pole of the patella. This may or may not demonstrate evidence of ossification at the time of the injury. In the former instance, the fragment(s) will demonstrate central high signal intensity of fat with a cortical margin of diminished signal intensity. When no ossification is present, the fragment(s) is of intermediate signal intensity on T1- and T2-weighted images, consistent with ossified cartilage. The fragment demonstrates perifocal high signal intensity edema or blood on T2-weighted images. As the lesion advances in age, the amount of perifocal edema will diminish and be replaced by a chronic fibrotic response of intermediate signal intensity. With healing, although not invariable, there is eventual incorporation of the fragment(s) within the patella, causing fibrous and/or cartilaginous partition.

OSTEOCHONDRITIS DISSECANS

Osteochondritis dissecans refers to posttraumatic osteochondral fragmentation with or without separation of the osteochondral fragment(s) from their donor site (63). Although osteochondritis dissecans may involve any articular surface that is exposed to trauma, the most common location is the distal femoral condyle, particularly the medial condyle (64–72). Most cases of osteochondritis dissecans in the knee involve the posterolateral articular surface of the medial femoral condyle. However, between 15% and 30% of cases involve the lateral femoral condyle, and a smaller percentage involves the medial facet of the inferior patella (73–76). Regardless of location of the osteochondritis dissecans within the knee, the average age of onset is between 15 and 20 years. However, with MRI the asymptomatic lesions are being identified at a much earlier age. Most lesions are unilateral, although bilaterality is seen in approximately 25–30% of cases. Men are affected more commonly than women.

Although there is no universal agreement on the etiology of osteochondritis dissecans, most investigators believe that it results secondary to shearing, rotatory, or malalignment impaction (traumatic) forces within the knee. The predominant location within the lateral articular aspect of the medial femoral condyle invokes one of three potential traumatic mechanisms. The most probable mechanism consists of patellofemoral impaction within a relatively flexed position. However, alternate mechanisms involve the femoral-tibial spine impingement during rotational valgus stress or tibial-femoral impingement during anterior femoral tibial dislocation with concomitant varus stress (Fig. 7-13) (63). However, reports demonstrating a potential familial factor in osteochondritis dissecans have been cited (77,78).

The size of the osteochondral fragment in osteochondritis dissecans is variable. In some instances the osteochondral fragments consist mainly of a chondral fragment with no associated cortical bone (67,68,79). The fate of such osteochondral fragments is variable. Fragments with time may be reincorporated into the donor site with reconstitution of the cortical margin with or without depression or elevation. Viability of the overlying cartilage varies, and premature osteo-

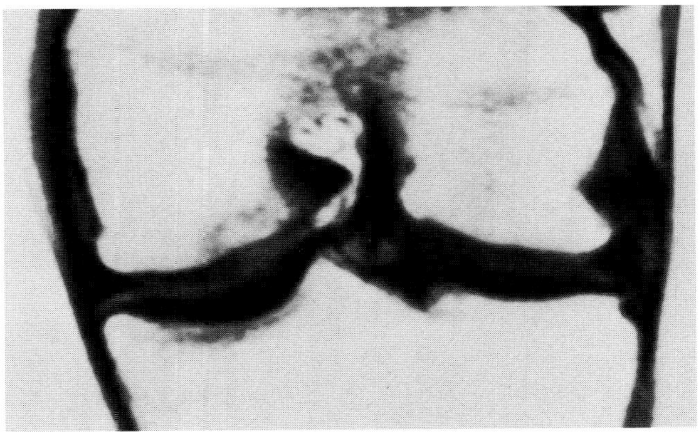

FIG. 7-13. Pathogenesis of osteochondritis dissecans: occult subcortical fracture. T1-weighted (SE 600/20) coronal image following acute posttraumatic hemarthrosis. There is a crescentic low signal intensity geographic subcortical fracture of the lateral articular surface of the medial femoral condyle. This is secondary to a shear impaction of the tibial spine upon the medial femoral condyle during a rotational valgus injury of the knee. The location corresponds to the predicted location of osteochondritis dissecans.

arthritic change invariably ensues. The osteochondral fragments may remain integral in situ, attached by a fibrous tissue union to the margin of the donor site. The articular cartilage remains viable over the fragment, but the fragment remains relatively mobile. Once fibrous separation occurs, reincorporation becomes less likely. Progressive fragmentation of the osteochondral fragment may occur, with a variable number of smaller fragments or a single large intra-articular osteochondral loose fragment. This leaves an osteochondral donor site that constitutes the early stage of progressive osteoarthritic change. The fate of osteochondral fragments depends on the degree to which lamellar new bone is deposited and cartilage growth is permitted. Once the fragment becomes free within the joint, further fragmentation may occur. The fragment may itself instigate further osteochondral injury or become sequestered.

MRI is valuable not only from a diagnostic point of view but also with regard to surveillance of patients with osteochondritis dissecans (80–83). Within both in situ and loose intra-articular osteochondral fragments, focal regions of osteonecrosis may be identified histologically. On MRI the appearances of osteochondritis dissecans depend on the age and the size of osteochondral fragments. Small, isolated osteochondral fragments may be difficult to appreciate, and their detection relies on the utilization of $T2^*$ gradient-echo imaging (Fig. 7-14). With increasing size, both in situ and loose intra-articular osteochondral fragments and osteochondritis dissecans, particularly when immature, may demonstrate a significant volume of viable epiphyseal marrow as an integral component of the osteochondral fragment (Fig. 7-15). The medullary margin of the osteochondral fragment often demonstrates a poorly defined region of T2-shortening in the immature state. With advanced age and increasing fibrous separation from the donor site, peripheral new bone formation occurs, resulting in an irregular, often prominent halo of T2 shortening. This may be separated from the donor site by an intermediate-signal-intensity interface demonstrated on both T1- and T2-weighted images. With intercurrent injury or intrusion of synovial fluid along this interface, the signal intensity may be low on T1-weighted images and of increasing intensity on T2-weighted images and gradient-echo images (Fig. 7-16). With progressive separation the width of the high signal intensity interface on T2-weighted images increases. With increasing age the appearances of osteochondral fragments become more complex, with a greater deposition of peripheral new bone. The articular cartilaginous surface also becomes more difficult to appreciate and there may be progressive loss of the central medullary fat signal (Fig. 7-17). The donor site may develop complex multicystic spaces within the subjacent epiphysis, demonstrating discrete demarcation from the adjacent trabecular marrow space (Fig. 7-18). When healing occurs, there is progressive bony bridging between the donor site and the osteochondral fragment, with T2-shortening obliteration of any fibrous tissue interspace (Fig. 7-19).

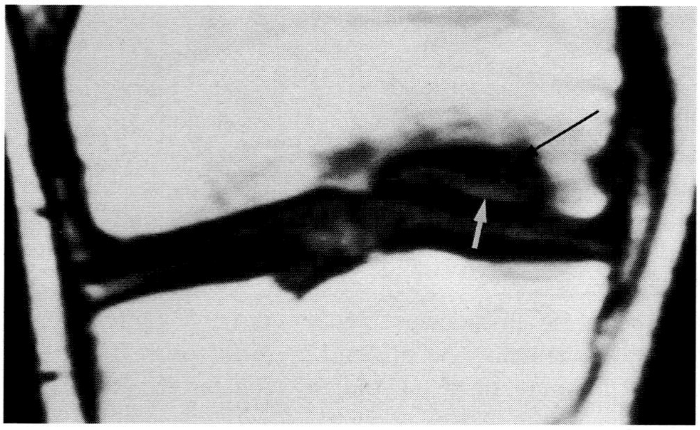

FIG. 7-15. Osteochondritis dissecans. T1-weighted (SE 600/20) coronal image demonstrates large focus of osteochondritis dissecans within the medial femoral condyle. There is a large, well-corticated fragment within an established donor site. The fragment is separated from the donor site by an intermediate signal intensity fibrous cleft *(long arrow)* and contains central marrow fat *(arrow).*

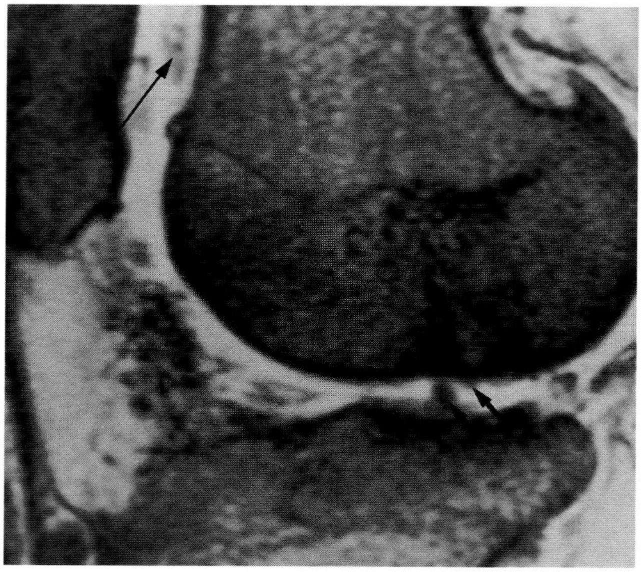

FIG. 7-14. Small chondral fracture. T2-weighted (SE 2000/70) sagittal image demonstrates a small free intra-articular chondral fragment *(arrow).* Note irregularity and punctate magnetic susceptibility of Hoffa's fat pad consistent with findings seen in posttraumatic synovitis.

MRI may prove valuable in identifying osteochondral fragments that fail to incorporate themselves within the donor site, and surgical intervention may be electively planned as progressive separation and fragmentation become evident on MRI (83). As osteochondral allograft becomes a more technically acceptable form of treatment for osteochondral pathology such as osteochondritis dissecans, MRI will play an increasingly important role in preoperative planning and postoperative surveillance.

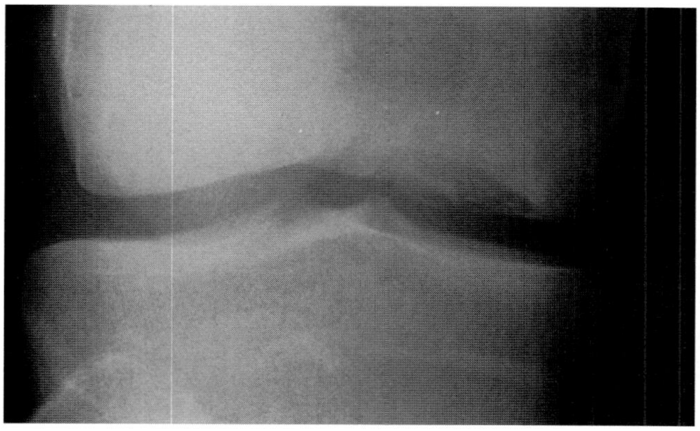

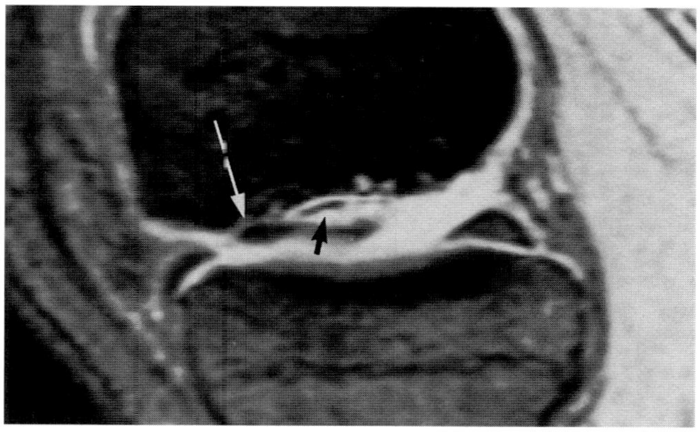

FIG. 7-16. **A:** Osteochondritis dissecans. AP plain film of fragmented osteochondritis dissecans osteochondral fragment. **B:** Osteochondritis dissecans. Corresponding sagittal gradient-echo (55/13/35°) images of chronic osteochondritis dissecans of the medial femoral condyle demonstrates fragmentation and collapse of the osteochondral fragment with extensive distraction of the posterior fragment from the donor site with intrusion of synovial fluid *(arrow)* between the fragments and the donor site. Apparent fibrous adherence *(long arrow)* is evident anteriorly. Some small subcortical high signal intensity cystic change is noted maximally at the site of fragment distraction.

OCCULT FRACTURES

Occult fractures of bone are defined as fractures of either cortical or medullary trabecular bone that are unsuspected clinically and unrecognized with conventional imaging techniques such as plain film, tomography, and computer tomography (CT), although they are detectable by nuclear medicine bone scan.

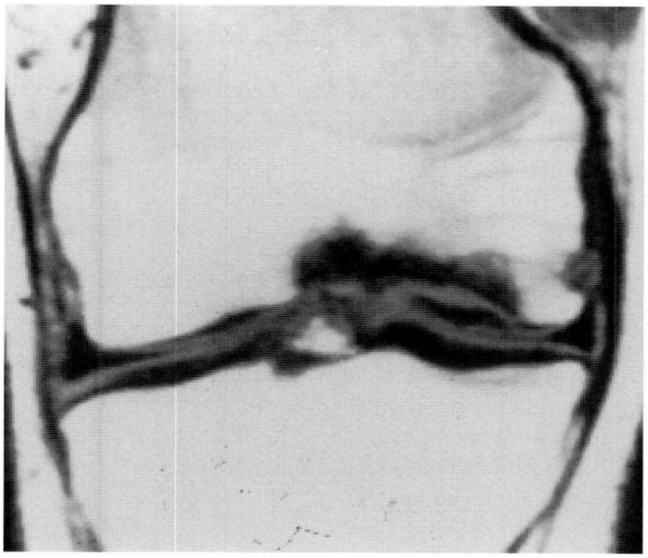

FIG. 7-17. Osteochondritis dissecans. T1-weighted (SE 600/20) coronal image of a collapsed osteochondral fragment within a chronic wide-based osteochondritis dissecans donor site. The roof of the donor site demonstrates a thick contour of endosteal T2 shortening consistent with reactive new bone formation.

Occult Medullary Fractures

An increasingly important group of recently identified acute posttraumatic occult medullary fractures has been reported on MRI (41,84–93). Through its ability to identify structural and morphologic abnormalities within the marrow component of bone, MRI has a unique capacity to demonstrate either directly or indirectly unsuspected occult injuries of trabecular bone. When trabecular bone is subjected to superphysiologic impactive and/or shear loading stresses, microfractures may ensue (93). Such fractures occur without evidence of cortical transgression. MRI has only recently afforded the means of characterizing and evaluating the natural history of such lesions.

Early Stage of Occult Medullary Fracture

The location, multitude, discreteness, and appearances of occult medullary fractures are directly related to the mechanism of their production. However, their signal characteristics are consistent at all stages of their evolution. Immediately following an inciting traumatic event, such lesions present as circumscribed or reticular regions of low signal intensity on T1- and T2-weighted images (Fig. 7-20). The diminished signal intensity at this stage on both T1- and T2-weighted images support the contention that the bulk of such lesions represent peritrabecular hemorrhage resulting from disruption of vascular channels intermittently related to trabeculae. The features of T2-weighted images reflect the T2-shortening characteristics of intracellular deoxyhemoglobin. The behavior of intramedullary blood at this stage depends on its compactness, its extent, and the degree to which it incites a local, low-grade inflammatory response. When

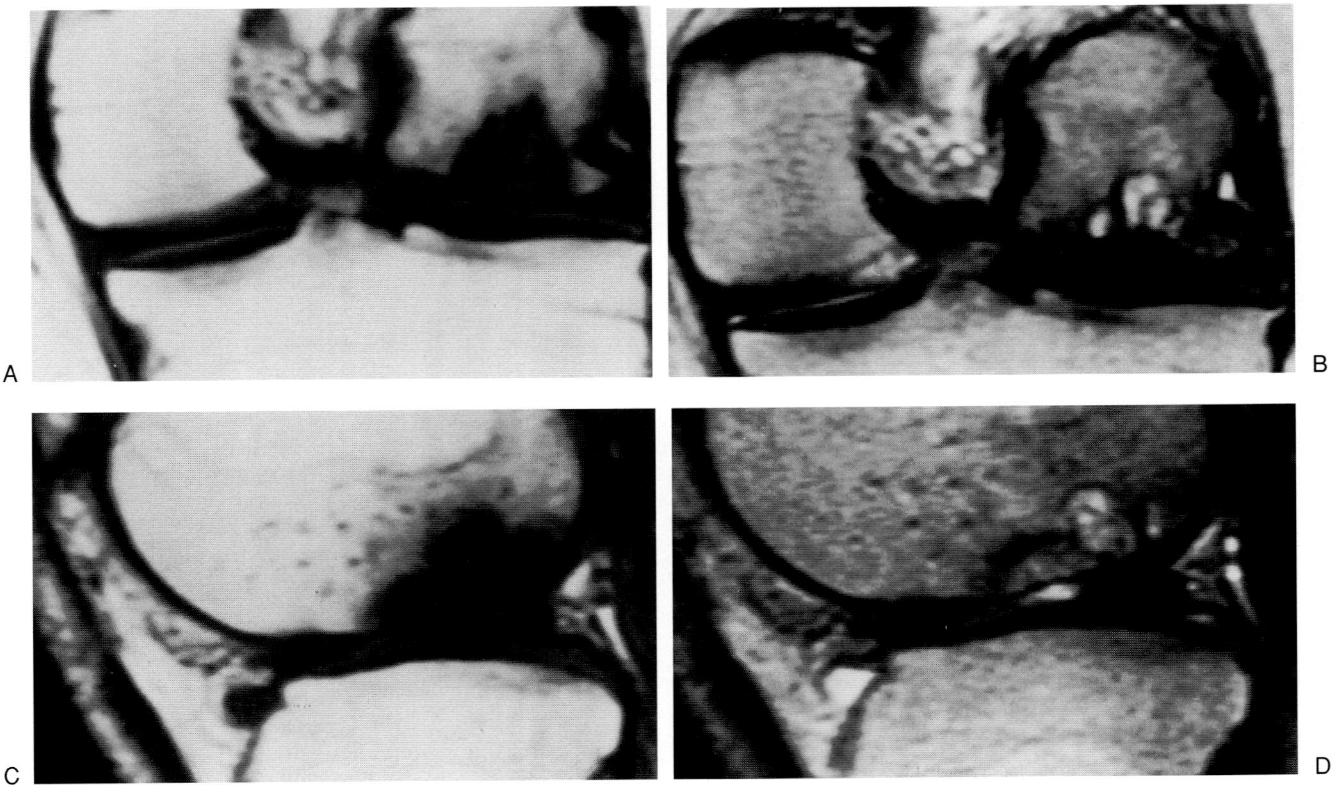

FIG. 7-18. A: Chronic osteochondritis dissecans. T1-weighted (SE 600/20) coronal image of chronic osteochondritis dissecans of the medial femoral condyle demonstrates a complex, multicystic region of low to intermediate signal intensity within the subarticular medial femoral condyle. There is a defect of the overlying osteochondral surface with no evidence of adherence of the distracted osteochondral fragment. **B:** Chronic osteochondritis dissecans. Corresponding T2-weighted (SE 2000/70) coronal image demonstrates multiple subcortical high signal intensity cysts above a well-corticated osteochondral defect. The margins of the cysts are defined by discrete regions of T2 shortening. **C:** Chronic osteochondritis dissecans. Corresponding T1-weighted (SE 600/20) sagittal image of chronic osteochondritis dissecans of the medial femoral condyle demonstrates a complex, multicystic region of low to intermediate signal intensity within the subarticular medial femoral condyle. There is a defect of the overlying osteochondral surface with no evidence of adherence of distracted osteochondral fragment. **D:** Chronic osteochondritis dissecans. Corresponding T2-weighted (SE 2000/70) sagittal image demonstrates multiple subcortical high-signal-intensity cysts above a well-corticated osteochondral defect. The margins of the cysts are defined by discrete regions of T2 shortening.

hemorrhage represents a diffuse reticular bleed, transition of intracellular deoxyhemoglobin to intracellular and inter- and extracellular methemoglobin is less apparent than that seen with hematomas. This partly reflects the rate of resolution of the hemorrhage and the associated inflammatory response. Consequently, reticular bleeds appear to remain of diminished signal intensity on T1-weighted images but to have increased signal intensity on T2-weighted images during this stage of evolution. In those regions in which the hemorrhage was initially more compact, the increased signal intensity on T1-weighted images due to T1 shortening of methemoglobin may be difficult to appreciate. This reflects the convergence of signal intensity of fat and methemoglobin on T1-weighted images and may only be perceived on fat-suppressed images.

Intermediary Stage of Occult Medullary Fractures

With more compact hemorrhage, usually subjacent to the endosteal cortical bone surface, mobilization of hemorrhage is slower and there is less central inflammatory response. Such hemorrhage undergoes similar, although less marked, evolution of concentric signal characteristics of hematoma in other body locations.

Late Stage of Occult Medullary Hemorrhage

Mobilization of medullary hemorrhage is aggressive, reflecting the disproportionate percentage of reticuloendothelial cells within the marrow compartment. As a result, re-

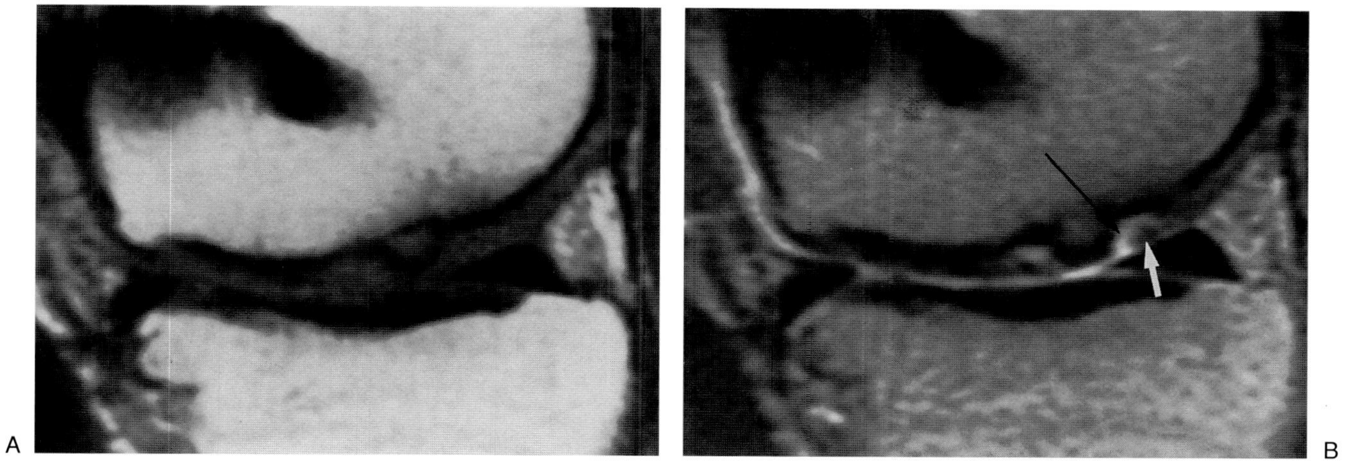

FIG. 7-19. A: Healing osteochondritis dissecans versus osteochondral sequelae of occult geographic subcortical fracture. T1-weighted (SE 600/20) sagittal image demonstrates reincorporation of osteochondral fragment at the site of suspected osteochondritis dissecans versus cortical remodeling following impactive subcortical fracture. The interface between the fragment and the donor site is identified by a discrete low signal intensity region consistent with bridging new bone formation. Note lateral femoral condyle metal artifact from neo-ACL repair. **B:** Healing osteochondritis dissecans versus osteochondral sequelae of occult geographic subcortical fracture. Corresponding T2-weighted (SE 2000/70) sagittal image demonstrates marked undercutting of the cartilage marginating the osteochondral fragment with intrusion of synovial fluid between cartilage and cortical bone *(long arrow)*. Fragmentation of the cartilage surface is noted *(arrow)*.

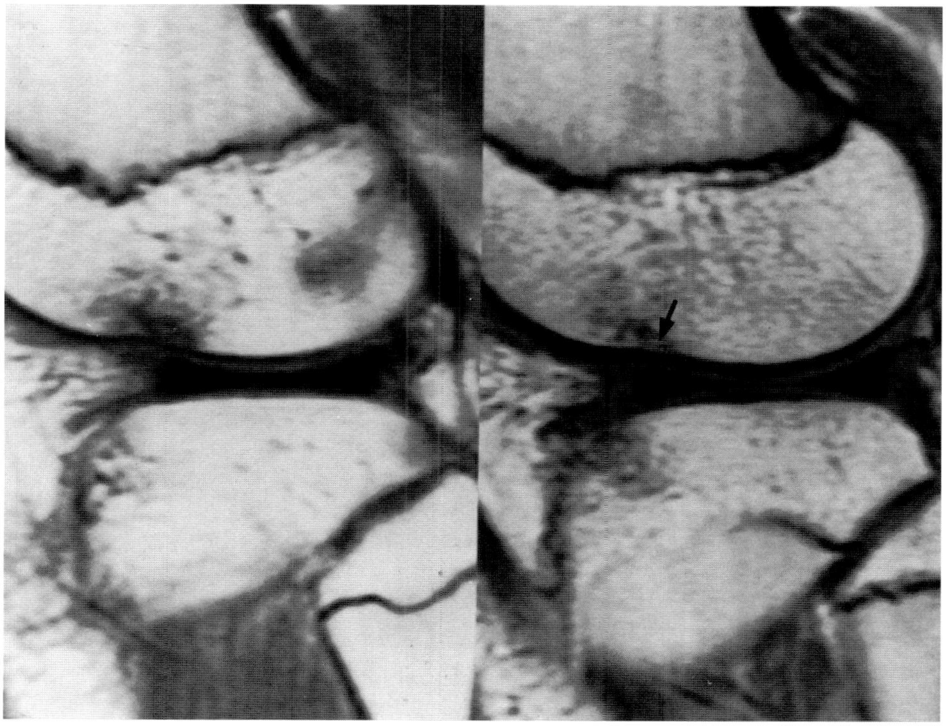

FIG. 7-20. Early occult subcortical fracture. T1-weighted (SE 600/20) sagittal image (L) and corresponding T2-weighted (SE 2000/60) image (R) demonstrating an acute reticular subcortical low signal intensity fracture *(arrow)* that is of diminished signal intensity on both pulse sequences.

gional deposition of hemosiderin is an unremarkable feature of the healing phase of such hemorrhage even when discrete. The residua of an occult microtrabecular fracture are dependent upon its location and category (see later). Most reticular fractures resolve within 6–8 weeks with no apparent residua. When fractures are more compact, particularly when geographic, there often is long-standing regional osteosclerosis resulting from endosteal and trabecular new bone formation, and fibrosis is evident as regions of diminished signal intensity on all pulse sequences corresponding to the trabecular architecture of the antecedent bone (Fig. 7-21). Such new bone formation will ultimately remodel if intercurrent injury does not occur and integrity of the osteochondral complex is maintained.

The incidence of such occult medullary fractures depends on the nature of the trauma. In patients with a history of significant trauma associated with hemarthrosis, occult fractures are seen in approximately 70%, with a significant number of patients presenting with multiple lesions (41,86–88). Such occult fractures demonstrate a preponderance for the lateral joint compartment, seen in approximately 75% of patients with acute hemarthroses (41,90,93).

The major categories of occult subcortical fractures are depicted schematically in Fig. 7-22 with corresponding T1-weighted images. Of the major categories demonstrated, geographic fractures demonstrate a significant incidence of short-term osteochondral sequelae. An incidence of approximately 65% of this category of occult fracture demonstrates osteochondral sequelae at 6 months follow-up. The changes ranged from subcortical osteosclerosis—which correlates with thickening of the osteochondral plate (10%), cartilage thinning or overt loss (62%), frank osteochondral defects (14%), and remodeling of the osteochondral surface (24%) (41,93). On longer-term MRI follow-up of both patients with reticular and geographic fractures, a significant number of patients in both categories show evidence of chondral and osteochondral sequelae of occult infractions (personal communication).

Pathogenesis of Occult Fractures

Most occult subcortical fractures occur within the lateral joint compartment, which is consistent with preexistent or induced valgus forces at the time of injury, whether or not they are associated with rotation or deceleration forces (41,90,95). The association of geographic occult fracture of the lateral femoral condyle with reticular, impactive, or geographic fracture of the posterior nonarticular aspect of the lateral tibial plateau is consistent with an associated, impactive, dislocative mechanism of injury (Figs. 7-22, 7-23).

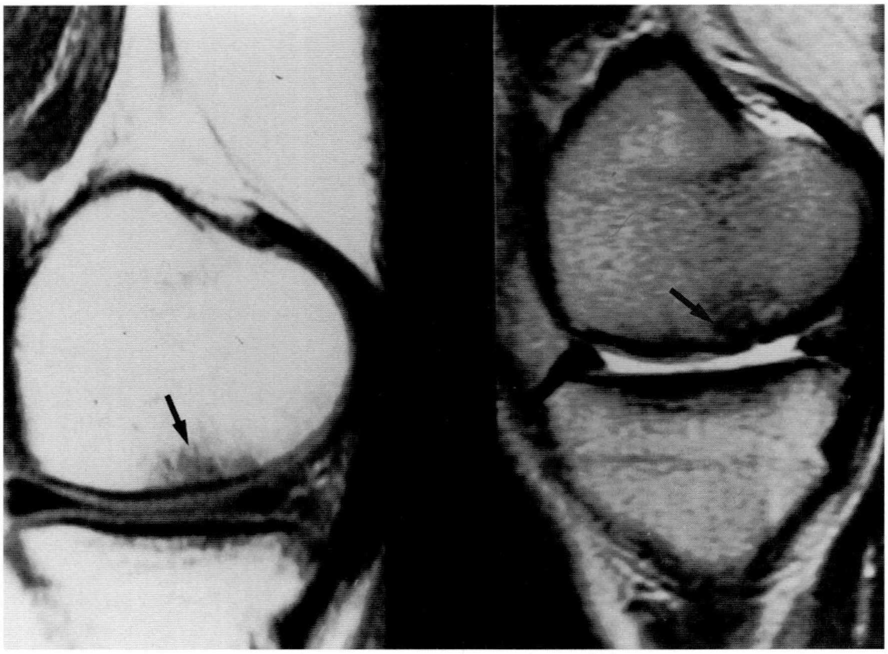

FIG. 7-21. Subcortical osteosclerosis following resolution of occult subcortical fracture. T1-weighted (SE 600/20) sagittal image (left) of lateral femoral condyle occult subcortical fracture at presentation and T2-weighted (SE 2000/70) images (right) corresponding to the site of the original fracture 8 months following the injury, demonstrates focal region of subcortical T2 shortening *(right arrow)* at the site of the original fracture *(left arrow).* There is grade 4 chondromalacia of the overlying cartilage surface, the combination of cortical remodeling and chondromalacia being consistent with osteochondral sequelae seen in majority of geographic occult fractures.

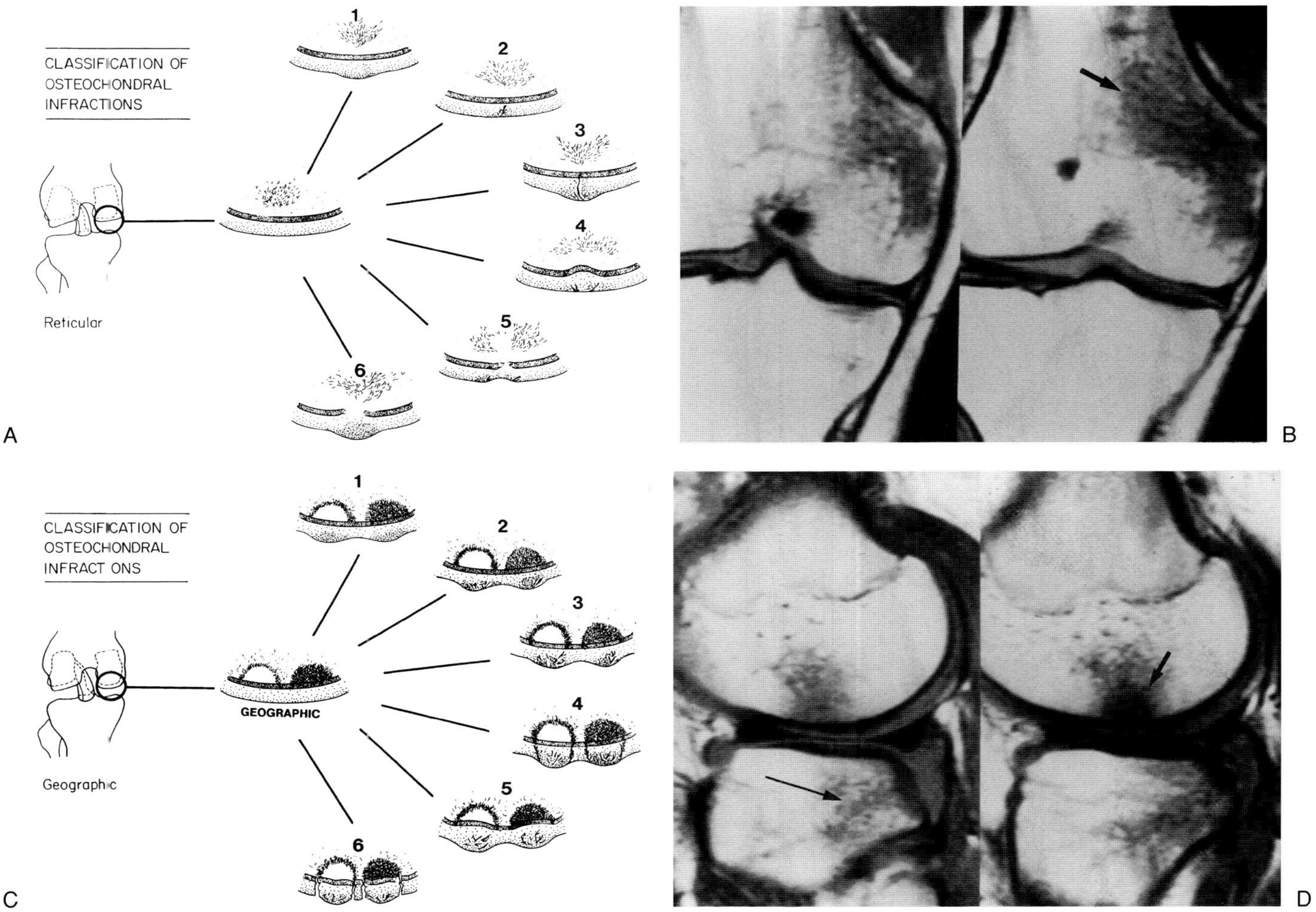

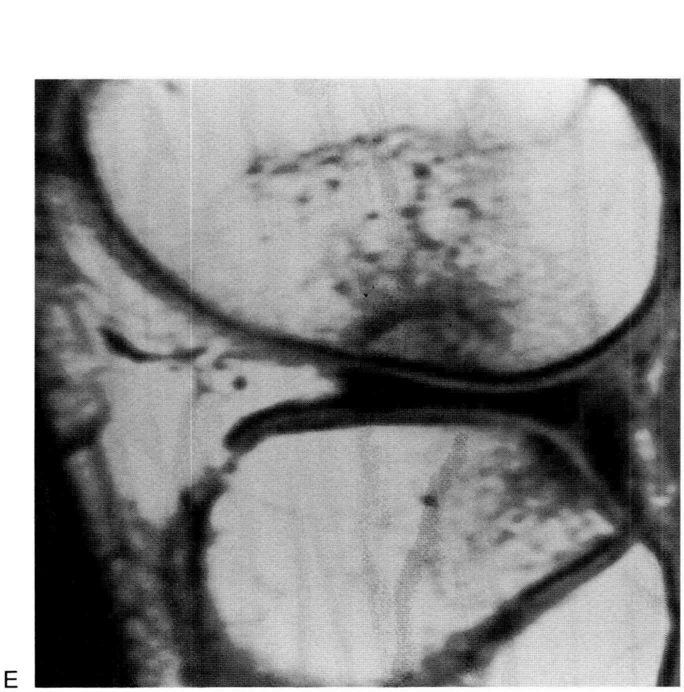

FIG. 7-22. **A:** Schematic representation of major subcategories of occult subcortical fractures. Schematic representation and diagram of reticular occult subcortical fracture. The theoretical concomitant osteochondral injuries incurred at the time of occult fracture are noted in a clockwise fashion in each instance. **B:** Corresponding reticular subcortical fracture. Contiguous coronal T1-weighted (SE 600/20) images of coalescent subcortical hemorrhage within lateral femoral condyle, remote from the articular surface. Reticulation of the hemorrhage is prominent at the periphery of the lesion *(arrow)*. **C:** Schematic representation of major subcategories of occult subcortical fractures. Schematic representation and diagram of geographic occult subcortical fracture. The theoretical concomitant osteochondral injuries incurred at the time of occult fracture are noted in a clockwise fashion in each instance. **D:** Corresponding coalescent geographic subcortical fracture. Contiguous sagittal T1-weighted (SE 600/20) images of discrete subcortical fracture abutting the cortical surface of the lateral femoral condyle *(arrow)* with some marginal reticulation. A corresponding fracture is noted within the posterior lateral tibial plateau *(long arrow)*. **E:** Corresponding crescentic geographic subcortical fracture. Sagittal T1-weighted (SE 600/20) image of crescentic arcuate geographic fracture abutting the femoral articular surface. Some central hemorrhage is evident but the bulk of the lesion demonstrates a central marrow fat component.

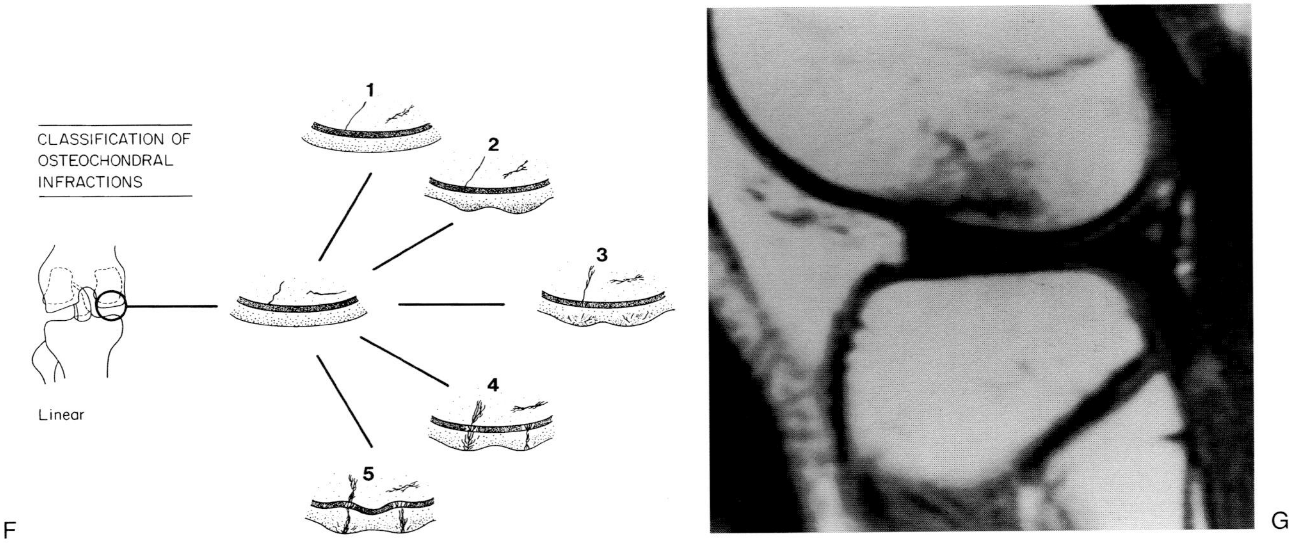

FIG. 7-22. *Continued.* **F:** Schematic representation of major subcategories of occult subcortical fractures. Schematic representation and diagram of linear occult subcortical fracture. The theoretical concomitant osteochondral injuries incurred at the time of occult fracture are noted in a clockwise fashion in each instance. **G:** Linear subcortical fracture. Contiguous T1-weighted (SE 600/20) image of linear subcortical fracture within the lateral femoral condyle.

Occult Cortical Fractures

Occult fractures of the cortical bone may present as linear transcortical fractures, subtle impaction fractures, or nondistracted osteochondral fractures (fracture planes transgressing both cortical bone and hyaline cartilage). Just as medullary trabeculae are susceptible to fracture when exposed to superphysiological loading, although more resilient, cortical bone is equally vulnerable. Occult cortical fracture may present as vertical linear fractures, particularly in osteopenic bone,

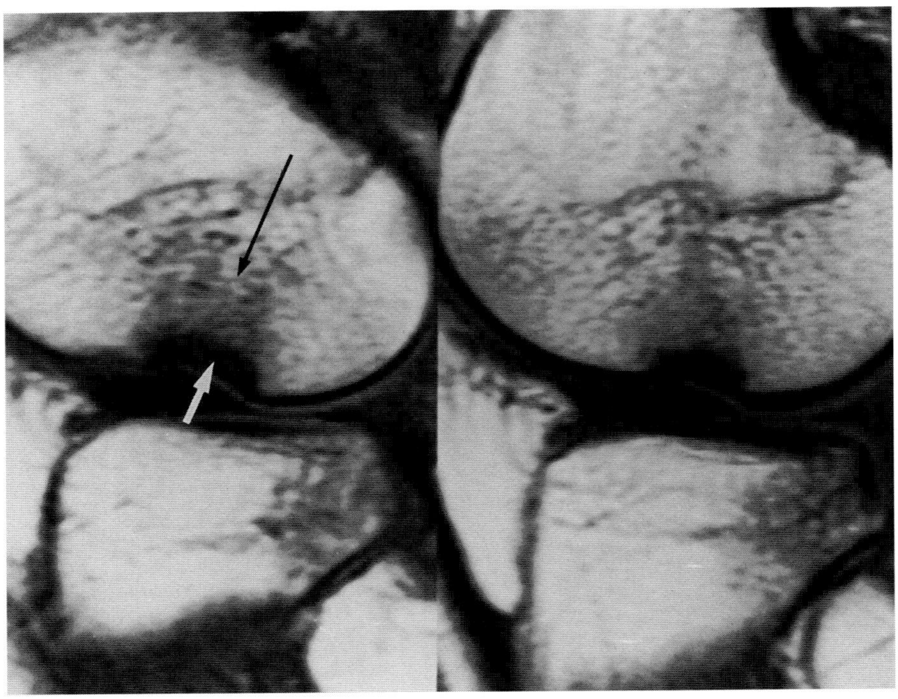

FIG. 7-23. Impaction osteochondral fracture. Contiguous T1-weighted (SE 600/20) sagittal images of impaction fracture of lateral femoral cortex *(arrow)* with associated geographic fracture of the subjacent epiphyseal trabeculae *(long arrow)*.

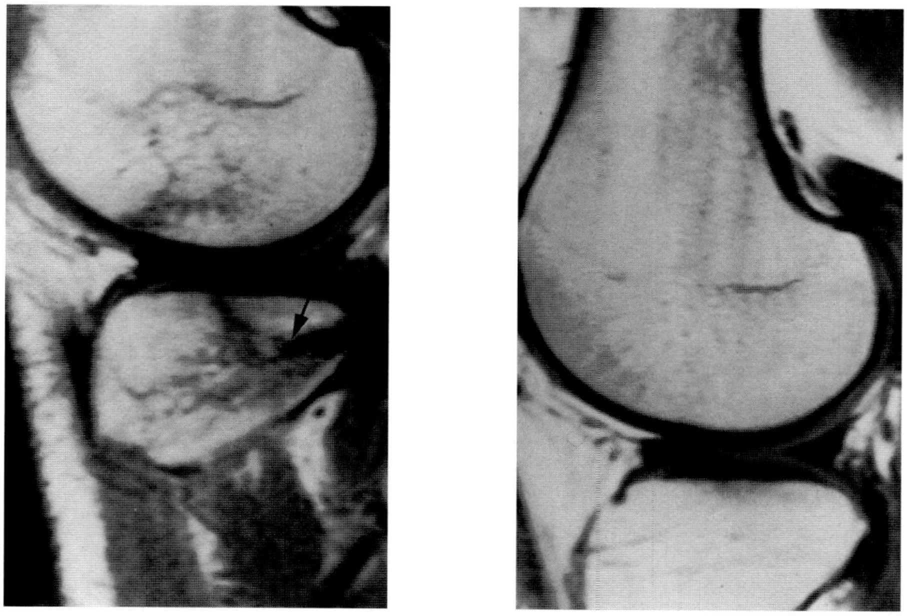

FIG. 7-24. Vertical linear occult fracture. Contiguous T1-weighted (SE 600/20) sagittal images demonstrating irregular linear fracture of both the lateral femoral condyle and tibial plateau (L), with a more discrete geographic occult fracture of the posterior tibial plateau *(arrow)*. Resolution of the fractures is evident at 8 months follow-up.

nondisplaced complete or incomplete osteochondral fractures, or impacted fractures (Figs. 7-23–7-25). Osteochondral and impaction fractures are invariably associated with occult medullary fractures in the first incidence. Impaction fractures present with variable degrees of depression of the articular cortical osteochondral surface. Discrete disruption of cortical bone may not be apparent at the site of impaction when the impaction only represents bowing of the signal void representing the cortical surface. Increasing degrees of compression occur at the point of cortical fracture. At this stage, distinction from a depressed, nondistracted osteochondral fracture may be somewhat arbitrary, although the mechanism of injury may be different. The natural course of such injuries depends on varying fractures. With healing, established reparative new bone appears as focal low signal intensity marginating the impaction on all pulse sequences. This leads eventually to a persistent, suboptimal remodeled cortical depression (Fig. 7-26). Progressive interactive loading, reinjury, or osteonecrosis results in nonhealing or defective remodeling. This process may result in progressive osteochondral settling, a nondistracted stable osteochondral fragment, an unstable osteochondral fragment, osteochondral fragmentation, or a free intra-articular osteochondral fragment. Resultant cortical defect is predisposed to progressive undermining of its margins or reinjury, with progressive expansion and deficient fibrocartilage resurfacing. It is becoming increasingly apparent that some osteochondral fractures are only visible at the time of MRI and may heal with no sequela. Osteochondral fractures are identified as discrete adherent or distracted circumferential cortical fractures asso-

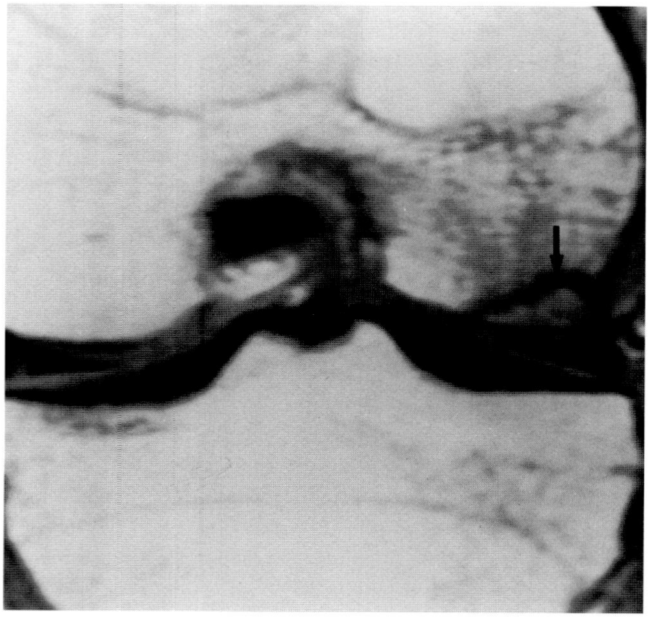

FIG. 7-25. Occult osteochondral fracture. T1-weighted (SE 600/20) coronal image demonstrates occult, nondistracted osteochondral fragment arising from the lateral femoral condyle *(arrow)*.

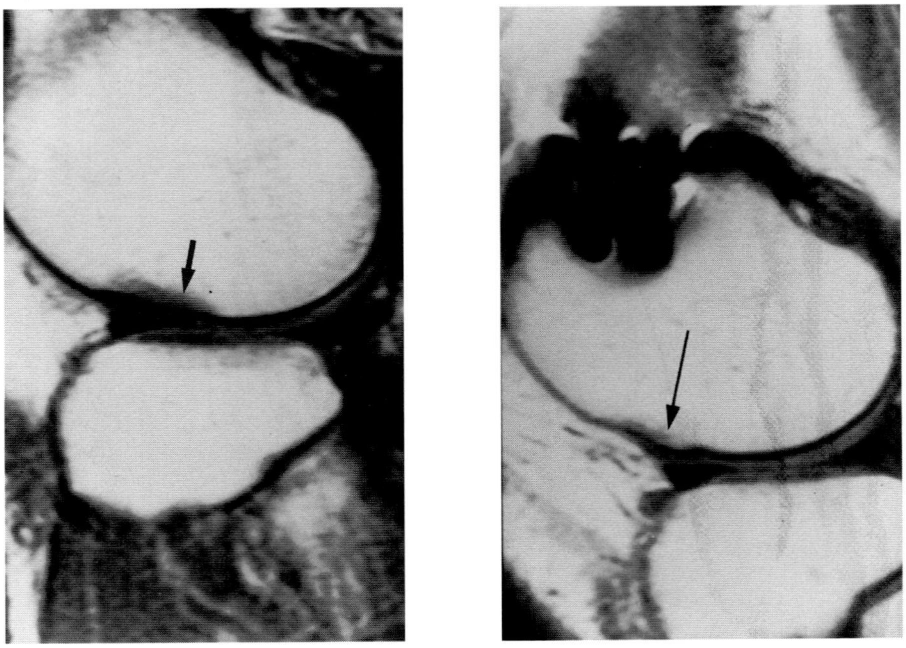

FIG. 7-26. Cortical remodeling following occult geographic subcortical fracture. Contiguous T1-weighted (SE 600/20) sagittal images demonstrate low-grade occult femoral geographic fracture *(left) (arrow)* with subtle cortical impaction. At follow-up at 12 months there is irregular corrugation of the femoral cortical surface *(right) (long arrow).*

ciated with variable quantities of marrow fat (see Fig. 7-25). These lesions contain an intact overlying cartilage surface. The low signal intensity interface with the donor site marginating such lesions on T1-weighted images is of increased signal intensity on T2-weighted images and may be seen to communicate freely with the joint space. A high incidence of meniscal ligamentous injury is reported in patients with occult subcortical fractures (41,46–93). The incidence of disruption of the anterior cruciate ligament and meniscal tears is higher in patients with occult fracture than in those without. This is a reflection of the higher magnitude of contributing forces at the time of the injury. The dominant mechanism of injury identified in patients with occult fractures consists of deceleration, rotation, and valgus stress as isolated mechanisms or in combination (41,88,93).

Original classification of occult fractures combined these injuries as bone bruises, suggesting that they resolved with few sequelae (86). Later modifications to this original classification demonstrated definite subgroups of occult fractures, described as geographic, which are associated with a significant incidence (approximately 65%) of osteochondral sequelae at short-term follow-up, including cartilage loss, persistent cortical settling with residual impaction with or without cartilage loss, overt cartilage loss (grade 4 chondromalacia), and cortical irregularity with cartilage loss due to overt osteochondral defects (Figs. 7-27, 7-28) (41,88,90,93). The importance of this finding cannot be overstated. The majority of such occult geographic femoral condylar fractures appear to result from impaction of the posterior tibial

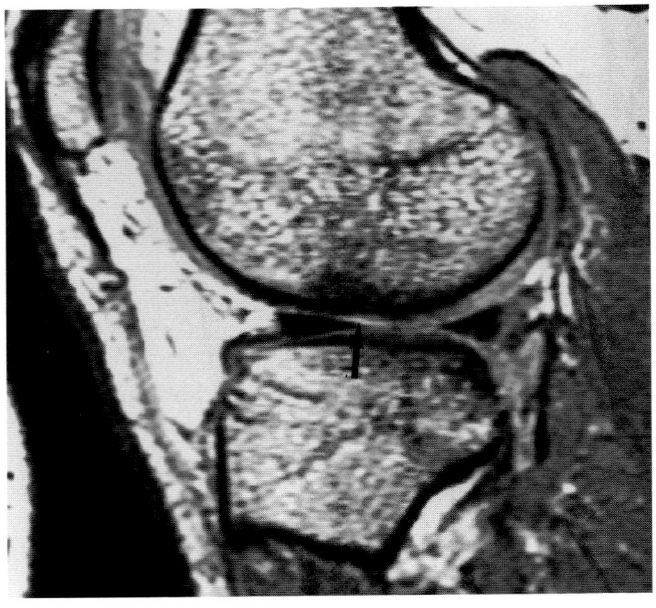

FIG. 7-27. Intermediate-term chondral sequelae of occult fracture. Sagittal volumetric grass (55/13/35°) demonstrates fenestrated loss of articular cartilage surface of the lateral femoral condyle, with heterogeneity of the residual cartilage surface consistent with early chondromalacia. Evidence of remodeling of the posterior tibial margin is consistent with the site of a previous occult fracture reflecting the site of tibial impaction upon the femur. More diffuse cartilage damage suggests greater breadth of original impaction, as seen in reticular fractures.

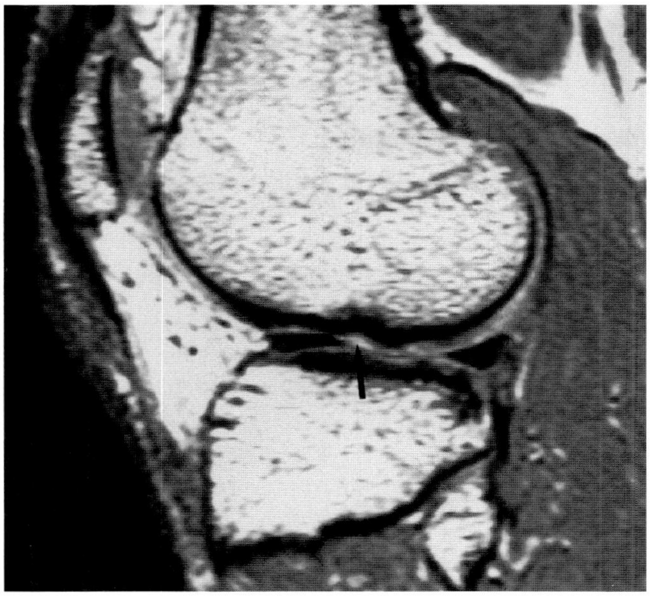

FIG. 7-28. Intermediate-term chondral sequelae of occult fracture. Sagittal volumetric grass (55/13/35°) demonstrates focal denuded cartilage defect of lateral femoral condyle. Evidence of remodeling of the posterior tibial margin is consistent with the site of a previous occult fracture reflecting the site of tibial impaction upon the femur. More focal nature of lesion suggests focal nature of original impaction as seen in geographic fractures.

margin on the articular surface of the femoral condyle. The finding of osteochondral sequelae complicating such lesions corroborates earlier studies performed in viable human subchondral bone–cartilage preparations and similar studies in an animal model (94,95). These studies demonstrated that when cartilage is exposed to impulsive loading pressures in excess of 25 MPa (below this threshold of overt fracture), fissuring and laceration of cartilage occurred and that such loading pressures are associated with evidence of subcortical microtrabecular fractures (94). With longer-term follow-up of both geographic and reticular occult fractures there is a greater incidence of osteochondral sequelae, with cartilage loss occurring in instances of apparently less significant reticular fractures (personal communication).

Recent studies performed to evaluate the distribution of impacted forces on cartilage surfaces demonstrated that a relatively large chondral surface area was subjected to pressures of more than 25 MPa when subjected to a blunt impactive loading (96). It can be assumed that when such impactive loading is directed to a focal point, forces well in excess of 25 MPa are imparted on the osteochondral complex. As suggested, the proposed mechanism of injury associated with the majority of occult geographic subcortical fractures relates to anterior dislocation of the tibia. The appearance of such geographic fractures relates to the concentration of the impactive forces, and in contradistinction to reticular lesions, which reflects a much wider surface area of impaction. Although osteochondral sequelae are identified relatively early in the follow-up of geographic lesions, the cartilage surface in reticular lesions is theoretically at risk, and given time and/or repetitive injury will develop changes consistent with osteoarthritis.

Consequently, although healing of microtrabecular fractures may occur readily, the chondral surface, which is less resilient, would theoretically undergo chondrolysis and death, proportionate to an impactive load and its distribution. Such an outcome would be a complex interaction of loading dynamics, such as force, duration, direction (such as shearing), elasticity of subchondral bone and cartilage, cartilage volume, and integrity of transcortical, basal cartilage vascularity.

The posttraumatic occult subcortical fractures represent a heterogeneous group of lesions, with different lesions associated with a high incidence of osteochondral sequelae. We believe that the subcategory of geographic occult fractures is undoubtedly associated with adverse osteochondral sequelae in the short term. Associated meniscal (particularly within the same joint compartment) and ligamentous injury would facilitate ongoing cartilage injury, consequently providing the early foundations for posttraumatic osteoarthritis. A sufficiently high frequency of such lesions would prompt modifications in immediate and rehabilitative management of such patients to ensure maintenance of the best possible chondral integrity.

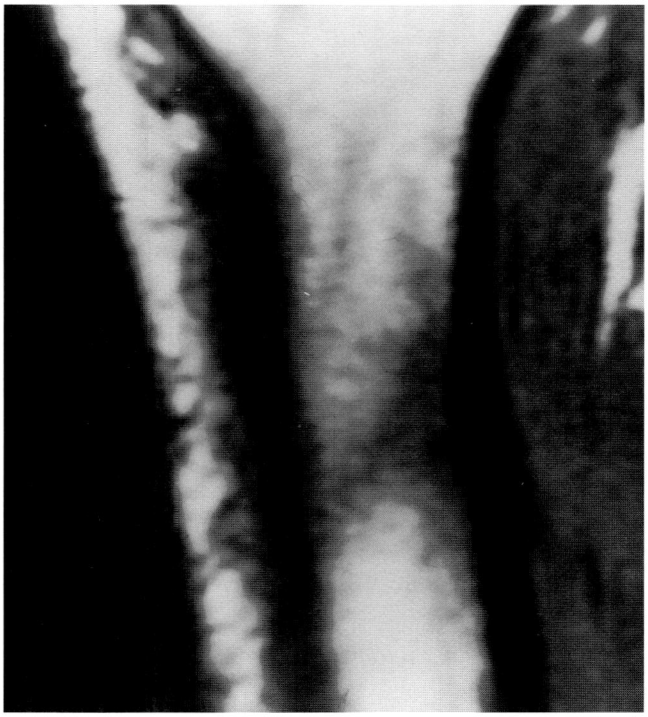

FIG. 7-29. Stress fracture. T1-weighted (SE 500/20) sagittal image of the proximal tibia demonstrates an irregular, eccentric wedge-shaped low-signal-intensity medullary focus. This is immediately subcortical, with no evidence of periosteal reaction or cortical pathology.

STRESS FRACTURES

Stress fractures occur in immature skeletons in adolescents and in adults. They usually result from repetitive loading stresses in the long bones of the lower limb, in particular the proximal tibia and femur, the smaller tubular bones of the feet, and the navicula (97–99).

Although such injuries are ideally evaluated using 99m technetium radionuclide bone scans and plain radiography, stress fractures may be identified incidentally, or one may be called on to perform MRI to exclude a neoplastic process when the periosteal reaction is florid or the fracture plane is not evident on radiograph or tomography (87,100,101).

The MRI appearance of stress fractures of the proximal tibia or distal femur depends on the age of the fracture (98,99). Acute stress fracture is characterized by abundant marrow edema adjacent to the fracture plane (Fig. 7-29), which may not be evident. This is seen as a poorly defined eccentric region of low signal intensity on T1-weighted images and of high signal density on T2- and T2*-weighted images. The underlying fracture may be seen as a focus of linear low signal intensity on T1-weighted images distinct from the edema; however, this is not invariable in early lesions. The fracture will be of high signal intensity on T2-weighted images, marginated by a parallel region of linear medullary T2* shortening. At this stage a poorly organized, indiscrete periosteal reaction will be evident as a region of periosteal low-signal-intensity T2 shortening on all pulsed sequences. With maturation there is a diminished amount of marrow edema but an increased organization of the periosteal reaction, resulting in a more discrete periosteal reaction seen as a region of masslike periosteal T2 shortening (Fig. 7-30). At this stage a fracture plane may demonstrate a fibrous union that is seen as a zone of intermediate signal intensity on all pulsed sequences with a broader zone of marginating new bone formation. In fact, the fracture plane may be difficult to appreciate on any MRI plane.

Although the appearance noted in most cases of stress fracture is characteristic, it may be difficult to characterize these lesions when florid.

FRACTURES AND POSTTRAUMATIC SEQUELAE

Just as MRI can detect subtle occult subcortical and cortical fractures, it can identify overt transcortical, intra-articular fractures evident on plain film and CT. The imaging characteristics depend on the age of the fracture. During the early stages the fracture is seen as a region of diminishing signal intensity on T1-weighted images and intermediate to increased signal intensity on T2-weighted images of variable complexity (Figs. 7-30, 7-31). With healing, reactive new

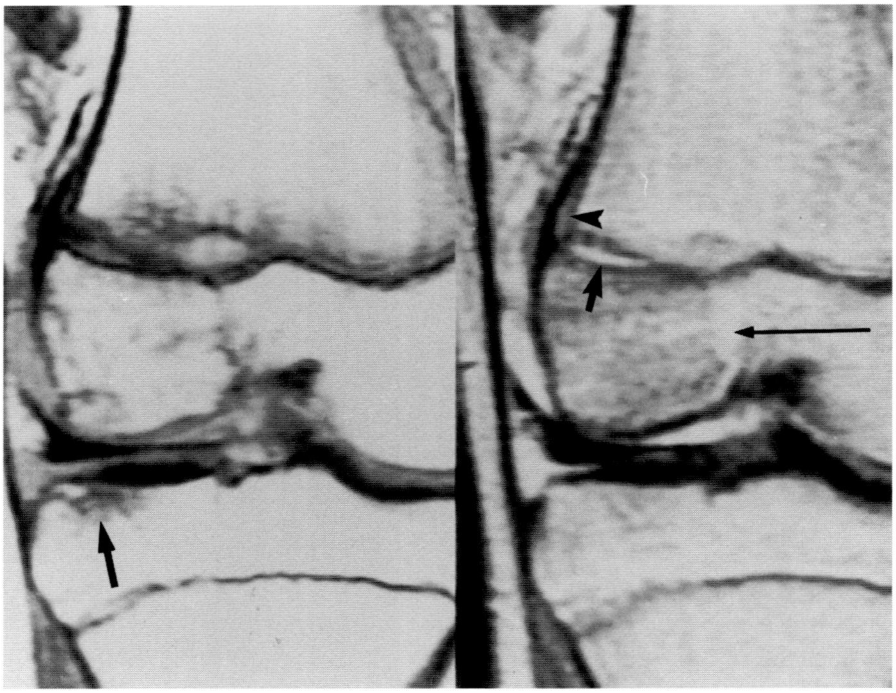

FIG. 7-30. Signal characteristics of acute fracture. T1-weighted (SE 600/20) coronal image (left) and corresponding T2-weighted (right) (SE 2000/60) image of Salter-Harris III fracture of lateral femoral epiphyseal-metaphyseal region. Accompanying reticular fractures of lateral tibial plateau are noted *(arrow)*. The fracture plains are of increased signal intensity on the T2-weighted images *(long arrow)*. The lateral periosteum is elevated by hematoma *(arrowhead)*, and high signal intensity is noted within the lateral physis *(short arrow)*.

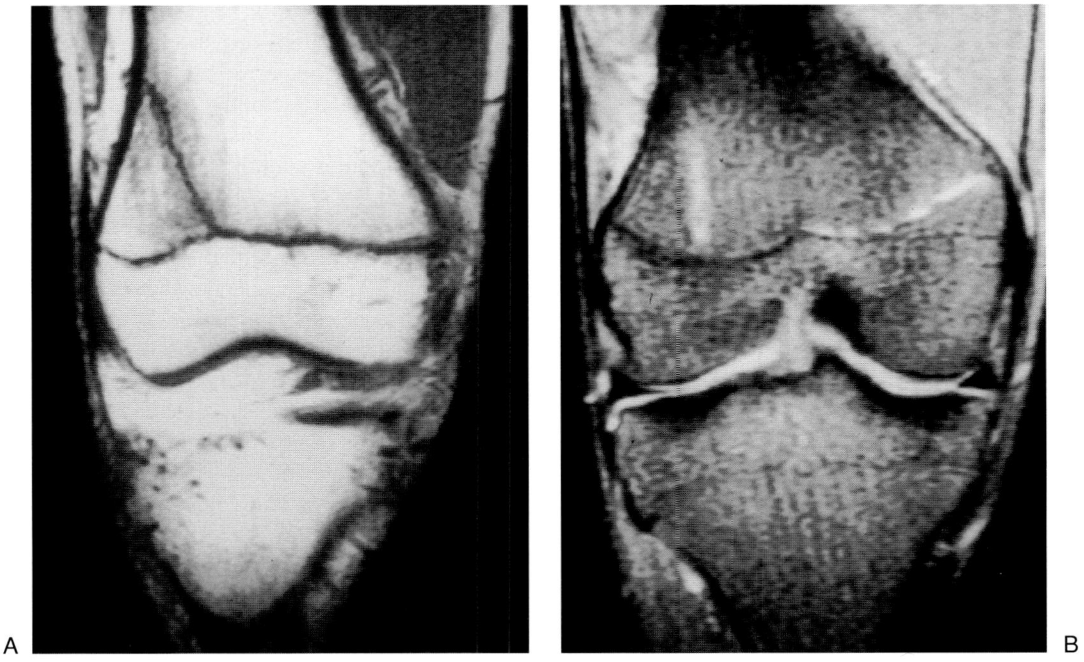

FIG. 7-31. A: Acute occult Salter-Harris fracture. Coronal T1 (SE 450/18) demonstrates an oblique region of diminished signal intensity extending vertically within the lateral femoral condyle to the plane of the distal femoral physis. The fracture extends along the physeal plane medially, directly cranially in its most medial metaphyseal extent. Some intermediate-signal-intensity reticulation of the epiphysis adjacent to the physis is noted consistent with microtrabecular infraction and ensuing hemorrhage. **B:** Acute occult Salter-Harris fracture. Corresponding coronal multiplanar grass (MPGR 400/20/20°) demonstrating high-signal-intensity edema and/or hemorrhage along the course of the fracture plane.

bone and callus bridge the intermediate to high signal intensity interface between fracture fragments. There is progressive obliteration of fracture planes by the diffuse T2 shortening of new bone, which persists throughout the phases of remodeling and resorption. The major role of MRI in overt trauma is the evaluation of peri- and intra-articular complications of such fractures, and osteochondral fracture sequelae. This includes the evaluation (a) intra-articular extension of fracture planes, (b) congruity of articular margins across the fracture plane, (c) the relationship of meniscal and crucial ligaments to the fracture planes and fragments, and (d) the presence of chondral or osteochondral fractures. This allows the surgeon to plan arthroscopic or open surgical management. Postoperative MRI permits surveillance of osteochondral integrity and evaluation for long-term osteochondral sequelae of such fractures. Through such an analysis MRI can provide a greater appreciation of the true extent of an intra-articular fracture and of its complications.

POSTTRAUMATIC OSTEOCHONDRAL COMPLICATIONS AND THE EVOLUTION OF OSTEOARTHRITIS

The role of MRI in evolving or established osteoarthritis remains unclear, although significant technical developments have improved the reported accuracy of MRI in the evaluation of the chondral surface in the radiology literature (102–107). Initial inaccuracy of MRI in the evaluation of the hyaline cartilage surface of many joints, but of the knee in particular, reflected technical limitations of MRI at the time (108–111). Multiple factors are responsible for limitations of conventional T1- and T2-weighted pulse sequences, but particularly contrast resolution between hyaline cartilage and joint fluid, independent of spatial resolution. Two independent avenues have been pursued to improve the evaluation of the chondral surface within the knee.

The first approach involves the optimization of pulse sequence development, in conjunction with the use of high-resolution three-dimensional gradient-echo images. At this time it appears that the optimum pulse sequence for the evaluation of hyaline cartilage consists of fat-suppressed three-dimensional spoiled GRASS, being superior to nonfat-suppressed three-dimensional gradient-echo and three-dimensional spoiled GRASS techniques (102,105–107).

The second approach involves the intra-articular administration of gadolinium. Studies have shown that the intra-articular injection of 15 ml of 1 mmol/L gadolinium provides high contrast between the intra-articular structures of the knee joint, including articular cartilage (Figs. 7-32, 7-33) (112). Such techniques are limited by their invasive nature, the unpredictable perfusion of intra-articular contrast, and diffusion of gadolinium into the hyaline cartilage. Thinning

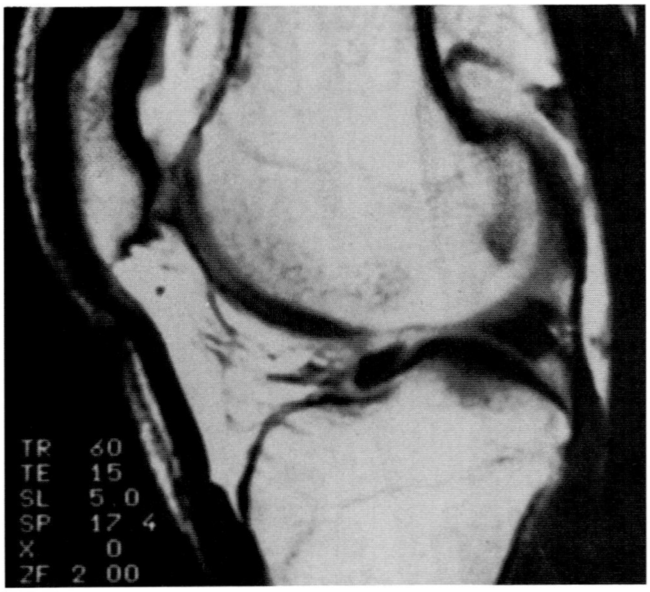

FIG. 7-32. Ulceration of the patellar cartilage. Sagittal T1-weighted spin-echo image after intra-articular administration of Gd-DTPA (1 mmol/L). The cartilage defect is filled with contrast media and clearly visualized.

of the cartilaginous layer may be diagnosed. In vitro as well as in vivo experiments show that diffusion of gadolinium depends on intra-articular concentration and the perfused tissue. No signal increase could be identified within meniscal fibrocartilage and cruciate ligaments. It was concluded from these studies that normal imaging is best performed immediately after intra-articular injection of gadolinium. To achieve homogeneous distribution of the contrast material within the joint, flexion and extension as well as valgus and varus stress maneuvers should be performed. However, with progressive refinement in MRI technique and a routine application of such technique in clinical imaging, the ultimate need for such intra-articular contrast administration is to a large extent obviated.

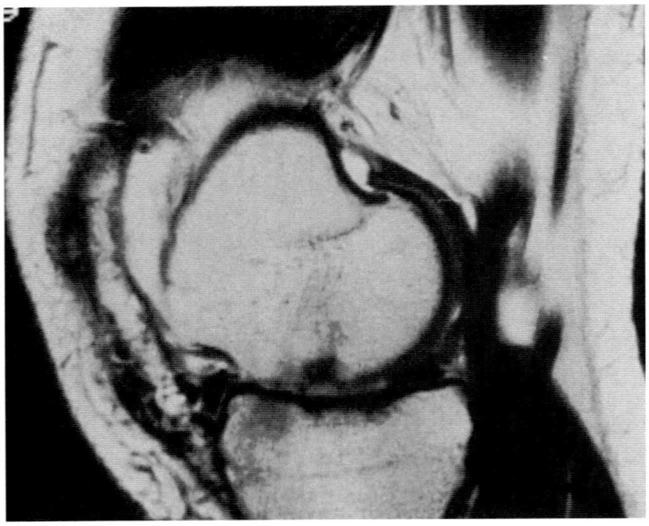

FIG. 7-33. Osteoarthritis of the knee joint. Sagittal T1-weighted spin-echo image after intra-articular administration of Gd-DTPA (1 mmol/L). High-grade thinning and erosions of the femoral cartilage are highlighted by the intra-articular contrast media.

With progressive experience with three-dimensional fat-saturation gradient-echo, fast spin-echo, and magnetization transfer technique, consistent, accurate MRI evaluation of chondral disease can be achieved, obviating the use of invasive procedures such as arthroscopy to evaluate chondral pathology. This will in turn result in the institution of standardized clinical trials to evaluate various surgical and medical therapies for osteoarthritis of the knee.

Time and greater clinical experience will determine the value of MRI in predicting outcome of the different pathologies described thus far. The ultimate goal must be to determine the role of MRI in elucidating the pathogenesis of posttraumatic osteoarthritis. Once it is established that MRI can identify definite pathogenic mechanisms such as occult subcortical fractures, it may be possible to minimize their eventual effect on the osteochondral complex at the time of their detection.

REFERENCES

1. Andersen H. Development, morphology and histochemistry of the early synovial tissue in human foetuses. *Acta Anat* 1964;58:90.
2. Gardner E, O'Rahilly R. The early development of the knee joint in staged human embryos. *J Anat* 1968;102:289.
3. Sledge CB. Structure, development, and function of joints. *Orthop Clin North Am* 1975;6:619.
4. O'Rahilly R, Gardner E. The timing and sequence of events in the development of the limbs in the human embryo. *Anat Embryol* 1975; 148:1.
5. Sledge CB. Developmental anatomy of joints. In: Resnick D, Niwayama G, eds. *Diagnosis of bone and joint disorders*, vol 1. Philadelphia: WB Saunders, 1981;3–20.
6. Hamerman D, Rosenberg LC, Schubert M. Diarthrodial joints revisited. *J Bone Joint Surg* 1970;52:725.
7. Ahlbach, S, Bauer, GCH, Bohne, WH. Spontaneous osteonecrosis of the knee. *Arthritis Rheum* 1968;9:705.
8. Megar DM, Martrepierre J, Durant J. Primary osteonecrosis in elderly subjects (11 cases). *Rev Rhum Mal Osteoartic* 1969;36:697.
9. Sutro CJ. Dentated inner femoral condyle. *Bull Hosp J Dis Orthop Inst* 1969;30:171.
10. Dupare J, Alnot JY. Primary osteonecrosis of the medial femoral condyle in elderly subjects. *Rev Chir Orthop* 1969;55:615.
11. Serrer H, Simon L Sany J, et al. Primary osteonecrosis of the knee in elderly subjects. *Presse Med* 1970;78:2119.
12. Muheim B, Bohne WH. Prognosis in spontaneous osteonecrosis of the knee. *J Bone Joint Surg* 1970;52B:617.
13. Fourrier P, Bert G. Bilateral aseptic osteonecrosis of the femoral condyles. *Lyon Chir* 1972;68:208.
14. Davis A, Carpenter Y. One case of isolated necrosis of both femoral condyles. *Acta Orthop Belg* 1972;38:611.
15. Blauth W, Edelman P. Spontaneous osteonecrosis of the knee joint in adults. *Z Orthop* 1973;111:503.
16. Williams JL, Cliff MM, Bonakdarpour A. Spontaneous osteonecrosis of the knee. *Radiology* 1973;107:15–19.
17. Steda A, Surra A. Osteonecrosis on postnecrotic films of the knee joint simulating post-traumatic condition. *Radiol Diagn (Berlin)* 1975; 16:603.

18. Gilula LA, Staple TW. Roentgen rounds osteonecrosis. *Orthop Rev* 1975;4:47.
19. Daumont A, DePlante JR, Bouvier M, et al. Osteonecrosis of the femoral condyles in adults: 30 original cases. *Rev Rheum Mal Osteoartic* 1976;43:27.
20. Cleland LG, Bowey RR, Henderson ORF, et al. Spontaneous osteonecrosis of the medial femoral condyle. *Med J Aust* 1976;2:92.
21. Lotke PA, Ecker ML, Alauc A. Painful knees in older patients: radionuclide diagnosis of possible osteonecrosis with spontaneous resolution. *J Bone Joint Surg* 1977;59:617.
22. Norman A, Baker ND. Spontaneous osteonecrosis of the knee and medial meniscal tears. *Radiology* 1978;129:653–656.
23. Bauer GCH. Osteonecrosis of the knee. *Clin Orthop* 1978;130:210.
24. Norman A, Baker ND. Osteonecrosis of the knee and medial meniscal tears (letter to the editor). *Radiology* 1979;133:828.
25. Rozing PM, Insall AJ, Bohne W. Spontaneous osteonecrosis of the knee. *J Bone Joint Surg* 1980;62:2–7.
26. Greyson ND, Lotem MM, Gross AE, Houpt JB. Radionuclide evaluation of spontaneous femoral osteonecrosis. *Radiology* 1982;142: 729–735.
27. Aglietti P, Insall JN, Buzzi R, Deschamps G. Idiopathic osteonecrosis of the knee—etiology, prognosis, and treatment. *J Bone Joint Surg* 1983;65:588–597.
28. Bayne O, Langer F, Pritzker KPH, Houpt J, Gross AE. Osteochondral allografts in the treatment of osteonecrosis of the knee. *Orthop Clin North Am* 1985;16:727–740.
29. Solomon L. Mechanisms of idiopathic osteonecrosis. *Orthop Clin North Am* 1985;16:655–667.
30. Lotke PA, Ecker ML. Osteonecrosis of the knee. *Orthop Clin North Am* 1985;16:797–808.
31. Lotke PA, Ecker ML, Alavi A. Painful knee in older patients. *J Bone Joint Surg* 1977;59:605.
32. Lotke PA, Abend JA, Ecker ML. The treatment of osteonecrosis of the medial femoral condyle. *Clin Orthop* 1982;171:109–116.
33. Koshino T. The treatment of spontaneous osteonecrosis of the knee by high tibial osteotomy with and without bone grafting or drilling of the lesion. *J Bone Joint Surg* 1982;64:47.
34. Burk DL, Kanal E, Brunberg JA, Johnsone GF, Swensen HE, Wolf GL. 1.5 T surface-coil MRI of the knee. *AJR* 1986;147:293–300.
35. Dey HM, Jaros RH, Swan CS II, et al. Spontaneous femoral osteonecrosis: correlation with MRI. *Clin Nucl Med* 1988;13:756.
36. Hartzmann S, Reicher MA, Bassett LW, Duckwiler GR, Mandelbaum B, Gold RH. Magnetic resonance of the knee joint. Clinical update II: Chronic disorders. *Radiology* 1987;162:553–559.
37. Pollack MS, Dalinka MK, Kressel HY, et al. MRI in the evaluation of osteonecrosis of the knee. *Skeletal Radiol* 1987;16:121.
38. Reicher MA, Bassett LW, Gold RH. High-resolution magnetic resonance imaging of the knee joint: pathologic correlations. *AJR* 1985; 145:903–909.
39. Kenzora JE, Steele RE, Yosipovitch ZH, et al. Tissue biology following experimental infarction of femoral heads. Part I: bone studies. *J Bone Joint Surg* 1969;51:1021.
40. Rosingh GE, James J. Early phases of avascular necrosis of the femoral head in rabbits. *J Bone Joint Surg* 1969;51:165–174.
41. Vellet AD, Marks P, Fowler P, Munro T. Occult post-traumatic osteochondral lesions of the knee: prevalence, classification and short-term sequelae. *Radiology* 1991;178:271–276.
42. Lotke PA, Ecker ML. Osteonecrosis-like syndrome of the medial tibial plateau. *Clin Orthop Rel Res* 1983;176:148–153.
43. Mink JH, Reicher MA, Crues IH, eds. *Magnetic resonance imaging of the knee*. New York: Raven, 1987.
44. Sweet DE, Madewell JE. Pathogenesis of osteonecrosis. In: Resnick D, Niwayama G, eds. *Diagnosis of bone and joint disorders*, vol 3. Philadelphia: WB Saunders, 1981;2780–2831.
45. Mitchell DG, Rao VM, Dalinka MK, et al. Femoral head avascular necrosis: correlation of MR imaging, radiographic staging, radionuclide imaging, and clinical findings. *Radiology* 1987;162:709–715.
46. Markisz JA, Knowles RJR, Altchek DW, et al. Segmental patterns of avascular necrosis of the femoral heads: early detection with MR imaging. *Radiology* 1987;162:717–720.
47. Mitchell MD, Kundell HL, Steinberg ME, et al. Avascular necrosis of the hip: comparison of MR, CT and scintigraphy. *AJR* 1986;147: 67–71.
48. Ehman RL, Berquist TH, McLeod RA. MR imaging of the musculoskeletal system: a 5-year appraisal. *Radiology* 1988;166:313–320.
49. Mitchell DG, Kressel HY. MR imaging of early avascular necrosis. *Radiology* 1988 169:281.
50. Ehman RL, Berquist TH, McLeod RA. MR imaging of early avascular necrosis: reply. *Radiology* 1988;169:282.
51. Mirra JM, Bullough PG, Marcove RC, Jacobs B, Huvos AG. Malignant fibrous histiocytoma and osteosarcoma in association with bone infarcts. Report of four cases, two in caisson worker. *J Bone Joint Surg* 1974;56:932.
52. Mirra JM, Gold RH, Marafiote R. Malignant (fibrous) histiocytoma arising in association with a bone infarct in sickle-cell disease: coincidence or cause-and-effect? *Cancer* 1977;39:186.
53. LaZerte GD, Rapp IH. Pathogenesis of Osgood-Schlatter's disease. *Am J Pathol* 1958;34:803.
54. Odgen JA. Southwick WO. Osgood-Schlatter's disease and tibial tuberosity development. *Clin Orthop Rel Res* 1976: 116:180.
55. Scotti DM, Sadhu VK, Heimberg F, O'Hara AE. Osgood-Schlatter's disease, an emphasis on soft tissue changes in roentgen diagnosis. *Skeletal Radiol* 1979;4:21.
56. D'Ambrosia RD, MacDonald GL. Pitfalls in the diagnosis of Osgood-Schlatter's disease. *Clin Orthop Rel Res* 1975;110:206.
57. Hartzman S, Reicher MA, Bassett LW, Duckwiler GR, Mandelbaum B, Gold RH. Magnetic resonance of the knee Joint. Clinical update II: chronic disorders. *Radiology* 1987;162:553–559.
58. Stoller DW. The knee. In: Stoller DW, Genant HK, Helms CA, Goumas CG, eds. *Magnetic resonance imaging in orthopaedics and rheumatology*. Philadelphia: JB Lippincott, 1989;168–171.
59. Bathfield CA, Beighton PH. Blount's disease: a review of etiological factors in 110 patients. *Clin Orthop Rel Res* 1978;135:29.
60. Golding JSR, McNeil-Smith JDG. Observations on the etiology of tibia vara. *J Bone Joint Surg* 1963;45B:320.
61. Resnick D. The Osteochondroses. In: Resnick D, Niwayama G, eds. *Diagnosis of bone and joint disorders*, vol 3. Philadelphia: WB Saunders, 1981;2874–2912.
62. Medlar RC, Lyne ED. Sinding-Larsen-Johansson disease: its etiology and natural history. *J Bone Joint Surg* 1978;60A:1113.
63. Hughston JC, Hergenroeder PT, Courtenay BG. Osteochondritis dissecans of the femoral condyles. *J Bone Joint Surg* 1984;66: 1340–1348.
64. Aichroth P. Osteochondritis dissecans of the knee: a clinical study. *J Bone Joint Surg* 1971;53B:440.
65. Milgram JW. Radiological and pathological manifestations of osteochondritis dissecans of the distal femur: a study of 50 cases. *Radiology* 1978;126:305.
66. Linden B, Telhag H. Osteochondritis dissecans: a histologic and autoradiograph study in man. *Acta Orthop Scand* 1977;48:682.
67. Lipscomb PR Jr, Lipscomb PR Sr, Bryan RS. Osteochondritis dissecans of the knee with loose fragments: treatment by replacement and fixation with readily removed pines. *J Bone Joint Surg* 1978;60A: 235.
68. Chiroff RT, Cooke CP. Osteochondritis dissecans: a histologic and microradiographic analysis of surgically excised lesions. *J Trauma* 1975;15:689.
69. Linden B. Osteochondritis dissecans of the femoral condyles: a long-term follow-up study. *J Bone Joint Surg* 1977;59A:769.
70. Linden B. The incidence of osteochondritis dissecans in the condyles of the femur. *Acta Orthop Scand* 1976;47:664.
71. Aichroth P. Osteochondral fractures and their relationship to osteochondritis dissecans of the knee: an experimental study in animals. *J Bone Joint Surg* 1971;53B:448.
72. Matthewson MH, Dandy DJ. Osteochondral fractures of the lateral femoral condyle: a result of indirect violence to the knee. *J Bone Joint Surg* 1978;60B:199.
73. Pantazopoulos T, Exarchou E. Osteochondritis dissecans of the patella: report of four cases. *J Bone Joint Surg* 1971;53A:1205.
74. Rombold C. Osteochondritis dissecans of the patella. *J Bone Joint Surg* 1936;18:230.
75. Rideout DF, Davis S, Navani SV. Osteochondritis dissecans patellae. *Br J Radiol* 1966;39:673.
76. Edwards DH, Bentley, G. Osteochondritis dissecans patellae. *J Bone Joint Surg* 1977;59B:58.
77. Stougaard J. The hereditary factor in osteochondritis dissecans. *J Bone Joint Surg* 1961;43B:256.

78. Hanley W, McKusick VA, Barranco FT. Osteochondritis dissecans with associated malformations in two brothers: a review of familial aspects. *J Bone Joint Surg* 1967;49A:925.
79. Chiroff RT, Cooke CP. Osteochondritis dissecans: a histologic and microradiographic analysis of surgically excised lesions. *J Trauma* 1975;15:689.
80. Mesgarzadeh M, Sapega AA, Bonakdarpour A, Maurer AH, Moyer RA. MR imaging of osteochondritis dissecans. *Radiology* 1986; 161(P):24.
81. Reicher MA, Bassett LW, Gold RH. High resolution magnetic resonance imaging of the knee joint: pathologic correlations. *AJR* 1985; 145,903–909.
82. Mink JH, Reicher MA, Crues JV III, eds. Osteonecrosis, osteochondrosis, and osteochondritis: magnetic resonance imaging of the knee. New York: Raven, 1987;113–122.
83. Mesgarzadeh M, Sapega AA, Bonakdarpour A, et al. Osteochondritis dissecans: analysis of mechanical stability with radiography, scintigraphy, and MR imaging. *Radiology* 1987;165:775–780.
84. Deutsch AL, Mink JH, Waxman AD. Occult fractures of the proximal femur: MR imaging. *Radiology* 1989;170:113–116.
85. Yao L, Lee JK. Occult intraosseous fracture: detection with MR imaging. *Radiology* 1988;167:749–751.
86. Mink JH, Deutsch AL. Occult cartilage and bone injuries of the knee: detection, classification, and assessment with MR imaging. *Radiology* 1989;170:823–829.
87. Deutsch AL, Mink JH. Magnetic resonance imaging of musculoskeletal injuries. *Radiol Clin North Am* 1989;27:983–1002.
88. Murphy BJ, Smith RL, Uribe JW, Janecki CJ, Hechtman KS, Mangasaria RA. Bone signal abnormalities in the posterolateral tibia and lateral femoral condyle in complete tears of the anterior cruciate ligament: a specific sign? *Radiology* 1992;182:221–224.
89. Marks PH, Goldenberg JA, Vezina WC, Chamberlain MJ, Vellet AD, Fowler PJ. Subchondral bone infractions in acute ligamentous knee injuries demonstrated on bone scintigraphy and magnetic resonance imaging. *J Nucl Med* 1992;33:516–520.
90. Nawata K, Teshima R, Suzuki T. Osseous lesions associated with anterior cruciate ligament injuries: assessment by magnetic resonance imaging at various periods after injuries. *Arch Orthop Trauma Surg* 1993;113:1–4.
91. Kapelov SR, Teresi LM, Bradley WG, et al. Bone contusions of the knee: increased lesion detection with fast spin-echo MR imaging with spectroscopic fat saturation. *Radiology* 1993;189:901–904.
92. Newberg AH, Wetzner SM. Bone bruises: their patterns and significance. *Semin Ultrasound CT MR* 1994;15:396–409.
93. Vellet AD. Magnetic resonance imaging of bone marrow and osteochondral injury. *MRI Clin North Am* 1994;2:413–423.
94. Radin EL, Parker HG, Pugh JW, Steinberg RS, Paul IL, Rose RM. Response of joints to impact loading-III: relationship between trabecular microfractures and cartilage degeneration. *J Biomechan* 1973;6: 51–57.
95. Repo RU, Finlay JB. Survival of articular cartilage after controlled impact. *J Bone Joint Surg* 1977;59:1068–1076.
96. Haut RC. Contact pressures in the patellofemoral joint during impact loading on the human flexed knee. *J Orthop Res* 1989;7:272–280.
97. Pavlov H. Athletic injuries. *Radiol Clin North Am* 1990;28:435–436.
98. Walz D, Craig BM, McGinnis KD. Bone imaging showing shin splints and stress fractures. *Clin Nucl Med* 1987;12:822.
99. Lynch TCP, Crues JVIII, Morgan FW, Sheehan WE, Harter LP, Ryu R. Bone abnormalities of the knee: prevalence and significance at MR imaging. *Radiology* 1989;171:761–766.
100. Stafford SA, Rosenthal DI, Gebhardt MC, Brady TJ, Scott JA. MRI in stress fracture. *AJR* 1986;6:10.
101. Lee JK, Yao L. Stress fractures: MR imaging. *Radiology* 1988;169: 217–220.
102. Peterfy CG, van Dijke CF, Janzen DL, et al. Quantification of articular cartilage in the knee with pulsed saturation transfer subtraction and fat-suppressed MR imaging: optimization and validation. *Radiology* 1994;192:485–491.
103. Fernandez-madrid F, Karvonen RL, Teitge RA, Miller PR, Negendank WG. MR features of osteoarthritis of the knee. *Magn Reson Imaging* 1994;12:703–709.
104. Karvonen RL, Negendank WG, Teitge RA, Reed AH, Miller PR, Fernandez-Madrid F. Factors affecting articular cartilage thickness in osteoarthritis and aging. *J Rheumatol* 1994;21:1310–1318.
105. Broderick LS, Turner DA, Renfrew DL, Schnitzer TJ, Huff JP, Harris C. Severity of articular cartilage abnormality in patients with osteoarthritis: evaluation with fast spin-echo MR vs arthroscopy. *AJR* 1994; 162:99–103.
106. Disler DG, Peters TL, Muscoreil SJ, et al. Fat-suppressed spoiled GRASS imaging of knee hyaline cartilage: technique optimization and comparison with conventional MR imaging. *AJR* 1994;163:887–892.
107. Blackburn WD, Bernreuter WK, Rominger M, Loose LL. Arthroscopic evaluation of knee articular cartilage: a comparison with plain radiographs and magnetic resonance imaging. *J Rheumatol* 1994;21: 675–679.
108. Speer KP, Spritzer CE, Goldner JL, Garrett WE Jr. Magnetic resonance imaging of traumatic knee articular cartilage injuries. *Am J Sports Med* 1991;19:396–402.
109. Chan WP, Lang P, Stevens MP, et al. Osteoarthritis of the knee: comparison of radiography, CT and MR imaging to assess extent and severity. *AJR* 1991;157:799–806.
110. Hodler J, Berthiaume MJ, Schweitzer ME, Resnick D. Knee joint hyaline cartilage defects: a comparative study of MR and anatomic sections. *JCAT* 1992;16:597–603.
111. Recht MP, Kramer J, Marcelis S, et al. Abnormalities of articular cartilage in the knee: analysis of available MR techniques. *Radiology* 1993;187:473–478.
112. Applegate GR, Flannigan BD, Tolin BS, Fox JM, Del Pizzo W. MR diagnosis of recurrent tears in the knee: value of intraarticular contrast material. *AJR* 1993;161:821–825.

MRI of the Knee, Second Edition,
edited by P. L. Munk and C. A. Helms.
Lippincott-Raven Publishers, Philadelphia © 1996.

CHAPTER 8

Arthritis and Inflammatory Knee Disease

A. Dale Vellet, Peter L. Munk, and Maximilian F. Reiser

ANATOMY AND PATHOLOGY OF SYNOVIAL STRUCTURES OF THE KNEE

The fundamental constituents of any synovial joint are an investing fibrous capsule with its superficial tendinous and ligamentous reinforcements (1). This in turn is lined by the synovial membrane. The opposed osteochondral surfaces and the fibrocartilaginous menisci are bathed by synovial fluid secreted by the intimal component of the synovial membrane, whereas the cruciate ligaments are extrasynovial, invested by a sheath of synovium (2). The purpose of this chapter is to illustrate the role of magnetic resonance imaging in the evaluation of synovial anatomy and inflammatory diseases of the synovium.

STRUCTURE AND ANATOMY OF THE SYNOVIAL MEMBRANE

The synovial membrane consists of a cellular intima and areolar connective tissue subintima (3–9). The cellular intima is of variable thickness (one to four cells) embedded in a granular matrix. The subintimal layer of the synovial membrane is loosely adherent throughout to the fibrous capsule and cruciate ligaments, particularly the anterior cruciate ligament, through its deep subintimal layer. The synovial membrane is deficient over the articular surfaces of the joint. This allows the cartilage surfaces to articulate with one another while being lubricated by the fluid elaborated by the synovial membrane. The synovium extends from the fibrous capsule to the adjacent periosteal bony surfaces at the level of the osteochondral junction. It is these regions that demonstrate the greatest degree of capsular and subintimal vascularity. In some areas where the synovial membrane is loosely bound to these underlying structures, the synovium may be seen to form small fibrovascular projections referred to as villi.

TECHNIQUE OF MRI EVALUATION OF THE SYNOVIUM

The imaging techniques applicable to the evaluation of different meniscal ligamentous, tendinous, and osteochondral structures are detailed in respective chapters of this text. Evaluation of synovial disease is an integral component of the assessment of these images.

Various methods have been used to evaluate synovial membranes in the knee joint. T1- and T2-weighted spin-echo imaging is routinely used in knee imaging, and when synovium is significantly thickened this can be observed with these sequences. In addition, gradient-echo techniques (both static and dynamic) have been particularly helpful in allowing thin-section high-resolution imaging. Three-dimensional Fourier transform (3DFT) sagittal and/or coronal pre- and postcontrast gradient-echo techniques are especially well suited to specific evaluation of the synovial membranes of the tibiofemoral joint and, to a degree, of the patellofemoral joint. This technique has the advantages of multiplanar reconstruction if required, high spatial resolution with maintained signal-to-noise ratio, and high contrast resolution, which is particularly helpful when contrast is utilized. Such spatial resolution is of special assistance when evaluating serial magnetic resonance images (MRIs) for the objective assessment of synovial and osteochondral changes following therapeutic interventions. When the patellofemoral joint and its synovial structures are being evaluated, axial scans are especially useful.

The extension of the inflammatory process into surrounding soft tissue (i.e., in the form of popliteal cysts) (10) as well as the anatomic relationship to muscle bundles, vessels,

A. D. Vellet: Department of Diagnostic Imaging, University of Calgary, Foothills Hospital, Alberta, Canada T2N 2T9.
P. L. Munk: Department of Radiology, University of British Columbia, Department of Diagnostic Imaging, British Columbia Cancer Agency, Vancouver, British Columbia, Canada V5Z 4E6.
M. F. Reiser: Department of Radiology, University of Munich, Munich, Germany.

and nerves can almost always be clearly visualized by using a combination of imaging planes.

When gradient-echo sequences are used, it should be remembered that the contrast of tissues is dependent not only on TR (repetition time) and TE (echo time) but, most important, on the chosen flip angle. With flip angles of 30–50°, hyaline cartilage, cruciate ligaments, and menisci can usually all be adequately evaluated (11–13). This is discussed in greater detail in the chapter on technique.

INTRAVENOUS PARAMAGNETIC CONTRAST AGENTS

On nonenhanced T1-weighted spin-echo images suboptimal contrast is obtained between the low signal intensity pannus and other low signal intensity structures of the knee joint such as menisci and cruciate ligaments. Depiction of pathological alterations of these structures is therefore limited. On T2-weighted images signal intensity of synovium is often increased but is frequently difficult to discriminate from that of surrounding fluid. Because of this fluid, pannus and cartilage may be difficult to differentiate from one another. In the more chronic phase of the disease pannus may be fibrotic and laden with hemosiderin, making differentiation between it and the menisci and ligaments unclear.

Following injection of intravenous gadolinium chelate, the contrast agent is transported through plasma and passes into the interstitial space at a rate dependent on local capillary permeability and tissue perfusion. These are in turn related to the degree of inflammation. A significant increase in signal intensity is therefore found within inflammatory tissue, and this enhancement is to some degree dose dependent (14). Gadolinium chelates do have toxic effects at levels greater than 5.0 mM/kg body weight; however, this is far higher than the doses normally used for diagnostic purposes (0.1–0.2 mM/kg body weight).

Direction of gadolinium enhancement is highly dependent on the imaging technique. For MRI evaluation of paraosseous inflammatory processes and intra-articular lesions, T1-weighted spin-echo sequences demonstrate excellent contrast enhancement and provide for good visualization of anatomic detail (Fig. 8-1). As mentioned earlier, contrast-enhanced gradient-echo sequences are also extremely useful; the best parameters at 1.5 T are in the vicinity of TR 30–40 msec, with T10–12 msec with a flip angle in the 70–90° range.

After administration of gadolinium, hypertrophic synovium exhibits a marked increase in signal intensity on T1-weighted spin-echo images. In contrast, the signal intensity on intra-articular fluid does not show any significant change, provided images were obtained within the first 15–20 minutes after injection (14–27). Gadolinium will, however, slowly leach into joint effusions, especially if synovium is very inflamed, and delayed imaging produces a "gadolinium arthrogram" effect. By virtue of the increased signal of the

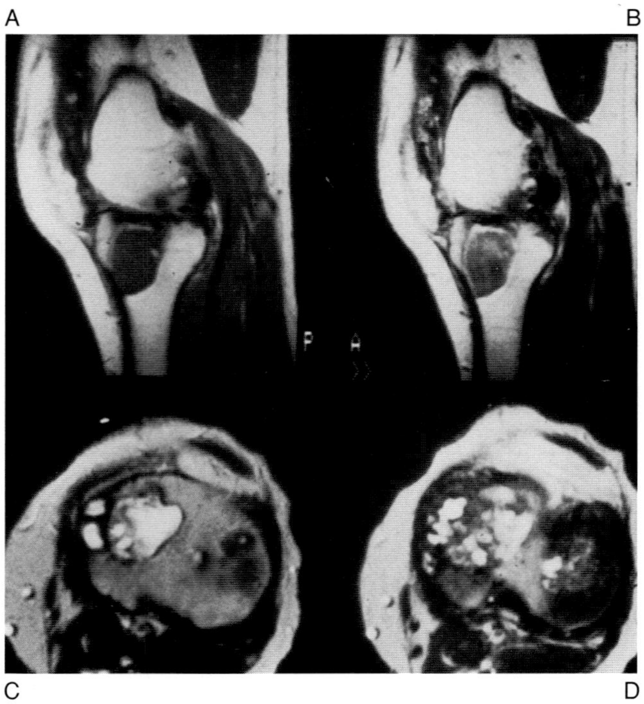

FIG. 8-1. Hemophilic arthropathy. **A:** Sagittal T1-weighted spin echo. Large, low-signal subchondral cysts are seen in the proximal epiphysis and metaphysis of the tibia. There is narrowing of the joint space and destruction of the menisci. The suprapatellar recess is widened by inhomogeneous soft-tissue proliferation. **B:** Sagittal T1-weighted spin echo after infusion of Gad-DTPA. Seen are rim enhancement of the synovial lining of the subchondral cyst within the tibia and differentiation of the soft-tissue components within the cystic lesion. There is an inhomogeneous signal increase of the pannus in the suprapatellar recess. **C,D:** T2-weighted spin echo, axial plane. Slices at the level of the tibial plateau. The subchondral cyst in the proximal tibia shows high signal intensity and is lined by a dark sclerotic margin.

enhancement synovium following injection of gadolinium, the low-signal-intensity menisci and cruciate ligaments can be visualized to great advantage (Fig. 8-2).

Dynamic postcontrast gadolinium imaging can be used for analysis of the rate of contrast enhancement within the proliferating synovium (17,19,21,28). Quantitative analysis demonstrates dramatic increase in the signal intensity of the synovial membrane. Following bolus injection of contrast, signal intensity can be plotted over time and provided the increment is sufficiently small (20 sec or less) the rate of enhancement can be studied (Fig. 8-3). Different studies have indicated that in patients with rheumatoid arthritis (19) absolute signal intensity increases in pannus can be up to 2–2.5 times that of baseline with both spin-echo and gradient-echo sequences that are T1-weighted. In comparison, muscle, fat, bone marrow, and joint effusion show minimal enhancement, usually being less than 20% of baseline signal intensity. If the signal intensity measurements are markedly delayed (i.e., 20 minutes or more) some evidence of gradual

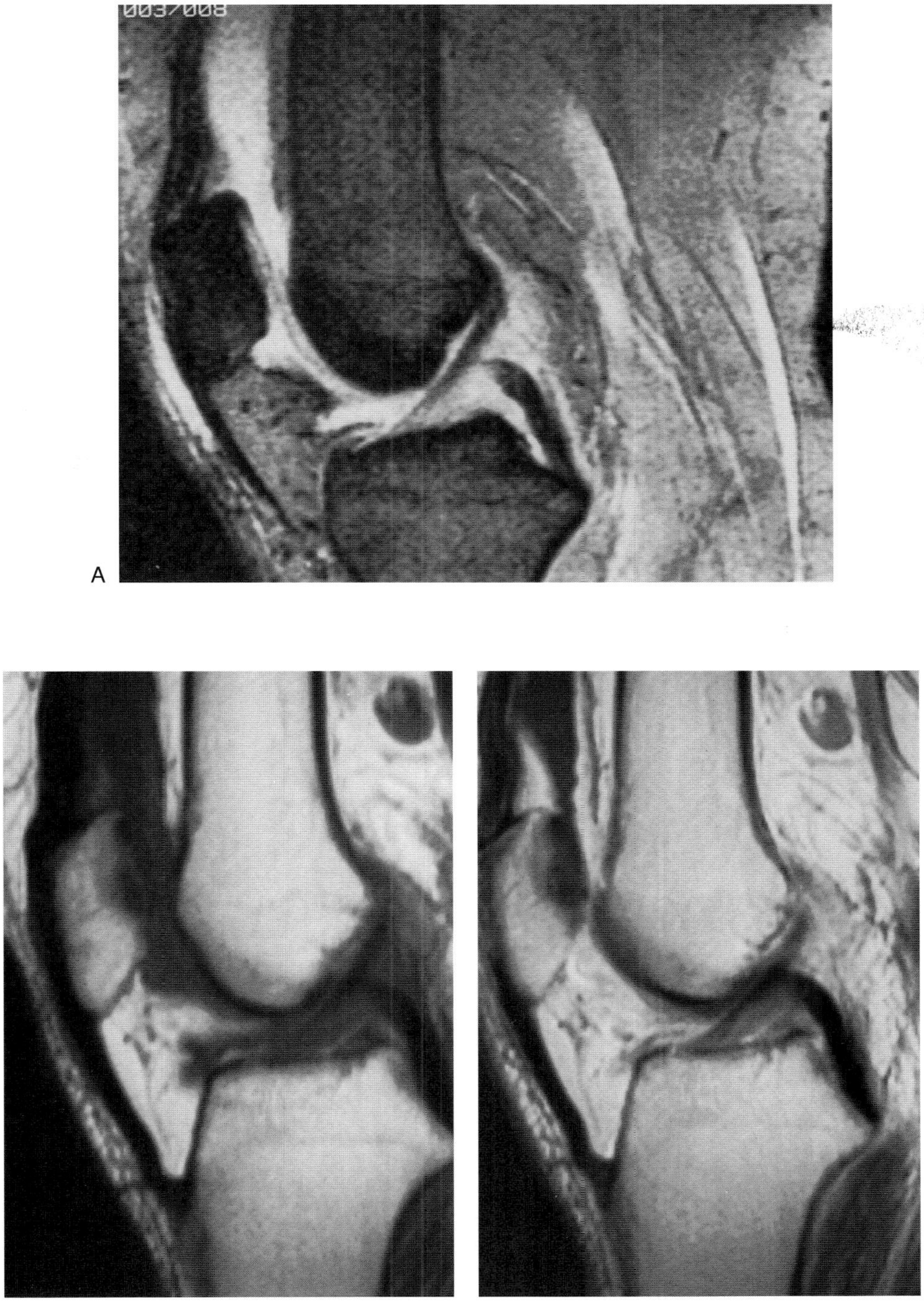

A B C

FIG. 8-2. A: Sagittal gradient-echo image of a patient with rheumatoid arthritis. The synovial proliferation and synovial effusion are both of high signal intensity with this sequence and cannot be readily differentiated one from the other. **B:** The T1-weighted spin-echo unenhanced image also shows better, but still poor discrimination between synovium and fluid. **C:** Following infusion of intravenous gadolinium, intense enhancement of synovium is apparent outlining the cruciate ligaments and showing that most of the volume of the knee joint is filled with synovium rather than with fluid. Some fluid is apparent in the suprapatellar recess.

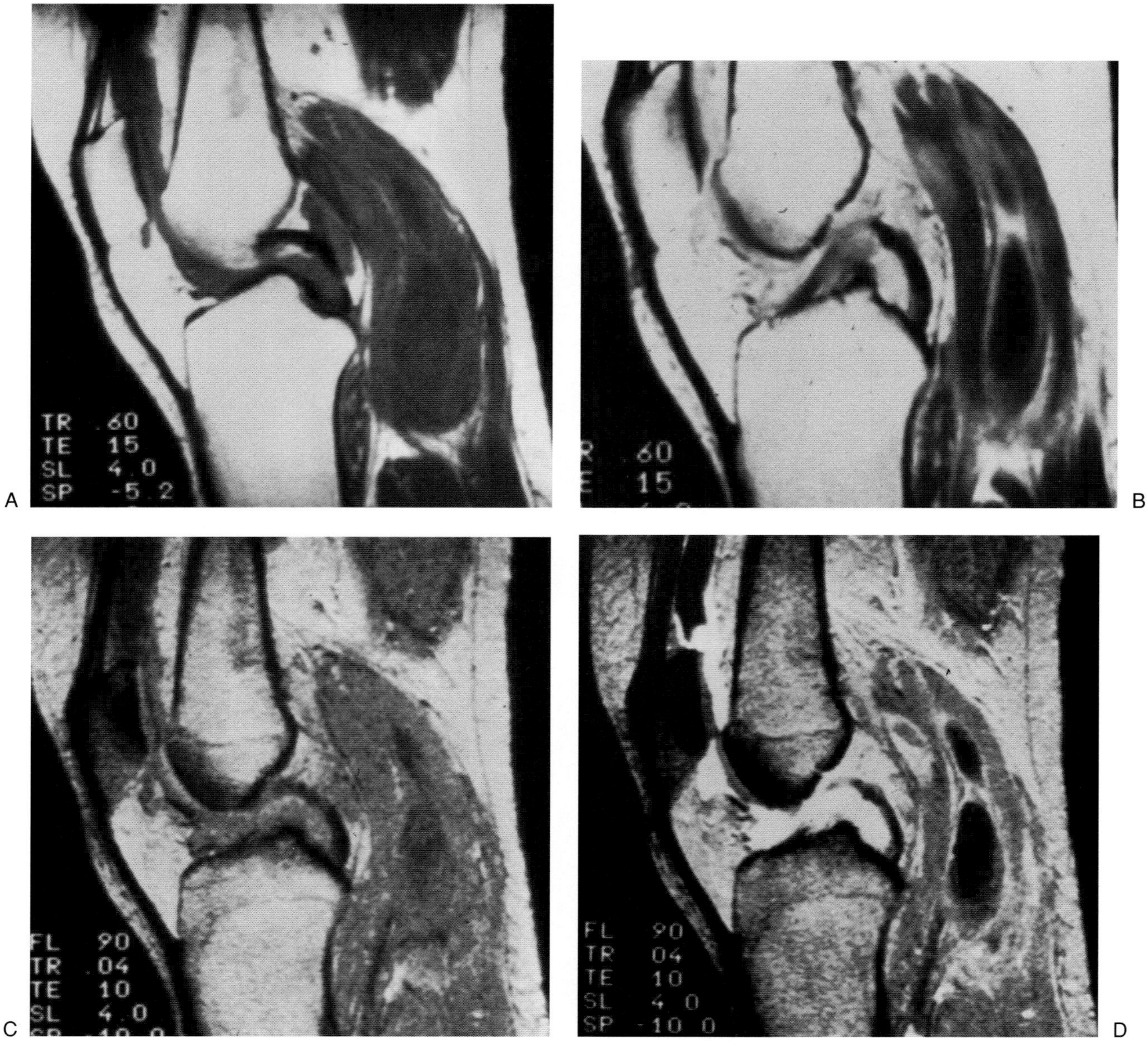

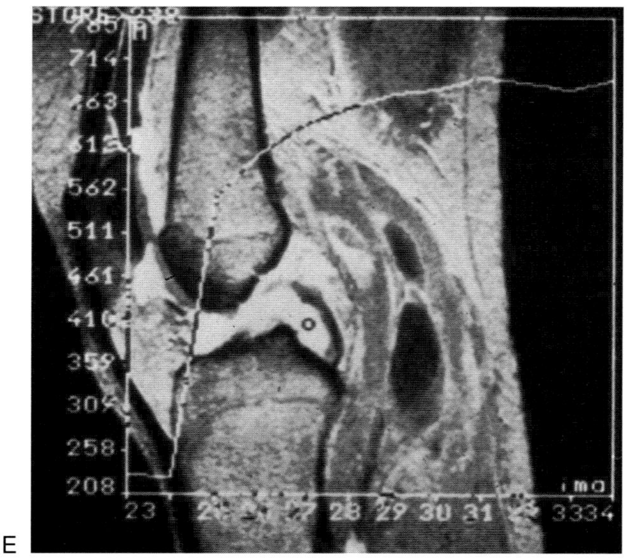

FIG. 8-3. Rheumatoid arthritis of the knee. **A:** T1-weighted spin-echo image. Intermediate and low signal intensity areas are visible within the knee joint, the suprapatellar recess, and the muscular bundles posterior to the knee joint. No bone erosions or bone marrow infiltrations can be appreciated. **B:** T1-weighted spin-echo image after injection of gadolinium. Improved contrast between pannus, cruciate ligaments, and fluid collections in the suprapatellar recess and within the Baker's cyst. **C:** T1-weighted gradient-echo image with a 90° flip angle obtained before injection of gadolinium. There is poor distinction between pannus, joint effusion, and joint structures. **D:** Less than a minute after injection of gadolinium, pannus shows a marked increase in signal intensity, whereas joint effusion does not exhibit an increase in signal intensity. Pannus and the posterior cruciate ligament are clearly visualized. A fluid-filled Baker's cyst with a thick wall of high signal intensity is detected. **E:** Signal intensity plot (vertical axis) against time postinjection (horizontal axis). A rapid increase in signal intensity can be appreciated reaching a plateau in approximately 2.5 minutes.

enhancement of the effusions that are present may be seen due to leaching of contrast into the fluid (29).

At the present time, it is still not clear if there is a correlation between the degree of contrast enhancement and/or the rate of contrast enhancement with clinical activity of the synovial inflammatory process. If a correlation can be proved to exist, it may provide an important tool for assessing the success of the medical therapy. It may also permit more sensitive tailoring of medical therapy early in the course of the disease before extensive and irreversible changes occur in the joint (30–32). Contrast-enhanced studies may also be helpful in staging patients who may be eligible for synovectomy because the distribution of abnormal synovium can be mapped out before the procedure.

MRI CHARACTERISTICS OF THE NORMAL SYNOVIUM

Normal tendons, joint capsule, menisci, and ligaments are visualized as low signal intensity structures on all spin-echo and gradient-echo sequences. The identification of these structures is facilitated by their contrast to the adjacent surrounding fat, muscle, cartilage, and joint fluid (11,25,33–40). The normal synovial membrane is not usually recognizable as a discrete anatomic structure on noncontrast-enhanced MRI. This is a reflection of the thinness of the normal membrane and its signal characteristics. If visible, synovium is seen as a very fine (approximately 1 mm) contrast-enhancing lining on T1-weighted spin-echo and gradient sequences with gadolinium.

MRI CORRELATES OF PATHOLOGY FINDINGS IN THE INFLAMMATORY ARTHROPATHIES

Inflammation of the synovial membrane results in progressive synovial proliferation. This proliferation or pannus and the consequent secretion of joint fluid (containing inflammatory cells and enzymes) underlie both the clinical and imaging manifestations of an inflammatory joint disease. Although untreated inflammatory arthropathy represents a continuum of clinical and imaging characteristics, for the purposes of this comparison, untreated arthropathy will be divided into three broad categories.

Early Phase

During the early phase of inflammation, synovial hyperemia and joint effusion predominate. This is a nonspecific manifestation of inflammatory arthritis, usually preceding microscopic evidence of synovial proliferation. It may be the only manifestation on MRI at this stage. Joint effusion demonstrates low signal intensity on T1-weighted spin-echo sequences, and poor meniscal contrast versus joint cartilage (Fig. 8-4) (33). On T2- or T2*-weighted sequences, joint fluid presents with high signal intensity, producing a so-called arthrographic effect, and is easily noticed even when relatively small because of its high signal relative to cartilage, capsule, menisci, ligaments, and fat (21). The signal characteristics of synovial fluid are nonspecific, precluding any pathologic correlation. Depending upon the aggressiveness of the synovitis and consequent synovial proliferation, this phase may be very short.

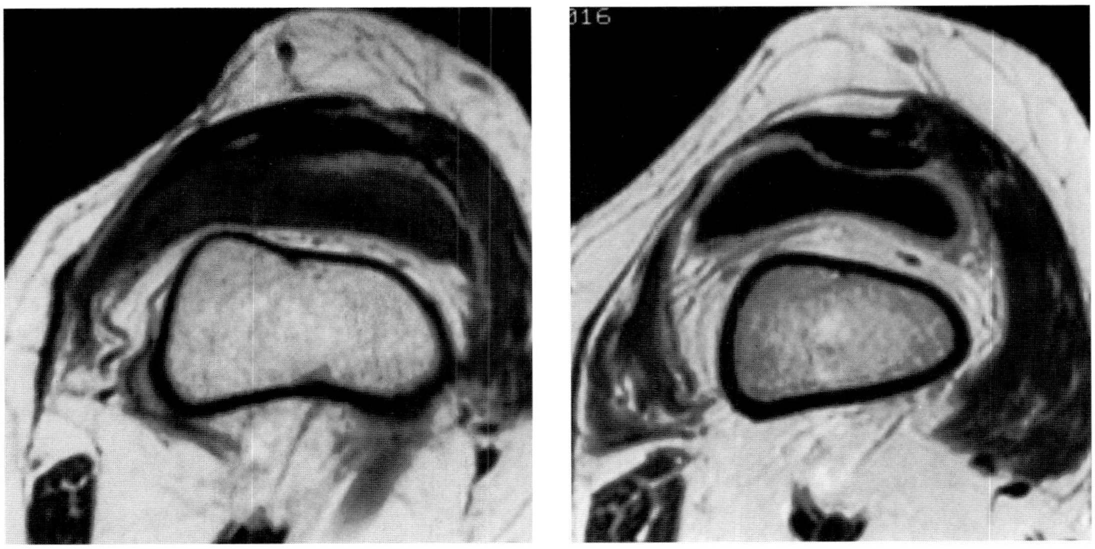

FIG. 8-4. A,B: Pre- and postcontrast T1-weighted spin-echo axial images through the suprapatellar bursa of the knee in a patient with rheumatoid arthritis. On the precontrast image, distention of the suprapatellar bursa is apparent by material of low signal intensity. Following infusion of gadolinium a peripheral band of enhancement is appreciated around the contours of the suprapatellar bursa representing the proliferating pannus within the joint. This early in the course of the examination no leaching of contrast into the effusion is apparent.

Intermediate Phase

There is increasing proliferation hypertrophy of the synovium, which is of variable thickness, depending on disease activity and chronicity. The initial regions of the most marked synovial proliferation or along the joint surface of the joint capsule, synovial reflections over the cruciate ligaments as well as the point at which the synovium extends from the fibrous capsule to the adjacent periosteal bony surfaces at the level of the periosteal/perichondral junction. Synovial proliferations in the knee demonstrate variable morphologic features (15–17,19,24,41). The synovium may be thickened and smooth or may show areas of irregular modularity. Cystic cavities, such as popliteal cysts (15), may show similar nodular changes and thickening of the membrane. Frequently, confluent areas of pannus are detected within the intercondylar notch in particular, with extension into the posterior portion of the joint cavity. At times, the volume of synovium is much greater than that of fluid within the joint and cystic cavities (Fig. 8-5) (19,20,40). In most instances, prominent synovial proliferation is identifiable on T1-weighted images as intermediate signal intensity thickening of the synovial lining, distinct from the lower-signal-intensity joint fluid (31). This distinction may be less clear on T2-weighted sequences because of the convergence of the signal intensity of joint fluid and high-signal-intensity acute synovial pannus. Very long TR images may help in this circumstance, allowing the two to be differentiated; however, this is at the expense of a poor signal-to-noise ratio. When the synovial proliferation is not substantial, the synovium may be easily distinguishable from the invariably associated joint effusion, because proliferating synovium is highly vascular and enhances markedly following administration of gadolinium. Focal areas of increased signal intensity may be seen on T1-weighted images that correspond to small areas of intersynovial hemorrhage, which are not uncommon. Small-foci of hemosiderin may also be detected as small punctate areas of low signal intensity, which are particularly prominent with gradient-echo sequences (Fig. 8-6) The MRI appearance may be similar to that of patients with very extensive chondrocalcinosis, although clinical history and plain films will usually clarify the situation (Fig. 8-7). At times, tiny fibrotic areas may also be visualized that do not show the same degree of blooming seen with hemosiderin on gradient-echo sequences. Occasionally, areas of high signal within the synovial proliferations may also be visible on T2-weighted images. These regions of increased signal intensity correspond to collections of fluid that are trapped or that are within cysts.

During this phase there is progressive destruction of periosteum and cortical bone in regions of synovial proliferation. Initially, there is thinning of the cortical bone, accompanied

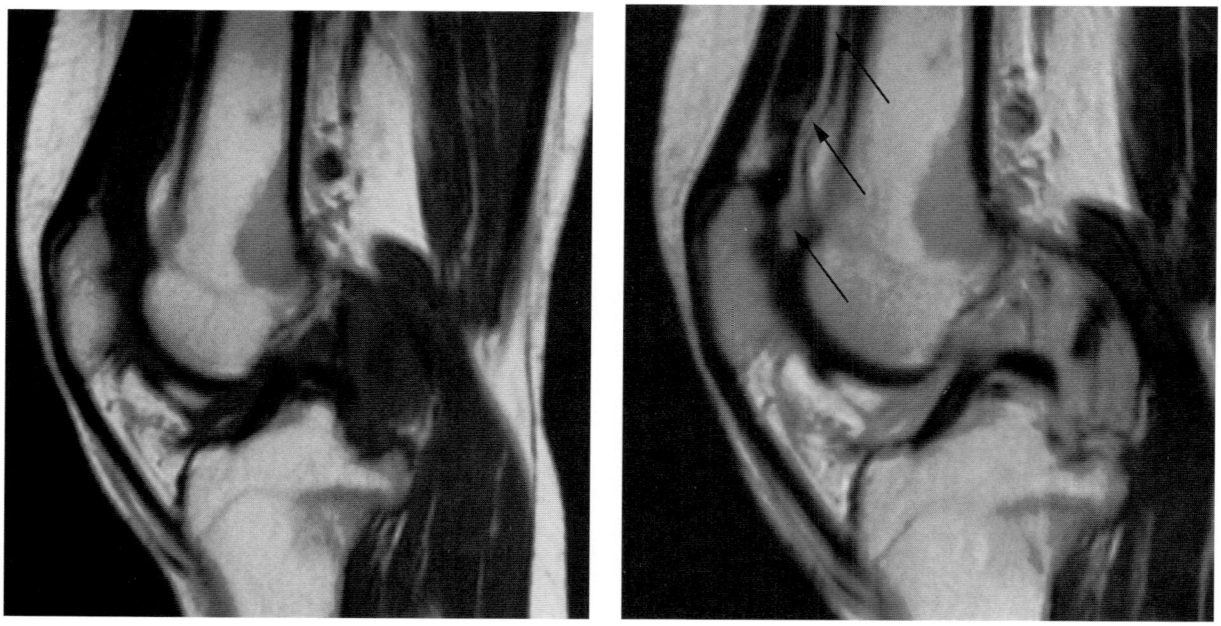

A B

FIG. 8-5. Sagittal T1-weighted spin-echo precontrast image shown in **(A)** with a large amount of low-signal-intensity material distending the suprapatellar bursa, the intercondylar notch, and the popliteal fossa. In **(B)** gadolinium has been injected and the pannus within the joint is noted to enhance. The lining of the suprapatellar bursa enhances in a thin linear fashion *(arrows)*. In the region of the intercondylar notch and popliteal fossa, diffuse enhancement is noted consistent with complete filling of the spaces by proliferating pannus. In this case, the amount of pannus greatly exceeds the amount of fluid within the joint, and the enhancing pannus serves to outline the cruciate ligaments and bridge the articular surfaces.

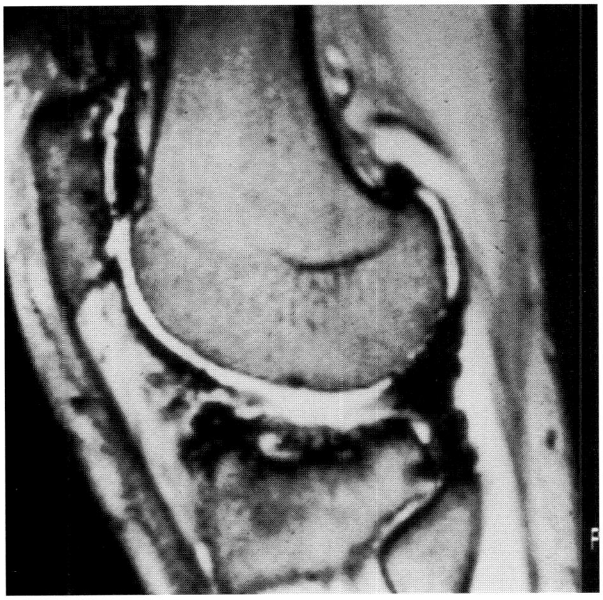

FIG. 8-6. Hemophiliac arthropathy of the knee, T1*-weighted gradient-echo image. The synovial proliferation in the posterior joint space and suprapatellar recess exhibit low signal intensity. Hemosiderin deposits within the pannus result in magnetic susceptibility artifacts and signal loss. Hyaline cartilage is depicted with high signal intensity. Areas of thinning and contour irregularities are demonstrated in the patellofemoral joint and in the posterior portion of the femorotibial joint. Subchondral cysts are visible in the tibial plateau.

by heterogeneous increase in the normal low signal intensity of the cortex (reflecting the areas of haversian tunneling) and bone marrow edema. Normal bone marrow exhibits high signal intensity on T1-weighted spin-echo imaging and reduced signal intensity on T2-weighted spin-echo imaging as well as T2*-weighted gradient-echo images (14,42,43). With bone marrow edema there is reduction in the signal intensity on T1-weighted images and an increase on T2-weighted and inversion recovery images. Marrow edema may preclude obvious evidence of cortical transgression by pannus. This may reflect the inflammatory hyperemia of the overlying pannus and does not necessarily represent actual invasion. This is important to remember when a septic joint is present, as underlying bone marrow changes do not invariably represent phrenic osteomyelitis. Fat suppression is helpful.

Once breech of the cortical bone has occurred, pannus may invade the marrow. This typically results in a relatively well demarcated area of low to intermediate signal intensity on T1-weighted images that are of high signal intensity as T2 weighting has increased. This area may be surrounded by a more poorly defined one of bone marrow edema. Regions of healing may be seen at sites of previous pannus invasion following treatment or in end-stage arthritis. These regions will be of low intensity on both T1- and T2-weighted imaging because of the fibrosis that occurs. The periarticular osteopenia that accompanies inflammatory arthropathy is difficult to appreciate on MRI. There may, however, be a subjective impression of a reduction in the degree of low signal intensity within the epiphyses and metaphyses, and thinning of the cortex may be apparent.

Late Phase

With chronic inflammation there is increasing fibrosis of the pannus. This results in regions of diminished signal intensity, which are often particularly well appreciated on T2-weighted sequences. By this phase, extensive cartilage abnormalities are usually present. Prior to arthritic changes, normal unaffected cartilage shows low to intermediate signal intensity on T1- and T2-weighted imaging, with high signal intensity on gradient-echo images that are T2*-weighted. Cartilage can usually be well differentiated from the low-intensity cortical bone and the low-intensity structures of the cruciate ligaments and menisci. As pannus progressively forms, synovial bridging of the articular surfaces may result; this is particularly well seen on postgadolinium imaging. At the same time, secretion of cells and fluid-containing enzymes occurs in gradual enzymatic resorption, and erosion of the cartilage surface takes place. This results in sometimes irregular thinning of the cartilage, which may be difficult to appreciate because of the similarity of the signal intensity of the cartilage and the fluid. The irregularity of the cartilage may be apparent because of the interdigitation of synovial pannus or fluid into the cartilage surfaces on T1-weighted imaging or on thin-section gradient-echo 3DFT imaging. With advancement of chondrolysis eventual pannus resorption of the underlying cortical bone results (20,36).

Ultimately, fibrous or osseous bridging of the joint space may result in ankylosis in the late stages of inflammatory joint disease, although this is less common in adults than in children

MRI CORRELATES OF CLINICAL AND RADIOGRAPHIC STAGES OF INFLAMMATORY ARTHROPATHY (WITH PARTICULAR REFERENCE TO RHEUMATOID ARTHRITIS)

MRI manifestations of inflammatory disorders are nonspecific (28). The goal of MRI is not to facilitate a diagnosis of the articular inflammatory disease, which may be done using laboratory and clinical parameters, but to assess both the extent of early soft-tissue and bone abnormalities and the presence of any accompanying internal derangement (30,44,45).

The most common inflammatory synovitis of the knee is rheumatoid arthritis. In the absence of a clinical history, the MRI features are insufficiently characteristic to differentiate between this and other inflammatory arthropathies. Because rheumatoid arthritis is the most prevalent disorder, correlations among the clinical (46), radiographic (46–49), and MRI features are given.

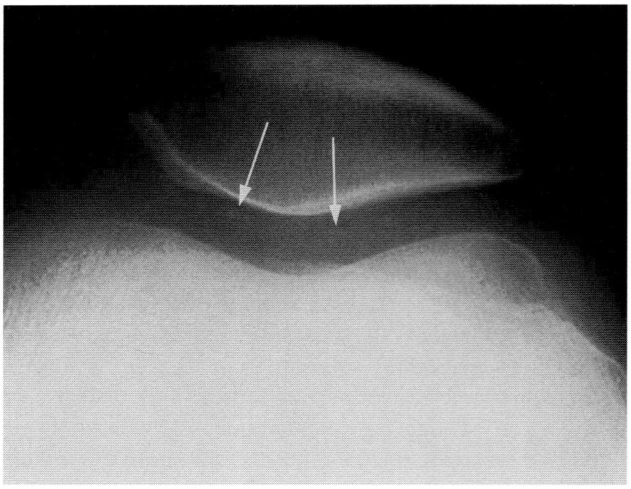

A

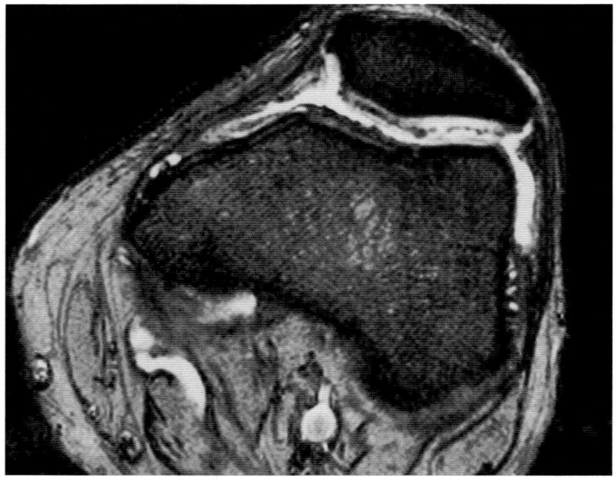

B

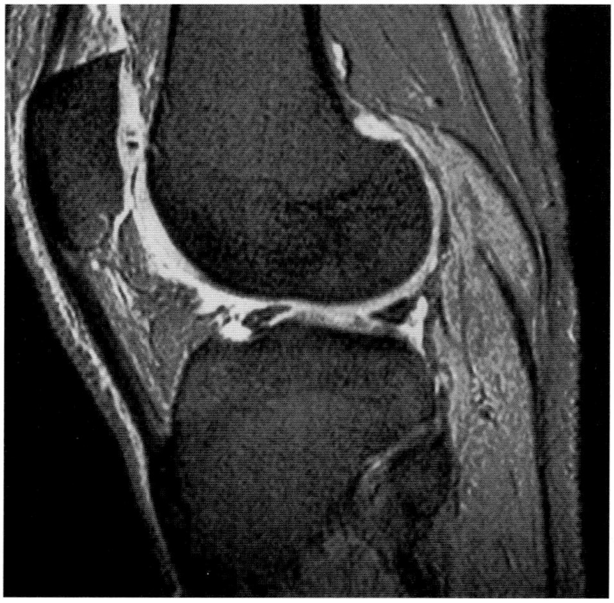

C

FIG. 8-7. Chondrocalcinosis. **A:** Skyline view of the patella shows small areas of calcification *(arrows)* within the cartilage of the patellofemoral joint. **B,C:** Axial and sagittal T2*-weighted gradient-echo images of the patellofemoral joint that show the chondrocalcinosis as punctate areas of signal dropout at the patellar face of the joint. The magnetic susceptibility of gradient-echo imaging highlights the small punctate areas of calcification within the cartilage making them far more obvious with this sequence.

Stage 1

In the initial phase of disease, periarticular soft-tissue swelling develops with variable symptoms of pain, stiffness, and joint dysfunction. Typical physical signs are articular swelling, tenderness, limitation of range of motion, and progressive instability of the joint. Radiographic evidence of periarticular osteopenia will become evident over time, although this will be preceded by evidence of a joint effusion. In its early phase, such osteopenia may only be evident as spotty demineralization of the patella on the lateral view as well as subchondral resorption zones along the edges of the femoral condyles on the anteroposterior view (31,47–49).

MRI will detect the presence of small volumes of intra-articular fluid before they are evident on radiographs and help distinguish pannus from fluid as detected clinically (50,51). At this stage, synovial proliferation will rarely be appreciated without contrast. Subchondral osteoporosis will not be perceptible at this time on MRI, although it is possible to detect early periosteal reaction as an alternative sign of early inflammatory arthritis, particularly in juvenile rheumatoid arthritis. This is best seen on gradient-echo imaging as regions of linear periosseous low-signal intensity.

Stage 2

Clinically, no joint deformities are present, although limitation of joint mobility and instability may be present. Extra-articular soft-tissue lesions, such as nodules and tenosynovitis, may well be present. Radiographically, periarticular osteoporosis is usually evident, and cartilage thinning may be apparent because of joint space narrowing, which may or may not be accompanied by marginal erosions. In the presence of a large effusion, cartilage thinning usually is not apparent because of joint distention.

Progression of synovial proliferation may be increasingly evident on MRI because of subtle contrast differentiation between synovium and joint fluid on T1- and T2-weighted images. A joint effusion is invariably present. There may be early cartilage thinning and foci of destruction that are very irregular. Progressive heterogeneity of the signal intensity of the synovium is not unusual.

Stage 3

Joint deformity, lateral subluxation, lateral deviation, or hyperextension without evidence of fibrous or bony ankylosis are present, often accompanied by extensive muscle atrophy and fatty infiltration of muscle. Extra-articular soft-tissue lesions, such as nodules and tenosynovitis, may be present. Over time a flexion contracture develops with progressive valgus deformity and external rotation. These changes are primarily related to hamstring spasm, quadriceps inhibition, and shortening of the fascia lata and posterior capsule. The medial collateral and the cruciate ligaments become lax, and the quadriceps muscle becomes weak (46). Radiographically, evidence of cartilage and bone destruction is often obvious, and osteoporosis may at times be profound.

MRI demonstrates the progressive joint deformity and malalignment. Typically, all three compartments show cartilage destruction, which may be quite variable, with one compartment being much more severely affected than another. Because of the cartilage thinning and destruction, redundancy, particularly of the medial collateral and cruciate ligaments, may be observed. Synovial thickening and/or joint effusion becomes increasingly dramatic.

Stage 4

In some instances, fibrous or bony ankylosis may occur by stage 4 (52). This may be reflected on radiographs.

MRI presents with criteria of stage 3 noted earlier. Furthermore, MRI reveals progressive muscle atrophy of the quadriceps and hamstring group and shortening of the posterior capsule. If fibrotic or bony ankylosis is present, bridging of the congruous, disorganized osteochondral surface will be present. If cartilage is present, this may or may not be incorporated within the fibrosis.

OTHER MRI MANIFESTATIONS OF INFLAMMATORY DISORDERS OF THE KNEE

Meniscal Ligamentous Structures

Inflammatory processes involving tendons, ligaments, menisci, and joint capsule may cause morphologic alterations (elongation, rupture, focal thickening or thinning) and/or signal intensity increase on T1- and especially T2-weighted spin-echo sequences due to edema and hemorrhage (53). The delineation of tendons, joint capsule, menisci, and ligaments may no longer be possible on T1-weighted images, and gadolinium is particularly helpful in evaluating these structures.

Synovial Cysts

Synovial cysts represent nonspecific accumulations of synovial fluid and/or abnormal synovium within the joint herniations or periarticular bursa (Fig. 8-8). Such synovial cysts

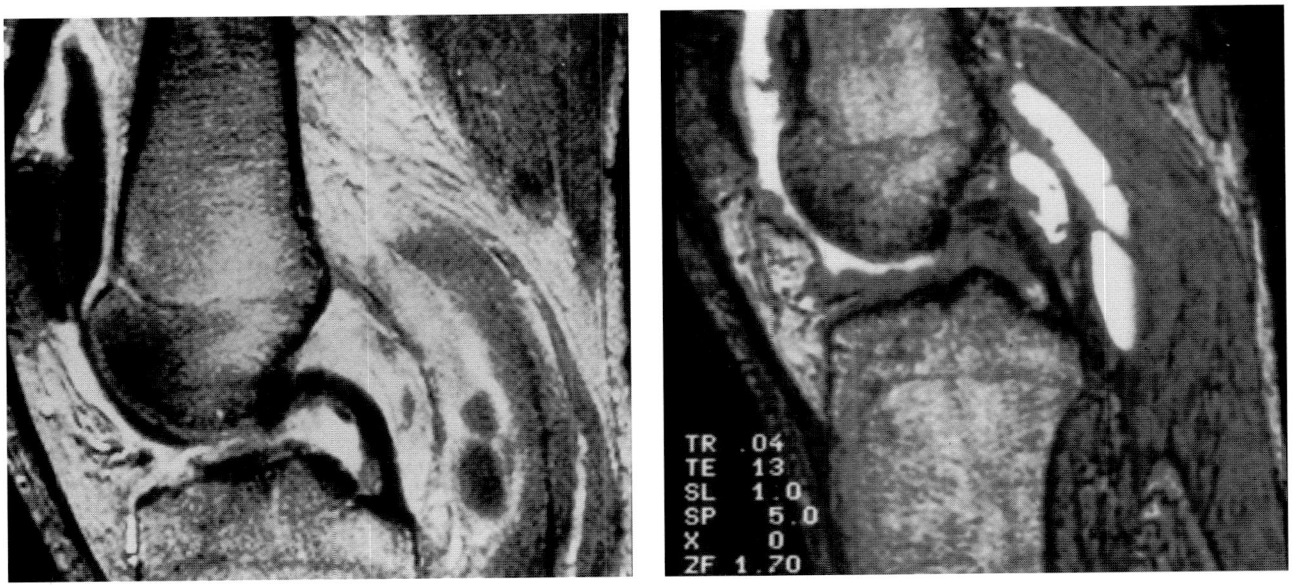

A B

FIG. 8-8. Rheumatoid arthritis. **A:** Sagittal T1-weighted gradient-echo contrast enhanced image showing diffuse enhancement in the suprapatellar bursa as well as in the popliteal fossa following infusion of gadolinium. **B:** Sagittal T1-weighted gradient-echo MRI arthrogram following injection of a dilute gadolinium solution into the joint outlines the fluid-filled recesses to better advantage and pushes coapted synovial membranes away from one another.

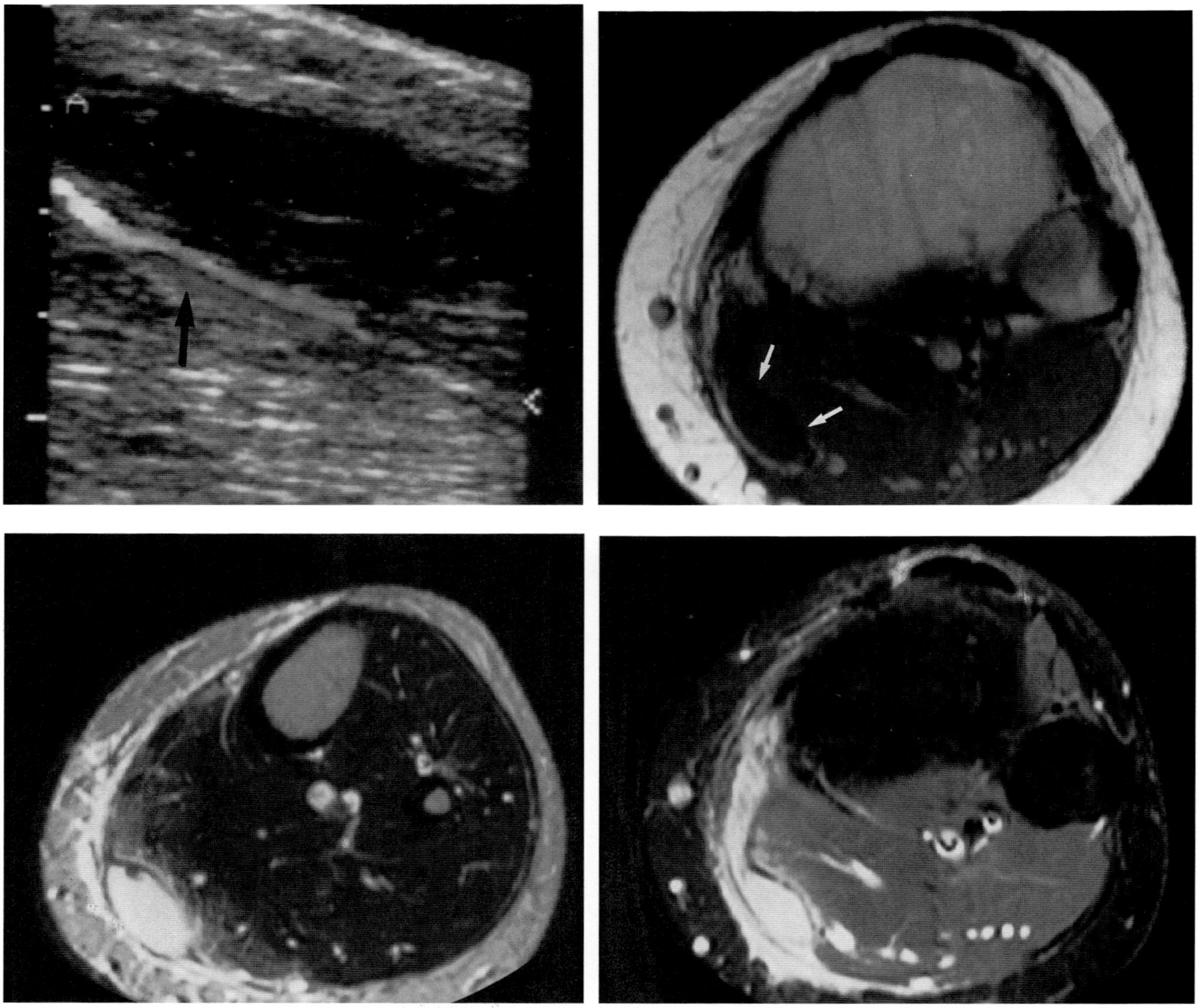

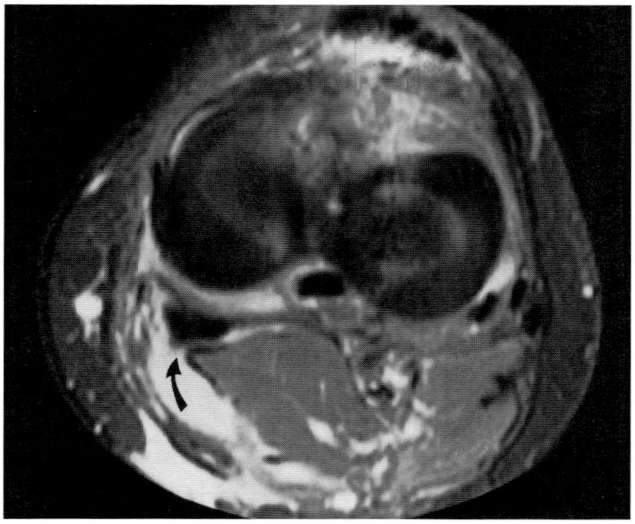

FIG. 8-9. Patient with leaking Baker's cyst that presented as a deep venous thrombosis. **A:** Image from color flow Doppler study of the calf demonstrates widely patent veins *(arrow)*. **B:** Axial T1-weighted image immediately below the level of the knee joint demonstrates an elliptic lesion with signal intensity similar to that of muscle *(arrows)*. The lesion lies between the gastrocnemius and the subcutaneous fat. **C:** T2-weighted image demonstrates the marked increase in signal intensity as T2 weighting is augmented. Feathery areas of increased signal intensity are present in the subcutaneous fat and adjacent muscle that represent inflammation secondary to leakage of cyst contents. **D:** The fat-suppressed inversion recovery (STIR) image shows to advantage the contents of the leaking cyst at the interface between the subcutaneous fat and the muscle tracking along the fascial plane. **E:** Image at the level of the knee joint demonstrates the neck of the Baker's cyst as it passes between the tendons and into the joint *(curved arrow)*. (Figures used courtesy of Munk PL, et al. *Can Assoc Radiol J* 1993;44(2):125–128.)

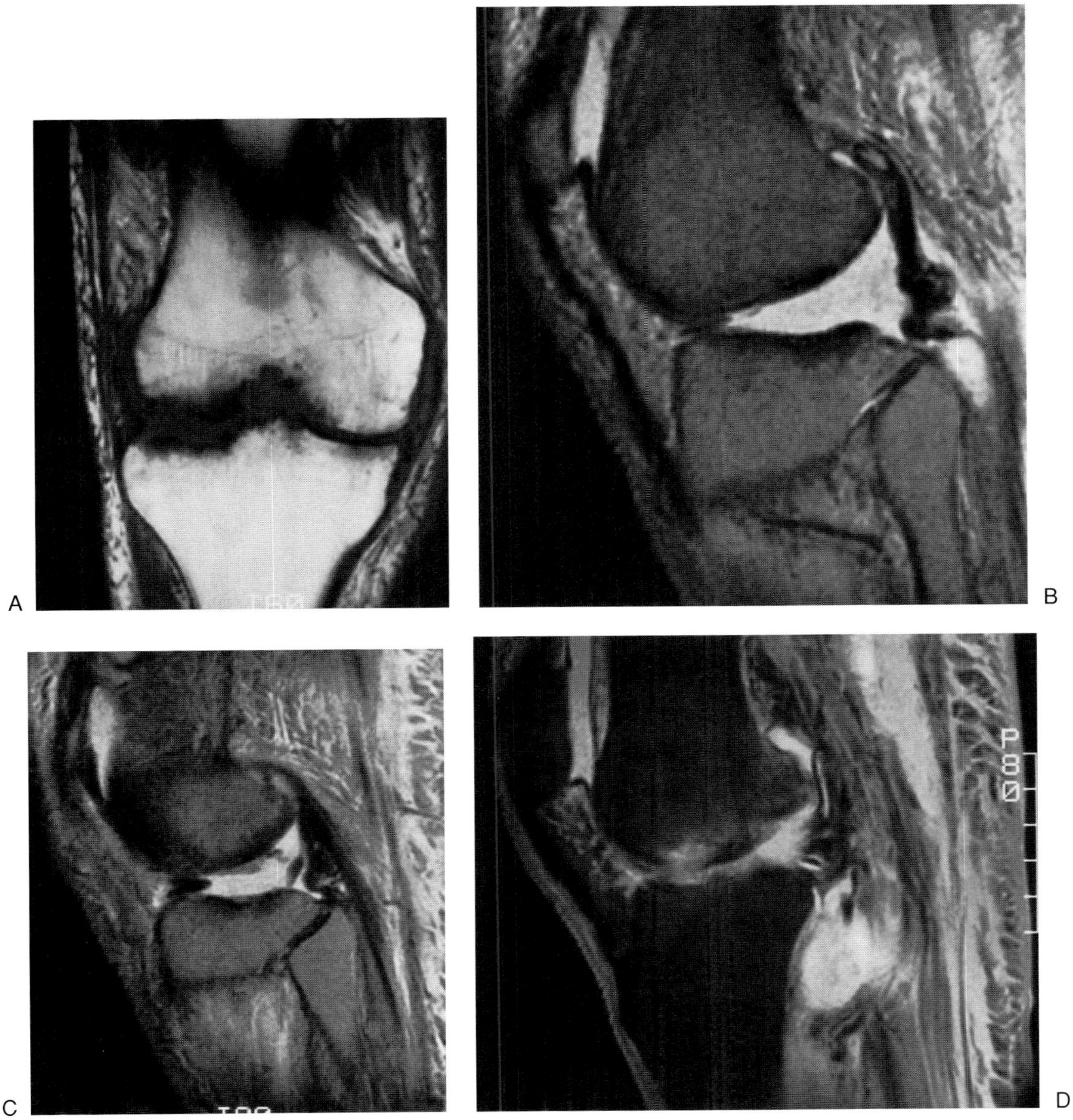

FIG. 8-10. Bacteroides septic arthritis. **A:** T1-weighted spin-echo coronal image demonstrates irregular widening of the joint space by intermediate to low signal intensity material with adjacent very low signal intensity material within the bone. The margins of the joint are extremely irregular; evidence of reticulation of the subcutaneous fat is also present. **B,C:** Adjacent T2*-weighted gradient-echo images on the same patient demonstrate extensive fluid within the joint which is of high signal intensity. The menisci have been partially destroyed and debris is evident within the joint. **D:** Fat-suppressed inversion recovery (STIR) image. High signal intensity within the suprapatellar bursa and the popliteal fossa are apparent, which is of slightly inhomogeneous signal intensity consistent with debris within the effusion. Also note areas of high signal intensity present subcortically within the distal femur consistent with early changes of osteomyelitis.

may be incidental or occur in association with traumatic or inflammatory synovial disorders. Whether in communication with the synovial lining of the knee joint or sequestered from it, the synovial membrane of such cysts will undergo inflammatory changes similar to those described under the rheumatoid arthritis section earlier; the changes will parallel these activities within the joint proper. Some synovial cysts (especially popliteal cysts) may rupture or leak and incite a pronounced inflammatory response that may mimic thrombophlebitis (pseudothrombophlebitis syndrome) (54). MRI in this instance will show high-signal-intensity tracking around fascia with edema affecting adjacent muscle bundles (Fig. 8-9).

Infectious Arthritis and Osteomyelitis

Septic joints are not frequently seen on MRI examination; however, when they are encountered they require urgent treatment. Commonly, *Staphylococcus aureus* is the organism in acute septic arthritis, although almost any organism may be found (Figs. 8-10 and 8-11). In a more chronic setting, tuberculosis and fungal organisms may be present; both have a considerably more indolent presentation and history (55–57). Common underlying clinical situations include septicemia, diabetes mellitus, immunosuppression, and trauma.

With pyogenic organisms the rapidity of the clinical course of infectious arthritis and the rate of osteochondral destruction are much more rapid than are seen with the inflammatory arthropathies such as rheumatoid arthritis. MRI cannot distinguish early infectious arthritis from inflammatory arthritis. With septic arthritis synovial proliferation may well be present, and this is especially common if a more

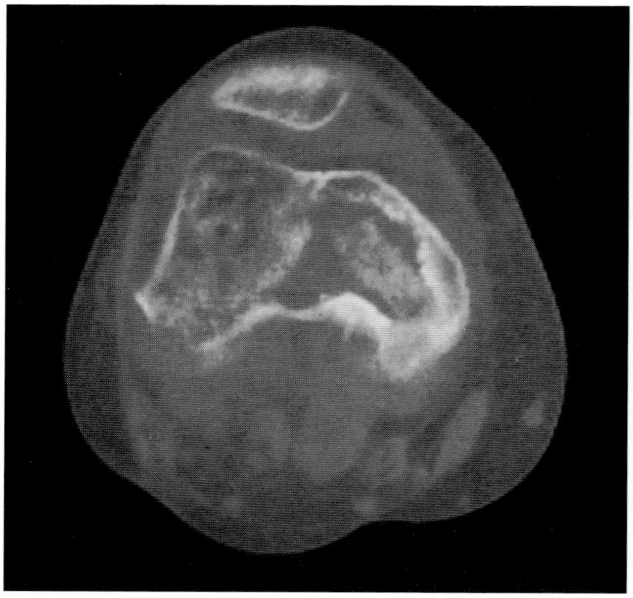
A

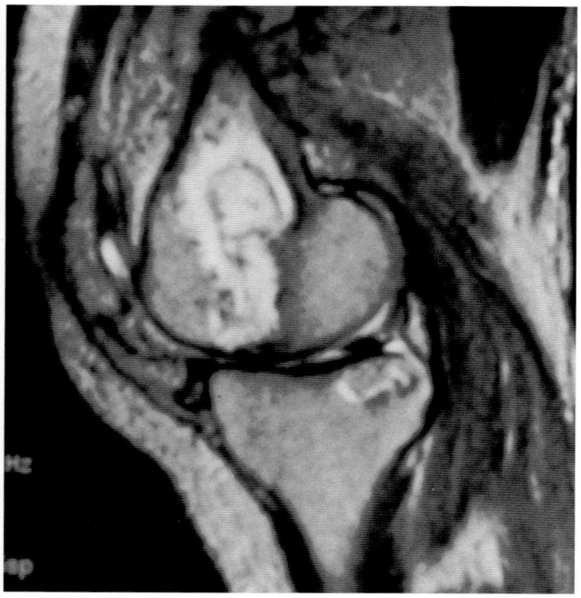
B

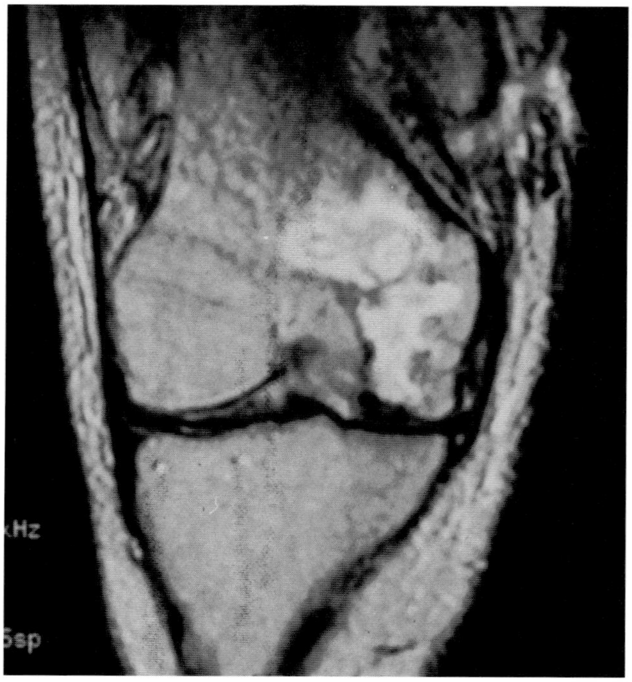
C

FIG. 8-11. *Staphylococcus aureus* septic joint and osteomyelitis. **A:** Axial CT image with bone windows demonstrating irregular destruction of the distal femur consistent with an aggressive infectious process. **B,C:** Sagittal and coronal proton density images on the same patient demonstrate well-demarcated areas of high signal intensity in the distal femur as well as in the posterior tibia consistent with regions of osteomyelitis associated with this septic joint. Note the marked narrowing of the joint spaces resulting from cartilage thinning. (Case courtesy of Dr. Joel Rubenstein, University of Toronto, Toronto, Ontario, Canada.)

indolent organism such as tuberculosis or fungus is present (Fig. 8-12). Regardless of the organism, some patients will show evidence of debris within the joint, and hemorrhage is not uncommon. Should the organism be more indolent, as is typical with fungus and myobacteria, the clinical course is more protracted and the rate of joint destruction is less rapid (32).

Not infrequently, osteomyelitis may be associated with a septic joint, and sepsis in the joint may reflect a previously established osteomyelitis that has extended into the joint, rather than the reverse.

Changes associated with acute osteomyelitis are typically visible on MRI long before they can be detected radiographically. Bone marrow edema will be seen as diminished signal intensity on T1-weighted imaging, usually with a poorly demarcated margin (Fig. 8-13). With T2-weighted imaging,

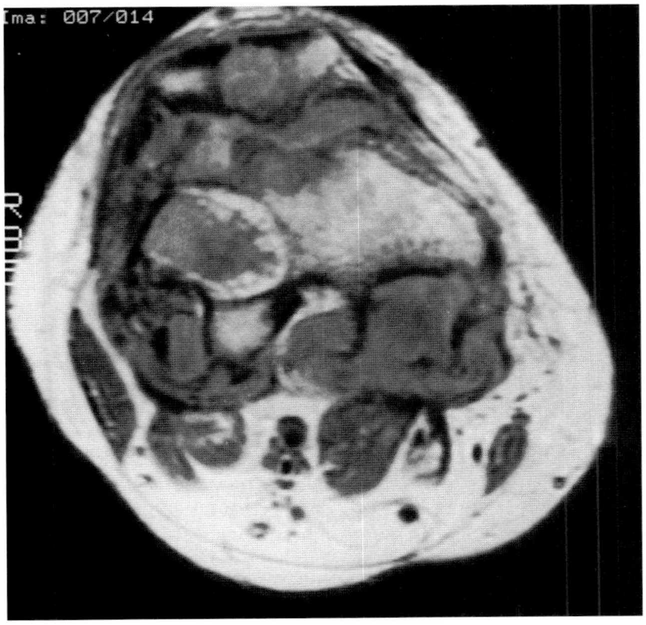

A

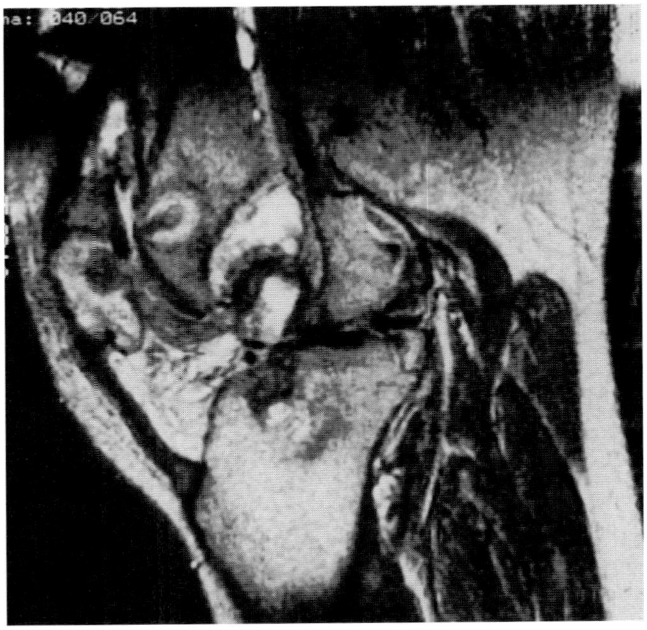

C

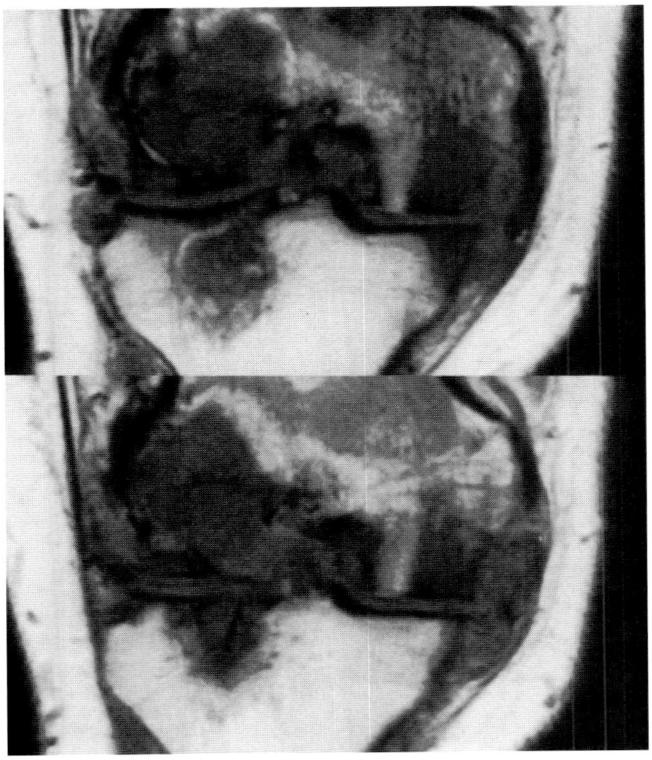

B

FIG. 8-12. Coccidioidmycosis of the knee joint. **A:** Axial T1-weighted spin-echo image demonstrates extensive destruction of the joint. A large focus of infection is present in the lateral femoral condyle as well as in the middle portion of the patella. Marked distention of the suprapatellar bursa is present. The coronal T1-weighted images in **B** show the extent of abnormal bone marrow and the distention of the joint capsule, which is filled with debris and hypertrophic synovium. In **C** a sagittal T2 spin-echo image the abnormal areas of high signal intensity within the marrow represent regions of infected bone interspersed with areas of low-signal-intensity debris and fibrosis. With these indolent infections, at times extensive desmoplastic reaction may occur, resulting in less augmentation of signal intensity as T2 weighting is increased than might otherwise be expected. Also the presence of heavy metals that may be sequestered by the organisms and of hemosiderin from bleeding decreases the signal intensity.

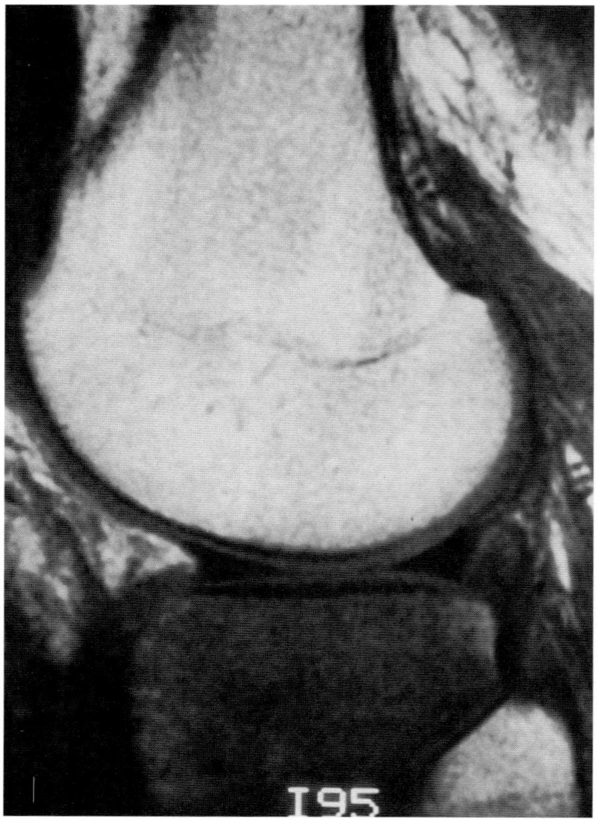

FIG. 8-13. *Nocardia* infection of the proximal tibia. On this sagittal T1-weighted image, the bone marrow has been replaced with low-signal-intensity edema, which has a relatively nonspecific appearance. (Used with permission from Munk PL, et al. *Can Assoc Radiol J* 1994;45(5):355–362.)

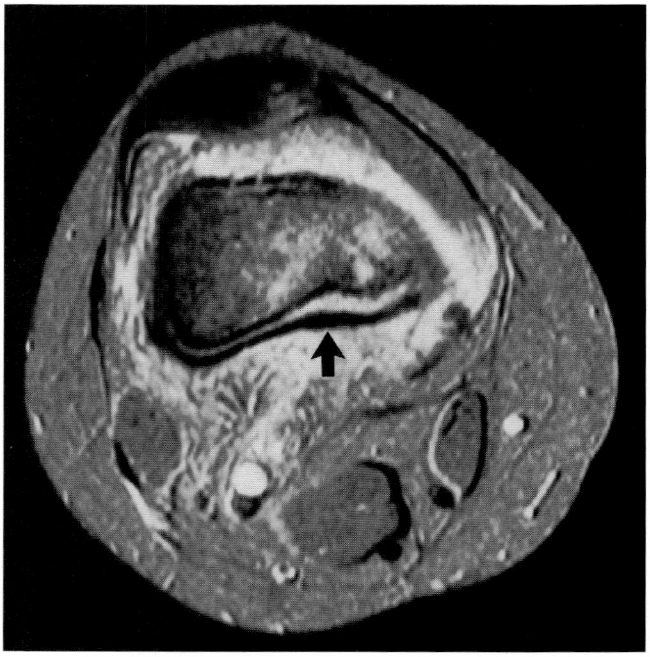

FIG. 8-14. Axial image through infected distal femur, T2*-weighted gradient-echo image. Early osteomyelitis with a subperiosteal abscess. High-signal-intensity soft-tissue edema is seen circumferentially around the bone, especially medially as well as within the bone marrow. In addition, elevation of the low-signal-intensity fibrous periosteum *(arrow)* is apparent, along with surgically proven high-signal-intensity subperiosteal pus between the periosteum and the low signal intensity cortex. The elevation of the periosteum by infected fluid collections is what is responsible for the periosteal "reaction" noted on radiographs. (Used with permission from Munk PL, et al. *Can Assoc Radiol J* 1994;45(5):355–362.)

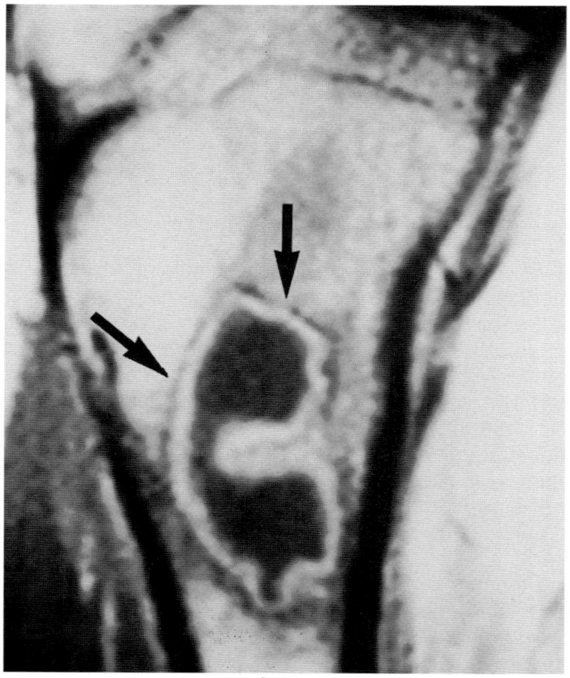

FIG. 8-15. Bone marrow abscess, sagittal T1-weighted spin-echo image, contrast enhanced. A well-circumscribed, lobulated lesion is apparent within the medulla of the proximal tibia. A thin enhancing rim *(arrows)* surrounds the fluid-filled nonenhancing core. (Used with permission from Munk PL, et al. *Can Assoc Radiol J* 1994;45(5):355–362.)

high signal intensity may be present, again poorly marginated and often patchy. It may be less apparent with T2*-weighted imaging because of the presence of magnetic septability artifact caused by trabeculae. Short-tau inversion recover (STIR) imaging or other fat-suppressed sequences are particularly helpful in that the suppression of the background high-signal-intensity fat will allow even subtle bone marrow changes to become vividly apparent (12,15,32,58,59).

Other fluid collections may also be present. For instance, subperiosteal pus may be seen adjacent to the low signal intensity cortex and is best appreciated with T2 weighting or fat suppression. The fibrous periosteal layer is usually of low signal intensity and is outlined dramatically in this situation (Fig. 8-14). Intraosseous abscesses may also be seen and typically are identified as well-demarcated areas that behave like typical fluid collections in that they are of low signal on T1-weighted sequences and of high signal on T2-weighted sequences (Fig. 8-15). Gadolinium administered to patients with acute osteomyelitis may improve delineation between perfused and devitalized tissues and may be extremely useful in planning surgical debridement. As the infection becomes more chronic, or if antibiotic therapy is administered, the demarcation between infected and noninfected tissue becomes more distinct. Early in osteomyelitis

A

B

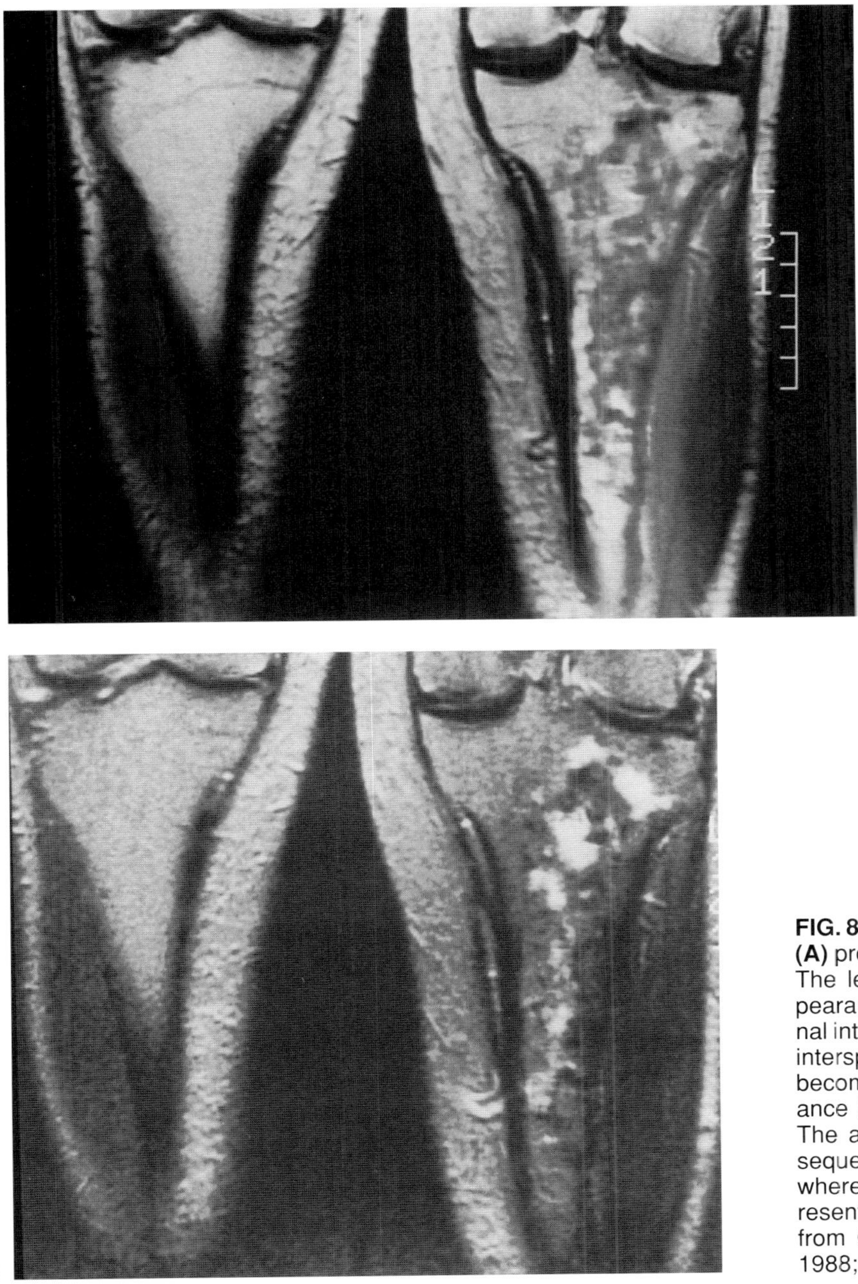

FIG. 8-16. Chronic Osteomyelitis. Coronal images **(A)** proton density and **(B)** T2-weighted spin echo. The left tibia has a mottled inhomogeneous appearance to its bone marrow with areas of low signal intensity that do not brighten with T2 weighting, interspersed with areas of low signal intensity that become brighter with T2 weighting. This appearance is typical of that of a chronic osteomyelitis. The areas that are of low signal intensity on all sequences represent fibrosis and calcification, whereas those that brighten with T2 weighting represent pus and/or edema. (Used with permission from Quinn SF, et al. *J Comput Assist Tomogr* 1988;12(1):113–117.)

the cortex is often preserved; however, as the process progresses, cortical margins become irregular, and areas of increased signal intensity develop in the cortex. Thin, low-signal-intensity bands may begin to form around the bone as a displaced periosteum attempts to elaborate a new shell of bone, referred to as an involucrum (15,32,60–66).

With chronic osteomyelitis the edematous bone marrow gradually becomes replaced either with fat, which has high signal intensity with T1-weighted imaging, or with fibrotic tissue, which has a more mottled, low signal intensity appearance (Fig. 8-16). Transition between normal and abnormal tissues is often better demarcated than in early acute osteomyelitis. The cortex usually becomes markedly thickened as an attempt to repair the destroyed tissues occurs. A thick shell of new bone may be present, representing the new bone elaborated by the displaced periosteum that has subsequently fused with the underlying cortex. At times, fragments of devitalized bone surrounded by fluid collections may be present, and these are referred to as sequestra (Fig. 8-17). The fluid collections may also drain spontaneously, extending out to the skin surface and producing a sinus (32,62,63,67).

Changes may be apparent in the soft tissues with or without accompanying bone changes in the setting of infection. If tissues are liquefied, an abscess is present and will behave as a fluid collection on MRI (low/intermediate signal on T1 weighting, high on T2 weighting) and will show rim enhancement with contrast. Contrast is therefore very helpful in delineating surgically drainable areas. Inflammation with or without actual infection produces increased signal on T1 and high signal on T2 weighting, with mild enhancement if contrast is administered. Inflamed tissue is often poorly delineated and has a feathery texture, especially when located in muscle. Subcutaneous fat when inflamed displays a reticulated appearance (15,32,43,64,65,68).

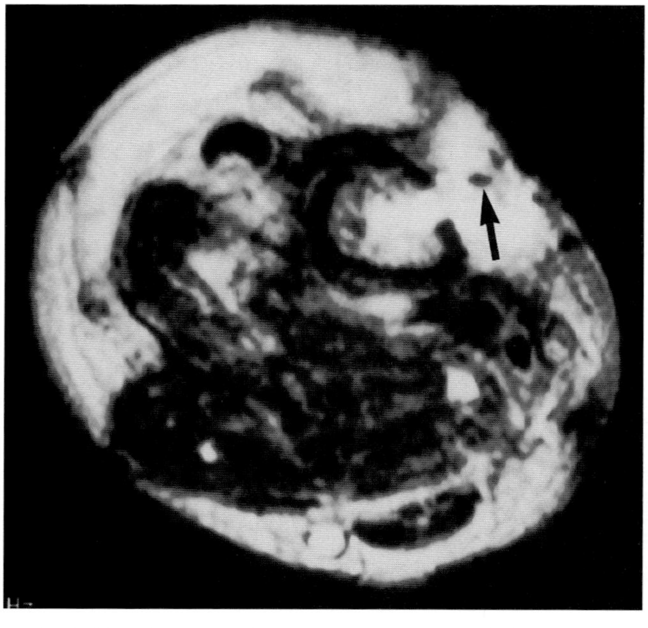

FIG. 8-17. Chronic osteomyelitis after joint fusion with sequestrum and chloaca. An axial T2-weighted spin-echo image through the femoral diaphysis immediately above the knee joint is shown. High signal intensity pus extends from the medullary space across a breach in the cortex to reach the skin surface. Low signal intensity debris (arrow) represents the sequestrum. (From Munk PL, et al., *Can Assoc Radiol J* 1994;45(5) (Oct. 1994):355–362.)

CLINICAL ROLE IN FUTURE APPLICATIONS OF MRI IN THE EVALUATION OF INFLAMMATORY DISORDERS OF THE KNEE

The role of MRI in the evaluation of inflammatory disorders of the knees is evolving. We are only beginning to appreciate the role of intravenous gadolinium in studying these disorders. It may well prove to be an extremely important research and clinical tool. The established and potential applications of MRI are as follows:

a. to accurately stage the extent of soft tissues and bone manifestations of the inflammatory processes
b. to enable differentiation of various pathologic entities (this is an ancillary role);
c. to evaluate complications of inflammatory disorders, including cartilage damage, intra-articular osteochondral loose bodies, supervening avascular necrosis, disruption of intra-articular and periarticular tendons and ligaments, and evaluation of surrounding periarticular bursa;

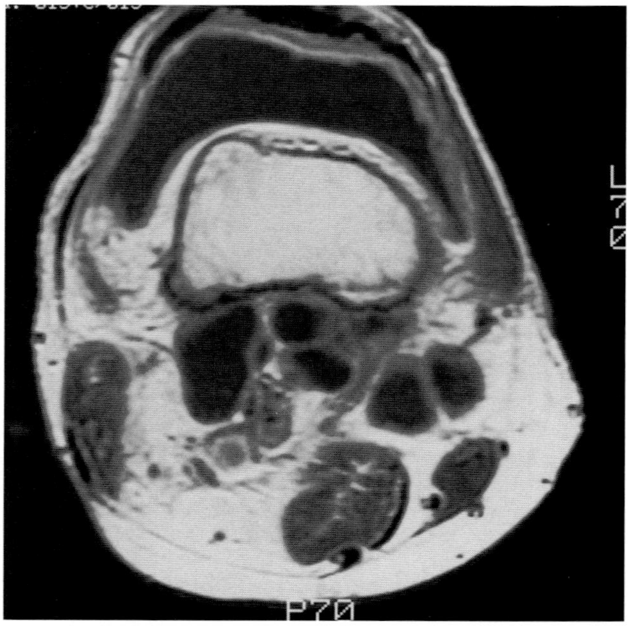

FIG. 8-18. Synovitis in osteoarthritic joint. Axial T1-weighted gadolinium-enhanced image. A thin rim of enhancement is apparent around the periphery of the fluid-distended suprapatellar bursa. Also note the septated popliteal fossa cyst, which shows a similar pattern of fluid and peripheral enhancement.

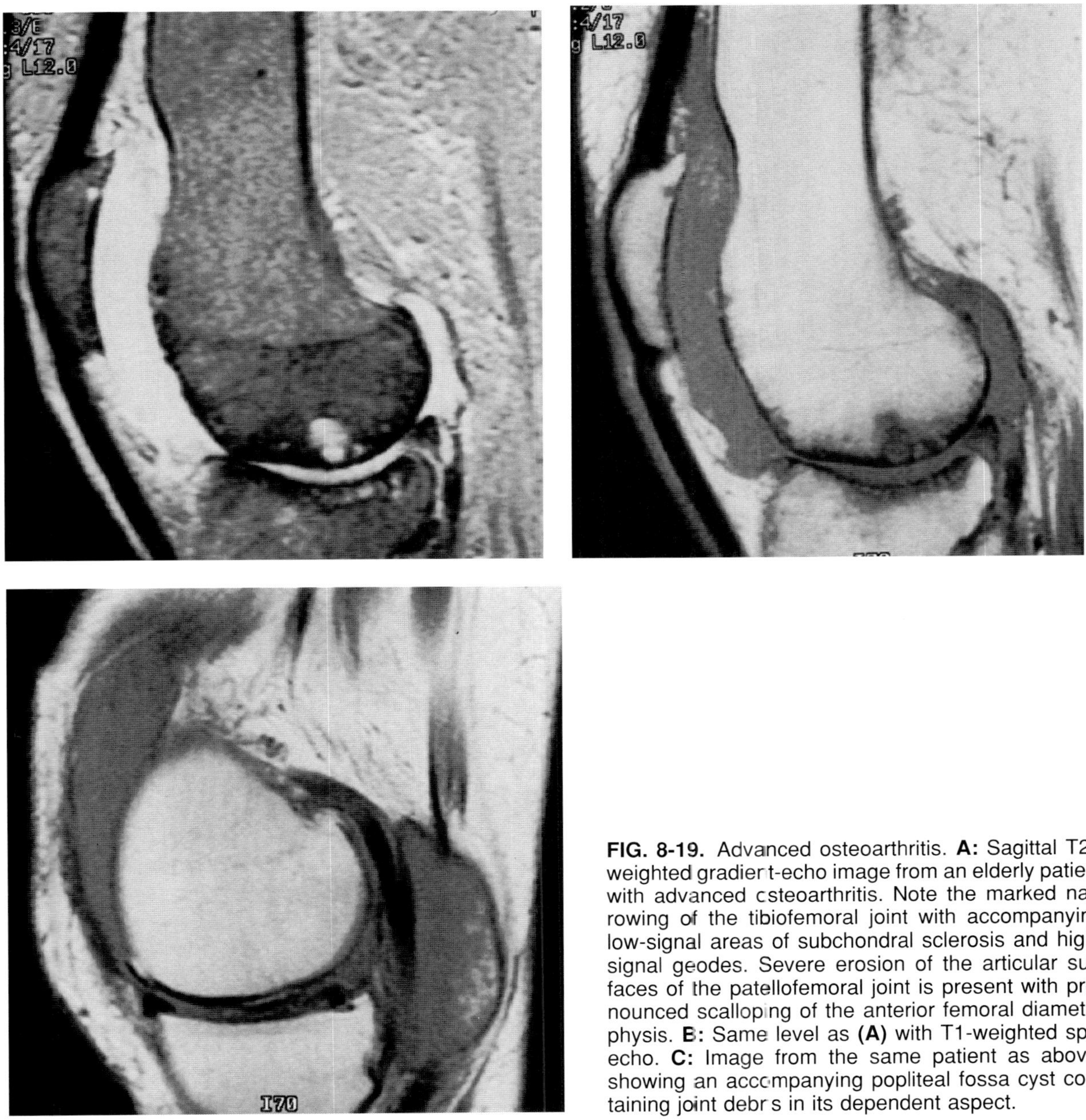

A B C

FIG. 8-19. Advanced osteoarthritis. **A:** Sagittal T2*-weighted gradient-echo image from an elderly patient with advanced osteoarthritis. Note the marked narrowing of the tibiofemoral joint with accompanying low-signal areas of subchondral sclerosis and high-signal geodes. Severe erosion of the articular surfaces of the patellofemoral joint is present with pronounced scalloping of the anterior femoral diametaphysis. **B:** Same level as **(A)** with T1-weighted spin echo. **C:** Image from the same patient as above, showing an accompanying popliteal fossa cyst containing joint debris in its dependent aspect.

d. surveillance of therapeutic response of inflammatory disorders to medical management or intra-articular injection of radiopharmaceuticals. Modification of therapeutic regimes may be possible based on the results of dynamic gadolinium MRI. Analysis of the progression or regression of pannus as well as distribution and enhancement characteristics may lead to early modification of therapy and presumably to better therapeutic outcomes.

MRI provides a valuable means of evaluating inflammatory disorders of the joints at the earliest possible stage in the evolution. Greater clinical experience with contrast-enhanced MRI should ensure an increasing role for MRI in the therapeutic management of inflammatory disorders of joints.

OSTEOARTHRITIS

Many of the changes of osteoarthritis and its related abnormalities are included in Chapter 7 and are discussed there in greater detail. Osteoarthritis is the result of a wear-and-tear phenomenon that may be aggravated by other superimposed disease or trauma and that causes joint narrowing, erosion, and destruction of cartilage.

As cartilage thins and bone becomes denuded, abnormal biomechanics occur, with abnormal stresses being created

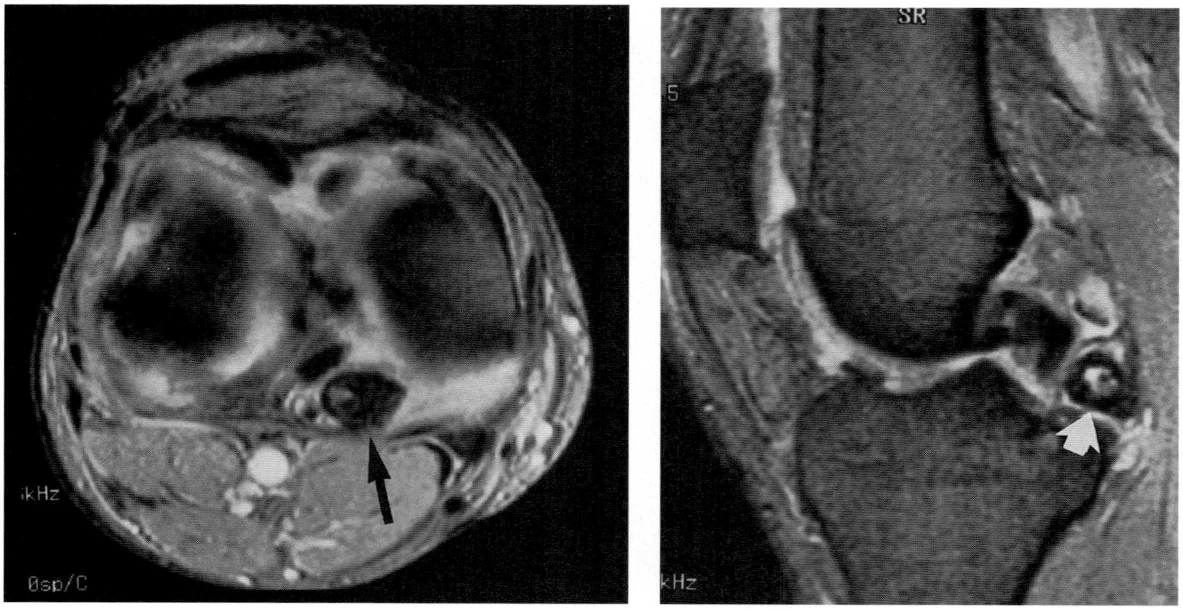

A B

FIG. 8-20. Loose body. **A:** Axial and **B:** sagittal gradient-echo images from a patient with osteoarthritis. Small osteophytes can be seen at the margins of the anterior femoral condyles and patella on the sagittal image, and both images show a low signal loose body (osteochondral fragment) posteriorly *(arrows)*. These often form from fragments from the joint surface or osteophytes, which break off into the joint and may continue to grow, receiving their nourishment from synovial fluid.

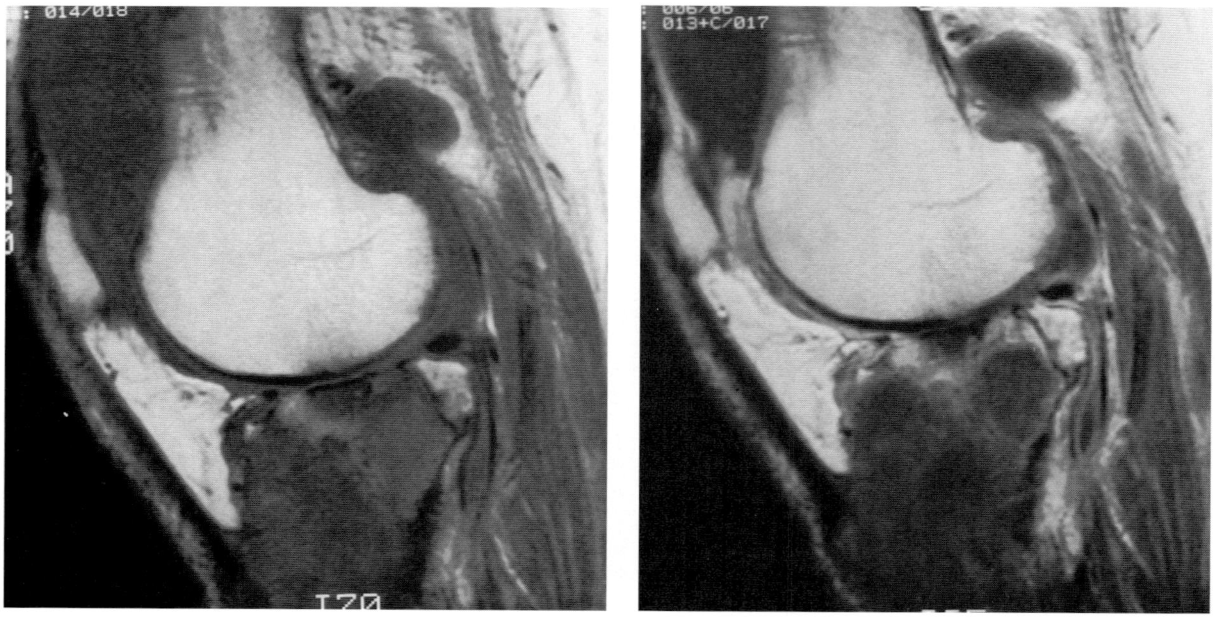

A B

FIG. 8-21. Giant geode. Axial **(A)** pre- and **(B)** postcontrast T1-weighted spin-echo images from a patient with osteoarthritis. The joint space is very narrow. A large low-signal-intensity lesion occupies most of the proximal tibia and shows a thin rim of peripheral enhancement with contrast. A large amount of fluid distends the suprapatellar bursa as well as a small popliteal cyst. At surgery a huge geode filled with myxoid debris and fluid was found in the tibia.

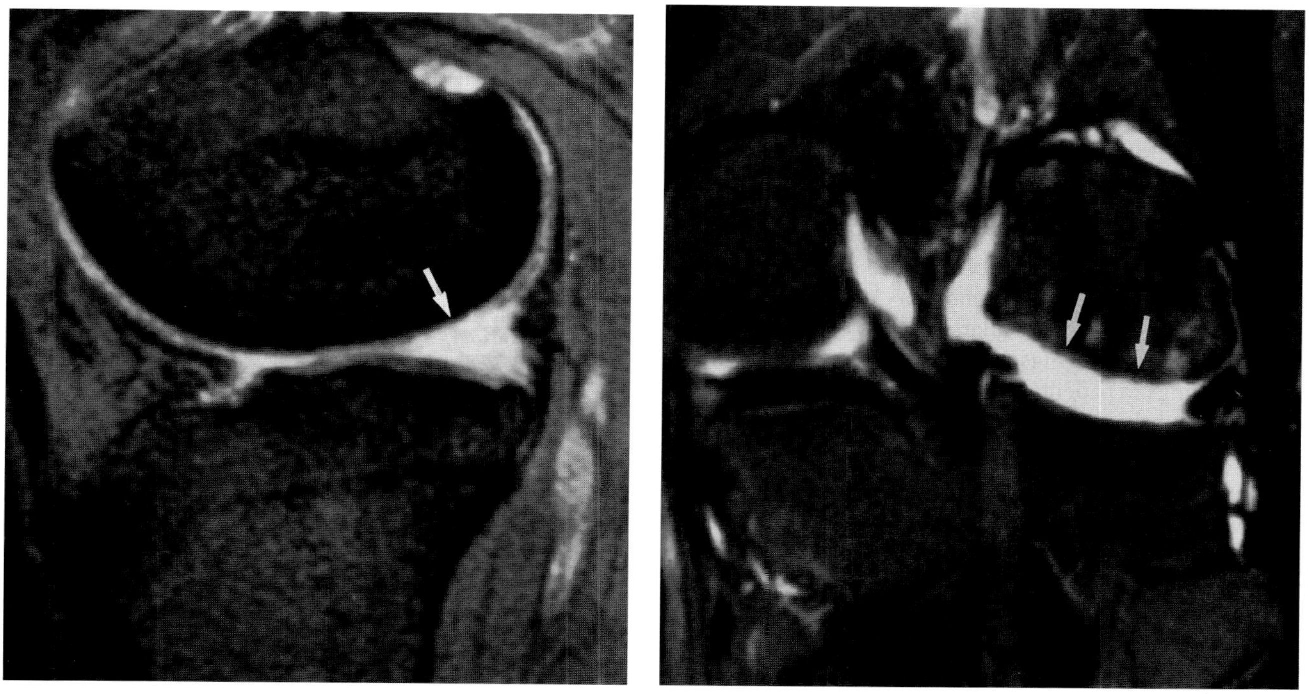

A B

FIG. 8-22. Sagittal **(A)** and coronal **(B)** fat-suppressed T2-weighted fast spin-echo images in a lateral meniscectomy patient with osteoarthritis show high-signal fluid outlining areas where cartilage is deficient and fluid is in contact with exposed bone *(arrows)*.

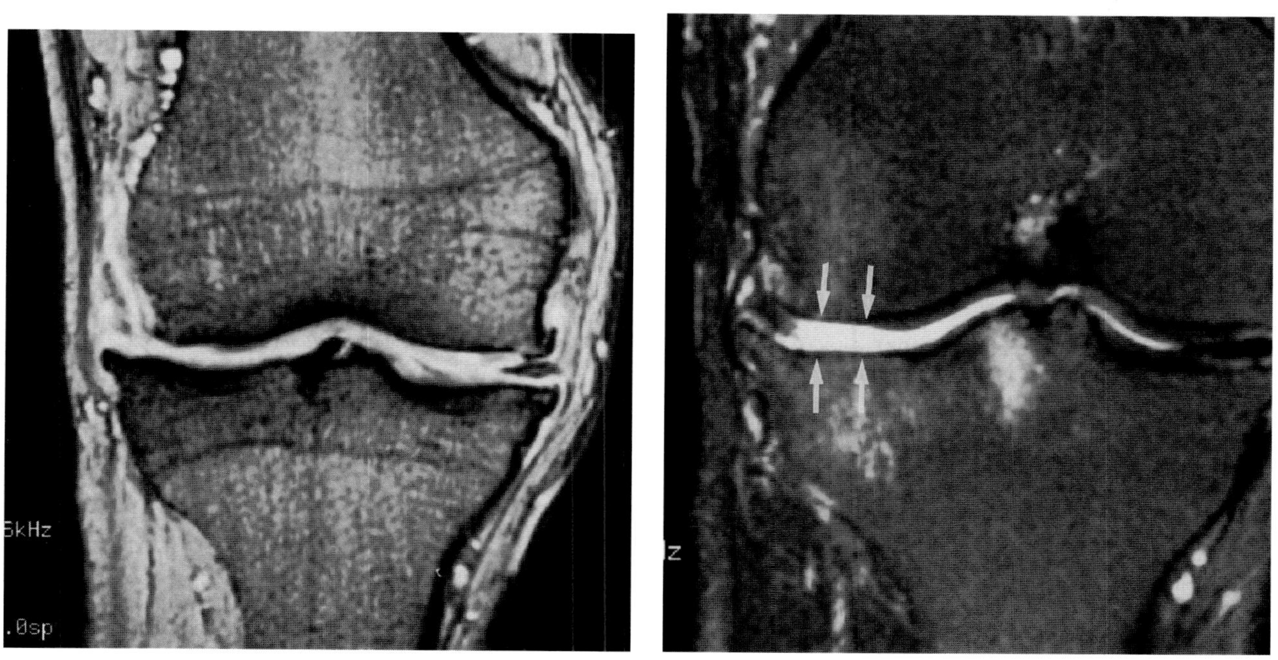

A B

FIG. 8-23. A: Coronal T2-weighted gradient-echo image in a patient with osteoarthritis. Osteophytes are clearly present at joint margins. Although joint appears narrow, the areas of deficient cartilage are difficult to appreciate. **B:** Coronal T2-weighted fast spin echo with fat suppression shows the zone of missing cartilage to better advantage *(arrows)*. Also note that regions of bone marrow edema are better appreciated.

A 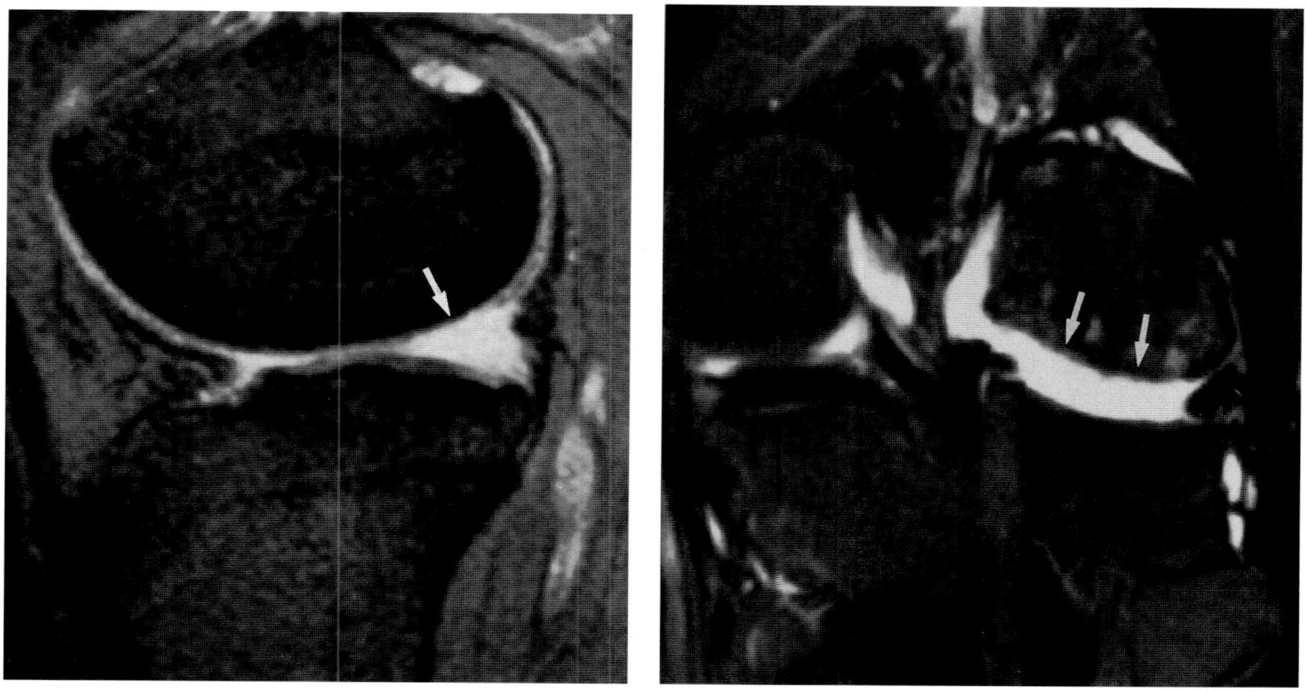 B

FIG. 8-22. Sagittal **(A)** and coronal **(B)** fat-suppressed T2-weighted fast spin-echo images in a lateral meniscectomy patient with osteoarthritis show high-signal fluid outlining areas where cartilage is deficient and fluid is in contact with exposed bone *(arrows)*.

A 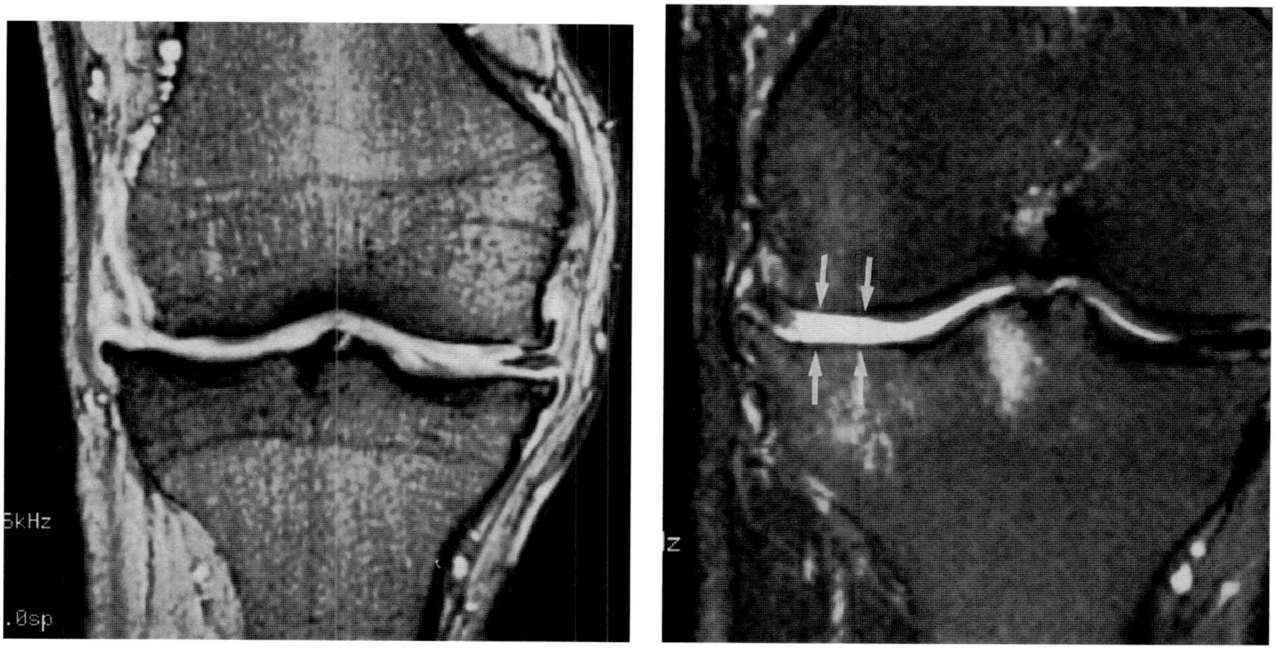 B

FIG. 8-23. A: Coronal T2-weighted gradient-echo image in a patient with osteoarthritis. Osteophytes are clearly present at joint margins. Although joint appears narrow, the areas of deficient cartilage are difficult to appreciate. **B:** Coronal T2-weighted fast spin echo with fat suppression shows the zone of missing cartilage to better advantage *(arrows)*. Also note that regions of bone marrow edema are better appreciated.

across the joint. This results in stiffening of underlying bone as it fractures and attempts to heal by buttressing itself with new osteoid and establishes an accelerating downward spiral that eventually results in severe joint damage. As in the inflammatory arthritides, an inflammatory response is almost invariably present in patients with osteoarthritis. If gadolinium-enhanced imaging is performed, enhancement of somewhat thickened synovium invariably will be seen (Fig. 8-18). The degree of synovial proliferation, however, is far less marked than that in the inflammatory arthritides. Small amounts of joint debris, particularly in a popliteal cyst, for instance, are common (Figs. 8-19 and 8-20). One of the frequent findings in patients with osteoarthritis is the formation of small subchondral pockets of synovium and granulation tissue known as geodes. These are particularly well seen on MRI as areas of low signal intensity on T1-weighted imaging that may show variable increased signal intensity as T2 weighting is augmented. Administration of gadolinium will show enhancement within the geodes. This may occur only at the periphery or throughout the entire geode, depending on its contents. These geodes may reach impressive size and produce bone weakening, which can lead to insufficiency fractures (Fig. 8-21). These geodes pathologically can be shown to communicate with the knee joint in some instances; however, the communication is impossible to demonstrate on MRI (69,70).

Often areas of low signal intensity will be present on T1- and T2-weighted sequences in the subchondral area, and these represent areas of sclerosis that are most frequently found in the weight-bearing areas of the joint. Cartilage thinning can be demonstrated to advantage by using either thin-section 3DFT or fat-suppressed imaging (Figs. 8-22 and 8-23).

REFERENCES

1. Beltran J, Noto AM, Mosure JC, Weiss KL, Zuelzer W, Christoforidis AJ. The knee: surface-coil MR imaging at 1.5 T. *Radiology* 1986;159: 747–751.
2. Haggar AM, Froelich JW, Hearshen DO, Sadasivan K. Meniscal abnormalities of the knee: 3DFT fast-scan GRASS MR imaging. *AJR* 1988; 150:1341–1344.
3. Arnett FC, Edworthy SM, Bloch DA. The 1987 revised ARA criteria for classification of rheumatoid arthritis. *Arthritis Rheumatol* 1988;31: 315–324.
4. Crues JV III, Mink JH, Levy TL, Lotysch M, Stoller DW. Meniscal tears of the knee: accuracy of MR imaging. *Radiology* 1987;164: 445–448.
5. Larsen A, Dale K, Eek M. Radiographic evaluation of rheumatoid arthritis and related conditions by standard reference films. *Acta Radiol Scand* 1977;18:481–491.
6. Reiser M, Bongartz G, Erlemann R, et al. Magnetic resonance in cartilaginous lesions of the knee joint with three-dimensional gradient-echo imaging. *Skeletal Radiol* 1988;17:465–471.
7. Yamayo M, Tamai K, Yamaguchi T, Ohno W. MRI of the knee in rheumatoid arthritis: Gd-DTPA perfusion dynamics. *J Comput Assist Tomogr* 1993;17:781–785.
8. Terrier F, Hricak H, Revel D, et al. Magnetic resonance imaging and spectroscopy of the periarticular inflammatory soft tissue changes in the experimental arthritis of the rat. *Invest Radiol* 1985;20:813–823.
9. Arthrology. In: Warwick R, Williams PO, eds. *Gray's anatomy,* 35th British ed. Philadelphia: WB Saunders, 1973;388.
10. Hamerman D, Rosenberg LC, Schubert M. Diarthrodial joints revisited. *J Bone Joint Surg* 1970;52:725.
11. Gylys-Morin VM, Hajek PC, Satoris DJ, Resnick D. Articular cartilage defects: detectability in cadaver knees with MR. *AJR* 1987;148: 1153–1158.
12. Tang JSH, Gold RH, Bassett LW, Seeger LL. Musculoskeletal infection of the extremities: evaluation with MR imaging. *Radiology* 1988;166: 205–209.
13. Carpenter TA, Everett JR, Hall LD, et al. High-resolution magnetic resonance imaging of arthritic pathology in the rat knee. *Skeletal Radiol* 1994;23:429–437.
14. Bjorkengren AG, Geborek P, Rydholm U, Holtas S, Petterson H. MR imaging of the knee in acute rheumatoid arthritis: synovial uptake of gadolinium-DOTA. *AJR* 1990;155:329–332.
15. Berquist TH, Brown ML, Fitzgerald RHJ, May GR. Magnetic resonance imaging: application in musculoskeletal infection. *Magn Reson Imaging* 1985;3(3):219–230.
16. Hull RG, Rennie JAN, Eastmond CJ, Hutchison JMS, Smith FW. Nuclear magnetic resonance (NMR) tomographic imaging for popliteal cysts in rheumatoid arthritis. *Ann Rheum Dis* 1984;43:56–59.
17. Konig H. Contrast enhanced dynamic MRI in the diagnosis of inflammatory knee joint disorders. *Acta Radiol* 1991;377S:50–53.
18. Palmer DG. Synovial villi: an examination of these structures within the anterior compartment of the knee and metacarpal phalangeal joints. *Ragum* 1967;10:451.
19. Reiser MP, Naegele M. Inflammatory joint disease static and dynamic gadolinium-enhanced MR imaging. *J Magn Reson Imaging* 1993;3: 307–310.
20. Kursunoglu-Brahme S, Riccio T, Weisman MH, et al. Rheumatoid knee: role of gadopentetate-enhanced MR imaging. *Radiology* 1990; 176:831–835.
21. Reiser M, Bongartz G, Erlemann R, et al. Gadolinium-DTPA in rheumatoid arthritis and related diseases: first results with dynamic magnetic resonance imaging. *Skeletal Radiol* 1989;18:591–597.
22. Adam G, Dammer M, Bohndorf K, Christoph R, Fenke F, Gunther RW. Rheumatoid arthritis of the knee: value of gadopentetate dimeglumine–enhanced MR imaging. *AJR* 1991;156:125–129.
23. Brown DG, Edwards NL, Greer JM, Longley S, Gillespy T III, Panush RS. Magnetic resonance imaging in patients with inflammatory arthritis of the knee. *Clin Rheumatol* 1990;9(1):73–83.
24. Yulish BS, Lieberman JM, Newman AJ, Bryan PJ, Mulopulos GP, Modic MT. Juvenile rheumatoid arthritis: assessment with MR imaging. *Radiology* 1987;165:149–152.
25. Beltran J, Caudill JL, Herman LA, et al. Rheumatoid arthritis: MR imaging manifestations. *Radiology* 1987;165:153–157.
26. Senac MOJ, Deutsch D, Bernstein BH, et al. MR imaging in juvenile rheumatoid arthritis. *AJR* 1988;150:873–878.
27. Murakami DM, Bassett LW, Seeger LL. Advances in imaging of rheumatoid arthritis. *Clin Orthop Rel Res* 1991;(265):83–95.
28. Tamai K, Yamato M, Yamaguchi T, Ohno W. Dynamic magnetic resonance imaging for the evaluation of synovitis in patients with rheumatoid arthritis. *Arthritis Rheum* 1994;37(8):1151–1157.
29. Drape J, Thelen P, Gay-Depassier P, Silbermann O, Benacerraf R. Intraarticular diffusion of Gd-DOTA after intravenous injection in the knee: MR imaging evaluation. *Radiology* 1993;188:227–234.
30. Munk PL, Vellet AD, Levin MF, Bell AD, Harth MM, McCain GA. Intravenous administration of gadolinium in the evaluation of rheumatoid arthritis of the shoulder. *J Can Assoc Radiol* 1993;44:99–106.
31. Konig H, Sieper J, Wolf K. Rheumatoid arthritis: evaluation of hypervascular and fibrous pannus with dynamic MR imaging enhanced with Gd-DTPA. *Radiology* 1990;176:473–477.
32. Munk PL, Vellet AD, Hilborn MD, Crues III JV, Helms CA, Poon PY. Musculoskeletal infection: findings on magnetic resonance imaging. *Can Assoc Radiol J* 1994;45(5):355–362.
33. Beltran J, McGhee RB, Shaffer PB, et al. Experimental infections of the musculoskeletal system: evaluation with MR imaging and Tc-99m MDP and Ga-67 scintigraphy. *Radiology* 1988;167:167–172.
34. Beltran J, Noto AM, Herman LJ, Mosure JC, Burk JM, Christoforidis AJ. Joint effusions: MR imaging. *Radiology* 1986;158:133–137.
35. Boden D, Quinn SF, Murray WT, et al. Magnetic resonance images of chronic patellar tendinitis. *Skeletal Radiol* 1988;17:24–28.
36. Greene WB, Yankaskas BC, Guilford WB. Roentgenographic classifications of hemophilic arthropathy. *J Bone Joint Surg* 1989;71A(2): 237–244.

37. Petterson H, Ahlberg A, Nilsson IM. A radiographic classification of hemophilic arthropathy. *Clin Orthop* 1980;149:153–159.
38. White ME. Magnetic resonance imaging in synovial disorders and arthropathy of the knee. *MRI Clin North Am* 1994;2:451–461.
39. Rominger MB, Bernreuter WK, Kenney PJ, Morgan SL, Blackburn WD, Alarcon GS. MR imaging of the hands in early rheumatoid arthritis: preliminary results. *Radiographics* 1993;13:37–46.
40. Herve-Somma CMP, Sebag GH, Prieur A, Bonnerot V, Lallemand DP. Juvenile rheumatoid arthritis of the knee: MR evaluation with Gd-DOTA. *Radiology* 1992;182:93–98.
41. Konig H, Sieper J, Wolf KJ. Dynamic MRI for the differentiation of inflammatory joint lesions. *Fortschr Roentgenstr* 1990;153:1–5.
42. Adams G, Dammer M, Bohndorf K, Christoph R, Fenke F, Gunther RW. Rheumatoid arthritis of the knee value of gadopentetate dimeglumine-enhanced imaging. *AJR* 1991;156:125–129.
43. Beltran J, Noto AM, McGhee RB, Freedy RM, McCalla MS. Infections of the musculoskeletal system: high-field-strength MR imaging. *Radiology* 1987;164:449–454.
44. Barnett CH; Davies DV; MacConaill MA. Thomas CC, eds. Synovial joints: their structure and mechanics. Springfield, IL: Charles C Thomas; 1961.
45. Tyrell RL, Gluckert K, Pathria M, Modic MT. Fast three-dimensional MR imaging of the knee: comparison with arthroscopy. *Radiology* 1988;166:865–872.
46. Sigurdson LA. The structure and function of articular synovial membranes. *J Bone Joint Surg* 1930;12:603.
47. Davis DUV. The structure and function of synovial membrane. *Br Med J* 1950;1:92.
48. Lehner KB, Rechl HP, Gmeinwieser JK, Heuck AF, Lukas HP, Kohl HP. Structure, function and degeneration of bovine hyaline cartilage: assessment with MR imaging in vitro. *Radiology* 1989;170:495–499.
49. Singson RD, Zalduondo FM. Value of unenhanced spin-echo MR imaging in distinguishing between synovitis and effusion of the knee. *AJR* 1992;159:569–571.
50. Gilkeson G, Polisson R, Sinclair H, et al. Early detection of carpal erosions in patients with rheumatoid arthritis: a pilot study of magnetic resonance imaging. *J Rheumatol* 1988;15:1361–1366.
51. Foley-Nolan D, Stack JP, Ryan M, et al. Magnetic resonance imaging in the assessment of rheumatoid arthritis: a comparison with plain film radiographs. *Br J Rheumatol* 1991;30:101–106.
52. Aisen AM, Martel W, Ellis JH, McCune WJ. Cervical spine involvement in rheumatoid arthritis: MR imaging. *Radiology* 1987;165:159–164.
53. Bloem JL, Reiser M, Vanel D. Magnetic resonance contrast agents in the evaluation of the musculoskeletal system. *Magn Reson Q* 1990;6(2):136–163.
54. Munk PL, Vellet AD, Levin MF. Leaking Baker's cyst detected by magnetic resonance imaging. *Can Assoc Radiol J* 1992;44:125–128.
55. Kulshrestha A Misra RN, Agarwal P, Gupta D. Magnetic resonance appearance of tuberculosis of the knee joint with ruptured Baker's cyst. *Australas Radiol* 1995;39:80–83.
56. Araki Y, Tsukaguchi I, Shino K. Tuberculous arthritis of the knee: MR findings. *AJR* 1993;160:664.
57. Sharif HS, Clark DC, Aabed MY, et al. Mycetoma: comparison of MR imaging with CT. *Radiology* 1991;178(3):865–870.
58. Dangman BC, Hoffer FA, Rand FF, O'Rourke EJ. Osteomyelitis in children: gadolinium-enhanced MR imaging. *Radiology* 1992;182:743–747.
59. Fletcher LD, Scoles PV, Nelson D. Osteomyelitis in children: detection by magnetic resonance. *Radiology* 1984;150:57–60.
60. Erdman WA, Tamburro F, Jayson HT, Weatherall PT, Ferry KB, Peshock RM. Osteomyelitis: characteristics and pitfalls of diagnosis with MR imaging. *Radiology* 1991;180:533–539.
61. Yuh TC, Corson JD, Baraniewski HM, et al. Osteomyelitis of the foot in diabetic patients: evaluation with plain film, 99m Tc-MDP bone scintigraphy, and MR imaging. *AJR* 1989;152:795–800.
62. Cohen MD, Cory DA, Kleiman M, Smith JA, Broderick NJ. Magnetic resonance differentiation of acute and chronic osteomyelitis in children. *Clin Radiol* 1990;41:53–56.
63. Unger E, Moloofsky P, Gatenby R, Hartz W, Broder G. Diagnosis of osteomyelitis by MR imaging. *AJR* 1980;150:605–610.
64. Wegener WA, Alavi A. Diagnostic imaging of musculoskeletal infection—roentgenography; gallium, indium-labeled white blood cell, gammaglobulin, bone scintigraphy; and MRI. *Orthop Infect* 1991;22(3):401–418.
65. Chandnani VP Beltran J, Morris CS, et al. Acute experimental osteomyelitis and abscesses: detection with MR imaging versus CT. *Radiology* 1990;174:233–236.
66. An HS, Vaccaro AR, Dolinskas CA, Cotler JM, Balderston RA, Bauerle WB. Differentiation between spinal tumors and infections with magnetic resonance imaging. *Spine* 1991;16(suppl 8):334–338.
67. Quinn SF, Murray W, Clark RA, Cochran C. MR imaging of chronic osteomyelitis. *J Comput Assist Tomogr* 1988;12(1):113–117.
68. Rahmouni A, Chosidow O, Mathieu D, et al. MR imaging in acute infectious cellulitis. *Radiology* 1994;192:493–496.
69. Bergman AG, Willen HK, Lindstrand AL, Petterson HTA. Osteoarthritis of the knee: correlation of subchondral MR signal abnormalities with histopathologic and radiographic features. *Skeletal Radiol* 1994;23:445–448.
70. Peterfy CG, van Dijke CF, Janzen DL, Gluer CC, Namba R, Majumdar S, Lang P, Genant HK. Quantification of articular cartilage in the knee with pulsed saturation transfer subtraction and fat-suppressed MR imaging: optimization and validation. *Radiology* 1994;192:485–491.

MRI of the Knee, Second Edition,
edited by P. L. Munk and C. A. Helms.
Lippincott-Raven Publishers, Philadelphia © 1996.

CHAPTER 9

Tumors and Tumorlike Conditions of the Knee

Dennis L. Janzen, Peter L. Munk, A. Dale Vellet, Malcolm M. M. Hayes, and Peter Y. Poon

The ideal imaging procedure for musculoskeletal tumor evaluation would provide accurate depiction of lesion location and extent; characterization of the tumor tissue type, grade, and stage; and assessment of tumor response to therapy. Magnetic resonance imaging (MRI) provides multiplanar images with high soft-tissue contrast sufficient to achieve many of these goals and has become the modality of choice for detection and staging of musculoskeletal tumors. Excellent reviews are available regarding the use of MRI in evaluation of musculoskeletal tumors (1–10). This chapter is organized into discussions of MRI imaging techniques and MRI characteristics of common bone, synovial, and soft-tissue tumors. Although this discussion will focus on the role of MRI in assessment of these conditions, it must be emphasized that other imaging modalities, particularly conventional radiography, are essential for accurate evaluation of bone and soft-tissue tumors. The features highlighted in this chapter attempt to place MRI in an appropriate complementary role to other imaging modalities.

IMAGING TECHNIQUE

Pulse Sequences and Imaging Planes

The MRI examination of a patient with a known or suspected musculoskeletal tumor must be tailored to the specific circumstances, particularly the tumor location and suspected diagnosis. In all patients, the examination should be performed in at least two orthogonal planes and include T1-weighted, T2-weighted, and fat-suppressed images. The T1- and T2-weighted spin-echo images are necessary to define the location of the tumor and to determine its composition (i.e., fat, fluid, tissue, calcification, etc.). Fat-suppression techniques such as short-tau inversion recovery (STIR) or frequency-selective presaturation techniques provide optimal contrast between tumor and adjacent normal tissues, and increase the conspicuity of peritumoral edema (11,12). Fat-suppressed sequences may show suppression of signal from the tumor: this provides definitive evidence of the fatty nature of a tumor. Gradient-echo images are especially useful to highlight the presence of hemosiderin, calcifications, or air bubbles within a mass. All these substances produce focal loss of signal due to magnetic susceptibility effects; this is especially well seen on gradient-echo images because of the absence of a 180° refocusing pulse (Fig. 9-1). The detection of hemosiderin on gradient-echo images is particularly helpful in establishing the diagnosis of giant cell tumor of tendon sheath, pigmented villonodular synovitis, and chronic hematoma, as these masses commonly contain hemosiderin (13,14).

The selection of imaging coil and pulse sequence parameters should be designed to optimize spatial and contrast resolution, while imaging the entire lesion within a reasonable amount of time. (For further discussion of these technical issues, see Chapter 1.)

Intravenous Contrast

Intravenous contrast enhancement with gadolinium chelates is useful in selected circumstances for the evaluation of patients with bone and soft-tissue tumors (13). In the majority of patients with untreated musculoskeletal tumors, the primary goals of lesion detection, staging, and characteri-

D. L. Janzen: Department of Radiology, Vancouver Hospital and Health Sciences Center, Vancouver, British Columbia, Canada V5Z 1M9.

P. L. Munk: Department of Radiology, University of British Columbia, Department of Diagnostic Imaging, British Columbia Cancer Agency, Vancouver, British Columbia, Canada V5Z 4E6.

A. D. Vellet: Department of Diagnostic Imaging, University of Calgary, Foothills Hospital, Alberta, Canada T2N 2T9.

M. M. M. Hayes: Department of Pathology, University of British Columbia, British Columbia Cancer Agency, Vancouver, British Columbia, Canada V5Z 4E6.

P. Y. Poon: Department of Diagnostic Imaging, British Columbia Cancer Agency, Vancouver, British Columbia, Canada V5Z 4E6.

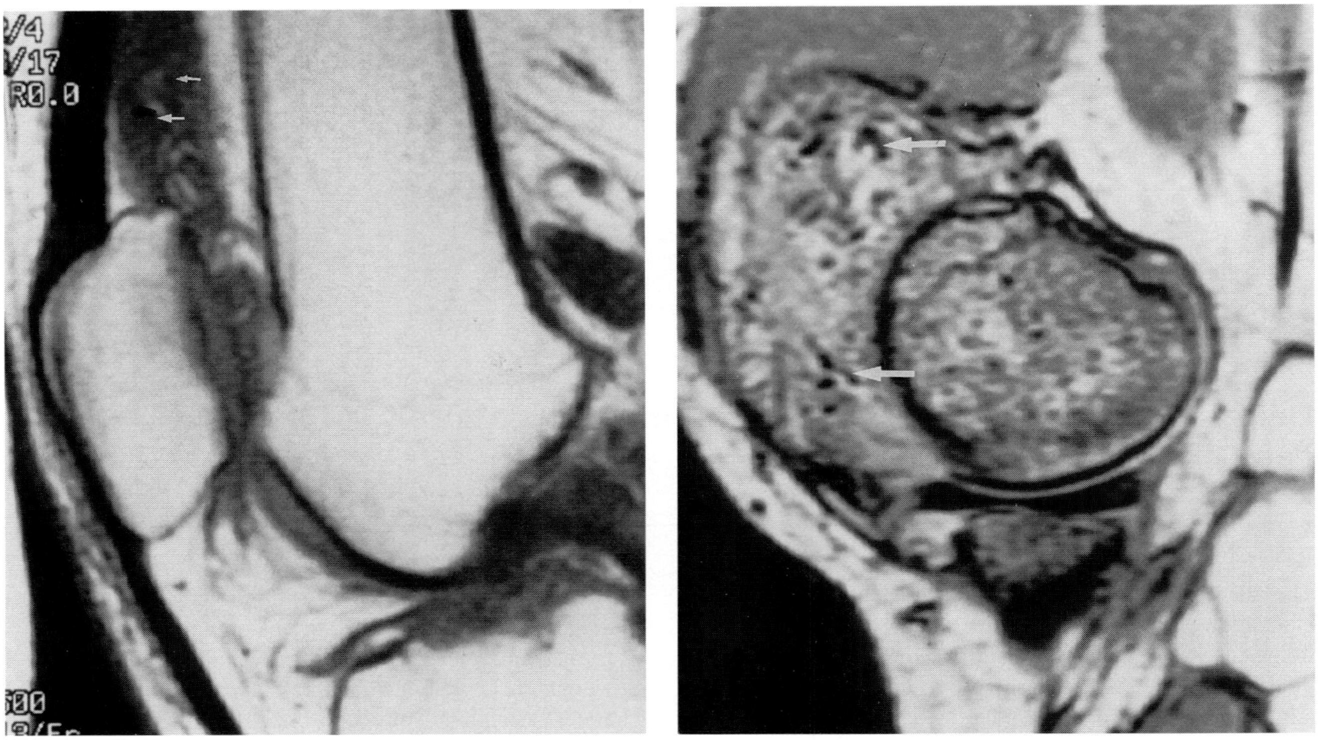

A B

FIG. 9-1. Magnetic susceptibility effects of hemosiderin on spin-echo and gradient-echo images. **A:** T1-weighted spin-echo image shows a few small punctate signal voids within the hypertrophied synovium of the suprapatellar recess *(arrows)*. **B:** Gradient-echo image shows larger and more numerous signal voids, caused by the "blooming" of signal voids around paramagnetic foci on gradient-echo images *(arrows)*. The synovial hypertrophy was due to pigmented villonodular synovitis.

zation can generally be accomplished without the use of intravenous contrast (14). The question of whether or not intravenous contrast administration improves diagnostic accuracy in determining the histologic nature of musculoskeletal tumors has not been clearly answered in the literature; our opinion is that intravenous contrast administration is generally unnecessary for the initial staging and characterization of musculoskeletal tumors (15,16). In preoperative patients, intravenous contrast enhancement may be useful to localize viable tissue versus necrotic or cystic areas, in order to guide biopsy (Fig. 9-2) (17,18). The rate and degree of tumor enhancement have been shown to be useful in assessing response of osteogenic sarcomas to chemotherapy (19). Intravenous contrast use has been described as helpful in detecting tumor involvement of adjacent joints, because contrast-enhanced T1-weighted images provide good delineation of high-signal-intensity enhancing tumor versus low-signal-intensity joint fluid (20). In this situation, T2-weighted or STIR images may not provide optimal delineation of tumor adjacent to high-signal-intensity joint fluid. Contrast enhancement is particularly helpful in postoperative patients, because it allows distinction between nonenhancing fluid collections (seromas, hematomas) and enhancing residual or recurrent tumor (21).

MRI CHARACTERISTICS OF BONE TUMORS

Tumor Signal Characteristics

Tumors of the musculoskeletal system are similar to tumors of other organ systems in that they are characterized by a relative increase in free water (22–24). There appears to be some correlation between free water content and the malignant characteristics of neoplasm, with higher-grade tumors showing higher signal intensity on T2-weighted images and more impressive perilesional edema, although this is far from absolute. With the exception of lipomatous tumors or tumors with myxomatous or fatty degeneration, the increase in tumor free water produces decreased signal intensity on T1-weighted images and increased signal intensity on T2-weighted and STIR images. Consequently, most tumors, regardless of their location, are of diminished signal intensity on T1-weighted images relative to muscle. Thus, the signal characteristics of tumor tissue usually do not allow accurate diagnosis of tumor histopathology (25–27). However, characteristic patterns of bone destruction, margination, matrix formation, and periosteal reaction may be identified on MR images and plain radiographs. These morphologic features allow considerable insight into the biological activity and

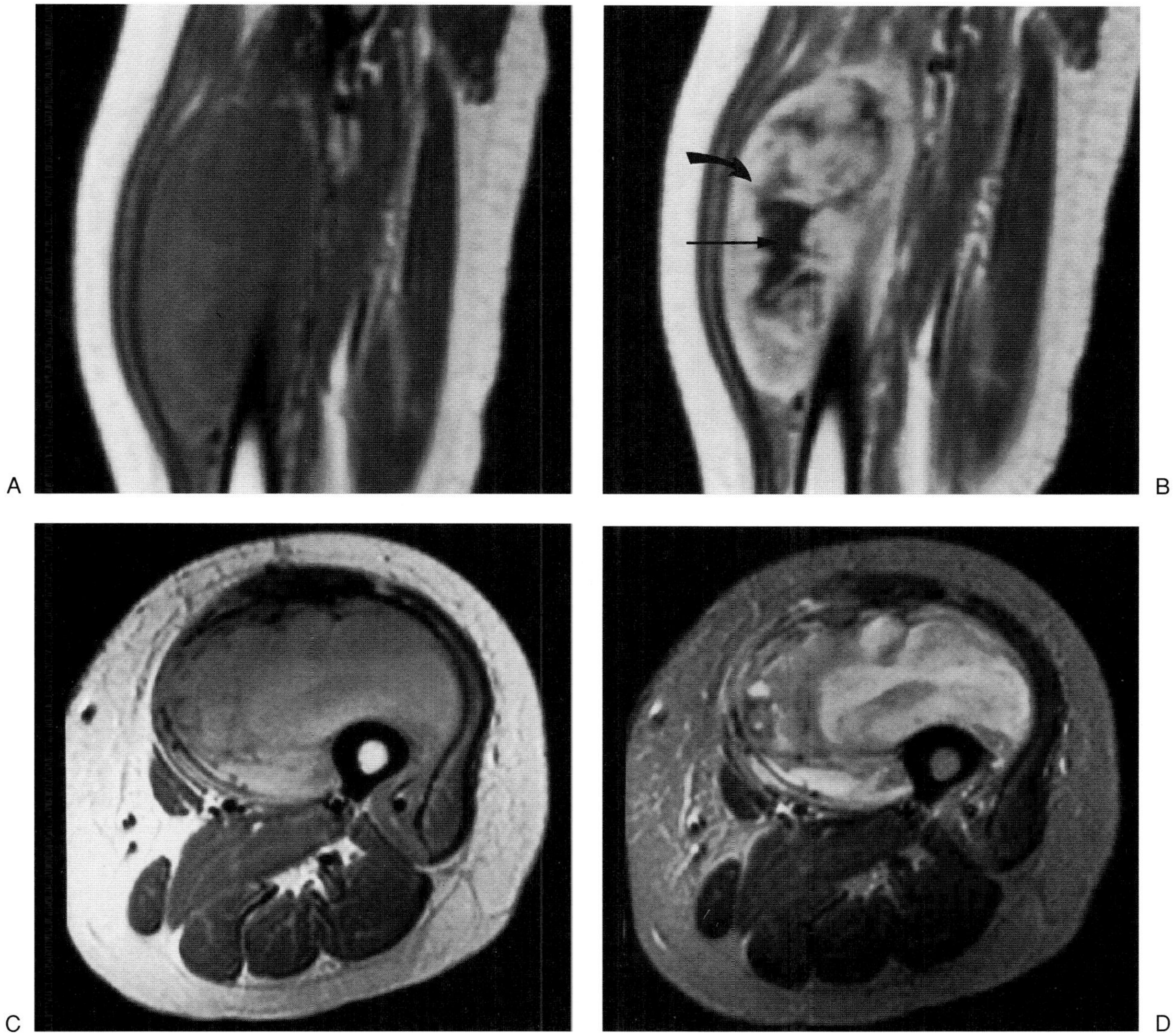

FIG. 9-2. Use of intravenous gadolinium enhancement to differentiate viable versus necrotic tumor prior to biopsy. **A:** Unenhanced T1-weighted sagittal image shows a large, mildly inhomogeneous soft-tissue tumor anterior to the femoral diaphysis. **B:** Enhanced T1-weighted sagittal image shows a central necrotic area *(long arrow)* surrounded by a thick rind of enhancing tumor *(curved arrow)*. Axial proton density **(C)** and T2-weighted **(D)** images did not allow differentiation of viable and necrotic tumor. Biopsy of the viable portion of the tumor showed spindle-cell sarcoma.

histopathology of bone tumors, and often allow a specific diagnosis to be made.

Patterns of Bone Destruction

Although MRI was originally believed to be relatively insensitive in the evaluation of trabecular and cortical bone, the improved spatial resolution and increasing application of gradient-echo and fat-suppression techniques have allowed MRI to accurately display pathologic conditions involving bone. With current techniques, MRI can show patterns of bone destruction analogous to recognized radiographic and CT patterns. MRI provides the added advantages of unsurpassed depiction of intramedullary tumor extent, soft-tissue tumor extent, and perilesional edema.

The classic radiographic and CT descriptions of bone destruction as geographic, moth-eaten, or permeative are equally appropriate to MRI (28). The classic descriptions of bone destruction as geographic, moth-eaten, or permeative are equally applicable to MRI. Since MRI is more sensitive than radiographs or CT in the identification of medullary lesions, it will detect such lesions at an earlier stage. Although the growth characteristics of most tumors are consistent throughout their evolution, it may be difficult to apply the MRI characteristics of bone destruction to smaller lesions.

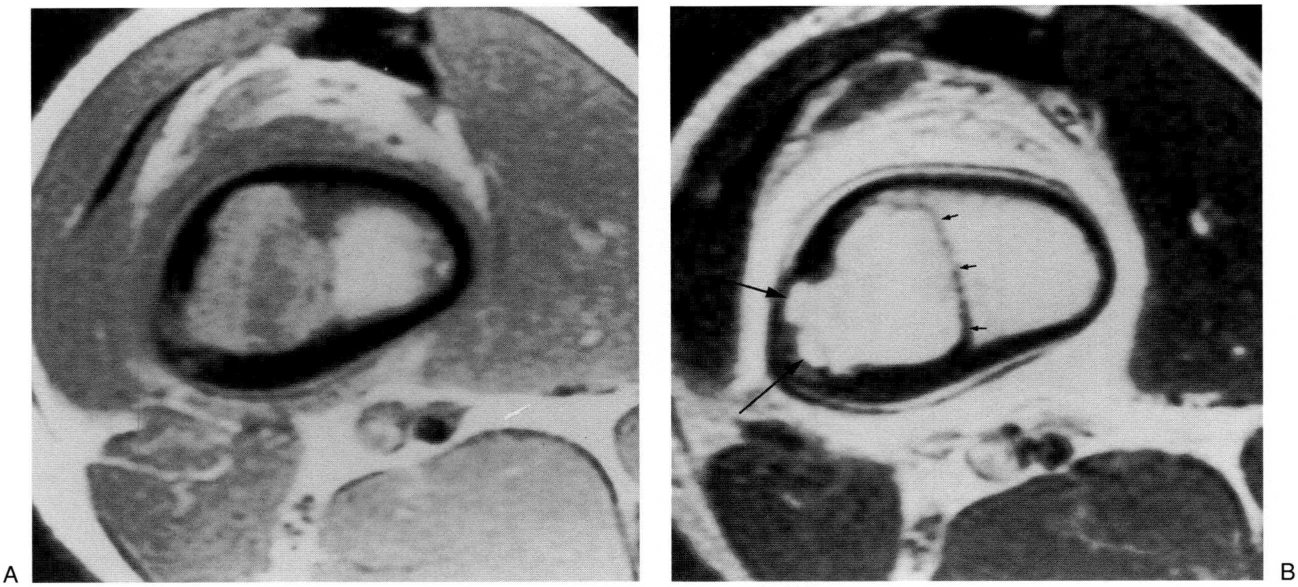

FIG. 9-3. Geographic pattern of medullary tumor growth contained by reactive medullary new bone. **A:** Proton density-weighted transverse image shows intermediate signal intensity eccentric, low-grade medullary osteosarcoma discretely demarcated from medullary fat. **B:** T2-weighted transverse image of same lesion shows a low-signal-intensity halo of reactive bone *(small arrows)* around the high-signal-intensity lesion. Endosteal scalloping is also noted along the lateral margin of the tumor *(long arrows).*

Geographic Bone Destruction

In geographic bone destruction, the intramedullary tumor is discretely demarcated by adjacent reactive cortical and trabecular bone or central medullary fat (Fig. 9-3). Reactive trabecular or cortical bone appears as a low-signal-intensity margin around the lesion on T1- and T2-weighted images. This pattern corresponds closely to the plain radiographic or CT appearance of a lytic lesion with a discrete, well-defined margin or reactive bone. No permeation of the adjacent marrow by tumor or reactive edema is present, and no high-signal-intensity tunneling of the cortical bone on T2-weighted or gradient-echo images is present.

More rapidly growing lesions, although geographically demarcated from trabecular bone and adjacent marrow fat, are not delineated by low-signal-intensity reactive new bone formation (Fig. 9-4). Such lesions consequently tend to demonstrate a more pronounced chemical shift artifact. Marrow edema is not a prominent feature in such lesions.

Moth-eaten Bone Destruction

As with plain radiographs and CT, the moth-eaten pattern on MRI is characteristic of a more aggressive lesion. The rapid growth rate of tumors with a moth-eaten pattern results in prominent intramedullary extension of tumor (Fig. 9-5). Although cortical bone may be spared, there is extensive destruction of trabecular bone. The medullary fat–tumor interface is often characterized by increased signal on T2-weighted images due to marrow edema. This corresponds to a region of diminished signal intensity on T1-weighted images. There is also growth of tumor along and between trabecular bone in advance of discrete trabecular bone destruction (Fig. 9-6). Extension of such a destructive pattern to the endosteal margin of cortical bone may occur. The consequence of such a pattern of growth is that the tumor size on MRI invariably exceeds that suggested by other imaging modalities (Fig. 9-7).

Permeative Bone Destruction

Permeative bone destruction on MRI is characterized by extensive medullary tumor burden disproportionate to the apparent extent of involvement on plain radiographs or CT. The growth rate of tumors with this pattern is extremely rapid, with intramedullary growth outstripping trabecular bone destruction and cortical tunneling. Endosteal cortical bone destruction and cortical permeation and thinning are usually present (Fig. 9-8). The endosteal tunneling is demonstrated as patchy, increased signal intensity within the cortical bone on gradient-echo and T2-weighted images.

Tumor Interface and Margination

Because MRI allows evaluation of the true intramedullary extent of a tumor, there are invariably two tumor margins to consider.

A 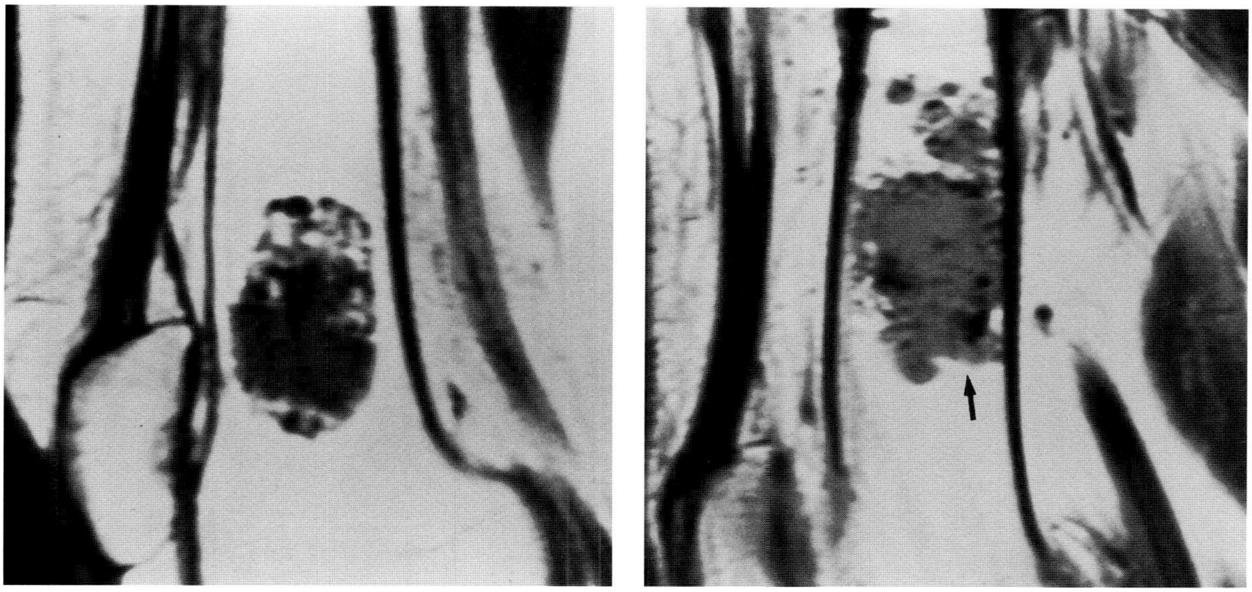 B

FIG. 9-4. Geographic pattern of medullary tumor growth without reactive medullary new bone formation. **A:** T1-weighted sagittal image of medullary chondrosarcoma demonstrates discrete demarcation of intermediate-signal-intensity medullary tumor from the adjacent fat. **B:** Proton-density-weighted sagittal image shows chemical-shift artifact at the tumor–fat interface, without reactive new bone *(arrow)*. The focal areas of low signal within the tumor represent chondroid calcifications.

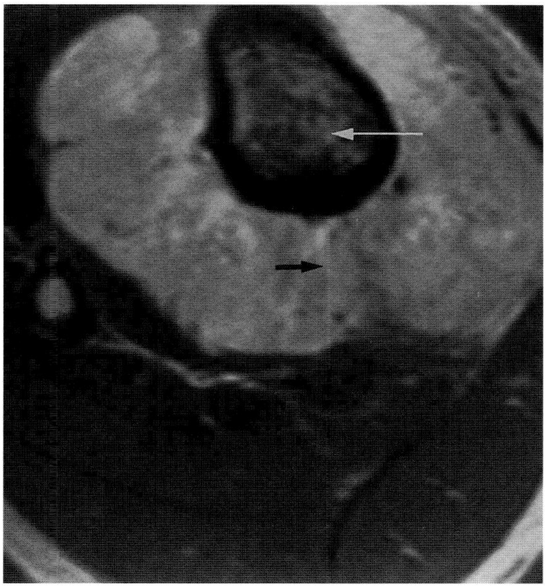

FIG. 9-5. Moth-eaten pattern of medullary tumor growth. T2-weighted transverse image of medullary osteosarcoma within the proximal tibial metaphysis demonstrates extensive periosseous extension, sunburst periosteal reaction *(black arrow)* and patchy intermediate- to high-signal-intensity medullary tumor interspersed within the heavily trabeculated metaphyseal marrow (*white arrow*). In this case, no reactive trabecular new bone is evident.

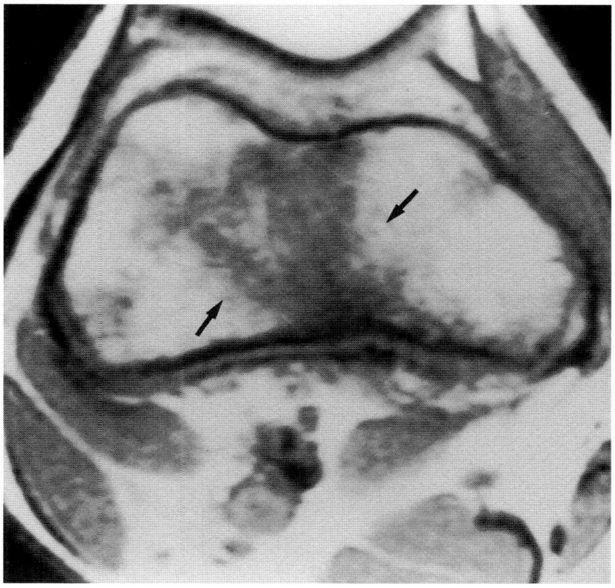

FIG. 9-6. Tumor–trabecular bone interface in moth-eaten pattern of medullary tumor growth. T1-weighted transverse image of a medullary osteosarcoma shows poorly defined islands of low-signal-intensity tumor intruding into the high-signal-intensity marrow fat *(arrows)*. The periosteum along the posterior aspect of the femoral cortex is elevated.

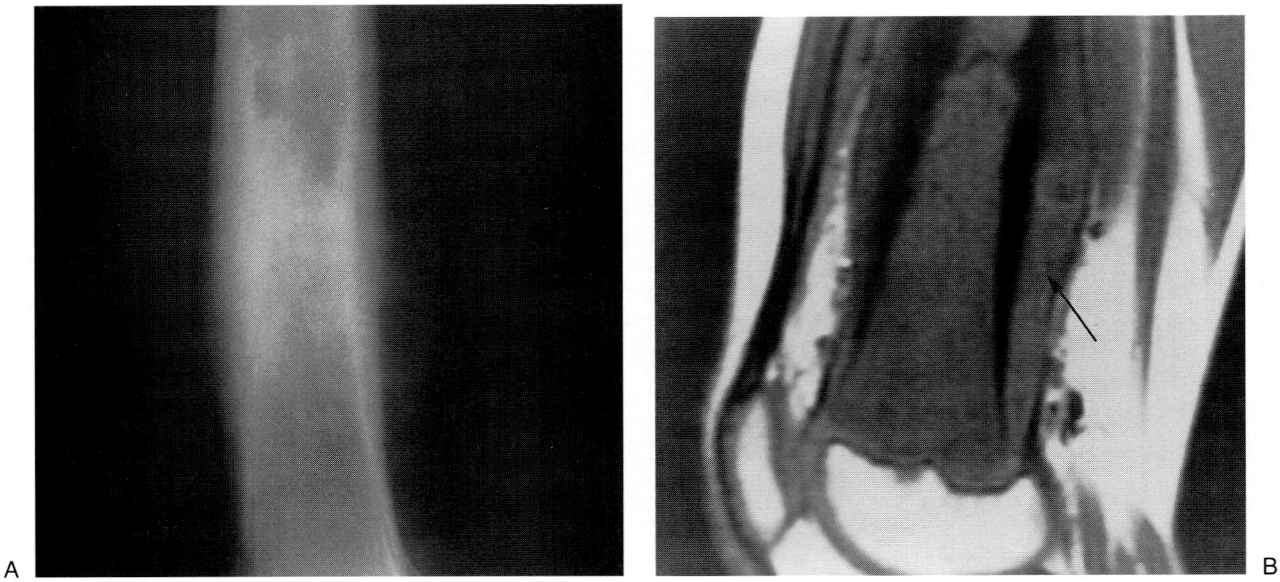

FIG. 9-7. Plain-film and MRI comparison of moth-eaten pattern of medullary tumor growth. **A:** Plain film shows a moth-eaten pattern of bone destruction at the superior and inferior borders of the sclerotic femoral osteosarcoma. **B:** Corresponding sagittal T1-weighted image shows tumor replacing the medullary fat, with extraosseous tumor extension *(arrow)*. Of note, the plain radiograph underestimates the extent of the tumor within the medullary space; this disproportional extent of tumor extent between plain films and MRI is characteristic of moth-eaten and permeative patterns of growth.

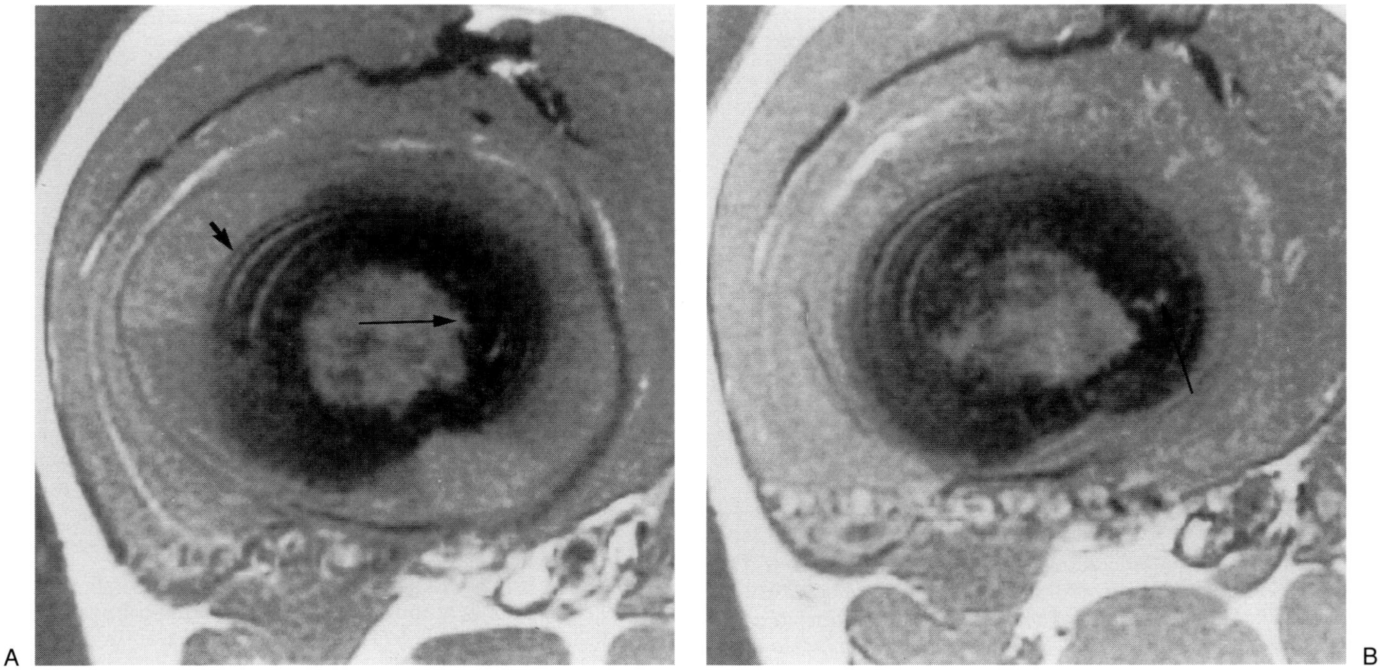

FIG. 9-8. Permeative pattern of bone destruction. **A:** T1-weighted transverse image of femoral osteosarcoma shows destruction and permeative invasion of the endosteal cortex *(long arrow)*. An onion-skin periosteal reaction is present *(short arrow)*. **B:** T1-weighted image at a different level of the same tumor shows intermediate-signal intensity-tumor tunneling through the bone cortex *(arrow)*.

Medullary Fat–Tumor Margin

Tumors with relatively benign growth patterns, but unassociated with evidence of medullary trabecular new bone formation, are characterized by a discrete demarcation between the advancing margin of tumor and fat (see Fig. 9-4). The rate of tumor growth is such that significant medullary edema is rarely present and consequently rarely evident on T2-weighted, gradient-echo, or fat-suppressed images. In more aggressive tumors, the fat–tumor interface becomes progressively less discrete and focal tumor extension into the adjacent marrow fat and trabecular bone is present (see Fig. 9-5). Such lesions are rarely associated with significant reactive trabecular bone formation.

Tumor–Endosteal Bone Interface

The cortical endosteal bone surface is invariably intimately related to the growing front of a tumor and provides the greatest resistance to tumor growth. On MRI the endosteal interface must be interpreted in conjunction with the extent of medullary tumor burden. Extensive intramedullary tumors may demonstrate little endosteal scalloping or erosive destruction. Discrete focal lesions associated with a scalloped margin of the low-signal-intensity endosteal margin are usually benign, the scalloping being indicative of a slow rate of growth. At this endosteal surface, progressive endosteal new bone may be deposited. This may be less compact than normal cortical bone and consequently has an inhomogeneous appearance on gradient-echo and T2-weighted images (Fig. 9-9). As the rate of local tumor growth increases, particularly if intramedullary extension is not a characteristic feature, there is a relative acceleration of cortical endosteal bony expansion (Fig. 9-10). Whereas slower-growing lesions are associated with multifocal lobulated regions of endosteal resorption leading to endosteal scalloping, more rapidly growing lesions tend to be associated with global cortical expansion. Such expansion will in turn be associated with variable periosteal buttressing. With increasing aggressiveness the cortical margin may become indistinct, and eventually endosteal tunneling will ensue (see Fig. 9-8).

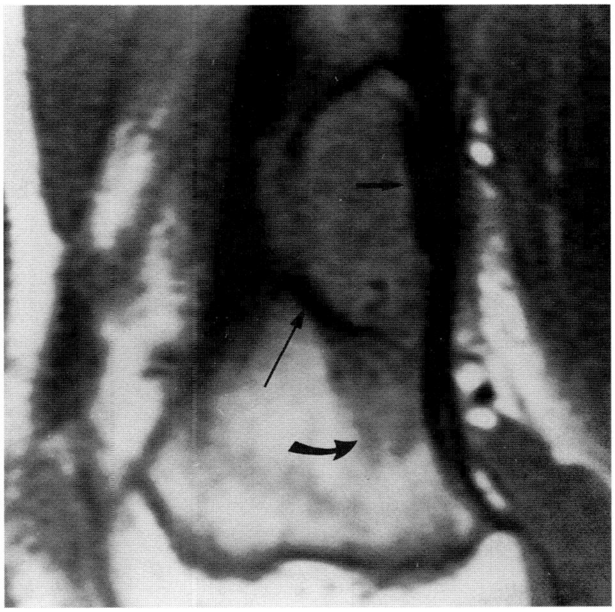

FIG. 9-9. Reactive endosteal new bone formation at tumor–endosteal bone interface. A T1-weighted sagittal image of an eccentric metaphyseal osteosarcoma shows low-signal-intensity new bone formation *(short arrow)* at the tumor margin. The tumor is partly confined by a halo of reactive trabecular new bone *(long arrow)* but demonstrates a more aggressive invasive inferior margin *(curved arrow).*

Tumor Matrix

Some tumors produce a chondroid or osteoid matrix that may calcify or ossify. Such regions of ossification or calcification will be seen as foci of diminished signal intensity on all pulse sequences. However, subtle regions of calcification or ossification may be apparent only on gradient-echo pulse sequences because of their sensitivity to magnetic susceptibility. It is difficult to differentiate such regions of T2 shortening from dystrophic calcification within the degenerative or necrotic lesions.

Central flocculent or flecklike chondroid matrix calcification may be found in enchondromas, chondroblastomas, chondromyxofibromas, chondrosarcomas, and, rarely, chondroblastic osteosarcomas. Such calcification will generally be found in the center of such lesions even when they are elongated (Fig. 9-11). The volume of such calcification is usually proportionate to the age and benignity of such lesions.

More complex regions of diminished signal intensity may be found within tumors capable of osteoid production. Such tumors include osteomas, osteoblastomas, ossifying fibromas, and osteosarcomas. In such tumors, new bone formation tends not to conform to a specific location within the lesion, is generally amorphous or conglomerate, and may have a bizarre appearance (Fig. 9-12).

Periosteal Response

MRI is unique in that it allows evaluation of the pathogenesis of different periosteal patterns. The normal periosteum is inseparable from cortical bone on MRI. However, when periosteum is elevated by tumor infiltration, hemorrhage, or bone marrow edema, it produces new bone that is evident on MRI as regions of T2 shortening adjacent to the periosteal surface of cortical bone. MRI was originally believed to be less sensitive than CT in its ability to detect periosteal new bone formation. However, with the use of gradient-echo imaging, MRI appears to be equally sensitive to CT in the identification and characterization of periosteal new bone.

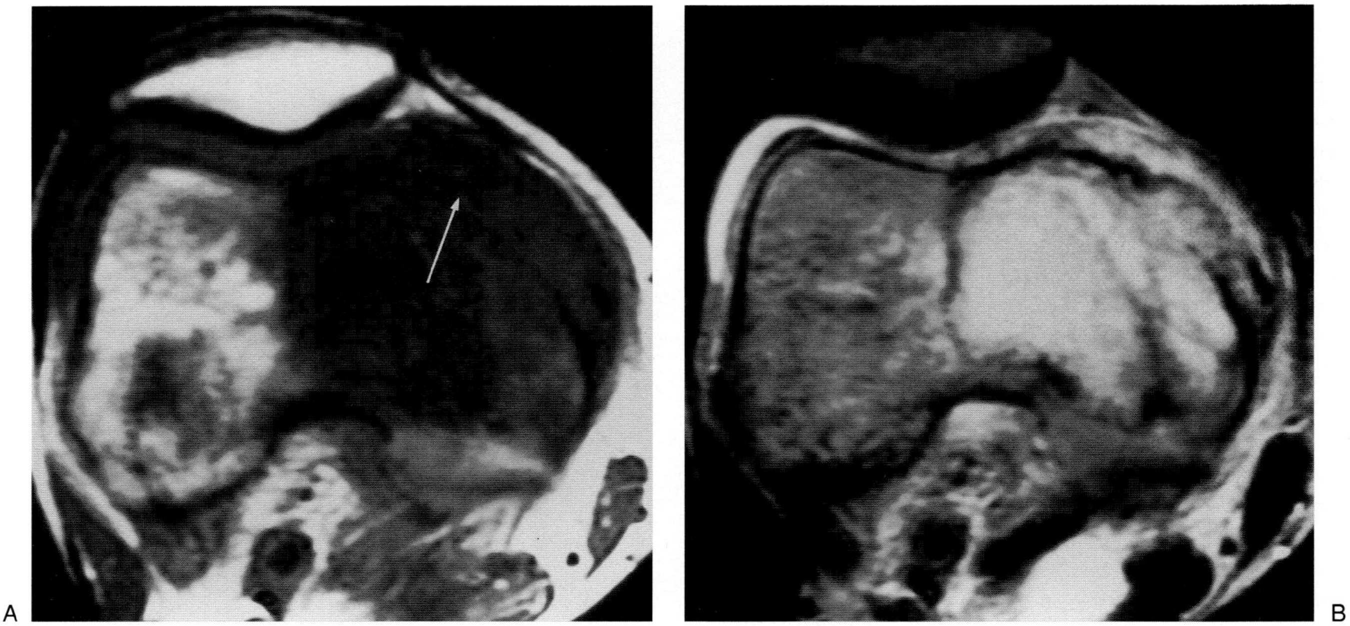

FIG. 9-10. Endosteal scalloping at tumor–endosteal bone interface. T1-weighted **(A)** and T2-weighted **(B)** transverse images of femoral osteosarcoma show endosteal scalloping *(arrow)*, focal cortical breach, and transcortical extension of tumor.

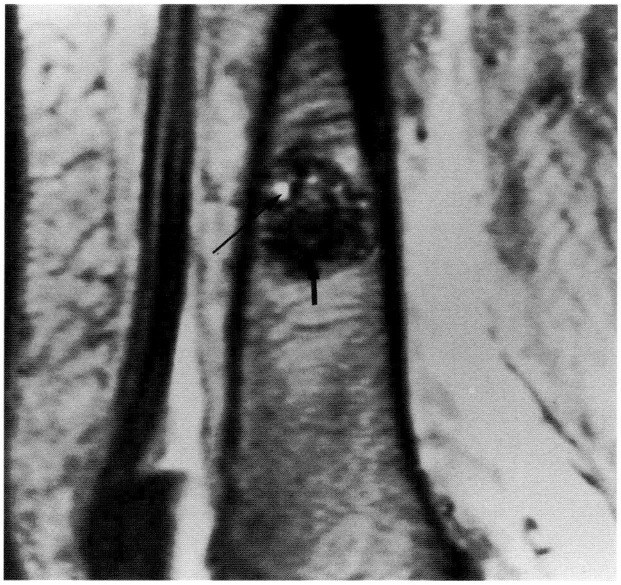

FIG. 9-11. Chondroid matrix calcification. A gradient-echo T2*-weighted sagittal image of an enchondroma shows flocculent low-signal-intensity areas *(short arrow)* within the tumor, typical of chondroid calcifications. The interspersed high-signal-intensity regions *(long arrow)* represent uncalcified hyaline cartilage. Note the sharp margins and lack of medullary edema around this benign lesion.

The incorporation of consecutive layers of periosteal new bone within the cortex results in periosteal buttressing, which is characteristic of benign bone tumors. MRI shows containment of the benign lesion by thickened low-signal-intensity endosteal and periosteal new bone. Lesions identified in an earlier phase of their evolution may be characterized by single or dual layers of periosteal new bone. When associated with benign bone lesions, tumor containment by endosteal and periosteal new bone is evident. However, when associated with lesions of greater aggressivity, tumor extension beyond the apparent confines of the single or dual periosteal layers may be seen (Fig. 9-13). This becomes more apparent when multiple layers of periosteal new bone are evident, producing the characteristic onion-skin pattern (Fig. 9-14). Such patterns are invariably associated with evidence of extraosseous extension of tumor. A progression of such extraosseous extension of tumor is production of a Codman's triangle (Fig. 9-15). Codman's triangle represents a layer or layers of elevated periosteum that is partially destroyed by transcortical extension of an aggressive tumor. The layers of periosteal new bone may be separated by high-signal-intensity tumor or reactive tissue on T2-weighted images. With increasing aggressivity, rapid subperiosteal tumor growth results in formation of periosteal new bone in an alignment perpendicular to the bone surface. This "sunburst" or "hair-on-end" periosteal pattern appears on T2-weighted images as low-signal-intensity strands of new bone within the subperiosteal tumor (Fig. 9-16).

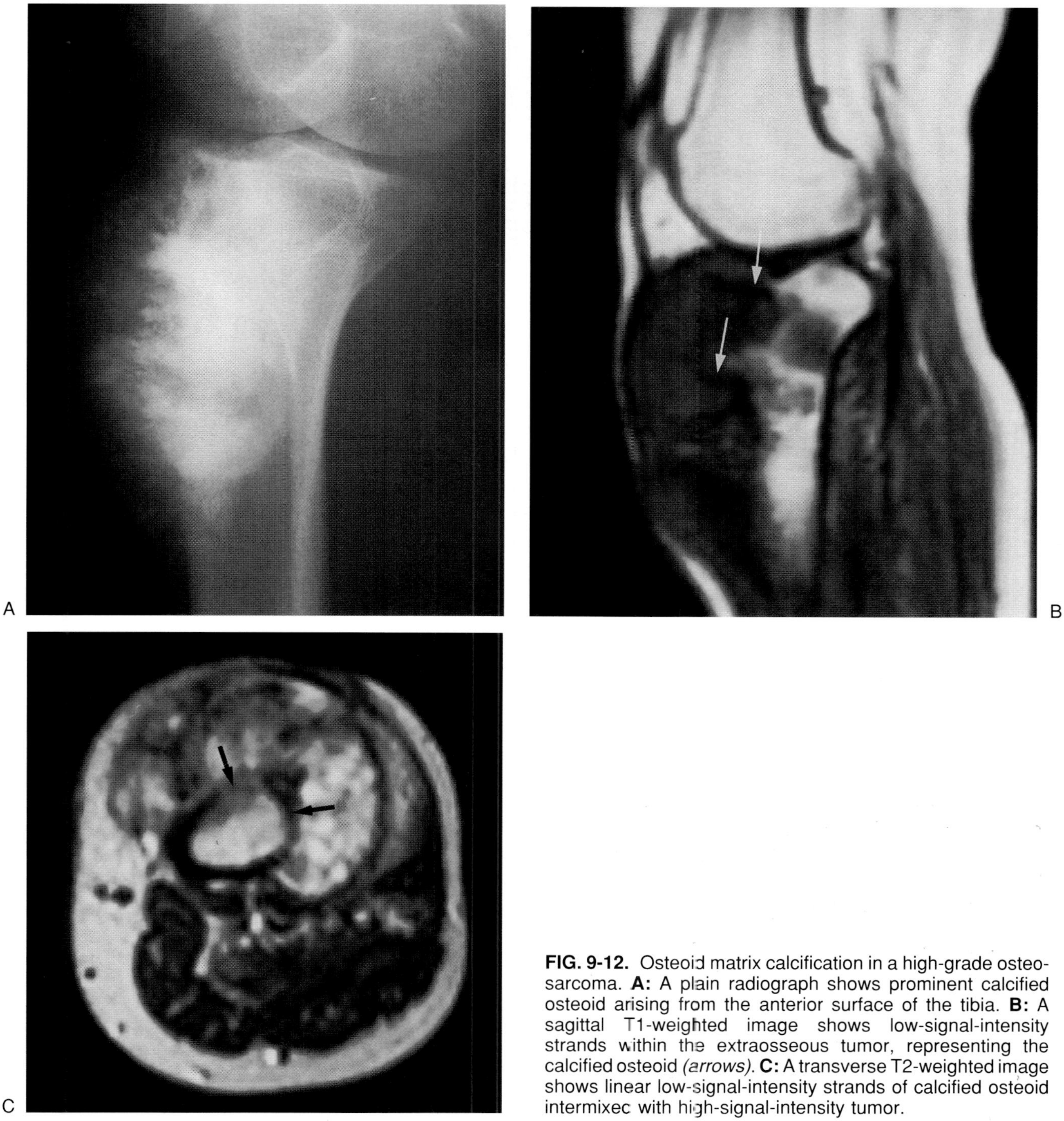

FIG. 9-12. Osteoid matrix calcification in a high-grade osteosarcoma. **A:** A plain radiograph shows prominent calcified osteoid arising from the anterior surface of the tibia. **B:** A sagittal T1-weighted image shows low-signal-intensity strands within the extraosseous tumor, representing the calcified osteoid *(arrows)*. **C:** A transverse T2-weighted image shows linear low-signal-intensity strands of calcified osteoid intermixed with high-signal-intensity tumor.

Axial Tumor Location

As with CT, MRI allows accurate evaluation of the position of the center of the lesion relative to the axis of the bone of origin. Characterization of lesions as central, eccentric, medullary, cortical, periosteal, or parosteal may be made. This analysis allows categorization of lesions according to location. The axial location of bone tumors is important, as many lesions have a predilection for specific axial locations.

Soft-Tissue Extension and Edema

Because of MRI's inherently superior soft-tissue contrast, it provides a unique ability to identify extracompartmental extension of primary bone tumors. Tumor extension, as shown by periosteal high signal intensity on T2-weighted images, can be easily identified in cases where CT and plain radiographs show no evidence of extraosseous extension. Recognition of subtle extraosseous tumor

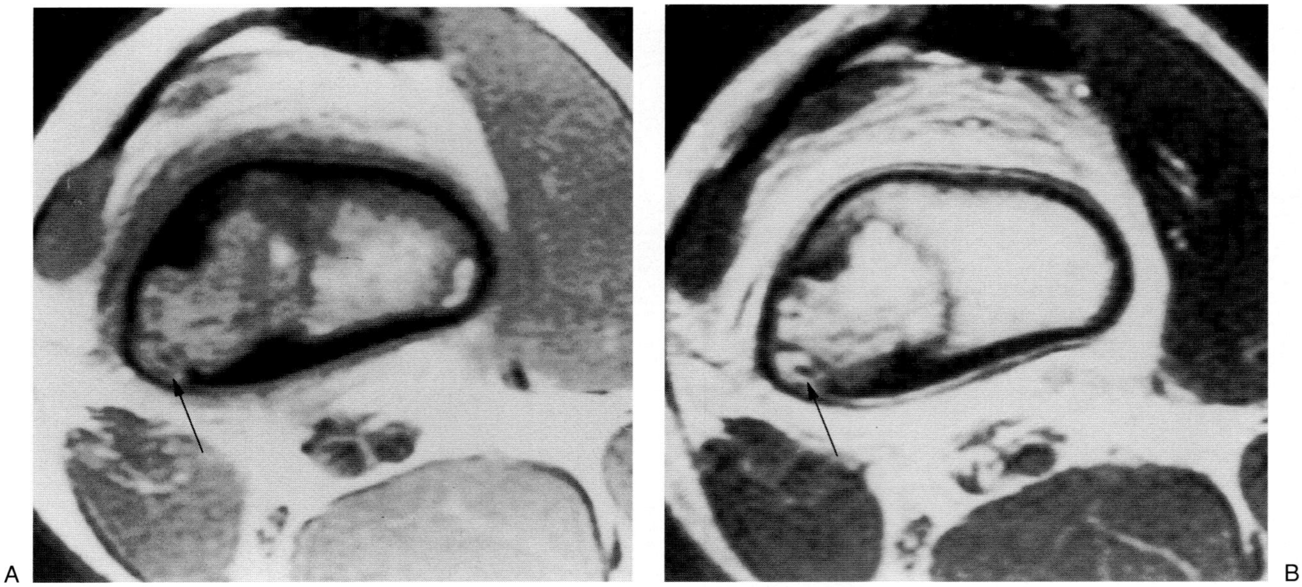

FIG. 9-13. Unilamellar periosteal reaction adjacent to medullary tumor. T1-weighted **(A)** and T2-weighted **(B)** transverse images of a femoral osteosarcoma show tumor extending through the cortex *(arrows)* confined by a single layer of low-signal-intensity thickened periosteum.

extension is of considerable importance in staging and surgical planning.

Many musculoskeletal tumors are associated with adjacent ill-defined infiltrating regions of high signal intensity on T2-weighted and STIR images. These regions of high signal intensity, commonly termed *edema*, are particularly

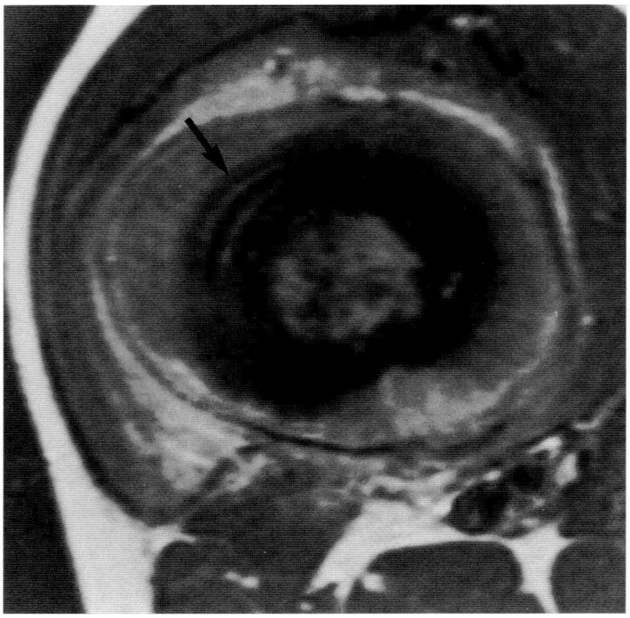

FIG. 9-14. Onion-skin periosteal reaction. A T2-weighted transverse image of osteosarcoma shows permeative invasion of the cortex with transcortical extension of tumor and a multilamellar low-signal-intensity periosteal reaction *(arrow)*.

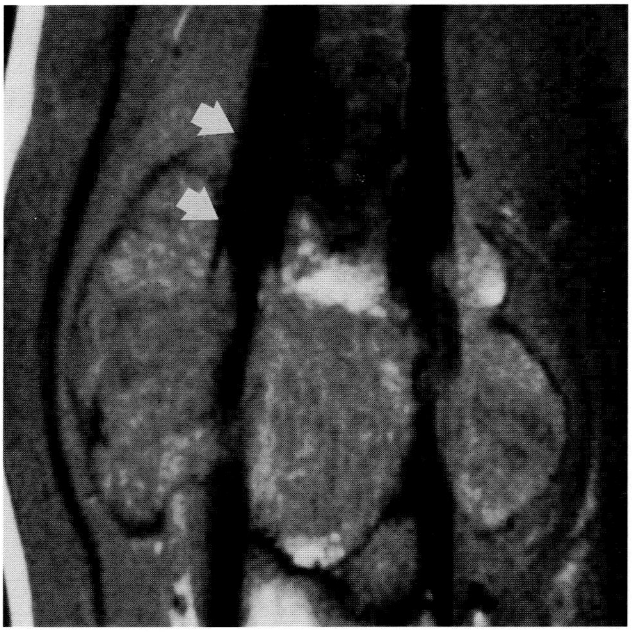

FIG. 9-15. Codman's triangle. A coronal T2-weighted image of an osteogenic sarcoma shows extensive intramedullary tumor that has broken through the cortex and invaded the adjacent soft tissues. Codman's triangle is shown as a triangle of elevated periosteum *(arrows)* that is truncated by tumor destruction. The presence of Codman's triangle indicates an aggressive process such as a malignant bone tumor or infection.

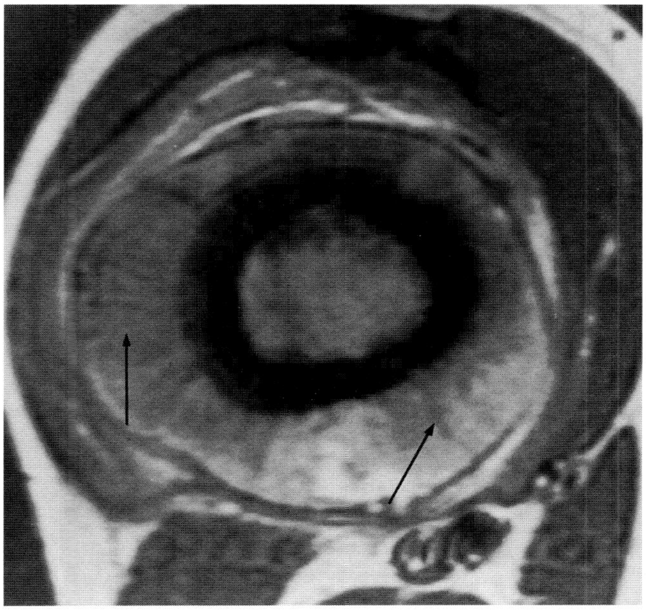

FIG. 9-16. Sunburst periosteal reaction. A proton-density-weighted transverse image shows aggressive extraosseous extension of tumor containing multiple linear radiating low-signal-intensity strands *(arrows)*, typical of sunburst periosteal reaction. Tumor permeation of the bone cortex is also present.

associated with malignant, inflammatory, or infectious tumors; however, many benign tumors can also produce impressive edema (e.g., osteoid osteoma, chondroblastoma) (29,30). In the setting of a malignant tumor, it is impossible to differentiate benign fluid exudate from malignant tumor infiltration, even with intravenous gadolinium chelate enhancement. Although some researchers have described more rapid enhancement in ''malignant'' edema than in ''benign'' edema on dynamic contrast-enhanced studies, this technique does not appear sufficiently accurate to alter the staging of individual patients (16,31–34). With regard to staging, the peritumoral edema should be assumed to be malignant and should be excised in any attempt at curative surgery (35). Preoperative chemotherapy or radiotherapy often causes significant regression of the peritumoral edema. Thus, reimaging after adjuvant treatment often displays a smaller region of tumor involvement and allows a more localized curative resection (36,37).

MRI CHARACTERISTICS OF TUMORS AND TUMORLIKE CONDITIONS THAT OCCUR ABOUT THE KNEE

Bone Tumors

It is not our intention to present a detailed discussion of all bone tumors; rather, we shall discuss common tumors that demonstrate a predilection for arising about the knee joint. Each tumor and its MRI characteristics will be described, because MRI is able to provide valuable information about the axial location and compartmentalization of primary bone tumors. These lesions will be subcategorized according to their anatomic location.

Epiphyseal Lesions

Epiphyseal lesions are discrete tumors arising within the epiphysis, to the exclusion of the metaphysis—usually chondroblastomas, lymphoma, or metastases. Giant cell tumors are characterized by their extension to the articular cortical margin of the epiphysis but at presentation invariably involve the adjacent metaphysis. Geodes, ganglia, and osteomyelitis may also produce focal lesions in the epiphysis.

Chondroblastoma

Chondroblastomas are relatively rare tumors arising in the second to third decades of life (29,38–41). These lesions affect men more often than women in a ratio of 2:1. Chondroblastomas demonstrate a predilection for the epiphysis of the proximal femur, humerus, and tibia. Although lesions tend to be confined to the epiphysis, rare extension to the metaphysis may occur (42).

Chondroblastomas are typically presented to the pathologist as multiple fragments of reddish-brown tissue obtained from curettage of the lesion. Microscopic examination reveals nodular deposits of chondroid matrix material that frequently calcifies in a characteristic ''chicken-wire'' form. The cellular component may predominate and matrix is sometimes scanty. The neoplastic cells are hapazardly arranged sheets of round, oval, and polygonal chondroblasts that contain eosinophilic cytoplasm. Mitotic figures are usually evident within the tumor cells, but atypical mitoses are exceptionally rare. Scattered osteoclastic giant cells are also present within the tumor (43–45).

On MRI, chondroblastomas appear as well-defined, circumscribed regions of low signal intensity on T1-weighted images and increased signal intensity on T2-weighted images (Fig. 9-17) (46). The lesion is geographic and may demonstrate evidence of marginal T2 shortening consistent with trabecular new bone formation. Chondroid matrix calcification is seen in approximately 50% of chondroblastomas and appears as focal regions of flocculent or flecklike T2 shortening on all pulse sequences (47). When such lesions are eccentric and subcortical, they may be associated with a focal region of periosteal new bone formation. A low-signal-intensity region on T1-weighted images transecting the lesion is consistent with a fracture complication. This may also be suggested when buckling occurs at the endosteal margin of the tumor. On rare occasions, chondroblastomas may demonstrate aggressive characteristics with breach of the overlying cortical bone and intra-articular invasion (48).

Clear-cell chondrosarcoma is a rare tumor that shares

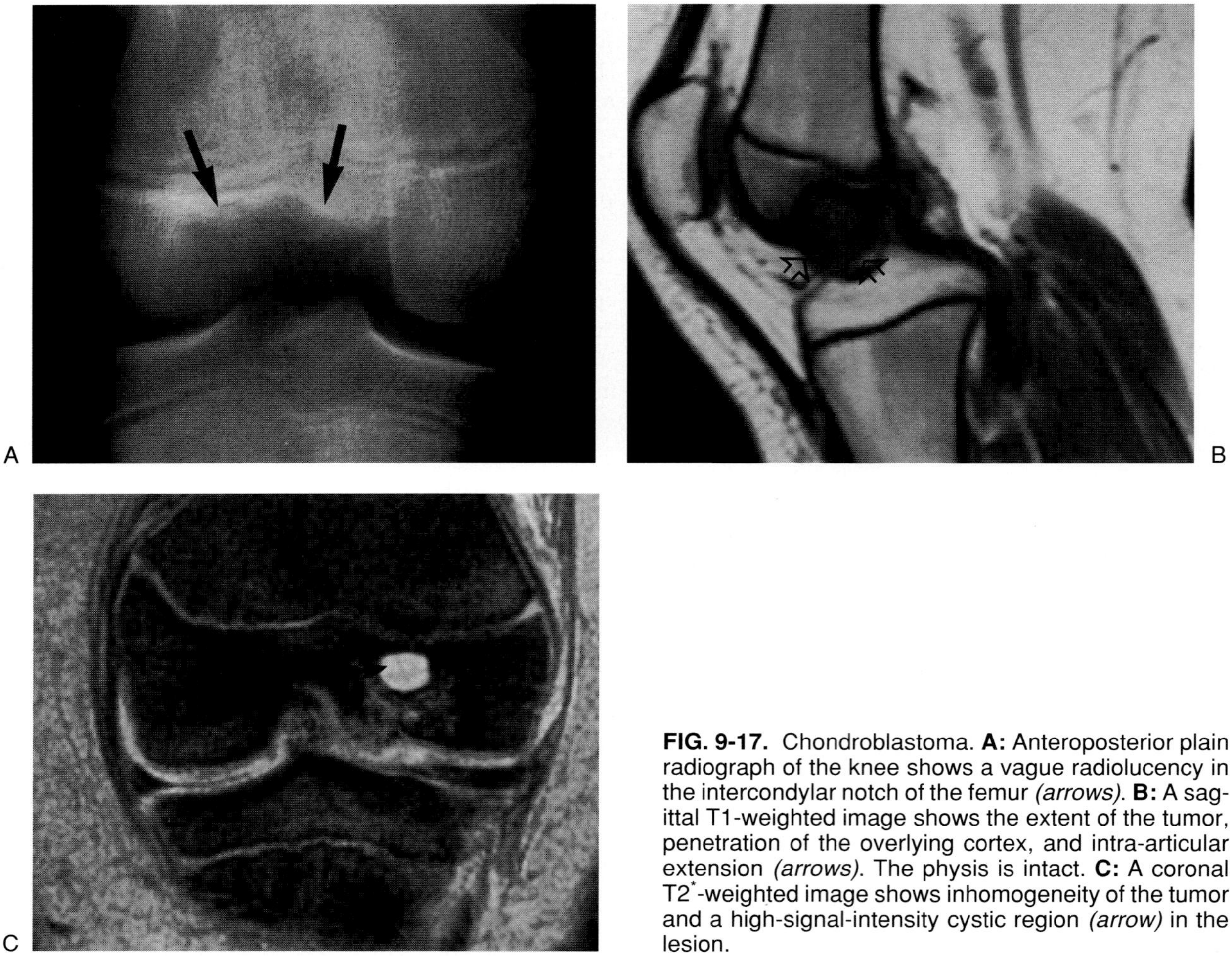

FIG. 9-17. Chondroblastoma. **A:** Anteroposterior plain radiograph of the knee shows a vague radiolucency in the intercondylar notch of the femur *(arrows)*. **B:** A sagittal T1-weighted image shows the extent of the tumor, penetration of the overlying cortex, and intra-articular extension *(arrows)*. The physis is intact. **C:** A coronal T2*-weighted image shows inhomogeneity of the tumor and a high-signal-intensity cystic region *(arrow)* in the lesion.

many of the characteristics of chondroblastoma; however, it tends to occur in older patients, with a mean age of 39 years at diagnosis. Clear-cell chondrosarcoma is most common in the proximal epiphyses of the femur and humerus (49). The tumor is geographic and lytic, with relatively little extraosseous extent. This tumor has a much better prognosis than classic chondrosarcoma (50).

Giant Cell Tumor

Giant cell tumors (GCTs) arise in the metaphysis, but almost invariably have progressed to contact the articular surface at the time of diagnosis (51). These common tumors have the following radiographic features that allow the correct diagnosis to be made in the majority of cases: a lytic lesion in the end of a long bone, extensive contact with the articular surface, no matrix calcification, eccentric location, and a nonsclerotic margin (52,53). MRI examination shows many of these features, plus such findings as intratumoral hemorrhage and cyst formation, which is common in giant cell tumors (51,54).

GCTs occur most commonly in the third and fourth decades of life with equal male and female incidence. The most common sites of origin are the distal femur and proximal tibia, with 50% of GCTs occurring around the knee (54). GCTs are often treated with curettage; however, local recurrence has been reported in up to 50% of cases. The use of adjuvant cryotherapy reduces the recurrence rate to approximately 10–15% by ablating residual tumor located beyond the curettage margin (55–57). Approximately 5% of GCTs are malignant, with most malignant GCTs developing many years after radiation treatment of an initially benign GCT. Very rarely, a histologically benign GCT can produce lung metastases (58,59). The risk of recurrence or malignant degeneration cannot be reliably predicted from radiographic or histologic analysis (57).

Histologically, GCT is characterized by numerous large osteoclast-like cells scattered throughout the tumor. These cells have numerous (often more than 20) uniform nuclei and abundant cytoplasm. The giant cells are located within sheets of spindle-shaped fibroblastic cells. Mitoses may be numerous in actively proliferating lesions. Thin-walled capillaries, vascular spaces, and hemorrhagic areas are common, frequently resembling the vascular spaces of an aneurysmal bone cyst. The differential diagnosis of giant cell tumor is vast, as a wide range of benign and malignant bone tumors contain giant cells. Therefore, it is especially important to correlate the clinical, radiographic, and surgical findings with the pathologic appearance before a final diagnosis is rendered (60–62).

GCTs are usually large at presentation and show diminished signal intensity on T1-weighted images and increased signal intensity on T2-weighted images (Fig. 9-18) (54,63,64). The medullary fat–tumor interface may be discrete or poorly defined, with evidence of invasive tumor stranding of the medullary fat. Lesions rarely demonstrate evidence of intramedullary or soft-tissue edema. There is a tendency to expand the overlying cortex, with evidence of relatively fine trabeculae arising from the endosteal interface extending within the tumor. Despite obviously aggressive behavior with transcortical extension and focal regional endosteal cortical tunneling, a discrete periosteal reaction is uncommon. The extension to the subarticular cortical bone surface is well appreciated on the multiplanar images provided by MRI (Fig. 9-19). Areas of hemorrhage or cystic necrosis are often seen within GCTs on MRI; these features may suggest degeneration into an associated aneurysmal bone cyst (65). Aggressive features such as cortical destruction, paraosseous tumor, and tumor invading an adjacent joint are occasionally seen and are easily recognized on MRI.

Metaphyseal Lesions

Chondrosarcoma

Chondrosarcomas consist of sarcomatous stroma with cartilaginous differentiation (66,67). Radiographically, chondrosarcomas can be classified by location as central (intramedullary) versus peripheral (arising from osteochondromas or cortical chondromas), and described as primary or secondary (arising from a preexisting lesion) (68). Histologically, chondrosarcomas are described by grade and by tissue type (myxoid, dedifferentiated, clear-cell, mesenchymal, etc.). Classic primary intramedullary chondrosarcomas occur most commonly in the fifth to sixth decades of life and affect men more frequently than women with a ratio of 1.5 to 2 : 1 (69). Secondary chondrosarcomas arise in preexisting benign lesions such as enchondromas, osteochondromas, or periosteal chondromas and occur over a broader age range.

Low-grade chondrosarcomas are characterized pathologically by multinodular masses of chondroid tissue that resemble hyaline cartilage. Higher-grade chondrosarcomas may exhibit areas of myxoid tissue, necrosis, or hemorrhage. Histologically, the chondroid tissue of a chondrosarcoma is more cellular than hyaline cartilage. The neoplastic tissue extends between and around adjacent bone trabeculae in an ''infiltrative'' pattern. Cytologic atypia and pleomorphism are common in higher-grade tumors. Chondrosarcomas are graded according to the degree of cellularity, cellular pleo-

A

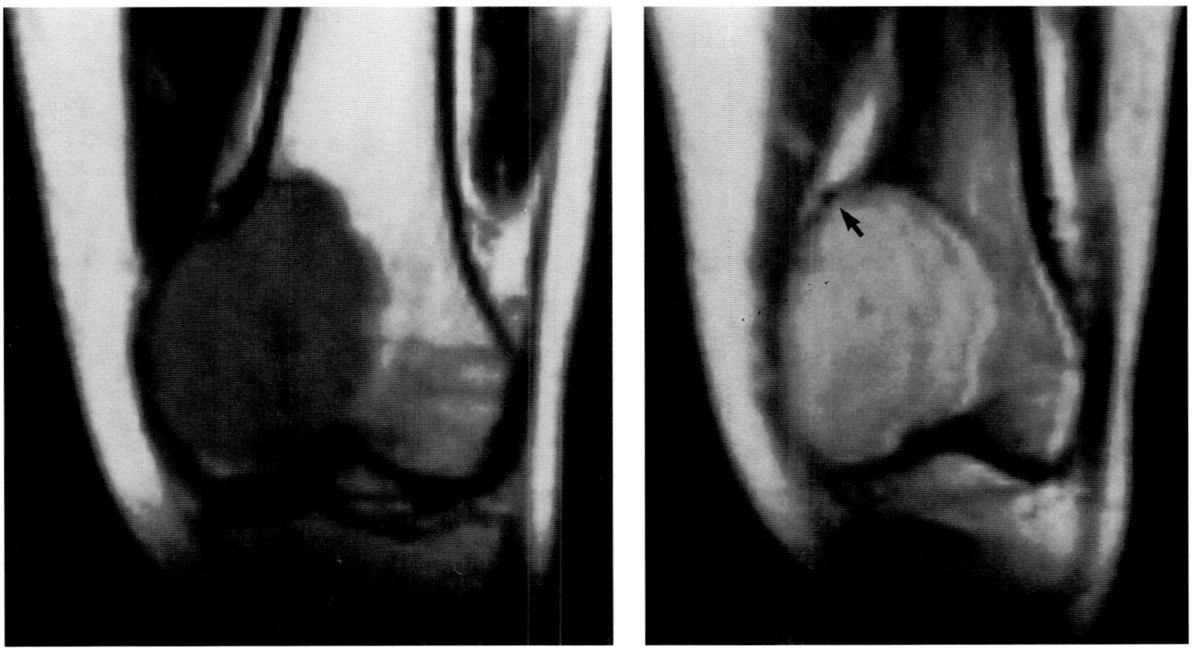

B

FIG. 9-18. Giant cell tumor. **A:** A T1-weighted coronal image shows a large mass in the metaphysis of the distal femur with extension to the articular surface of the medial femoral condyle. The tumor–medullary fat interface is geographic, with no reactive trabecular new bone; this type of margin is typical of giant cell tumor. **B:** A T2-weighted coronal image shows inhomogeneous high signal intensity in the lesion with ballooning of the overlying cortex and endosteal scalloping *(short arrow)*. Peritumoral edema and periosteal reaction are absent, typical of giant cell tumor.

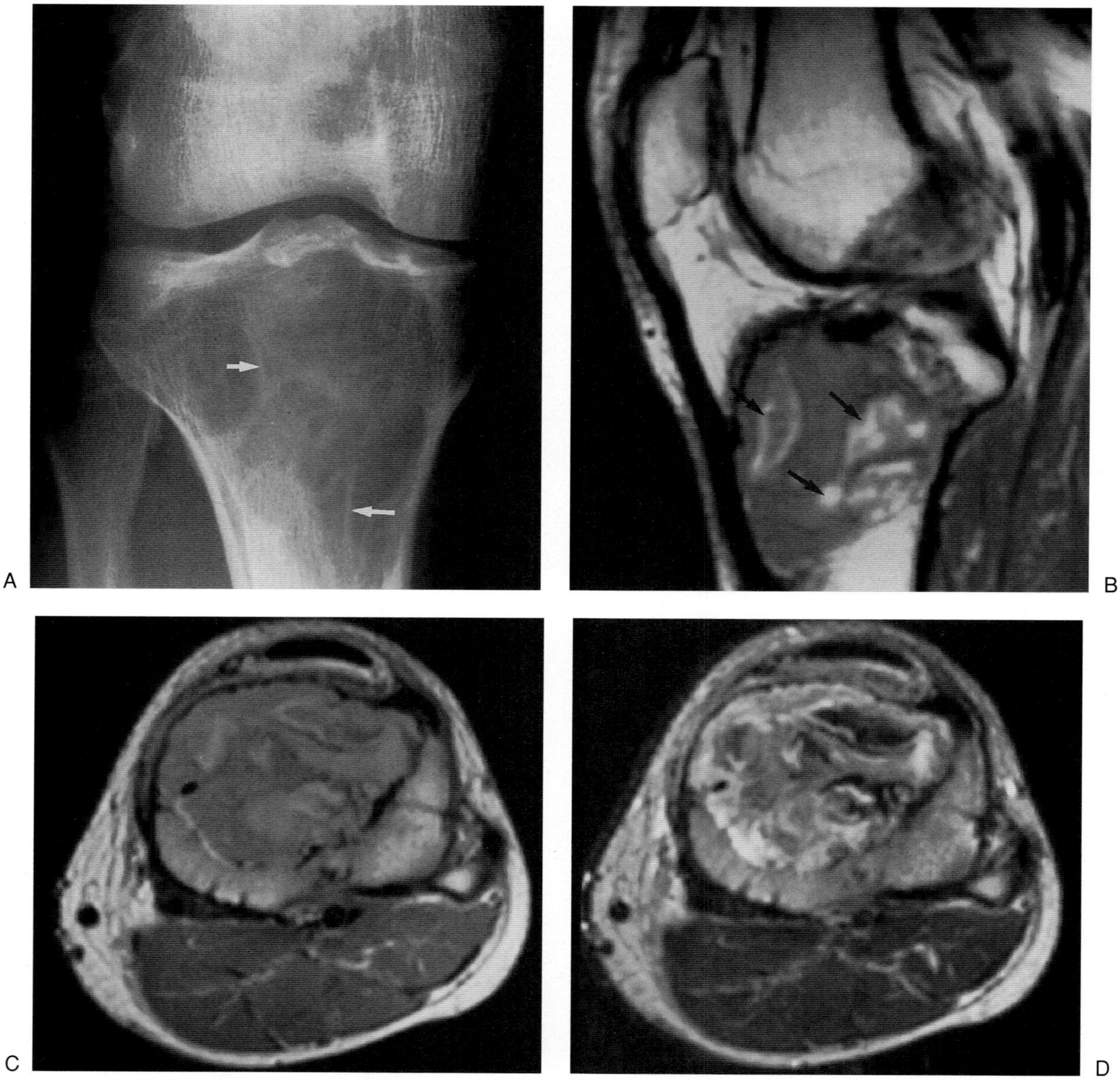

FIG. 9-19. Intratumoral hemorrhage within giant cell tumor. **A:** A plain radiograph shows a typical appearance of giant cell tumor, with extension to the articular surface, well-defined nonsclerotic margins, and lack of matrix calcification. Pseudotrabeculation is present *(arrows)*, representing strands of normal reactive bone at the margin of the tumor, rather than true intratumoral trabeculae. **B:** Sagittal T1-weighted image clearly shows the tumor extent to the articular surface. High-signal-intensity foci of methemoglobin are present in the tumor *(arrows)*. Transverse proton density **(C)** and T2-weighted **(D)** images show a complex signal appearance caused by multiple foci of intratumoral hemorrhage.

morphism and mitotic rate and are described by tissue type (myxoid, dedifferentiated, clear-cell, mesenchymal, etc.). The major differential diagnosis of low-grade chondrosarcoma is enchondroma; low-grade chondrosarcomas are identified on the basis of an infiltrative growth pattern and radiologic evidence of bone destruction (70,71).

Primary chondrosarcomas originate within the medullary cavity of the metaphysis, but with progression will involve the epiphyseal and diametaphyseal marrow spaces. High-grade lesions often demonstrate poor fat–tumor margination within the medullary cavity, reflecting the underlying aggressiveness of the tumor. Evidence of endosteal destruction, cortical tunneling, and transcortical extension is often present at the time of presentation. Chondrosarcomas appear on MRI as lobulated lesions of low signal intensity on T1-weighted images and very high signal intensity on T2-

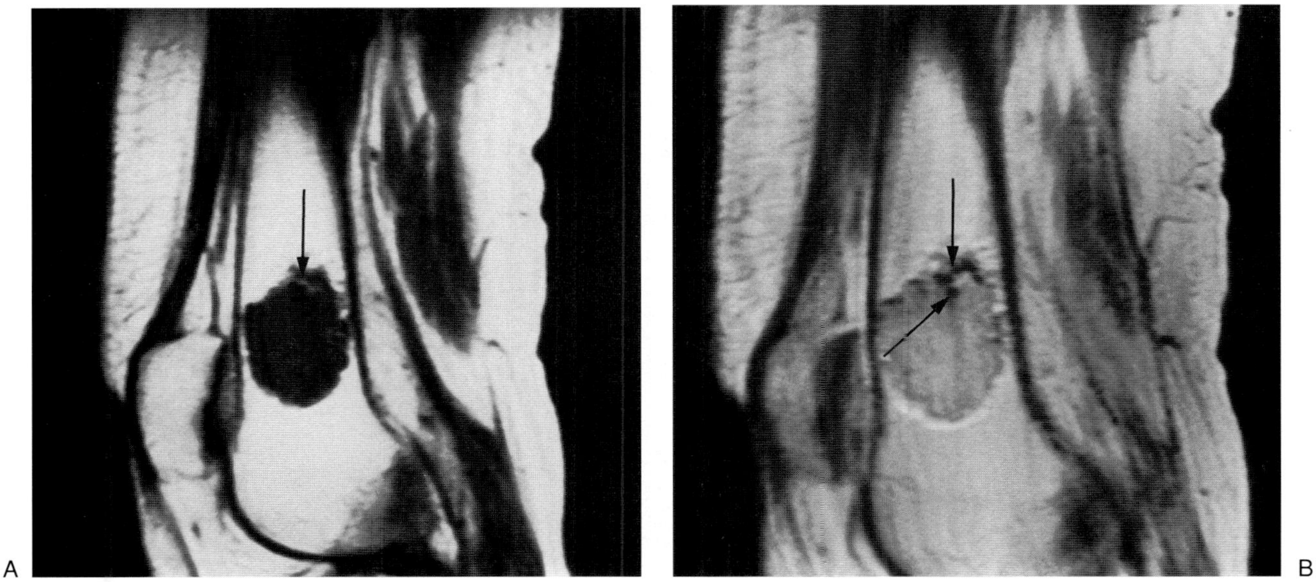

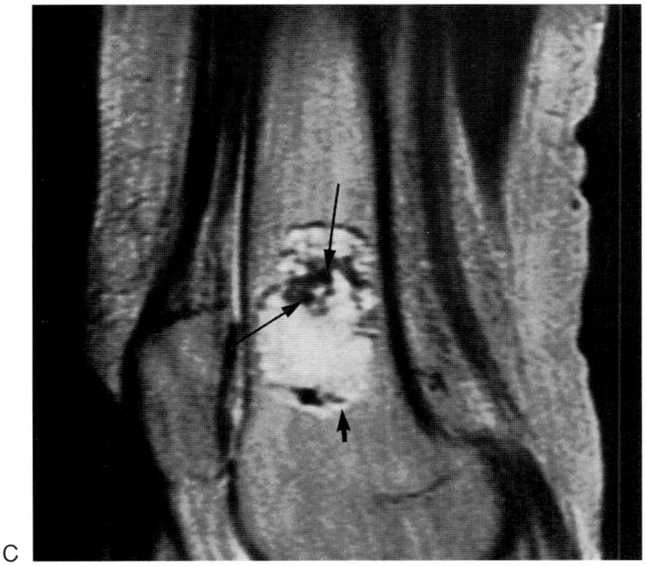

FIG. 9-20. Secondary central chondrosarcoma. **A:** A T1-weighted sagittal image shows a discrete, low-signal-intensity intramedullary chondrosarcoma. The inferior pole of the tumor represents chondrosarcoma, whereas the inhomogeneous appearance of the superior pole of the tumor *(arrow)* is typical of an enchondroma. **B:** A proton-density-weighted sagittal image shows flocculent low-signal-intensity chondroid calcifications in the superior pole of the tumor *(arrows)*. The chondrosarcoma displaces the chondroic calcification. **C:** A T2-weighted sagittal image clearly shows the bimorphic nature of the mass, with high signal intensity present in the chondrosarcoma and calcifications *(long arrows)* present in the residual portions of the enchondroma. Prominent chemical-shift artifact is noted at the inferior boundary of the tumor *(arrow)*.

weighted images (68,72–74). These signal characteristics are nonspecific; however, detection of chondroid matrix calcification is often diagnostically helpful. This appears as regions of flocculent or flecklike T2 shortening on gradient-echo or T2-weighted images (Fig. 9-20). In most cases, the finding of typical ''chondroid-type'' calcifications is a reliable indicator of a cartilaginous tumor, although this pattern of calcification has also been reported in plasmacytomas (75). Although it was originally suggested that tumors of hyaline cartilage origin have a characteristic septated lobular appearance on T2-weighted images due to lobular fibrous septation, these features are not invariable, and other malignant primary bone tumors may have this appearance (76). A typical pattern of septal and marginal enhancement has been described after intravenous administration of gadolinium chelates (77,78).

Secondary Chondrosarcomas

Malignant degeneration into a chondrosarcoma may occur in osteochondromas, enchondromas, or periosteal chondromas (79–81). Some authors believe that the majority of chondrosarcomas arise in this fashion; however, it is often impossible to prove or exclude the presence of an underlying benign lesion once a destructive chondrosarcoma has developed (69). Uncommonly, serial imaging studies are available that display expansion and destructive change superimposed upon a previously quiescent lesion. The development of a malignant tumor within an enchondroma or superimposed on an osteochondroma is characterized by disorganization of the preexisting lesion, destruction of the bony stalk, and enlargement of the cartilage cap (Fig. 9-21). A cartilage cap thickness greater than 2 cm is highly suggestive of malignant degeneration (82).

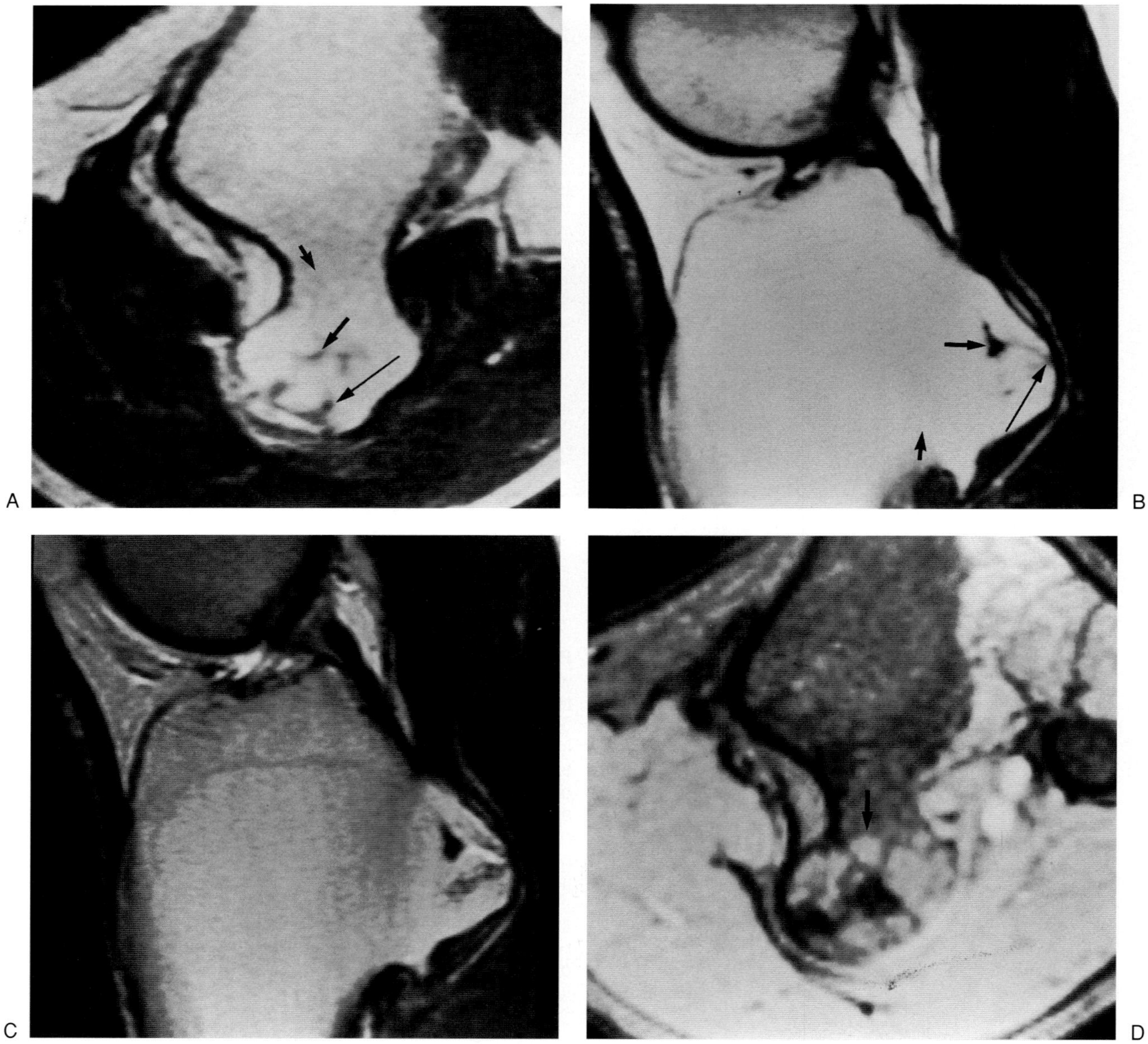

FIG. 9-21. Secondary peripheral chondrosarcoma. T1-weighted transverse **(A)** and sagittal **(B)** images of the proximal tibia show a sessile osteochondroma located on the posterior surface of the tibia. The medullary canal of the tibia is confluent with the stem of the osteochondroma *(short arrow).* The cartilage cap appears as a region of complex high signal intensity. Focal regions of low signal intensity are present centrally and peripherally *(long arrows)* in the cartilage cap, representing chondroid calcifications. No destructive or invasive features are present. **C:** A T2-weighted sagittal image shows clear distinction between the high-signal-intensity cartilage cap and the lower-signal-intensity medullary fat. **D:** A $T2^*$-weighted transverse image shows the interface *(arrow)* between the fat in the stalk of the osteochondroma and the cartilage cap. The cartilage cap exceeds 2 cm in thickness; this finding is strongly suggestive of malignant transformation.

With enchondromas, displacement of the central chondral calcification is a useful sign of malignant degeneration (see Fig. 9-20). The displacing lesion invariably demonstrates evidence of diminished signal intensity on T1-weighted images and increased signal intensity on T2-weighted images. It may, however, be difficult to differentiate between a relatively cellular enchondroma and chondrosarcomatous transformation within a preexisting enchondroma on signal characteristics alone (Fig. 9-22); histologic differentiation of enchondroma from low-grade chondrosarcoma can also be difficult (70). Evidence of interval change on imaging studies or a clinical history of pain is strongly suggestive of

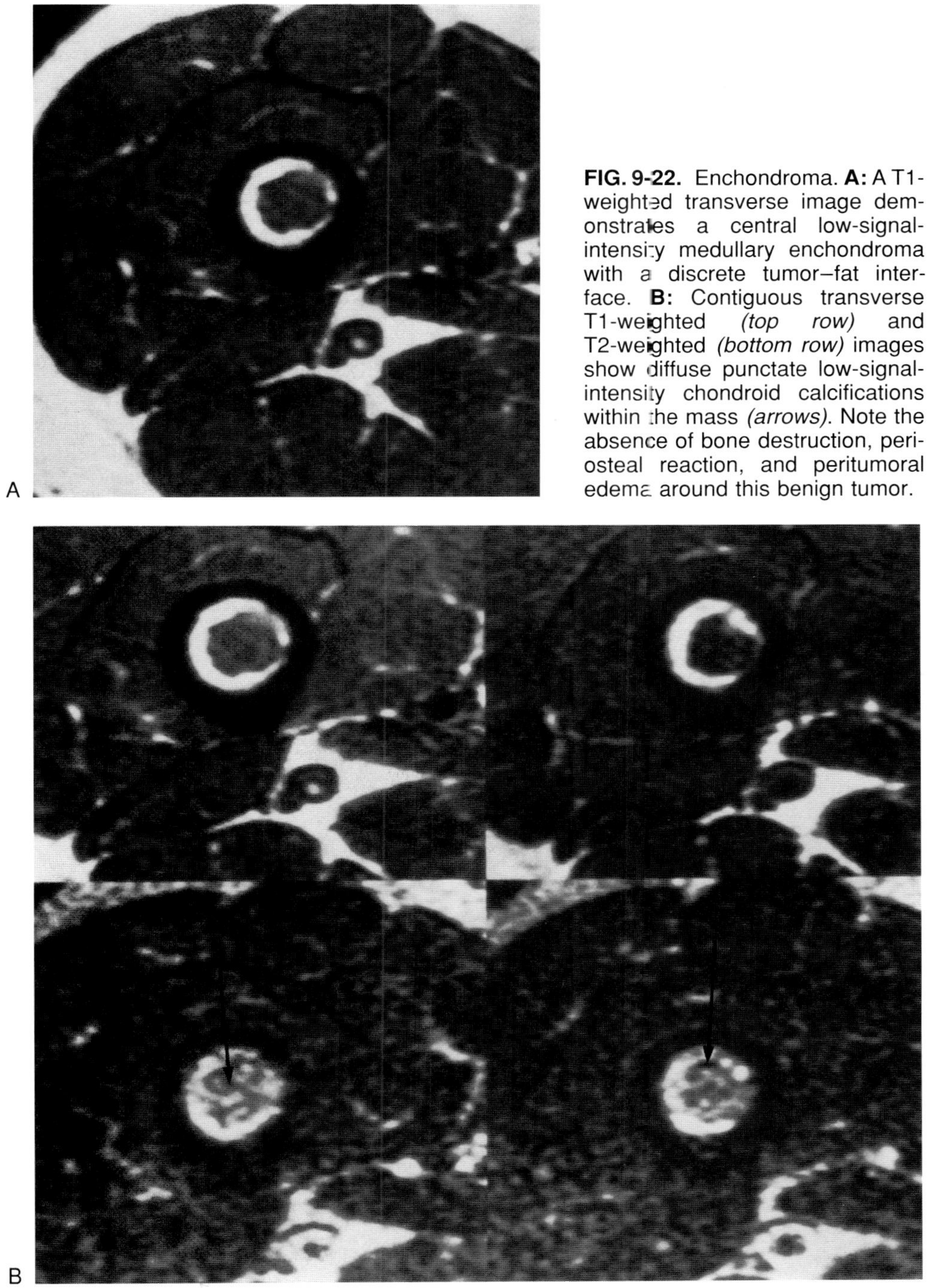

FIG. 9-22. Enchondroma. **A:** A T1-weighted transverse image demonstrates a central low-signal-intensity medullary enchondroma with a discrete tumor–fat interface. **B:** Contiguous transverse T1-weighted *(top row)* and T2-weighted *(bottom row)* images show diffuse punctate low-signal-intensity chondroid calcifications within the mass *(arrows)*. Note the absence of bone destruction, periosteal reaction, and peritumoral edema around this benign tumor.

malignancy. On MRI the supervening chondrosarcoma may have fewer foci of chondral calcification than the preexisting enchondroma and may be more inhomogeneous.

Identification of chondrosarcomatous degeneration within an antecedent enchondroma or osteochondroma may be aided by using intravenous gadolinium chelates. Higher-grade tumors are characterized by increased vascularity and will consequently enhance disproportionately to the relatively hypovascular benign cartilage (77).

Fibrosarcoma

Fibrosarcoma is a rare malignant primary bone tumor arising from fibrogenic precursors and is characterized by variable proportions of fibrous tissue and fibroblasts, with no osteoid or chondroid matrix (83,84). These tumors occur with equal frequency in men and women, most frequently between the fourth and sixth decades of life. Long tubular bones are the site of origin in approximately 50% of cases, with the distal femur and proximal tibia being the most frequent locations (84). Twenty-five to 30% of fibrosarcomas are secondary to preexisting lesions such as bone infarcts, radiation necrosis, fibrous dysplasia, osteomyelitis, or Paget's disease (85–87).

Fibrosarcomas are characteristically intramedullary, metaphyseal lesions with variable degrees of transcortical and medullary extension, depending on the aggressivity of the lesion. Fibrosarcomas show low signal intensity on T1-weighted images and variable signal intensity on T2-weighted images; the low-grade lesions tend to have low to intermediate signal intensity on T2-weighted images because of a predominantly fibrous tissue matrix, whereas high-grade lesions usually have high signal intensity on T2-weighted images as a result of cellularity and edema (88). No chondroid or osteoid matrix is produced; however, fibrosarcomas do have an unusual propensity to contain sequestra (87). Permeative destruction of the adjacent cortex, with ballooning of the cortex, transcortical extension, and soft-tissue mass formation are common in these aggressive tumors.

Histologically, fibrosarcomas contain bundles of spindle-shaped fibroblasts with a variable degree of nuclear pleomorphism and atypica. Regions of necrosis and hemorrhage are common in higher grade tumors. In contrast with MFH, giant cells are uncommon. Low-grade fibrosarcoma may resemble aggressive fibromatosis or desmoplastic fibroma. Fibrosarcomas are graded on the basis of cellularity, number of mitoses, degree of nuclear pleomorphism, and presence of necrosis (85,89).

Malignant Fibrous Histiocytoma

Malignant fibrous histiocytoma (MFH) is an uncommon primary bone tumor, in contradistinction to its frequent occurrence as a soft-tissue neoplasm. This tumor is characterized histologically by varying degrees of dense collagen fiber formation, differentiated fibrocytes, and mixed inflammatory cellular infiltrate (90,91). The vast majority of MFH cases are high-grade tumors with destructive and invasive features.

MFHs are more common in men, with a peak incidence in the sixth decade of life. These tumors usually arise de novo, but up to 25% of cases occur secondary to underlying conditions, such as radiation, avascular necrosis, fibrous dysplasia, osteomyelitis, or Paget's disease (Fig. 9-23) (84,86,87). The femur and the tibia are the most common sites of origin (90).

Grossly, MFHs show a destructive pattern of growth, often with extension through the cortex into adjacent soft tissues. Histologically, the most common appearance of MFH is a pleomorphic storiform pattern comprised of bundles of spindle cells. A characteristic feature is the presence of numerous bizarre giant cells that impart a histiocytoid appearance. Areas of hemorrhage, necrosis, and cyst formation are common. No osteoid or chondroid matrix is present.

The histologic differential diagnosis of MFH includes high-grade osteosarcoma, high-grade fibrosarcoma, dedifferentiated chondrosarcoma, and metastatic sarcomatoid carcinoma of renal, pancreatic, or pulmonary origin (91).

On MRI, MFHs are typically centered within the medullary cavity of the metaphysis with aggressive intramedullary extension and cortical destruction seen in most cases (90). The medullary–tumor interface demonstrates variable degrees of definition, with aggressive lesions demonstrating epiphyseal and diaphyseal extension, with a poorly defined fat–tumor interface and marginating marrow edema. Transcortical extension with paraosseous soft-tissue mass formation is seen in the majority of cases; however, periosteal reaction is often lacking (89,92).

The signal characteristics of MFH have not been well described in the literature; in our experience, these tumors often have areas of whorled low-signal intensity on T2-weighted and gradient-echo images consistent with central collagen matrix. This feature is likely more common in low-grade tumors, because these tumors histologically show more collagen formation. MFHs rarely contain calcification.

The benign intraosseous counterparts of MFH are benign fibrous histiocytoma, intraosseous desmoid, and desmoplastic fibroma. Benign fibrous histiocytoma usually appears as a well-defined lesion with no destructive or infiltrative features (84,93). Desmoplastic fibromas have a more aggressive appearance with bone destruction and expansion; however, distant metastases do not occur (94,95). In our limited experience with these rare lesions, a central whorled region of low signal intensity may be seen, representing the dominant fibrous matrix (Figs. 9-24 and 9-25).

Osteosarcoma

Osteosarcoma is the second most common primary malignant bone tumor after myeloma. These tumors are characterized histologically by the production of osteoid or bone matrix by the tumor (96). Osteosarcomas occur most commonly during the second and third decades of life, with a male to female ratio of 1.5:1. Approximately 40–50% of lesions occur about the knee (97). Osteosarcomas are described by a number of features, including origin (primary, secondary), location (intraosseous, periosteal, parosteal, extraosseous), and histologic features (telangiectatic, small-cell, low-grade, etc.) (98). The most common subtype of osteosarcoma is the primary intraosseous type; this is commonly referred to as "classic" or "conventional" osteosarcoma.

All types of osteosarcoma are characterized histologically by the production of osteoid and woven bone. These tumors contain spindle cells, polygonal cells, and often osteoclastic giant cells. Areas of necrosis and hemorrhage are common. A variety of histologic subtypes have been described: (a) osteoblastic—characterized by the production of abundant osteoid and woven bone; (b) chondroblastic—characterized by production of cartilage with minimal osteoid formation;

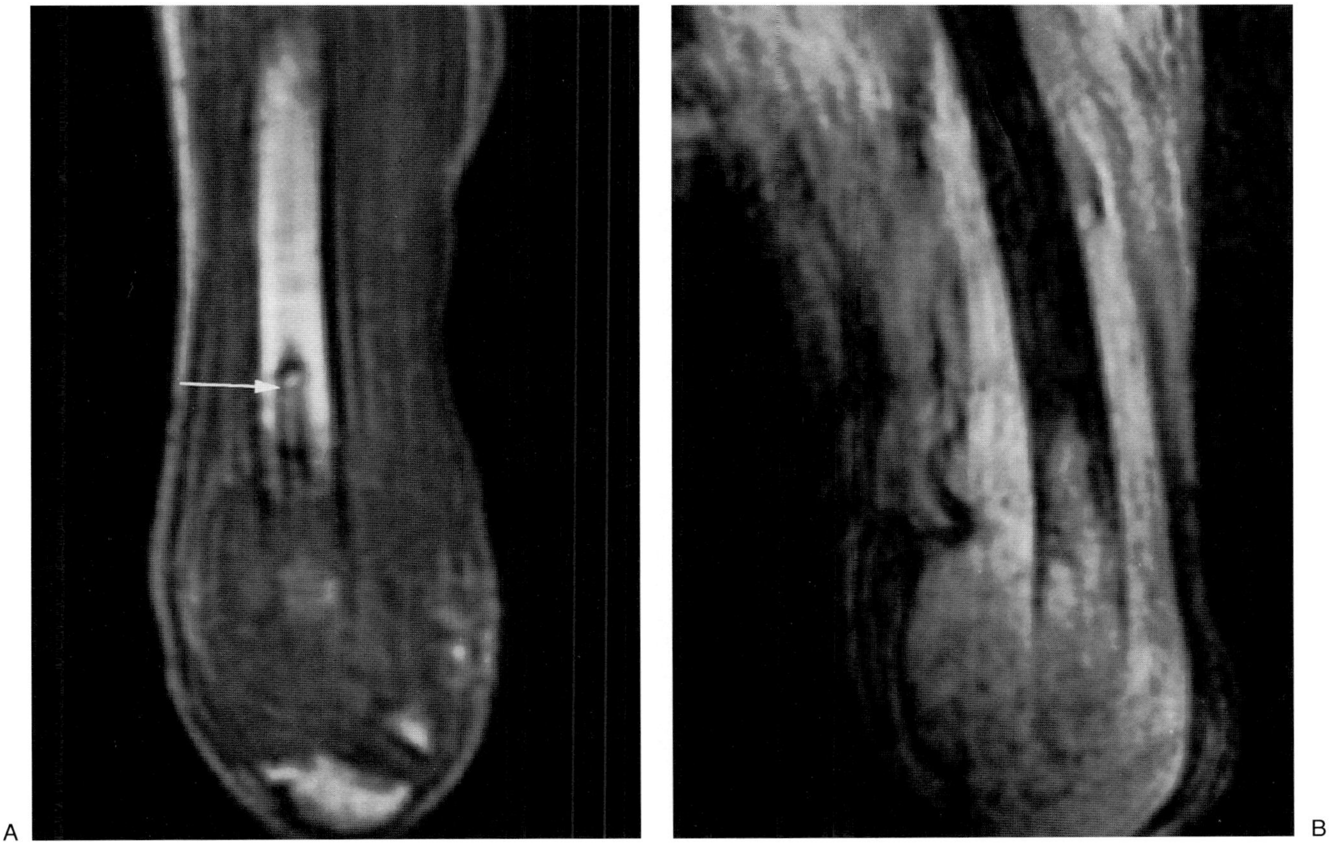

FIG. 9-23. Malignant fibrous histiocytoma secondary to an underlying chronic bone infarct. **A:** A coronal T1-weighted image shows a destructive mass in the distal femur with extraosseous extension. The low-signal-intensity rim of a chronic bone infarct is visible in the femoral diaphysis *(arrow)*. **B:** A sagittal T2*-weighted gradient-echo image shows marked bone destruction and periosseous tumor extension.

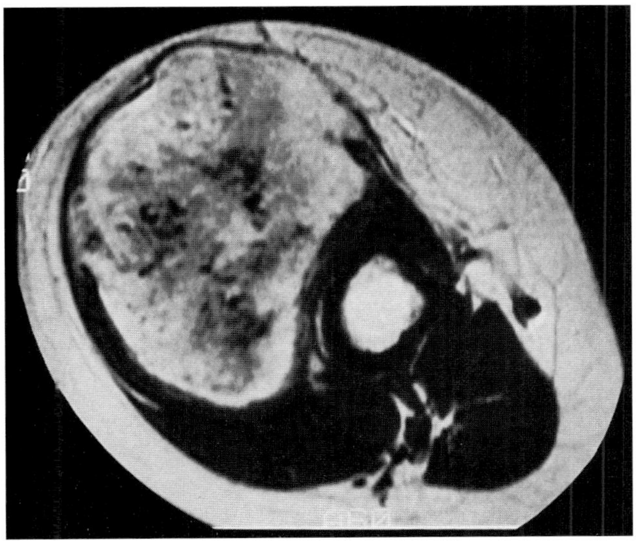

FIG. 9-24. Extraosseous desmoid. A T2-weighted transverse image shows a large extraosseous desmoid in the muscles of the distal arm. The tumor is of predominantly increased signal intensity, with focal whorled low-signal-intensity regions representing collagen tracts.

(c) fibroblastic—characterized by the production of a dense collagenous matrix; (d) telangiectatic—characterized by the presence of large vascular spaces and hemorrhagic areas; (e) small cell—characterized by sheets of monotonous small, polygonal cells with minimal osteoid production; (f) giant cell–rich osteosarcoma—this subtype may resemble giant cell tumor of bone. Osteosarcomas are graded on the basis of cellularity, mitotic rate, and nuclear pleomorphism (99–102).

Osteosarcoma is the primary bone tumor most widely studied by MRI (102–106). Osteosarcomas characteristically appear as eccentric metaphyseal regions of low- to intermediate-signal intensity on T1-weighted images and increased signal intensity on T2-weighted images (Fig. 9-26). Variable degrees of axial and longitudinal growth are present within the metaphyseal marrow compartment. The marrow fat–tumor interface may have a range of appearances: in low-grade tumors the margin may be geographic, with or without marginal trabecular new bone formation; higher-grade tumors often show infiltrative margins. Osteosarcoma is characterized by relatively aggressive permeative destruction of the adjacent cortical bone, leading to extension of tumor into the soft tissues. The finding of a relatively small

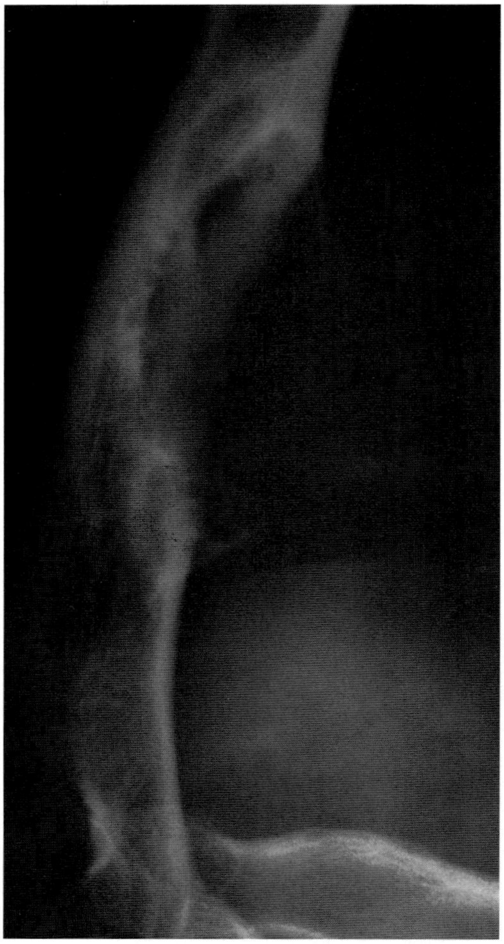

A

FIG. 9-25. Desmoplastic fibroma. **A:** A lateral plain radiograph of the humerus shows an intraosseous tumor with bone destruction and deformity. Marked ballooning of the anterior cortex of the humerus is present. The endosteal margins are thickened and scalloped. T1-weighted **(B)** and T2-weighted **(C)** transverse images show an inhomogeneous intermediate-signal-intensity mass *(arrow)* in the humeral diaphysis, with surrounding cortical thickening. The inhomogeneous low-signal-intensity areas in the mass correspond histologically to dense collagenous tracts.

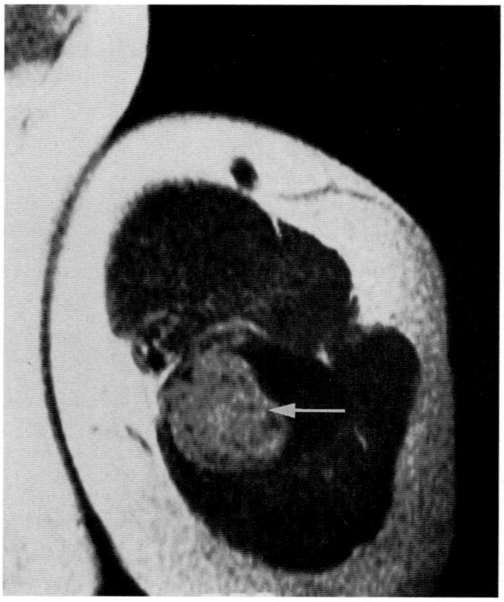

B

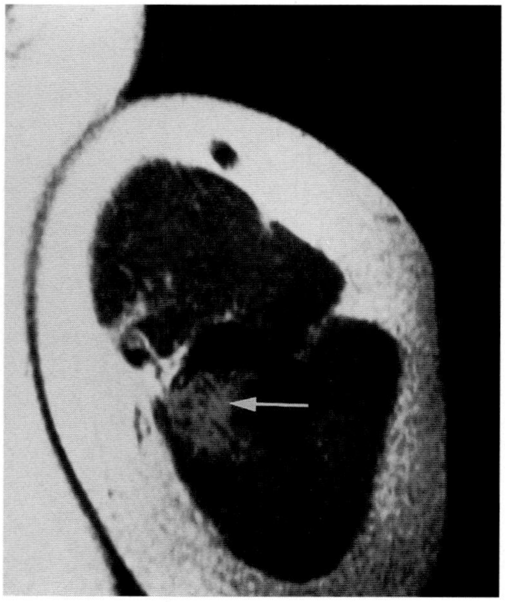

C

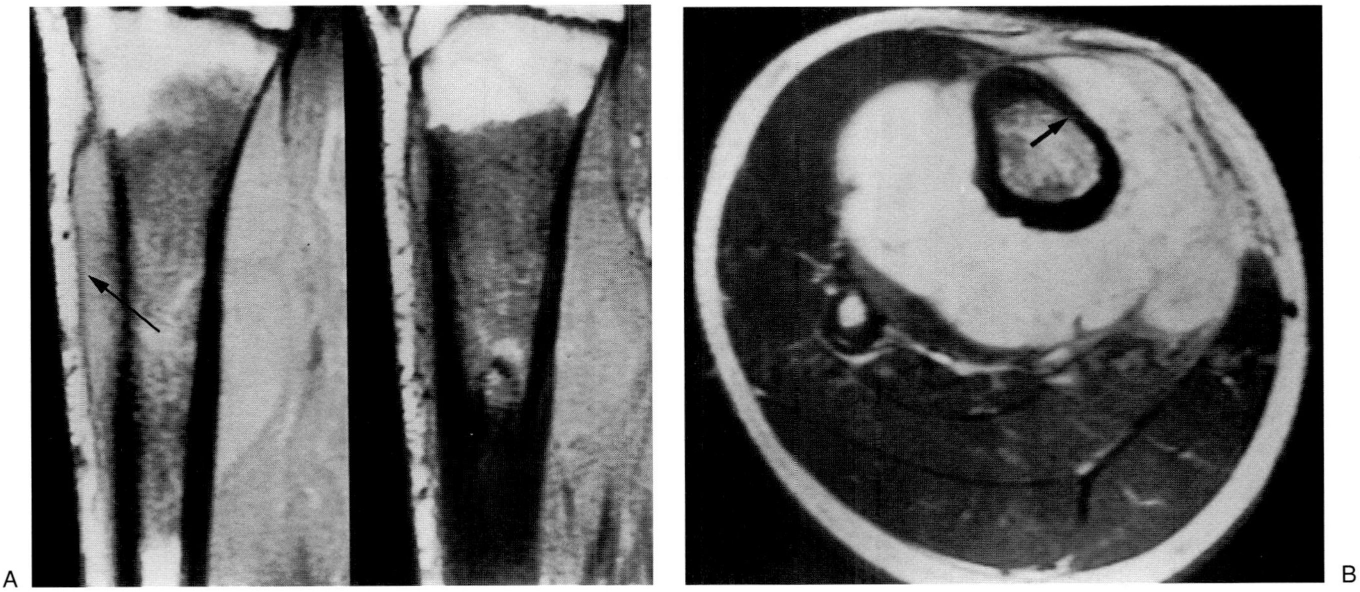

FIG. 9-26. Osteogenic sarcoma. **A:** T1-weighted sagittal images of the proximal tibial metaphysis show an intramedullary mass with extraosseous extension *(arrow)*. The tibial cortex is thinned and permeated by tumor. **B:** A T2-weighted transverse image shows increased signal intensity in the intramedullary and paraosseous tumor. Cortical permeation and endosteal scalloping are visible.

intraosseous tumor with prominent bone destruction and soft-tissue mass is characteristic of osteosarcoma. Circumferential subperiosteal extension may produce a unilamellar periosteal cloak around the affected bone (see Fig. 9-26). Transperiosteal extension may result in bilaminar, multilaminar, or sunburst periosteal reaction, depending on the rate of tumor growth and its induction of periosteal or tumor new bone formation. Osteosarcomas demonstrate varying degrees of ossification evident as regions of diminished signal intensity on all pulse sequences (Fig. 9-27). Such tumor new bone formation may be flocculent, flecklike, or amorphous and may extend to involve the parosteal soft-tissue mass.

The MRI appearance of the medullary tumor may vary, depending on the histologic subtype. For example, sclerosing osteosarcomas have prolific trabecular, endosteal, periosteal, and tumor new bone formation, which appears as diminished signal intensity on T1-weighted images and increased signal intensity on T2-weighted images. A peculiar form of osteosarcoma described as telangiectatic osteosarcoma presents as a relatively discrete eccentric metaphyseal lesion, with a multicystic appearance, demonstrating complex signal characteristics (Fig. 9-28). The cystic cavities have low-signal-intensity margins corresponding to trabecular bone, fibrosis, and hemosiderin (107). Such cavities represent aneurysmal blood-filled spaces that may show as regions of relatively intermediate or increased signal intensity on T1-weighted images and increased signal intensity on T2-weighted images, often containing fluid–fluid levels. Regions of increased signal intensity on T2-weighted and gradient-echo images may be identified consistent with flow-related enhancement of relatively slow-flowing blood within cavernous telangiectatic channels. Telangiectatic osteosarcomas tend not to be associated with significant tumor new bone formation; consequently, extensive regions of T2 shortening would not be a characteristic feature. Approximately 5% of osteosarcomas are of the telangiectatic subtype (99).

Approximately 50% of lesions demonstrate evidence of chondroid or fibroblastic differentiation and are rarely characterized by significant new bone formation. When more than 90% of the tumor is composed of chondroid material, the tumor is designated as a chondroblastic osteosarcoma. These tumors often show the typical lobulated, septated appearance of chondroid matrix (98).

Periosteal Osteosarcoma

Periosteal osteosarcomas comprise 1–2% of all osteosarcomas. These lesions occur with an age and sex distribution similar to that of medullary osteosarcoma (100,108,109). The knee again is the most common location for such tumors. These lesions are characterized by an eccentric periosteal or cortical location in the diaphysis of a long bone and are usually relatively small at time of diagnosis. They rarely demonstrate invasion or destruction of the medullary canal or endosteal cortex. Although periosteal osteosarcomas are usually less aggressive than conventional osteosarcomas, transcortical and/or medullary extension may occur, resulting in a parosteal soft-tissue mass with a discrete, often prominent, periosteal reaction. Such lesions demonstrate diminished signal on T1-weighted images and increased signal

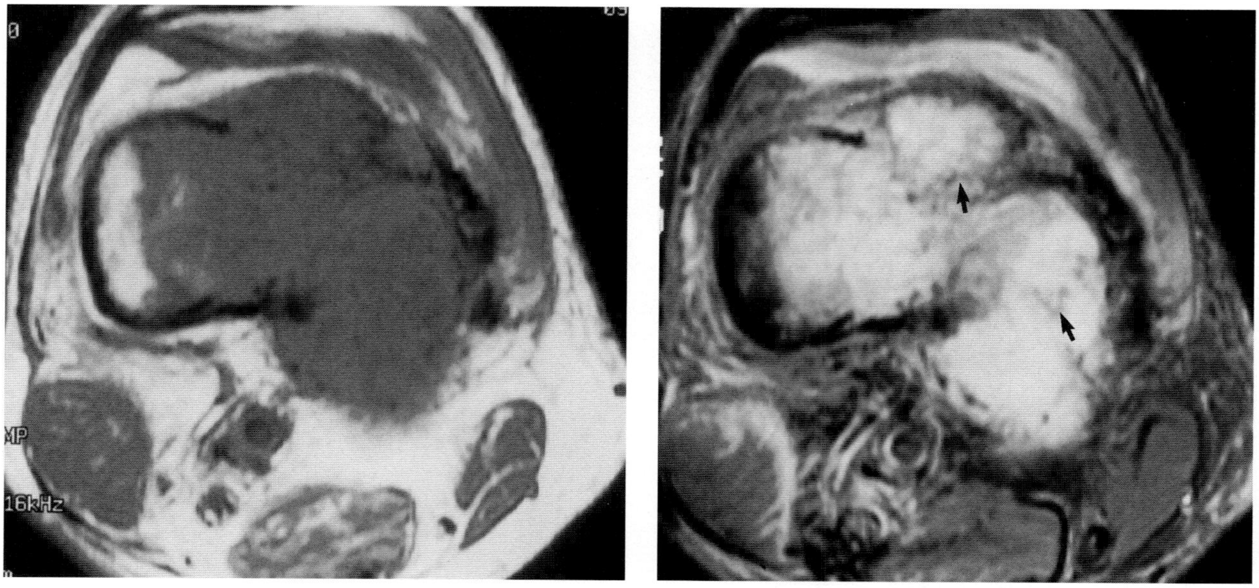

FIG. 9-27. Tumor new bone formation within osteogenic sarcoma. Transverse T1-weighted **(A)** and T2*-weighted **(B)** images show a destructive tumor in the distal femoral metaphysis. The low-signal-intensity strands *(arrow)* within the tumor represent tumor new bone formation.

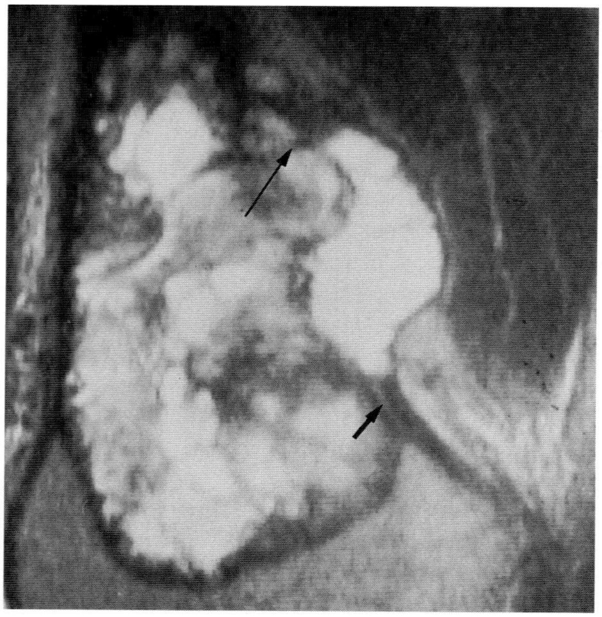

FIG. 9-28. Telangiectatic osteogenic sarcoma. A coronal T2-weighted image of a metaphyseal telangiectatic osteogenic sarcoma shows a large multilocular tumor with complex signal characteristics. The locules of high-signal intensity represent blood within cavernous vascular spaces. Transcortical extension is present *(long arrow)* and an incomplete Codman's triangle is noted inferiorly *(short arrow).*

intensity on T2-weighted images. They are characterized by a fairly high incidence of calcification and/or ossification, prominent chondroid components, and periosteal reaction. The prognosis for patients with periosteal osteosarcoma is better than that for those with conventional osteosarcoma (98).

Parosteal Osteosarcoma

Parosteal osteosarcomas comprise 5% of all osteosarcomas and occur in an older age group, most commonly in the third to fourth decades of life. They occur with equal frequency in men and women, and their location is predominantly about the knee (110,111). The classic location is along the posterior surface of the distal femoral metaphysis, with more than 50% of all parosteal osteosarcomas occurring at this site (98).

These lesions are characterized histologically by low-grade malignant tissue containing a mixture of fibrous, osseous, and cartilaginous elements (101,112,113). These tumors appear to arise from the outer surface of the periosteum or periosteal connective tissue and grow by continuity along the periosteal surface of bone from their site of origin. Although the degree of ossification depends on the relative proportion of fibrous, osseous, or cartilaginous elements, regions of dense ossification are usually present. The ossified regions appear as cloaklike areas of T2 shortening adjacent to the periosteum (Fig. 9-29). The mature ossification may be separated from the underlying periosteum by an intervening region of intermediate-signal intensity on T1-weighted images and intermediate- to high-signal intensity

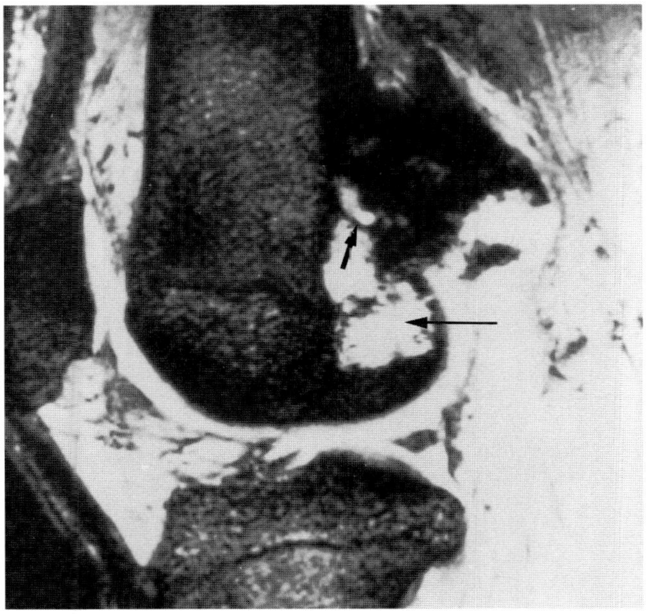

FIG. 9-29. Parosteal osteogenic sarcoma with tumor new bone formation. A sagittal T2*-weighted image shows an extensive cloak of paraosseous low-signal-intensity new bone formation adjacent to the posterior surface of the femoral metaphysis. The high-signal-intensity components *(arrows)* represent nonossified portions of the tumor.

on T2-weighted images, which often represents cellular tumor tissue (Fig. 9-29). Tumors that show minimal ossification and prominent invasion of the underlying bone are usually histologically high grade and have a worse prognosis than heavily ossified noninvasive parosteal osteosarcomas (Fig. 9-30) (113). Cases with extensive invasion and destruction of the underlying bone may be impossible to distinguish from conventional osteosarcomas with transcortical extension. Of note, a significant minority of parosteal osteosarcomas undergo dedifferentiation to high-grade sarcoma; this event significantly increases the likelihood of bone destruction and distant metastases and worsens the patient's prognosis (114).

Desmoplastic Fibroma

Desmoplastic fibromas are very rare benign tumors of fibrous origin, analogous to soft-tissue desmoids (115–117). These lesions occur most commonly in the second and third decades of life, with similar frequency in both men and women. Although they are found less commonly about the knee than elsewhere, when they occur in this location they most commonly involve the proximal tibial metaphysis. Histologically, desmoplastic fibromas consist of small fibroblasts interspersed between thick bundles of mature collagen, which resembles aggressive fibromatosis of soft-tissue origin. Desmoplastic fibroma is differentiated from fibrosarcoma and MFH by the absence of abnormal mitoses, nuclear pleomorphism, and cellular atypia (117,118).

Little information is available on the MRI characteristics of desmoplastic fibromas. They tend to occur eccentrically within bone and have an aggressive expansile appearance (84). Lesions are of inhomogeneous intermediate-signal intensity on T1-weighted images. On T2-weighted and gradient-echo images, regions of dense collagenization are of diminished signal intensity within the lesion, which is generally of intermediate to increased signal intensity (see Fig. 9-25). The endosteal margin is usually geographic, with varying degrees of endosteal new bone formation. This endosteal margin varies in thickness, depending on the growth rate of the tumor (95).

Diametaphyseal Lesions

Enchondroma

Enchondromas within the appendicular skeleton may occur as solitary or multiple lesions. Solitary lesions are most common and occur predominantly between the fourth and sixth decades of life (119,120). In solitary enchondromas there appears to be no predilection for either sex. Multiple lesions occur in patients with Ollier's disease and are associated with soft-tissue or intra-osseous hemangiomata in Maffucci's syndrome. Solitary enchondromas are most common in the hands and feet; the diametaphyseal regions of the femur and tibia are the next most common sites of origin.

Histologically, enchondromas consist of lobules of mature hyaline cartilage separated by fibrovascular septations (70,72,78). These tumors have well-defined margins and do not infiltrate the adjacent bone trabeculae, as is common in low-grade chondrosarcomas. Myxoid change and necrosis are uncommon in enchondromas and should raise suspicion of chondrosarcoma. Immature lesions, lesions occurring in pregnant patients, and lesions located in the hands or feet may show increased cellularity and thus be difficult to differentiate histologically from low-grade chondrosarcoma (67,69,70,121).

The MRI and radiographic features of enchondromas depend largely on their maturity. When immature, enchondromas appear as well-marginated intramedullary lucencies with no visible chondroid calcifications. On MRI, immature enchondromas appear as slightly lobular masses of low signal intensity on T1-weighted images and very high signal intensity on T2-weighted images (2). With progressive skeletal maturation migration away from the physis into the diametaphyseal region occurs, but the lesions retain their central intramedullary location. With increasing maturity, progressive diffuse calcification occurs in the cartilage matrix, resulting in flocculent or flecklike regions of T2 shortening (Figs. 9-22 and 9-31), which is particularly evident on gradient-echo imaging. Extensive calcification and/or osseous metaplasia may obscure the signal characteristics of the un-

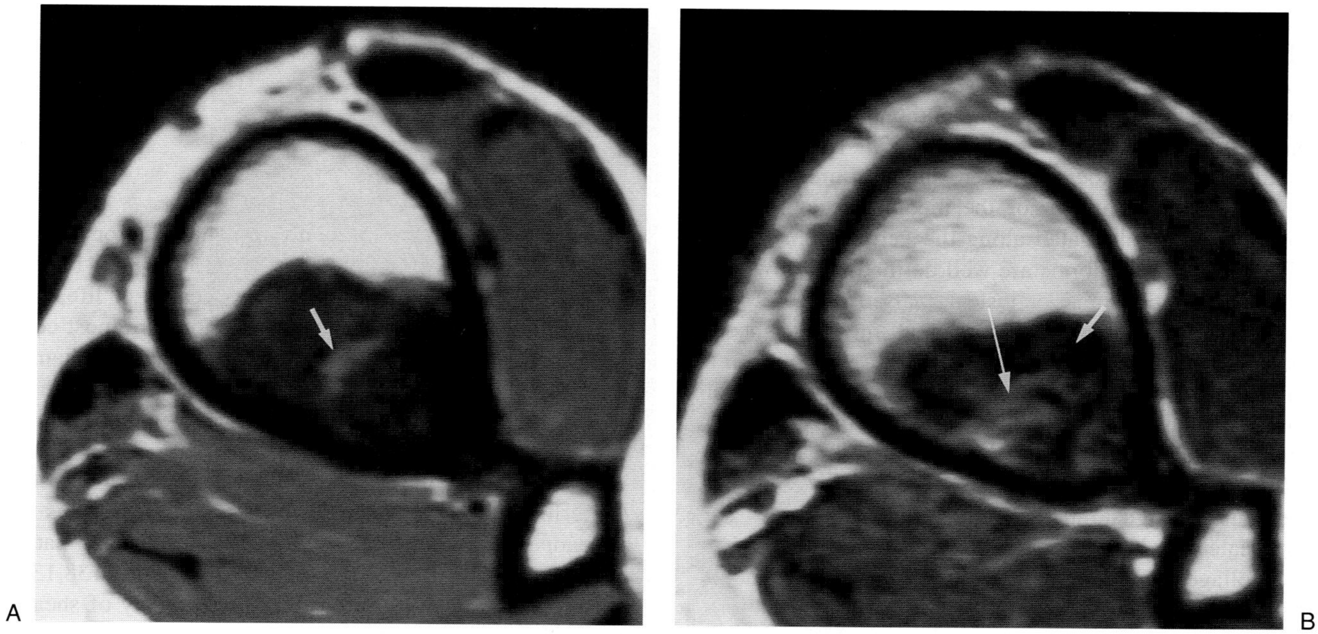

FIG. 9-34. Fibroxanthoma (nonossifying fibroma). **A:** A transverse T1-weighted image shows an eccentric lesion with a well-defined tumor–fat interface. The tumor contains predominantly low-signal-intensity material consistent with hemosiderin deposition in fibrous tissue. A crescent of high-signal-intensity lipid *(arrow)* is present. **B:** A transverse T2-weighted image shows low-signal-intensity hemosiderin-stained tissue *(short arrow)* and intermediate-signal-intensity collagenous regions *(long arrow)* within the fibroxanthoma.

thomas may contain regions of ossification, hemosiderin, or lipid; these findings are very unusual in chondromyxoid fibroma.

Osteochondroma

Osteochondromas are benign tumors of cartilage and bone that may occur as solitary or multiple lesions in diaphyseal aclasis (multiple hereditary exostosis syndrome) (144,145). Osteochondromas are the most common benign bone tumor. Lesions occur most commonly in the first and second decades of life and are most commonly found arising from long tubular bones.

Pathologically, osteochondromas consist of sessile or pedunculated protuberances from the metaphyseal region of the involved bone. These lesions are thought to arise from fragmentation of the physeal margin, with subsequent growth of a detached fragment (146). Osteochondromas have been shown to occur secondary to trauma or radiation; however, most cases are idiopathic (147–150). The cortex and medulla of the stem of the osteochondroma are in continuity with those of the parent bone. The end of the osteochondroma is capped by hyaline cartilage. The junction between the cartilage cap and the underlying stem contains a discrete zone of enchondral ossification; thus, the growth of the osteochondroma is a result of enchondral bone formation. The entire exostosis is covered by periosteum, which is in continuity with that of the parent bone. The appearance of an exostosis on both conventional imaging and MRI is predominantly dependent on the characteristics of the stalk and the age of the osteochondroma (72,151). Osteochondromas are morphologically described as pedunculated or sessile; the pedunculated type has a narrow stem, whereas the sessile type has a broad base of contact with the parent bone (69).

Immature osteochondromas have a relatively short stalk, whether they are sessile or pedunculated. The MRI signal characteristics of the marrow in the stalk are identical to those of the adjacent medullary cavity (152). The medullary space may contain irregular bone trabeculae that appear as linear low-signal-intensity structures on all pulse sequences. In immature lesions, the cartilage cap is of intermediate to high signal intensity on both T1- and T2-weighted pulse sequences and may vary in thickness from 1 to 10 mm. The region of enchondral ossification is evident as an irregular region of signal transition between the cartilage cap and the medullary space of the exostosis. When the medullary space of the exostosis contains fatty marrow, the low-signal-intensity interface represents the transition between irregular flocculent enchondral ossification and the ossification of poorly organized cortical bone. With maturation, calcification and involution of the cartilage cap result in diminished conspicuity of the cartilage cap (Fig. 9-35). Calcification of the cartilage cap appears as punctate or confluent regions of T2 shortening. Focal islands of intermediate signal intensity on both

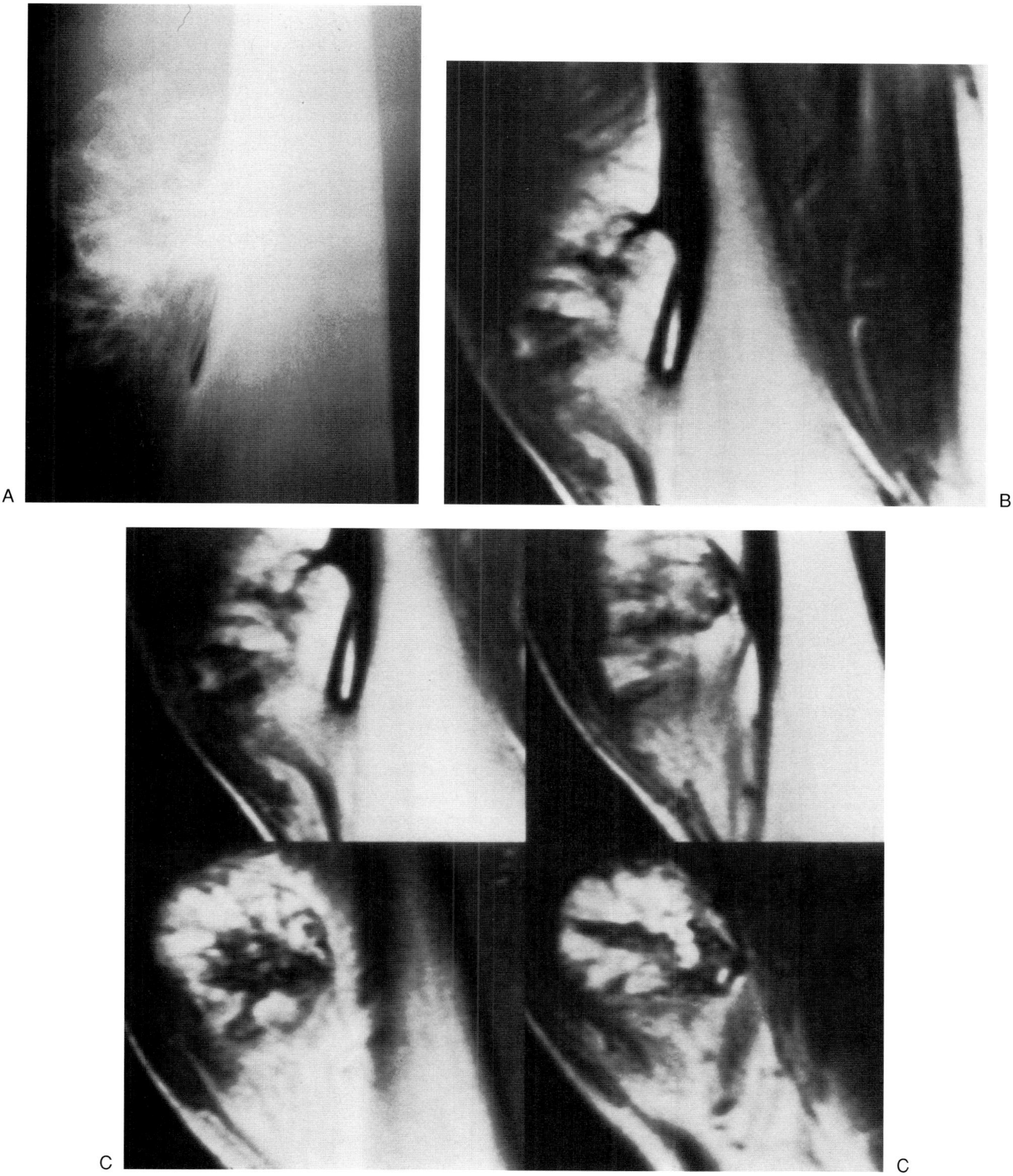

FIG. 9-35. Osteochondroma. **A:** An anteroposterior plain radiograph of the distal femoral metaphysis shows a large mature osteochondroma. The peripheral contour of the osteochondroma is smooth, and no destructive features are present. **B:** A T1-weighted coronal image shows continuity of the medullary space between the femur and osteochondroma stalk. The peripheral surface of the osteochondroma is lined by a lobulated and septated cap of hyaline cartilage. **C:** Contiguous coronal T1-weighted images of the same lesion show complex signal characteristics in the cartilage cap, representing a mixture of hyaline cartilage, chondroid calcification, and fibrous septae.

T1- and T2-weighted images represent residual mature hyaline cartilage. At this stage, the distinction between the periosteal and exosteal surface may be more apparent. Complete involution of the cartilage cap may occur, such that it is not apparent on MRI.

Malignant transformation rarely occurs in solitary osteochondromas, with an estimated frequency of 1% or less (69,145). The rate of malignant transformation in patients with multiple exostoses (also known as diaphyseal aclasia) is controversial, with reported rates ranging from 1% (150,153,154) to 30% (69,152). Lesions in the pelvis and shoulder regions are more prone to malignant degeneration than peripherally located lesions. Malignant degeneration almost invariably occurs in the cartilage cap, resulting in chondrosarcoma. The major signs of malignant degeneration are pain, growth of the osteochondroma after skeletal maturity, thickening of the cartilage cap, destruction of the bony component, and development of a soft-tissue mass. MRI is particularly well suited to evaluate cartilage cap thickness, bone destruction, and adjacent soft-tissue changes. A cartilage cap thickness of greater than 3 cm is strongly suggestive of malignant degeneration, particularly in a skeletally mature patient with fused epiphyses (152).

Periosteal Tumors

Various types of benign and malignant tumors may arise from the periosteum. Periosteal and parosteal osteogenic sarcomas are the most common malignant tumors arising in this location and are described in the section on osteogenic sarcomas. Chondrosarcomas may also arise on the bone surface, likely from dedifferentiation of a sessile osteochondroma (69,155). The benign periosteal tumors include chondromas, fibromas, and lipomas. Parosteal lipomas appear as fatty masses adjacent to the bone surface that contain a spur of ossification produced by the elevated periosteum (156). These rare lesions will not be discussed further.

Periosteal Desmoid

Periosteal desmoid is not a true neoplasm; it represents instead a periosteal response to adductor magnus traction at its posteromedial femoral insertion (157–159). This lesion is seen most commonly in males in the latter part of the second decade of life.

The lesion is characterized by subperiosteal fibrosis at the site described. MRI demonstrates low to intermediate signal intensity on T1- and T2-weighted images. When acute, a parosteal region of increased signal intensity may be seen on T2-weighted images. The adjacent cortex demonstrates irregular cortical thickening consistent with new bone formation.

Parosteal (Juxtacortical) Chondroma

Parosteal (juxtacortical) chondroma is an uncommon lesion of mature hyaline cartilage arising subjacent to the periosteum, rarely occurring about the knee (87,130,160,161). Lesions are characterized by relatively small size, discrete saucerization of the underlying cortical surface, and matrix calcification in approximately 50% of cases.

There are no specific MRI reports concerning such tumors. However, like other lesions of mature hyaline cartilage, they should demonstrate intermediate to high signal intensity on T1- and T2-weighted images. Such an appearance may be difficult to differentiate from a subperiosteal hematoma or ganglion. Central flocculent regions of T2 shortening, as seen in enchondromas, may be identified in lesions demonstrating calcification.

Lesions with No Specific Site of Predilection

Aneurysmal Bone Cyst

Aneurysmal bone cysts (ABCs) represent idiopathic, aggressively expansile benign lesions of bone. These lesions are not neoplastic; rather, they likely result from hemorrhage or arteriovenous fistula formation within a preexisting bone lesion (162,163). Aneurysmal bone cysts have been described as secondary changes in many types of benign bone tumors; an association of giant cell tumor with ABC is frequently described (57,164,165). In pathologic series, 30–36% of ABCs coexist with other tumors. The remainder are described as ''primary'' and may be posttraumatic or idiopathic in etiology (165–168).

ABCs occur most commonly in the second and third decades of life and are uncommon in patients over 30 years of age. The lower extremities, particularly the metaphyseal or diametaphyseal regions of long bones, are the most common sites of origin (169).

Histologically, ABCs consist of multilocular, cystic, blood-filled spaces separated by delicate fibro-osseous septa (132). The septa may calcify or ossify. The septa serve as conduits for a poorly organized vascular arcade and contain hemosiderin within macrophages. The lesions are invariably expansile and are contained by an expanded periosteal shell (162). the most important histologic differential diagnosis is telangiectatic osteogenic sarcoma, which can be recognized on the basis of cellular atypia and frequent mitoses (165).

On MRI, ABCs present as eccentric, expansile lesions of bone. The margins are well defined, usually with a low-signal rim representing sclerotic bone. The internal signal characteristics depend on the composition of the hematinic elements. The center of the ABC contains poorly defined locules of variable signal intensity, representing blood products in different stages of degradation (Fig. 9-36). These locules are separated by septations of intermediate signal intensity on T1- and T2-weighted images that may demonstrate focal regions of T2 shortening on T2-weighted or gradient-echo images as a result of hemosiderin, calcification, or ossification. In long-standing ABCs, some of the locules may fill in with fibrous tissue or marrow fat, and the contents

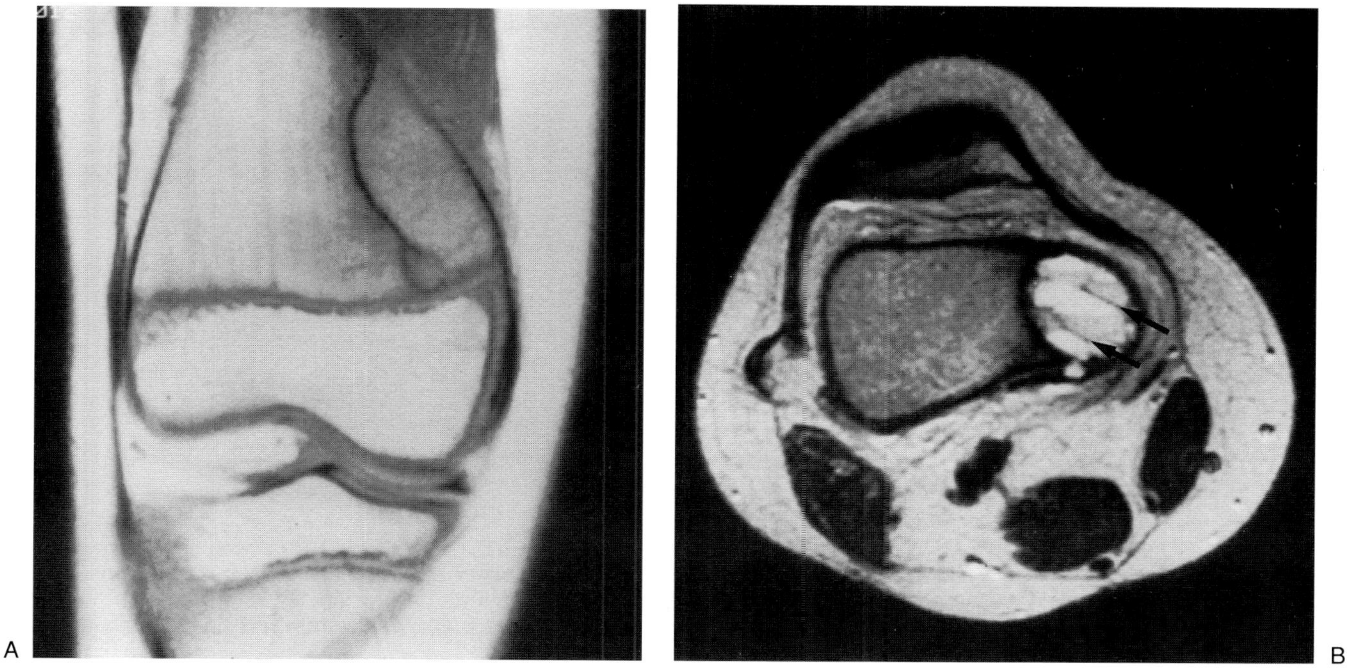

FIG. 9-36. Aneurysmal bone cyst. A: A T1-weighted coronal image of the distal femur shows an eccentric well-demarcated lesion in the metaphysis, with thinning and expansion of the overlying cortex. B: A T2-weighted transverse image shows multiple fluid–fluid levels *(arrows)*; a finding typical of but not exclusive to aneurysmal bone cysts. (Reprinted with permission from Munk PL, et al. MRI imaging of aneurysmal bone cysts. *AJR* 1989;153:99–101. Copyright 1989, American Roentgen Ray Society.)

of the fluid-filled spaces may become more homogeneous (Fig. 9-37). Periosteal reaction is usually absent, and breach of the periosteum may be associated with a parosteal soft-tissue mass similar to a hematoma (Fig. 9-38) (170–174).

Fluid–fluid levels are often seen within the locules, particularly if the patient is allowed to lie still for a few minutes prior to the MRI examination. The supernatant component of fluid–fluid levels may demonstrate a high-signal intensity on T1- and T2-weighted images, because of methemoglobin, or may be of low to intermediate signal intensity on both T1- and T2-weighted images because of fibrinous debris or suspended acute clot. The dependent portion may appear as high-signal-intensity fluid containing methemoglobin, linear intermediate-signal-intensity fibrinous strands, and dependent layering demonstrating T2 shortening representing hemosiderin. Although initially thought to be a fairly specific feature of ABC, fluid–fluid levels appear to be less specific than originally believed. Fluid–fluid levels may be seen in telangiectatic osteosarcomas, giant cell tumors, fibrous dysplasia, unicameral bone cysts, and chondroblastomas (72,175).

Osteoid Osteoma

Osteoid osteomas are painful benign tumors that occur most commonly in the second and third decades of life. This tumor is found more commonly in men, with a male to female ratio of approximately 2:1. The classical clinical history of focal dull pain that is worst at night and relieved by salicylates is found in approximately half of patients. Osteoid osteomas are most commonly located in the femur (50%); other common sites include the hands and feet (21%), tibia, vertebral column (13%), and humerus (98). These lesions are nonprogressive and nondestructive and tend to resolve spontaneously with time (176).

Histologically, these tumors consist of a central, highly vascular nidus of osteoid with varying degrees of disorganized central trabecular new bone formation, surrounded by florid sclerotic new bone formation (132,177). The osteoblasts lining the trabecular new bone contain large nuclei with frequent mitoses, but show no atypia or abnormal mitoses (178). The nidus ranges from 1 to 15 mm in diameter and may contain internal calcifications (179,180). The nidus contains many nerve fibers, which likely explains the painful nature of these lesions.

Osteoid osteomas differ in appearance, depending on whether they are cortical, medullary, or intra-articular. The majority of osteoid osteomas are cortical or subperiosteal in location; at these locations, the classic features of an intracortical nidus with prominent surrounding bone sclerosis, cortical thickening, and periosteal reaction are seen. In an intramedullary location, less sclerosis and periosteal reaction is seen (179). Intra-articular osteoid osteomas have a radically different appearance, being characterized by osteopenia, with no bone sclerosis, cortical thickening, or periosteal

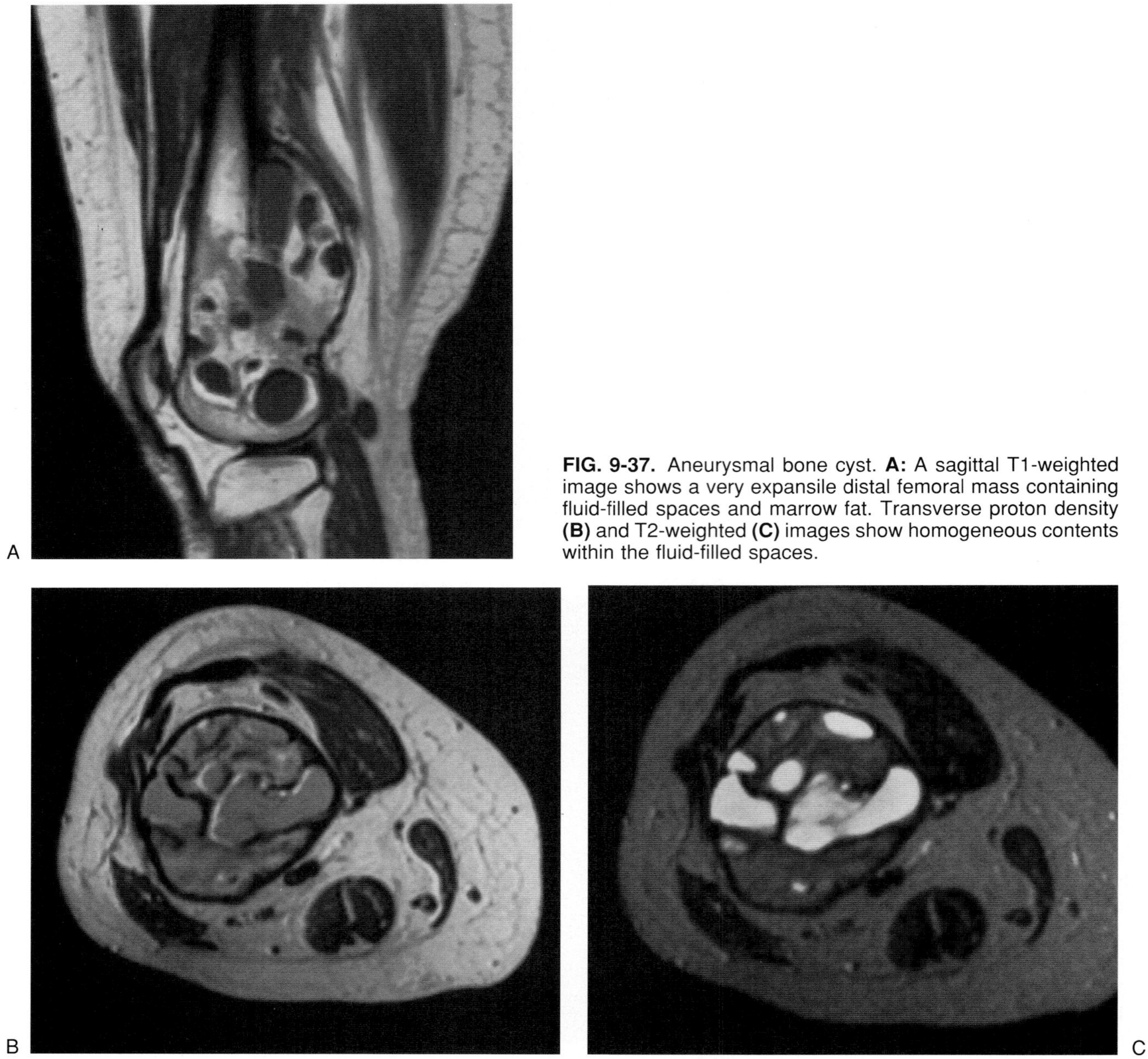

FIG. 9-37. Aneurysmal bone cyst. **A:** A sagittal T1-weighted image shows a very expansile distal femoral mass containing fluid-filled spaces and marrow fat. Transverse proton density **(B)** and T2-weighted **(C)** images show homogeneous contents within the fluid-filled spaces.

reaction. A joint effusion and lymphofollicular synovitis are common. Thus, these lesions may mimic a septic or inflammatory monoarthritis (181–184).

On MRI, the nidus is of low signal intensity on T1-weighted images and usually of very high signal intensity on T2-weighted images. Extensive calcification of the nidus may cause it to be less conspicuous on T2-weighted images. The surrounding bone sclerosis appears as low-signal-intensity thickening of the cortex on all pulse sequences (Fig. 9-39). Extensive intramedullary and subperiosteal edema is often present, which may produce a misleading aggressive appearance (3,185,186). CT is generally accepted as being more accurate than MRI for detection of the nidus. MRI is superior in the depiction of associated soft-tissue and bone marrow changes (30).

Osteoid osteomas often require excision for alleviation of pain. Preoperative localization of the nidus with CT is often helpful, because the surgeon may have considerable difficulty locating the nidus in the midst of the dense reactive bone (187). Techniques of percutaneous ablation under CT guidance have also been described (188,189).

Diffuse Marrow Tumors and Infiltrations

Diffuse neoplastic disorders involving the marrow compartment of the appendicular skeleton are well appreciated

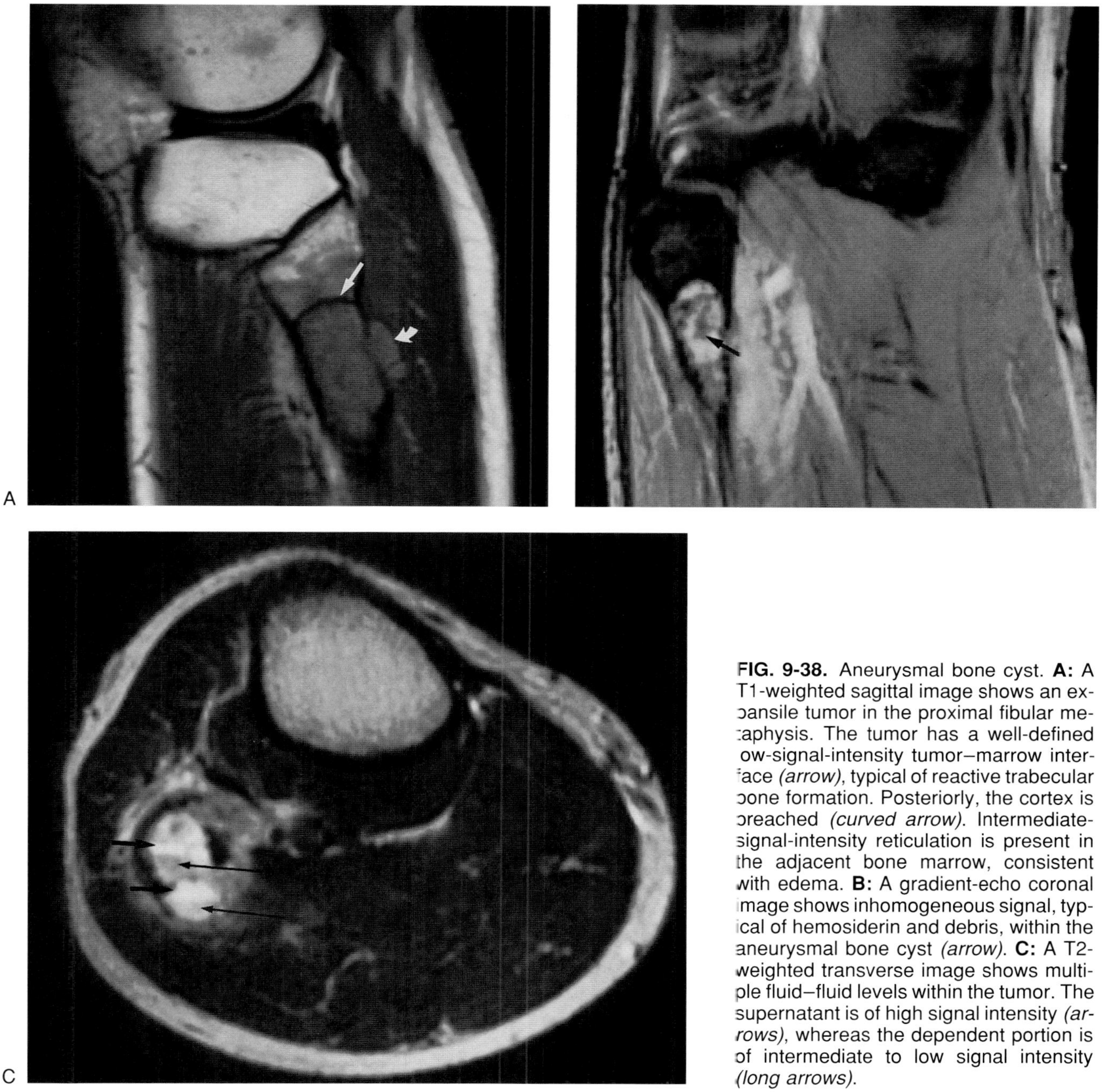

FIG. 9-38. Aneurysmal bone cyst. **A:** A T1-weighted sagittal image shows an expansile tumor in the proximal fibular metaphysis. The tumor has a well-defined low-signal-intensity tumor–marrow interface *(arrow)*, typical of reactive trabecular bone formation. Posteriorly, the cortex is breached *(curved arrow)*. Intermediate-signal-intensity reticulation is present in the adjacent bone marrow, consistent with edema. **B:** A gradient-echo coronal image shows inhomogeneous signal, typical of hemosiderin and debris, within the aneurysmal bone cyst *(arrow)*. **C:** A T2-weighted transverse image shows multiple fluid–fluid levels within the tumor. The supernatant is of high signal intensity *(arrows)*, whereas the dependent portion is of intermediate to low signal intensity *(long arrows)*.

on MRI (190–199). An understanding of the MRI appearance of normal bone marrow at various stages of maturity is necessary to avoid misdiagnosis, because age-related or reactive marrow processes can mimic neoplasm. At birth, almost all the marrow is occupied by hematopoietic (''red'') marrow. During childhood and adolescence, a gradual transition from hematopoietic to fatty (''yellow'') marrow occurs. This transition begins in the epiphyses and then progresses from the diaphyses to the metaphyses of long bones. In normal adults, red marrow persists in the proximal metaphyses of the femur and humerus and in the spine, skull, sternum, pelvis, and ribs. Streaks of red marrow are frequently seen in the distal femoral metaphyses of normal adults; this finding may be more prominent in smokers, obese patients, premenopausal females, and endurance athletes (200,201). In the elderly, fatty regions may be seen amid the red marrow in the vertebral bodies and pelvis. If the hematopoietic marrow is stimulated by anemia or hypoxia, reconversion of red to yellow marrow will occur in the reverse progression of normal marrow maturation (202–206).

On MRI, yellow marrow appears as high signal intensity on T1-weighted images and intermediate to low signal inten-

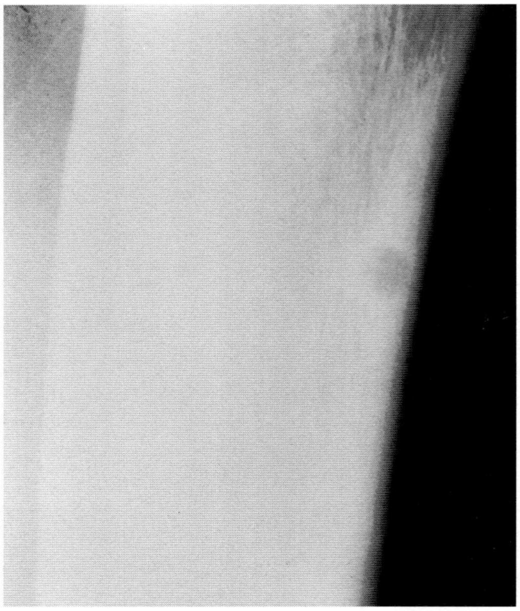

A

FIG. 9-39. Cortical osteoid osteoma. **A:** A lateral radiograph of the proximal femur shows a cortical lucency with mild surrounding sclerosis. **B:** A T2-weighted transverse image shows a discrete cortical nidus of high signal intensity *(arrow)* contained by thin endosteal and periosteal cortical margins. **C:** A transverse gradient-echo image shows a peripheral ring of low-signal-intensity calcification *(arrow)* within the nidus.

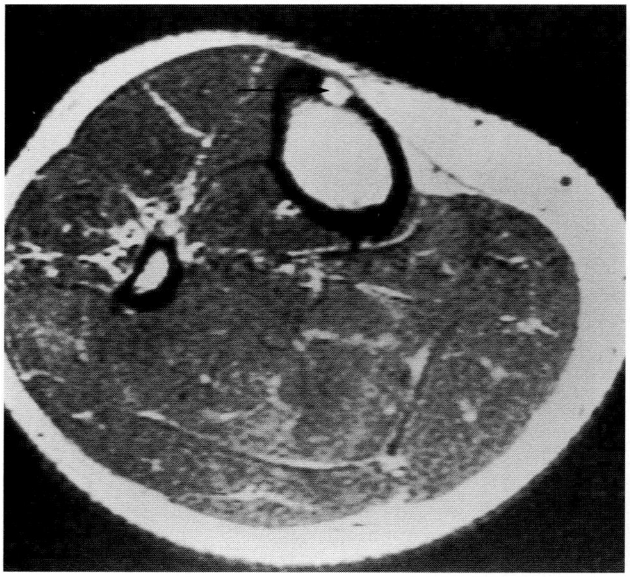

B

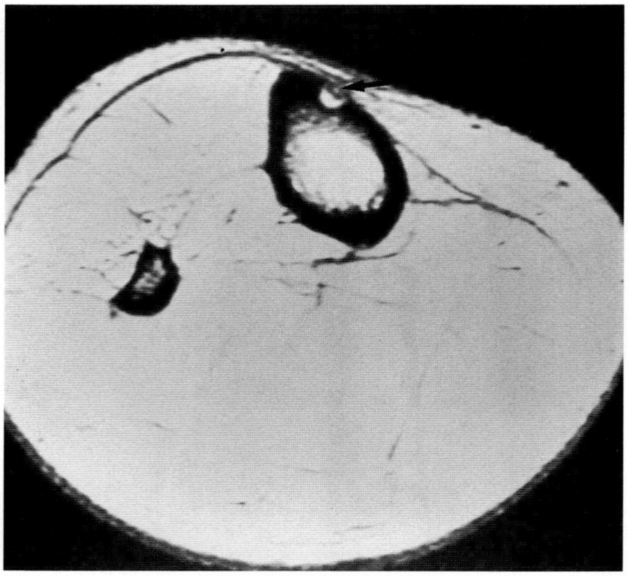

C

sity on T2-weighted images, identical to subcutaneous fat. Fine, linear, low-signal-intensity bone trabeculae are seen in the metaphyses and epiphyses. Fat-suppressed or STIR images show very low signal intensity in fatty marrow. Red marrow is similar in signal characteristics to muscle, being hypointense relative to fat on both T1- and T2-weighted images. Red marrow is of intermediate signal intensity on STIR images. Of note, normal red marrow in long bones can be differentiated from tumor by its typical bilateral patchy or streaky nongeographic distribution and by the lack of destructive features (202). On STIR images, normal red marrow is usually of similar signal intensity to muscle, whereas tumor is usually of higher signal intensity approaching that of fluid. Both normal red marrow and tumor will enhance with intravenous contrast administration.

Diffuse neoplastic proliferation within the marrow compartment is best appreciated on T1-weighted or STIR images. The characteristic appearances are those of diffuse or patchy diminished signal intensity on T1-weighted images. Such marrow changes are best appreciated in adults in the diametaphyseal marrow due to the high contrast between fatty marrow and tumor. In children, differentiation between normal red marrow and malignant infiltrate may be difficult, particularly if the tumor burden is small. Lymphoma, myeloma, and metastases may also be seen as multiple focal nodular marrow infiltrates of low to intermediate signal intensity on T1-weighted images and high signal intensity on T2-weighted images (Fig. 9-40). Gradient-echo images are less sensitive than T1-weighted or STIR images for visualization of nondestructive marrow infiltration or tumor, be-

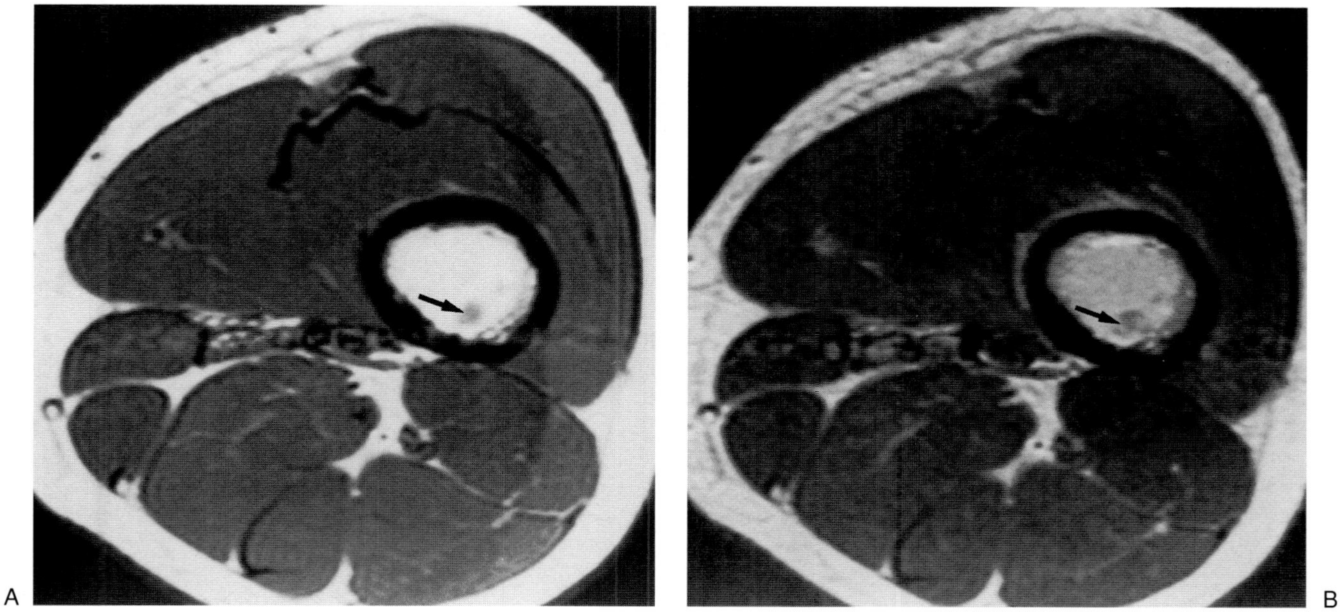

FIG. 9-40. Diffuse non-Hodgkin's lymphoma of bone. T1-weighted **(A)** and T2-weighted **(B)** transverse images of the distal femur show intermediate-signal-intensity nodular deposits *(arrow)* within the medulla. The lymphomatous deposits are discretely marginated from adjacent marrow fat.

cause magnetic susceptibility effects diminish the abnormal signal arising from the tumor (Fig. 9-41).

With the exception of nodular marrow infiltrative pathologies, the changes noted within the marrow compartment are not specific for malignant infiltrative disorders, nor do they allow differentiation from benign hyperplastic marrow disorders such as hemoglobinopathies. Although bone marrow biopsy is often necessary for definitive diagnosis, MRI is helpful for assessment of extent of disease and response to treatment. In focal or multifocal disease, MRI is helpful to locate the optimal site of biopsy (202).

Non-Hodgkin's Lymphoma of Bone

Primary lymphoma of bone comprises 3% of primary bone tumors; with approximately 40% of bone lymphoma

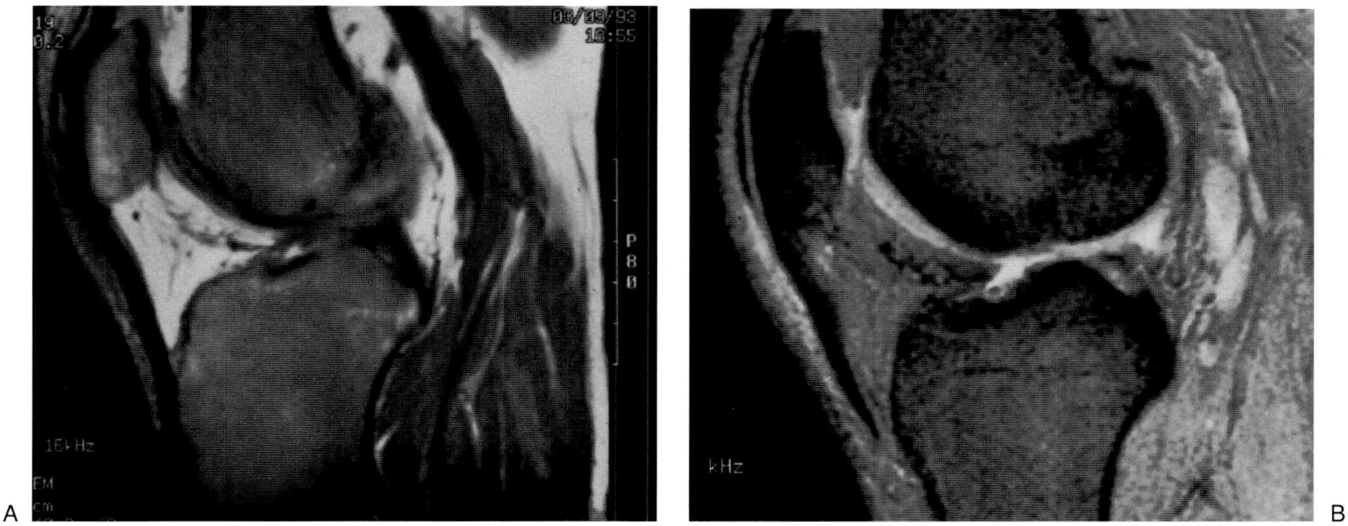

FIG. 9-41. Non-Hodgkin's lymphoma of bone. **A:** A sagittal T1-weighted image shows extensive replacement of the high-signal-intensity normal marrow fat by low-signal-intensity tumor. This marked abnormality is very inconspicuous on a T2*-weighted gradient-echo image **(B)**. Gradient-echo images are relatively insensitive to nondestructive bone marrow abnormalities.

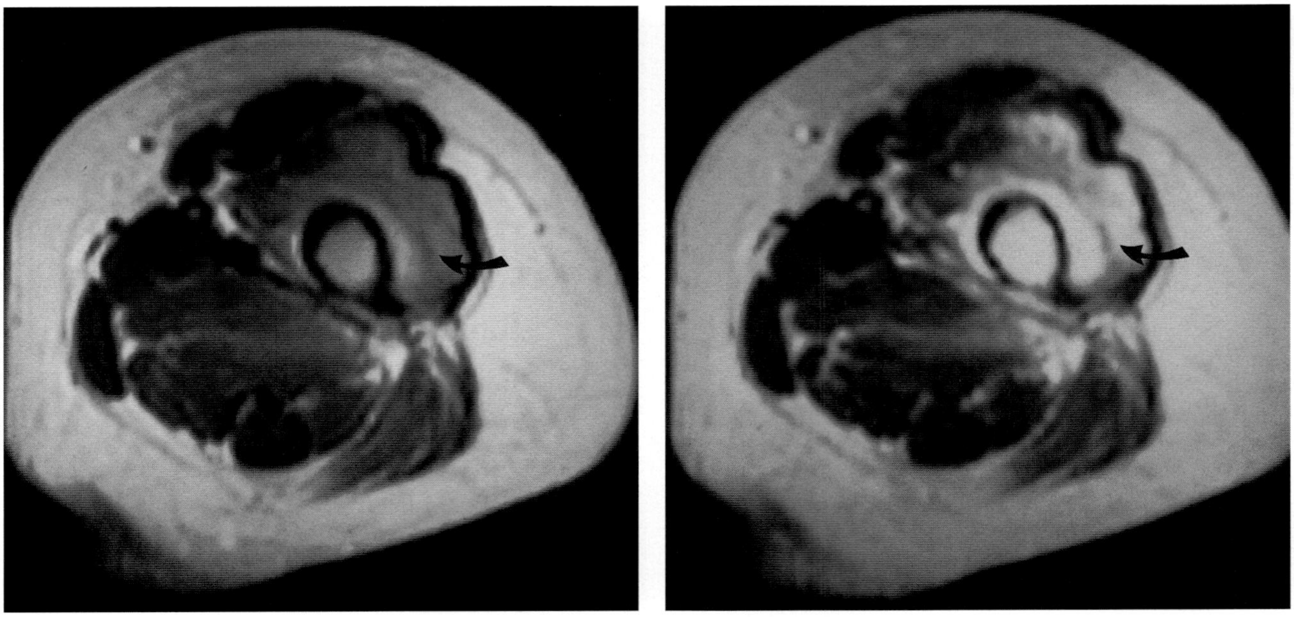

A B

FIG. 9-42. Non-Hodgkin's lymphoma with destructive features. Transverse proton-density **(A)** and T2-weighted **(B)** images show replacement of the marrow fat and extensive cloaking of the femur by soft-tissue extension of lymphoma *(arrows)*. The cortex is thinned and permeated.

being due to primary non-Hodgkin's lymphoma (NHL) (207,208). Any bone may be involved, although there is a predilection for long bones; when the knee is involved the distal femur is the most common site. NHL of bone usually occurs in patients in their fourth decade of life (although it may occur from the second through seventh decades) with no male or female predilection. NHL may also involve bone as part of multifocal or diffuse lymphoma. NHL is rare in children (209,210).

The histologic features of primary and secondary non-Hodgkin's lymphoma are similar. The neoplastic cells have a permeative growth pattern between preexisting bone trabeculae with limited destruction of bone. The cell morphology varies with the subtype of lymphoma; most lymphomas of bone are B-cell lymphomas, with large-cell being the most common subtype. Some of the large-cell lymphomas are associated with the production of abundant. Reticulin between the tumor cells, a feature that explains the designation of reticulum cell sarcoma in the older literature (211,212).

Non-Hodgkin's lymphoma may appear as an infiltrative process, with extensive replacement of the marrow fat and little evidence of bone destruction or periosteal reaction (see Fig. 9-41) or as an aggressive mass with prominent bone destruction (Fig. 9-42). The aggressive appearance is more common in cases of primary NHL of bone. MRI shows a geographic region of intermediate signal intensity on T1-weighted images and increased signal intensity on T2-weighted images. Inhomogeneous areas may be due to residual marrow fat, hemorrhage, or fibrosis within the tumor (202,213). Although less commonly associated with medullary new bone formation than Hodgkin's disease, a significant percentage of NHLs are associated with reactive trabecular new bone, both marginating and within the tumor. This will appear as poorly defined regions of T2 shortening on T2-weighted and gradient-echo images. However, tumors are rarely discretely demarcated by a complete halo of diminished signal intensity and tend to have an irregular, poorly defined tumor–fat interface.

NHL is often associated with transcortical extension and an extensive parosteal soft-tissue mass with signal characteristics similar to those of the intraosseous tumor. A classic appearance of NHL is that of a lytic destructive tumor extending along a considerable length of a long bone, with a surrounding soft-tissue mass.

Hodgkin's Disease

Primary Hodgkin's disease of bone is extremely rare (209). Consequently, clinically evident Hodgkin's disease of bone is usually a manifestation of systemic disease. This is reported to occur in approximately 10–15% of patients in clinical series (214,215), although prevalence of bone involvement on MRI may be higher because of its ability to detect medullary disease earlier, reflecting more closely the nearly 100% incidence of bone involvement at autopsy (216,217). The MRI characteristics of Hodgkin's disease are not well described; however, marrow infiltration and replacement similar to that of other diffuse marrow disorders is expected.

Metastases

Metastasis most commonly occurs in red marrow areas of the skeleton but may be found at any skeletal site and thus

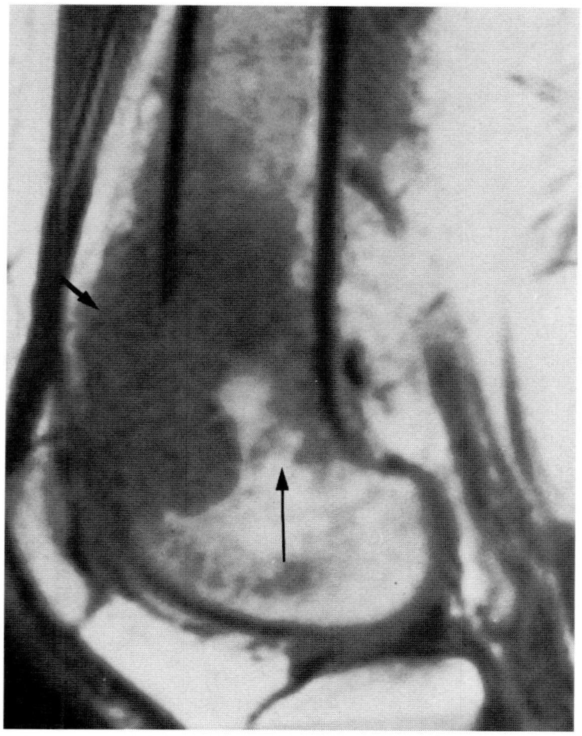

FIG. 9-43. Metastasis. A T1-weighted sagittal image of the distal femur shows an intermediate-signal-intensity metastatic renal cell carcinoma. The tumor–medullary fat interface is moth-eaten *(long arrow)* and transcortical extension of tumor is present anteriorly *(short arrow).*

must be considered in the differential diagnosis of epiphyseal lesions (218). Metastasis may occur at any age, most commonly in the fifth to seventh decades of life. With the exception of melanotic melanoma and hemorrhagic metastases, most metastases show diminished signal intensity on T1-weighted images and increased signal intensity on T2-weighted images (Fig. 9-43) (219,220). Bone marrow metastases frequently have a small region of perilesional edema (202). Osteoblastic metastases may demonstrate trabecular and endosteal T2 shortening in relation to the tumor consistent with tumor-induced new bone formation. With melanotic melanoma, the presence of melanin in sufficient concentration may result in paramagnetic relaxation enhancement and consequently T1 shortening. Consequently, melanotic melanoma metastases may demonstrate evidence of high signal intensity on T1-weighted and T2-weighted images (Fig. 9-44). The degree to which the previously mentioned changes are apparent is a reflection of the concentration of melanin within the individual metastatic lesion (221). Similar increased signal on T1-weighted images may be evident in hemorrhagic metastases due to the presence of methemoglobin within these lesions.

Solitary metastases may be relatively well-defined discrete lesions, although they rarely demonstrate evidence of marginating T2 shortening suggestive of endosteal new bone formation. With increasing aggressivity, metastases may demonstrate evidence of a poorly defined medullary fat–tumor interface with aggressive permeative destruction and tunneling of endosteal and cortical bone. Periosseous extension and complex periosteal new bone formation may be evident.

In the situation of bone metastases from an unknown primary tumor, biopsy of a bone metastasis is often useful because microscopic and immunohistochemical analysis may suggest or establish the primary tumor site.

TUMORS AND TUMORLIKE CONDITIONS OF SYNOVIUM

The synovial membrane consists of a cellular intima and areolar connective-tissue subintima (222–224). The cellular intima varies in thickness (one to four cells) and is embedded in a granular matrix. The synovial membrane is loosely bounded through its subintima to the overlying joint capsule, tendons, and intra-articular ligaments. In some areas where the synovial membrane is loosely bound to these underlying structures, the synovium may be seen to form small fibrovascular projections referred to as villi. The synovial membrane does not cover the hyaline cartilage or menisci within the joint. Benign and malignant tumors and tumorlike disorders of the synovium occurring in the knee will be discussed.

Synovial Osteochondromatosis

Synovial osteochondromatosis is due to chondroid metaplasia of the synovial membrane of joints, bursae, and tendon sheaths (132). This disorder occurs most commonly in men in the third through fifth decades of life. The most common site of synovial osteochondromatosis is the knee (50% of cases), the elbow, shoulder, and hip other commonly involved joints (28,225,226). Interestingly, approximately 10% of cases are bilateral (227).

Histologically, synovial osteochondromatosis consists of metaplastic production of mature hyaline cartilage within the synovial subintima. The cartilage bodies are more cellular than normal articular cartilage and may not show a nested pattern of chondrocytes. The cartilaginous bodies may subsequently calcify or ossify and may detach to form loose intra-articular bodies. There is a tendency for the initially sessile chonromata to become pedunculated. The surrounding synovium shows reactive changes of hypervascularity, fibrosis, and villus formation (226,228).

On MRI, synovial osteochondromatosis usually appears as multiple intra-articular bodies surrounded by a joint effusion (227,229). Immature cartilaginous fragments are of low signal intensity on T1-weighted images and of high signal intensity on T2-weighted images, typical of hyaline cartilage. Calcification of the chondroma produces a low-signal-intensity rim on all pulse sequences (Fig. 9-45). Mature ossified chondromata can be recognized by the presence of high-

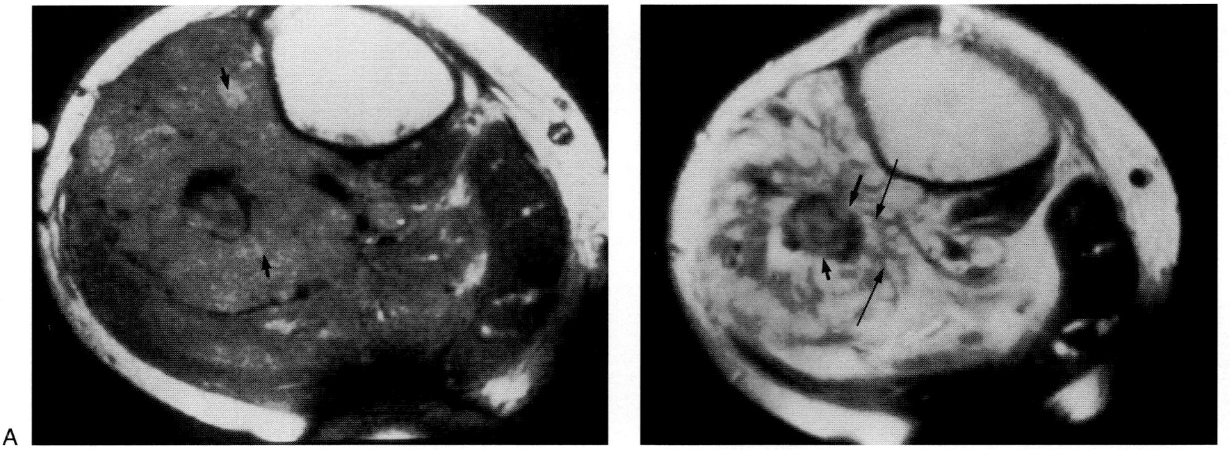

FIG. 9-44. Metastatic melanoma. **A:** A T1-weighted transverse image of the proximal fibula shows a grossly expansile inhomogeneous mass of intermediate signal intensity. Focal areas of increased signal intensity *(arrows)* are present in the lesion, corresponding to regions of melanin deposition and/or hemorrhage (methemoglobin). **B:** A T2-weighted transverse image shows patchy increased signal intensity throughout the intra- and extraosseous components of the tumor. Permeative destruction of the fibular cortex is noted *(short arrows)*, with extensive sunburst periosteal new bone formation within the extraosseous tumor *(long arrows)*.

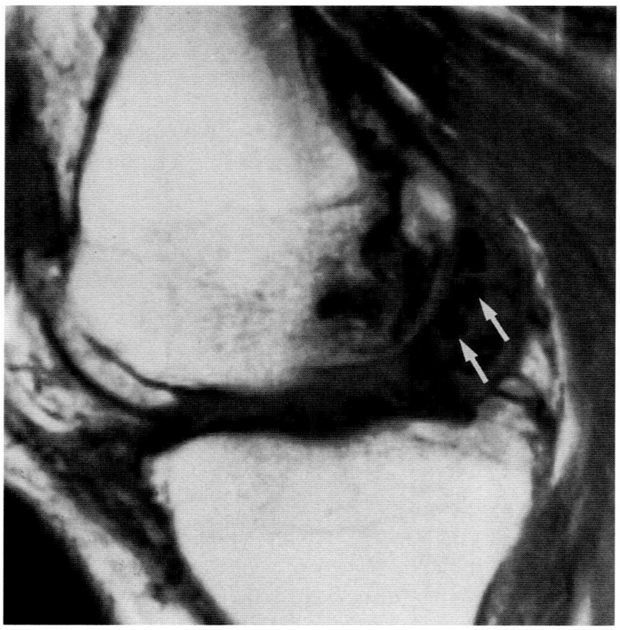

FIG. 9-45. Synovial osteochondromatosis. A T1-weighted sagittal image shows multiple low-signal-intensity loose bodies within the posterior recess of the knee joint *(arrows)*. These represent calcified cartilaginous bodies. (Reprinted with permission from Munk PL. Magnetic resonance of the knee: an overview. *J Can Assoc Radiol* 1989;40:296–303. Copyright, Canadian Association of Radiologists.)

signal-intensity marrow fat within the chondroma on T1-weighted images (230). The commonly associated joint effusion serves to silhouette the chondromata (Fig. 9-46). Malignant transformation rarely complicates synovial osteochondromatosis. Bone erosions are not commonly seen in synovial osteochondromatosis of the knee but may be seen in joints with less capacious capsules.

Pigmented Villonodular Synovitis

Pigmented villonodular synovitis (PVNS) is a localized or diffuse idiopathic benign proliferation of synovium. This condition is thought by most authors to be a reactive process, rather than a neoplasm; however, the inciting agent has not been established. This usually occurs as a monoarthropathy, with the knee being the most commonly involved site. PVNS occurs most commonly in the third to sixth decades of life and is slightly more common in men than in women (231–235).

The histologic evolution of PVNS is complex (235). In the initial stages, diffuse proliferation of stromal histiocytic cells is found within the subintima, with associated deposition of fibrous tissue, hemosiderin, and a reactive inflammatory cell infiltrate. Marked synovial villous hypertrophy occurs with villous overgrowth and cleft formation within fibrotic proliferative synovium. Involution may occur with dense fibrosis of the synovial membrane with residual hemosiderin deposition. Erosion of underlying cortical bone may be seen at the site of synovial proliferation secondary to extrinsic pressure effects. Diffuse hyperemia often produces osteopenia around the involved joint (234,236).

The MRI appearances depend on the stage of evolution

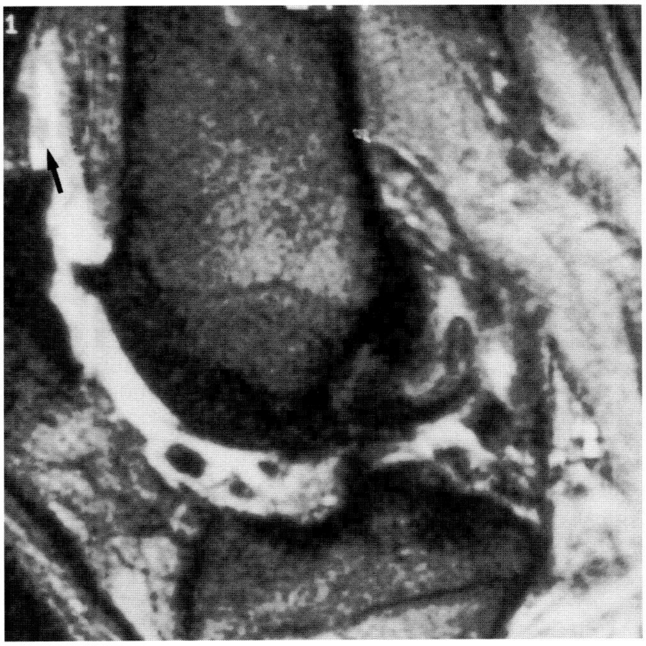

FIG. 9-46. Synovial osteochondromatosis. A sagittal gradient-echo image shows multiple free and adherent marginal nodular foci of low signal intensity consistent with calcified synovial osteochondromata. The "target" appearance of ossified osteochondromata is not present; however, some noncalcified cartilaginous bodies are present in the suprapatellar recess *(arrow)*. A joint effusion is also present.

of PVNS (237–239). In the early proliferative stage, the hypertrophied synovium is seen as a cloak of diminished signal intensity on T1-weighted images and increased signal intensity on T2-weighted images marginating the synovial membrane (Fig. 9-47). This is punctuated even in its early stages by the presence of focal regions of T2 shortening consistent with hemosiderin deposition. The signal voids produced by the hemosiderin deposits are more obvious on gradient-echo images than on spin-echo images, because of the magnetic susceptibility effects of hemosiderin. With increasing synovial villous hypertrophy and hemosiderin deposition, the proliferative synovium may demonstrate heterogeneous signal intensity on T2-weighted images, because of their high-signal-intensity villous clefts interdigitating with low-signal-intensity hemosiderin deposits (240). Intravenous gadolinium enhancement may be helpful in defining the extent and location of the synovial proliferation prior to synovectomy (Fig. 9-48). Of note, chronic severe rheumatoid arthritis or hemophilic arthritis can produce synovial hypertrophy, hemorrhage, and hemosiderin deposition that very closely resemble PVNS; these conditions are easily differentiated by clinical history.

Focal erosions of cortical bone in PVNS appear as geographic, nonarticular, subcortical regions of low signal intensity on T1-weighted images and intermediate to high signal intensity on T2-weighted images, marginated by a discrete region of focal T2 shortening consistent with trabecular new bone (Fig. 9-49).

The occurrence of a PVNS-like reaction in the synovium of a tendon sheath is termed *giant cell tumor of tendon sheath*. The signal characteristics of this condition are similar to those of PVNS; the conditions are differentiated mainly by the anatomic site of involvement (241,242).

Lipoma Arborescens

Lipoma arborescens is a very rare condition characterized by proliferation of fat and synovial tissue. This benign condition arises most commonly in the knee, usually in the suprapatellar bursa, and produces symptoms of slowly progressive knee swelling and limitation of motion. The preferred treatment is complete synovectomy. On MRI, a lobulated mass of predominantly fatty tissue is seen in the knee joint, associated with a joint effusion (Fig. 9-50) (243). Bone erosion is usually minimal or absent in lipoma arborescens. Hemosiderin deposition has not been described in this condition; this feature allows easy differentiation of lipoma arborescens from PVNS (244).

CYSTIC MASSES AROUND THE KNEE JOINT

A variety of cystic lesions are commonly encountered on routine knee MRI examinations. Recognition of these lesions is important, because they may produce symptoms and require specific therapy. Also, correct identification of the nature of a cystic lesion may allow avoidance of unnecessary biopsy or arthroscopy, because some cystic masses produce clinical findings that may mimic a soft-tissue tumor or internal derangement of the knee (230,245).

Bursal Fluid Collections

A variety of bursae are present around the knee joint that protect moving structures such as tendons and muscles from excessive friction against underlying bony structures. These bursae normally contain a minimal amount of fluid and are not visible on MR images unless the bursa is inflamed and distended with fluid. The most common sites of bursal distention and inflammation are the pes anserine bursa, the prepatellar bursa, the deep and superficial infrapatellar bursae, and the iliotibial bursa. Bursitis generally presents with focal pain, swelling, and erythema over the involved site. Most cases are due to friction and overuse and are treated with ice, rest, and anti-inflammatory medications. Refractory cases occasionally require aspiration and corticosteroid injection (230). Prepatellar bursitis is occasionally due to infection, because skin penetration may contaminate the superficially located prepatellar bursa; *Staphylococcus aureus* is the most common organism (246). Gout occasionally causes bursitis around the knee; this condition tends to occur in older pa-

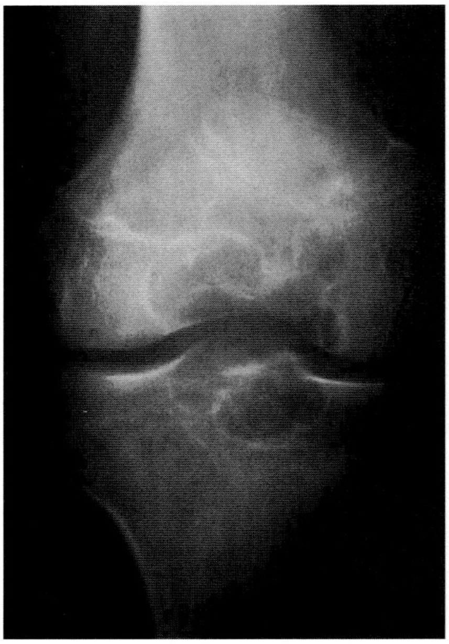

A

FIG. 9-47. Pigmented villonodular synovitis (PVNS). **A:** An anteroposterior plain radiograph shows extensive discrete radiolucencies in the femur and tibia corresponding to erosions of the bone surface. **B:** A proton-density-weighted sagittal image shows a large joint effusion with heterogeneous masses of intermediate signal intensity lining the synovial margins *(arrows)*. Small, frondlike nodules are noted in the suprapatellar bursa *(small arrow)*, whereas larger lesions are present in the posterior recess of the knee *(large arrow)*. Diffuse low-signal-intensity hemosiderin deposition is present in the infrapatellar fat pad *(long arrow)*. **C:** A T2-weighted sagittal image shows enlargement or "blooming" of the signal voids around the hemosiderin deposits in the infrapatellar fat pad.

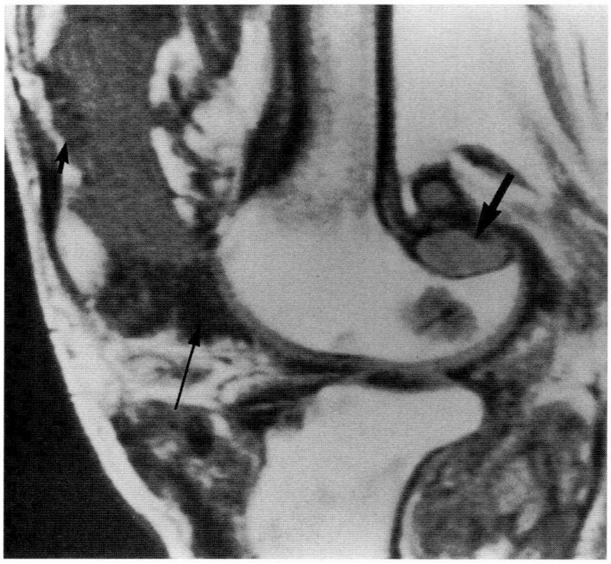

B

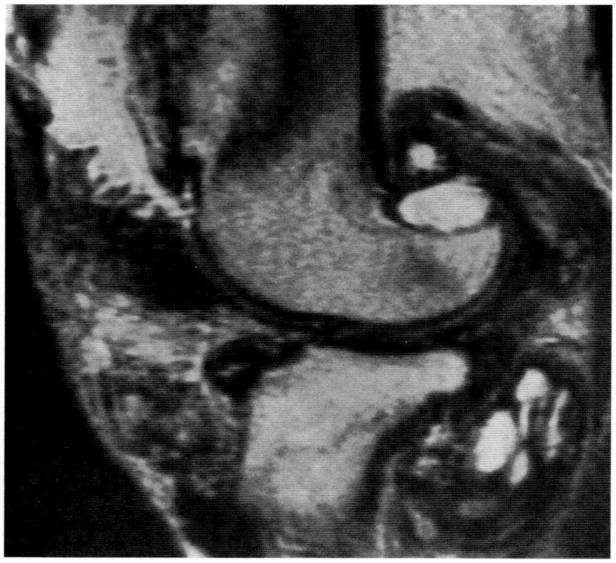

C

tients with an established diagnosis of gout and can be confirmed by finding uric acid crystals in fluid aspirated from the bursa (Fig. 9-51).

Pes Anserine Bursitis

The pes anserinus consists of the tendons of the sartorius, gracilis, and semitendinosus muscles and is so named because of the resemblance of the tendon insertion to the shape of a goose's webbed foot. The pes anserine bursa separates the pes anserinus tendons from the underlying bony surface of the medial tibial metaphysis and the distal end of the tibial collateral ligament. On MR images, a distended pes anserine bursa appears as an ovoid fluid collection adjacent to the medial aspect of the proximal tibia, which does not communicate with the knee joint (Fig. 9-52) (245). The pes anserinus tendons are often visible deep to the fluid collection. The bursa may extend superiorly to the level of the knee joint; thus, it is crucial to assess the medial meniscus carefully, because a medial meniscal tear with a parameniscal cyst could also occur in this location. Pes anserine bursitis is usually due to overuse, often in runners, and may present with medial knee pain and swelling suggestive of medial meniscal or collateral ligament damage (247). Correct identification of pes anserine bursitis may allow avoidance of unnecessary arthroscopy for the investigation of medial knee pain (245).

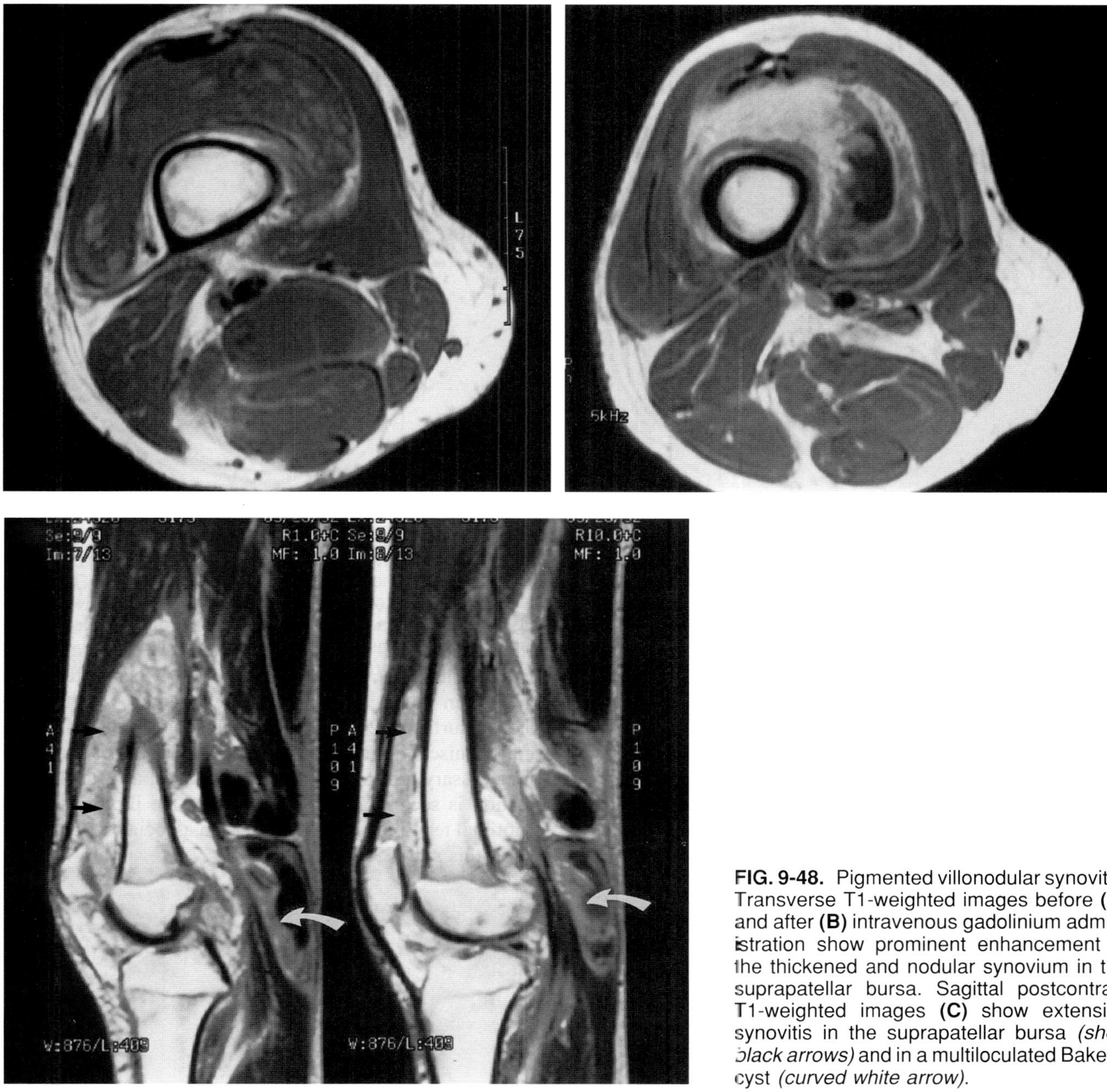

FIG. 9-48. Pigmented villonodular synovitis. Transverse T1-weighted images before **(A)** and after **(B)** intravenous gadolinium administration show prominent enhancement of the thickened and nodular synovium in the suprapatellar bursa. Sagittal postcontrast T1-weighted images **(C)** show extensive synovitis in the suprapatellar bursa *(short black arrows)* and in a multiloculated Baker's cyst *(curved white arrow).*

Prepatellar Bursitis

The prepatellar bursa is located between the anterior surface of the patella and the skin, and functions to reduce friction between these structures. Inflammation and hemorrhage in this bursa is often due to occupational (''housemaid's knee'') or recreational (''wrestler's knee'') kneeling and crawling; however, infectious bursitis is not uncommon. MR imaging shows a multiloculated fluid collection between the patellar surface and the overlying skin (see Fig. 3-13). The fluid collection is often heterogenous and poorly defined due to hemorrhage and inflammation in the bursa (230).

Superficial and Deep Infrapatellar Bursitis

Two bursae are present near the distal insertion of the patellar tendon: The superficial infrapatellar bursa is located between the tibial tubercle and the overlying skin, and the deep infrapatellar bursa is located between the distal end of the patellar tendon and the subjacent anterior tibial cortex (see Fig. 9-51). The superficial infrapatellar bursa may become inflamed and distended after direct trauma; however, this is not a common site of bursitis (247). On MR images, the deep infrapatellar bursa often contains a small amount of fluid in asymptomatic knees; thus, this is likely a normal

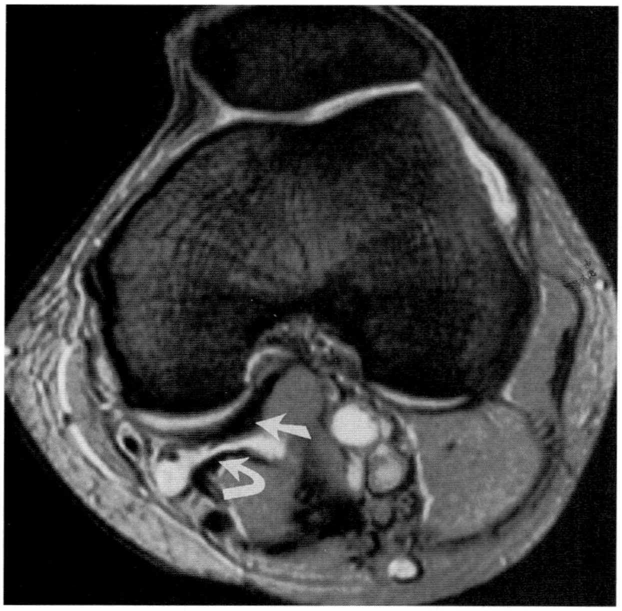

FIG. 9-53. Baker's cyst. A transverse gradient-echo image shows a small Baker's cyst projecting between the tendon of the medial head of the gastrocnemius muscle *(arrow)* and the semimembranosus tendon *(curved arrow)*.

Meniscal Cysts

Meniscal cysts, by definition, result from extrusion of joint fluid through a horizontal meniscal tear into the surrounding tissues (248,251,252). These cysts present with symptoms of knee pain, locking, and a palpable mass adjacent to the joint line. Correct diagnosis of meniscal cysts is important, because these cysts will require meniscal repair for successful treatment and will usually recur if aspiration or resection is attempted (253). Lateral meniscal cysts are three to four times more common than medial meniscal cysts (230).

MR imaging of meniscal cysts shows a fluid collection contacting the periphery of the meniscus, adjacent to a horizontal meniscal tear. Medial meniscal cysts tend to be large and show extensive dissection through tissue planes, because these cysts often penetrate the joint capsule and extend into the adjacent tissues (Fig. 9-56). Lateral meniscal cysts are generally smaller and are contained within the joint capsule (Fig. 9-57) (248).

Ganglion

Ganglia are cystic structures that contain fluid or mucoid material and are lined by flat, spindle-shaped cells. Ganglia may arise from joint capsules, tendon sheaths, bursa, bone, or connective tissue and generally do not communicate with the joint (254). Ganglia are thought to arise from degeneration or trauma to connective tissues. Superficial ganglia present clinically as a palpable small mass.

On direct inspection, ganglia are unilocular or multilocular cysts filled with thick mucoid material. They have well-circumscribed borders and appear encapsulated by a layer of dense fibrous tissue. Histologically, the walls of the cyst are composed of dense collagen, and no atypical cells or mitotic figures are present. The internal mucinous material stains intensely with Alcian blue stain (255,256).

In the knee, the most common site of ganglion formation is adjacent to a cruciate ligament; these intra-articular ganglia are likely secondary to degeneration of the ligament. If large, intra-articular ganglia may produce restricted knee flexion, locking, and pain. In the series of Brown and colleagues (257) the tibial end of the anterior cruciate ligament was the most common site, whereas in the series of Recht and colleagues the posterior cruciate ligament was the most common site (258). Another common site of ganglion formation is at the proximal tibiofibular joint. Ganglia at this site may compress the common peroneal nerve, resulting in atrophy of the anterior compartment muscles. Simple excision of the ganglion is usually curative.

On MR images, ganglia appear as well-defined fluid collections, often with prominent septations (Fig. 9-58). Bone erosion and dissection along tissue planes are not unusual (230). Ganglia can be easily distinguished from meniscal cysts by the absence of connection to a horizontal meniscal tear.

Intraosseous Cyst

Small intraosseous cysts are occasionally seen in the subchondral bone near the insertion of the cruciate ligaments or meniscotibial attachments. These asymptomatic cysts have been reported in 1% of routine knee MR examinations and are more common in older patients (259). Although the origin of these cysts has not been proven, they likely arise from bone resorption due to repeated avulsive stress (230,255,260).

On MR images, intraosseous cysts appear as small fluid-filled lesions within the subchondral bone of the proximal tibia. A small amount of bone marrow edema may be seen around the cyst on fat-suppressed T2-weighted images (Fig. 9-59). The imaging features are similar to those of a geode; however, geodes occur in association with significant degenerative joint disease, are not usually sited near the cruciate and meniscal attachments to tibia, and often contact the subchondral bone cortex.

SOFT-TISSUE TUMORS

The goals of imaging in patients with suspected soft-tissue masses include lesion detection and localization, staging, and noninvasive characterization of histologic type (261). MRI, by virtue of its excellent soft-tissue contrast and multiplanar imaging capacity, is the modality of choice for evaluation of soft-tissue tumors. Although this discussion will

A

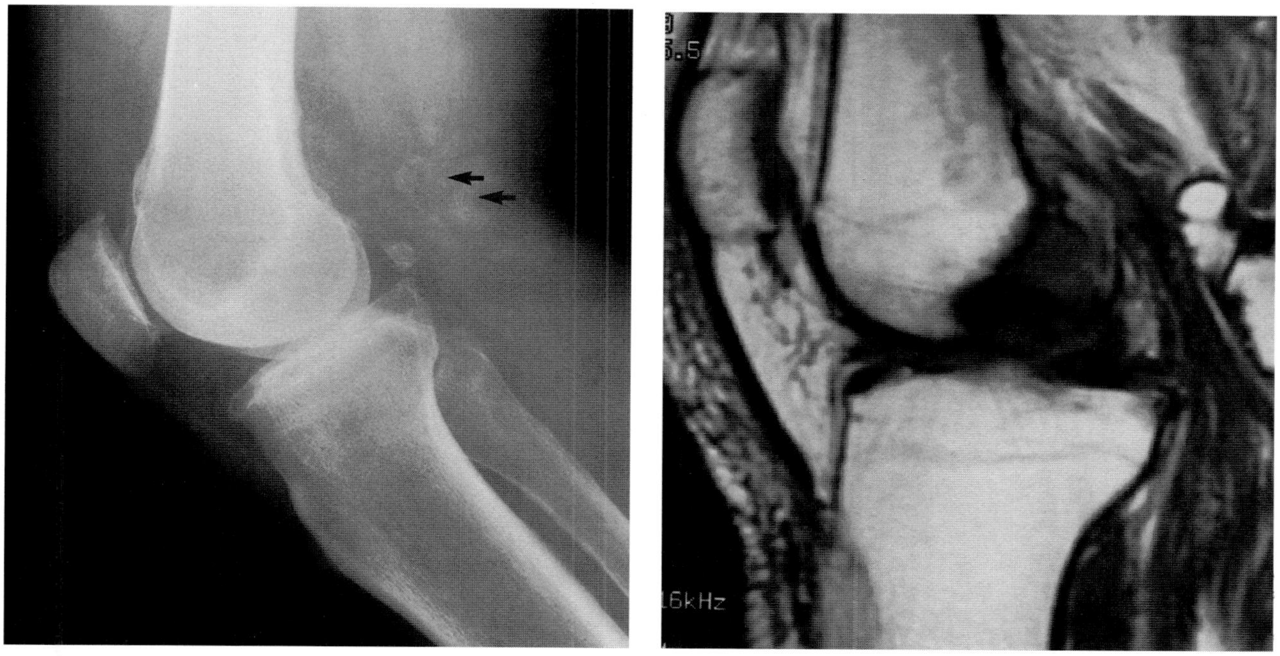

B

C

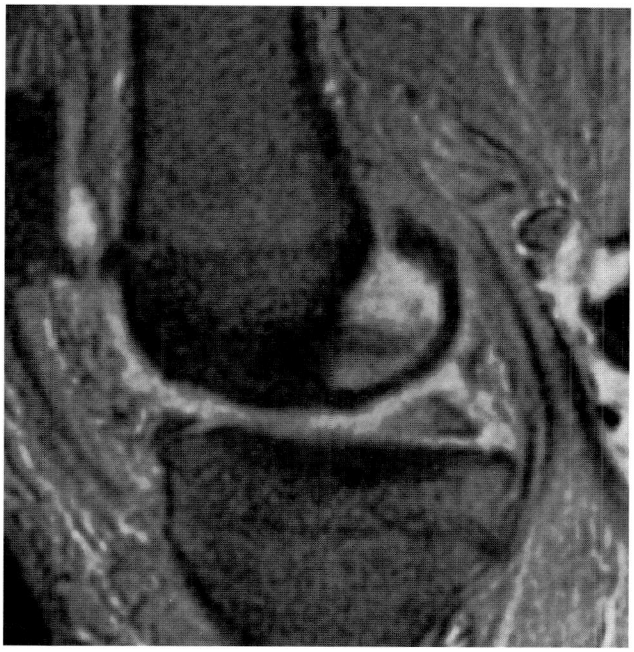

FIG. 9-54. Ossified loose bodies in a Baker's cyst. **A:** A lateral plain radiograph shows amorphous calcification in the popliteal fossa *(arrows)*. Sagittal T1-weighted **(B)** and T2*-weighted **(C)** images show a large ossified loose body in a Baker's cyst. The loose body contains central marrow fat and peripheral calcification.

highlight the role of MRI, it must be emphasized that MRI is best used in conjunction with other modalities. For example, plain radiographs are necessary to assess for calcification or ossification in a mass, CT is extremely useful for assessment of fatty tumors or detection of bony involvement, and sonography is useful for evaluation of cystic or vascular masses (262,263). This section is not intended as an exhaustive catalogue of all soft-tissue lesions; rather, it presents an overview of imaging technique and MRI findings in various soft-tissue tumors that may occur in the region of the knee. Those tumors are emphasized that are common or have characteristic MRI appearances.

Basic Clinical Considerations

The most common soft-tissue tumors are benign lesions, such as lipomas and ganglions, which generally do not require MRI or biopsy procedures for management. More ominous lesions—such as those that are large, painful, enlarging, or deep-seated—are more likely to be malignant, and require thorough investigation and staging prior to surgical or nonsurgical therapy. It is imperative that the imaging evaluation be completed prior to any attempt at biopsy or excision, because hemorrhage and edema resultant from the biopsy or excision will make accurate staging difficult or impossible (4,264). Bi-

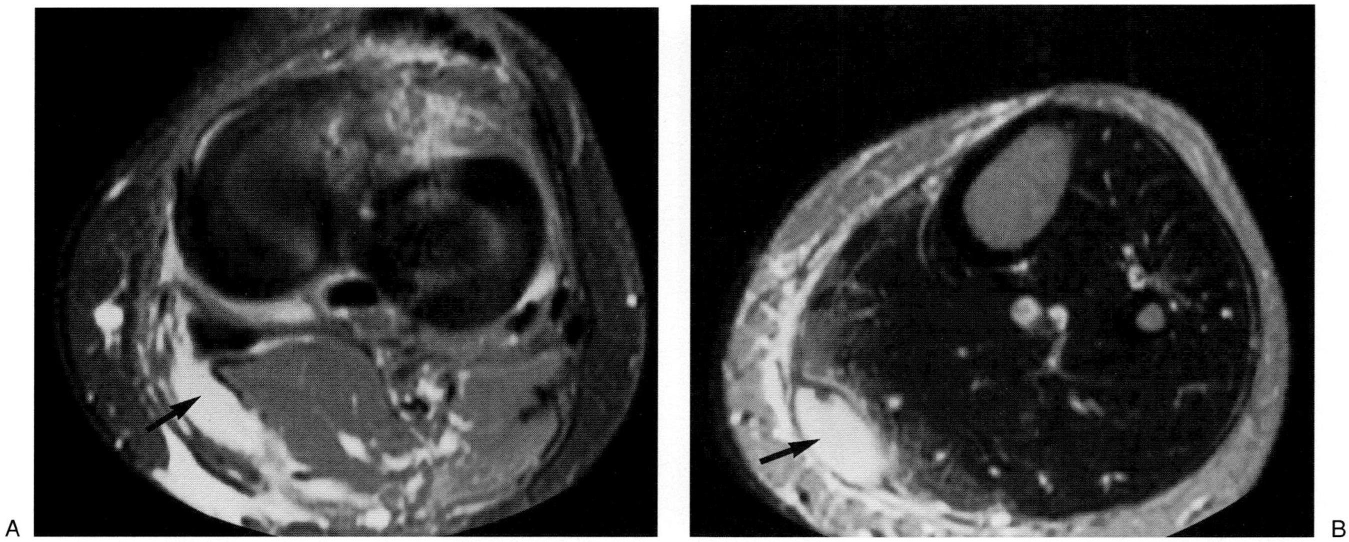

FIG. 9-55. Ruptured Baker's cyst. Transverse T2-weighted images at the level of the knee joint **(A)** and the midcalf **(B)** show a partially collapsed Baker's cyst *(arrows)* with extensive dissection of fluid between tissue layers. This patient presented with an acutely tender swollen calf.

opsy routes should be planned in conjunction with the surgeon responsible for tumor resection, because biopsy tracks crossing uninvolved tissue compartments may necessitate more extensive local resection. Evaluation and successful treatment of patients with suspected sarcomas require expertise in imaging, pathology, radiation therapy, chemotherapy, and orthopedic and reconstructive surgery (265). A team approach at a tumor center is recommended and has been shown to reduce the number of necessary surgical procedures and to improve patient outcome (266).

The major role of imaging in soft-tissue sarcoma management is anatomic staging (267,268). Precise definition of the boundary of abnormal tissue is essential for planning surgical resection, because negative tumor margins must be obtained to minimize the risk of local recurrence (269). Definition of tumor boundaries is also necessary to plan local radiotherapy and to minimize irradiation of normal tissue. Successful surgical therapy of soft-tissue and bone sarcomas requires that all involved tissue compartments, including those contaminated by biopsy tracks, be completely resected (35). The relationship of tumor to neurovascular structures is critical, because encasement or infiltration of these structures may make complete resection impossible, resulting in amputation or incomplete local resection. Recognition of tumor invasion of bone is also critical, as bone involvement may necessitate bone resection and reconstruction with bone grafts or prostheses. MRI often allows definitive identification of many nonneoplastic entities that may clinically mimic soft-tissue sarcomas, such as asymmetric or accessory muscles, ganglia, and hematomas (Fig. 9-60) (270).

Imaging Technique

The MRI examination of a patient with a suspected soft-tissue neoplasm should be tailored to the specific clinical situation. As a general rule, T1- and T2-weighted spin-echo images should be obtained (usually in the transverse plane), with short-tau inversion recovery (STIR) sequences in one plane (usually coronal or sagittal) and gradient-echo images in the third orthogonal plane. This basic strategy must be modified for each individual case; for example, depiction of the relationship of tumor to important neurovascular and bony structures in some anatomic sites may be aided by use of nonorthogonal planes. T1- and T2-weighted spin-echo images are necessary to assess signal intensity characteristics of the tumor tissue. STIR images provide optimal contrast and conspicuity of tumor and edema relative to normal tissues, and they give the best assessment of tumor extent. $T2^*$-weighted gradient-echo images are particularly sensitive to the presence of hemosiderin or calcifications within the tumor and may occasionally display the vascular elements as a result of flow-related enhancement effects.

The detection of fat or hemosiderin within a tumor is important, because these diagnostic findings often limit the differential diagnosis. The presence of fat within a tumor can be recognized by comparing the signal intensity characteristics of the tumor with those of surrounding normal fat. STIR images or frequency-selective fat presaturation techniques can be used to identify fatty components definitively. These techniques should be used to confirm the presence of fat within a tumor whenever the spin-echo images or other imaging studies are suggestive of intratumoral fat. Hemosiderin may be found in soft-tissue masses as a result of spontaneous hemorrhage or surgical intervention. On $T2^*$-weighted gradient-echo images, hemosiderin produces a prominent signal void as a result of magnetic susceptibility effects. This effect is more obvious on gradient-echo images than on spin-echo images because of the absence of a 180° refocusing pulse. Focal signal voids on $T2^*$-weighted gradient-echo im-

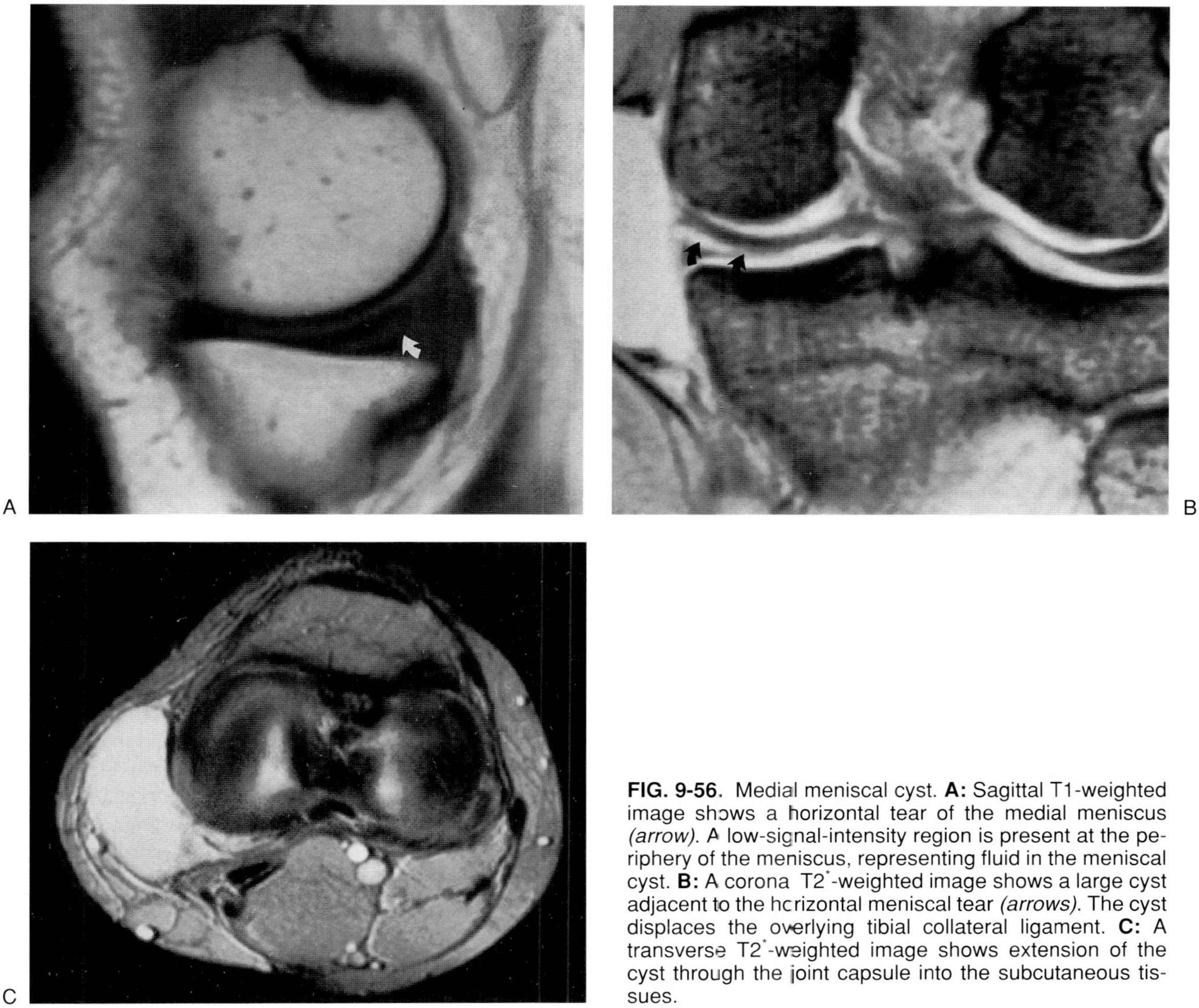

FIG. 9-56. Medial meniscal cyst. **A:** Sagittal T1-weighted image shows a horizontal tear of the medial meniscus *(arrow)*. A low-signal-intensity region is present at the periphery of the meniscus, representing fluid in the meniscal cyst. **B:** A corona T2*-weighted image shows a large cyst adjacent to the horizontal meniscal tear *(arrows)*. The cyst displaces the overlying tibial collateral ligament. **C:** A transverse T2*-weighted image shows extension of the cyst through the joint capsule into the subcutaneous tissues.

ages may also be due to surgical clips or calcifications; thus, correlation with plain radiographs is essential for correct interpretation (271).

Tumor Characterization

Many studies have addressed the ability of MRI to provide a specific histologic diagnosis of soft-tissue tumors, with variable results. Many of these studies have attempted to use "global criteria" such as tumor size, tumor margins, and internal homogeneity to predict the benign or malignant nature of a soft-tissue tumor. These studies have shown accuracies ranging from 55% to 100% (26,27,272–275). The global criteria most strongly associated with malignancy are large size (over 3 cm in diameter), irregular or infiltrative margins, and inhomogeneous internal signal. However, malignant soft-tissue tumors are occasionally small and well defined, and benign lesions such as abscesses and hematomas may be large, infiltrative, and inhomogeneous. In our experience, the global criteria listed earlier do not allow characterization of soft-tissue masses with enough accuracy to obviate biopsy and histologic diagnosis (261). However, some benign soft-tissue masses often have characteristic features that allow a confident and accurate diagnosis to made, thus obviating further investigation and biopsy. Common tumors with specific MRI characteristics include hemangiomas, lipomas, ganglia, neurofibromas, schwannomas, and pigmented villonodular synovitis. In our referral population, MR imaging allows a specific diagnosis in 10–30% of cases referred with a clinical diagnosis of "soft-tissue tumor." MR phosphorus-31 spectroscopy may prove to be a useful noninva-

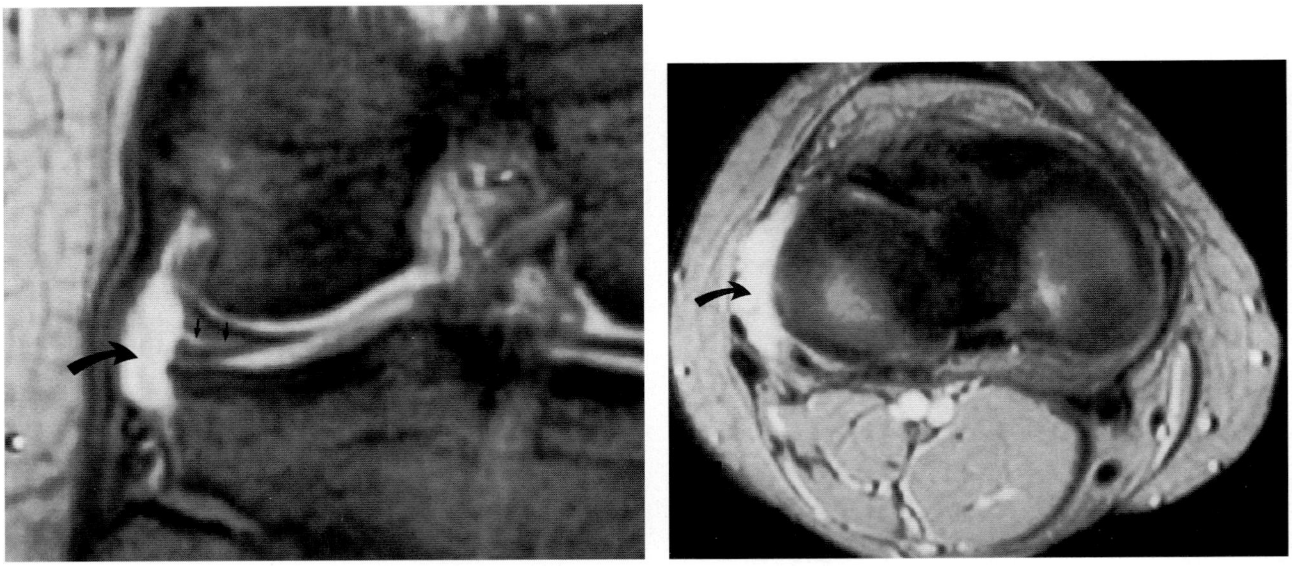

A B

FIG. 9-57. Lateral meniscal cyst. Coronal **(A)** and transverse **(B)** T2*-weighted images show a cyst *(curved arrow)* adjacent to a horizontal tear *(small arrows)* of the lateral meniscus.

sive method of differentiating benign from malignant soft-tissue masses, because this modality offers information on the metabolic activity of the tumor (276–279).

The signal intensity characteristics of a soft-tissue tumor can be used to identify specific tissue types, such as fat, hemosiderin, dense fibrous tissue, or hemorrhage. Most soft-tissue sarcomas have low signal intensity on T1-weighted sequences and high signal intensity on T2-weighted sequences (4). Substances with high signal intensity on T1-weighted images include fat, subacute hemorrhage (methemoglobin), or proteinaceous fluid. Identification of fat in a soft-tissue tumor is very important, because this finding limits the differential diagnosis to lipoma, hemangioma, arteriovenous malformation, or well-differentiated liposarcomas. Most high-grade liposarcomas do not contain macroscopic fat (280). Subacute hemorrhage also produces high signal intensity on T1-weighted images, because of the presence of methemoglobin. Soft-tissue hematomas may occur as a result of trauma, anticoagulation, vasculitis, or hemorrhage into a preexisting mass. Synovial sarcomas have a particular

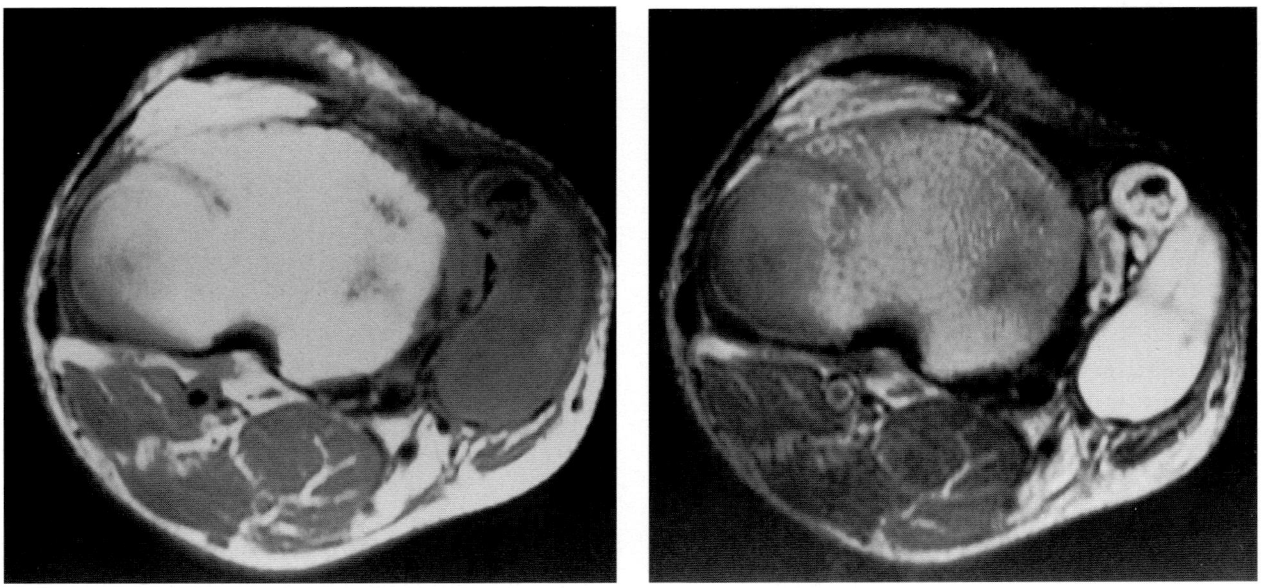

A B

FIG. 9-58. Soft-tissue ganglion. T1-weighted **(A)** and T2-weighted **(B)** transverse images show a multiloculated fluid collection encircling the medial collateral ligament. The adjacent tibia is normal.

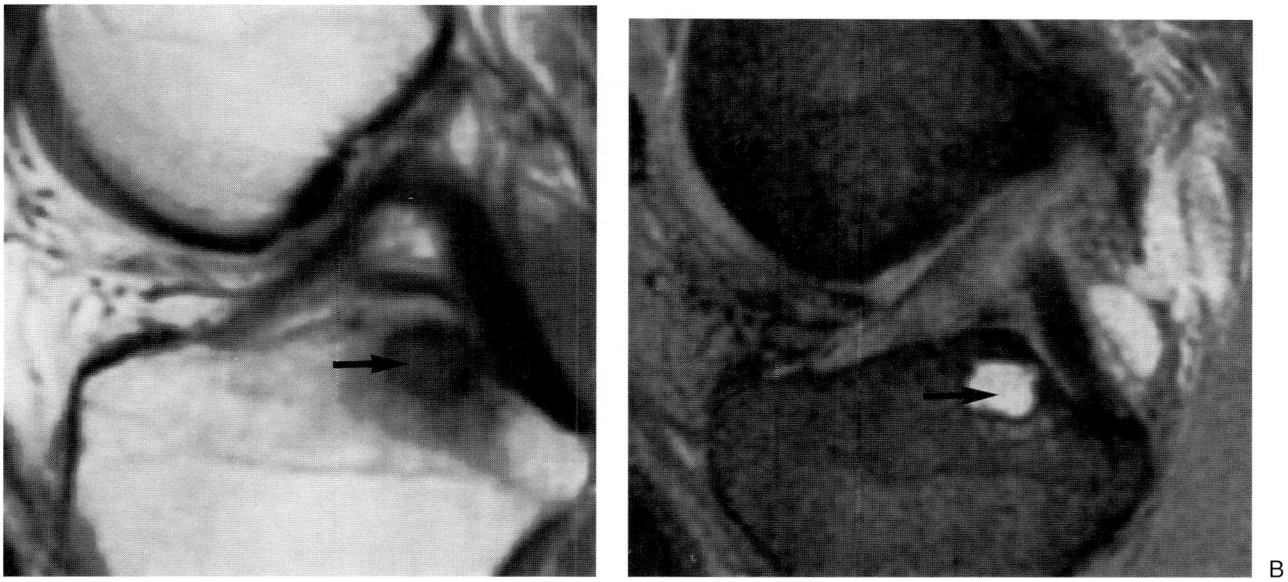

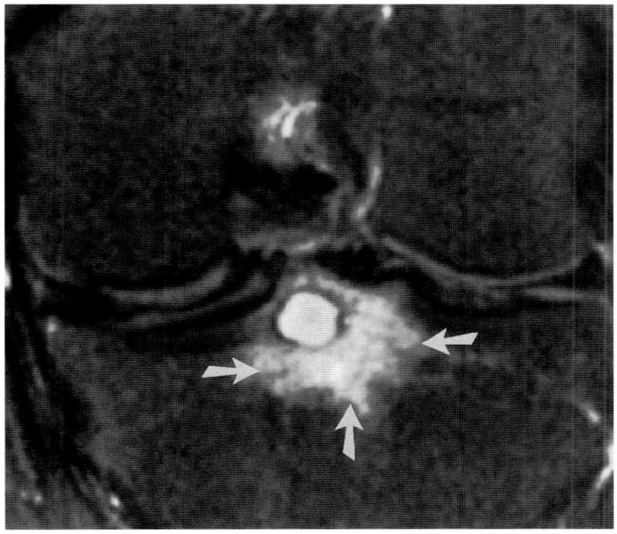

FIG. 9-59. Intraosseous cyst at site of posterior cruciate ligament insertion. Sagittal T1-weighted **(A)** and T2*-weighted **(B)** images show a focal intraosseous cyst *(arrow)* near the insertion of the posterior cruciate ligament, with a well-defined sclerotic margin. A coronal fat-suppressed fast spin-echo T2-weighted image **(C)** shows bone marrow edema surrounding the cystic lesion *(arrows).*

propensity for intratumoral hemorrhage; this finding was observed in 44% of cases in a recent series (281).

The finding of decreased signal intensity on T1- and T2-weighted images suggests the presence of dense fibrous tissue, calcification, ossification, or hemosiderin deposition. Correlation with plain radiographs is essential for detection of calcification or ossification within a soft-tissue tumor. Low signal intensity due to dense fibrous tissue is most commonly seen in benign fibrous lesions such as fibromas and desmoids but has also been described in malignant fibrous histiocytoma, fibrosarcoma, and malignant nerve sheath tumors (27,282). Gradient-echo images are useful for detection of hemosiderin, because the signal void will enlarge (''bloom'') on gradient-echo images relative to the size of the signal void on spin-echo images, because of the paramagnetic properties of hemosiderin. Tumors that often contain hemosiderin include pigmented villonodular synovitis (237–240,283), giant cell tumor of tendon sheath (242,273,284), and hematomas (see Figs. 9-48, 9-49, and 9-60).

Lipomatous Tumors

Benign Fatty Tumors

Lipomas are benign tumors containing encapsulated mature fat and a few fibrous septations. Lipomas are the most common soft-tissue tumor in most reported clinical series (271,285). Superficial lipomas are easily recognized clinically in most cases, and generally do not require further investigation, imaging, or resection. Deep-seated lipomas may present as nondescript soft-tissue masses, thus requiring further investigation to exclude malignancy (1).

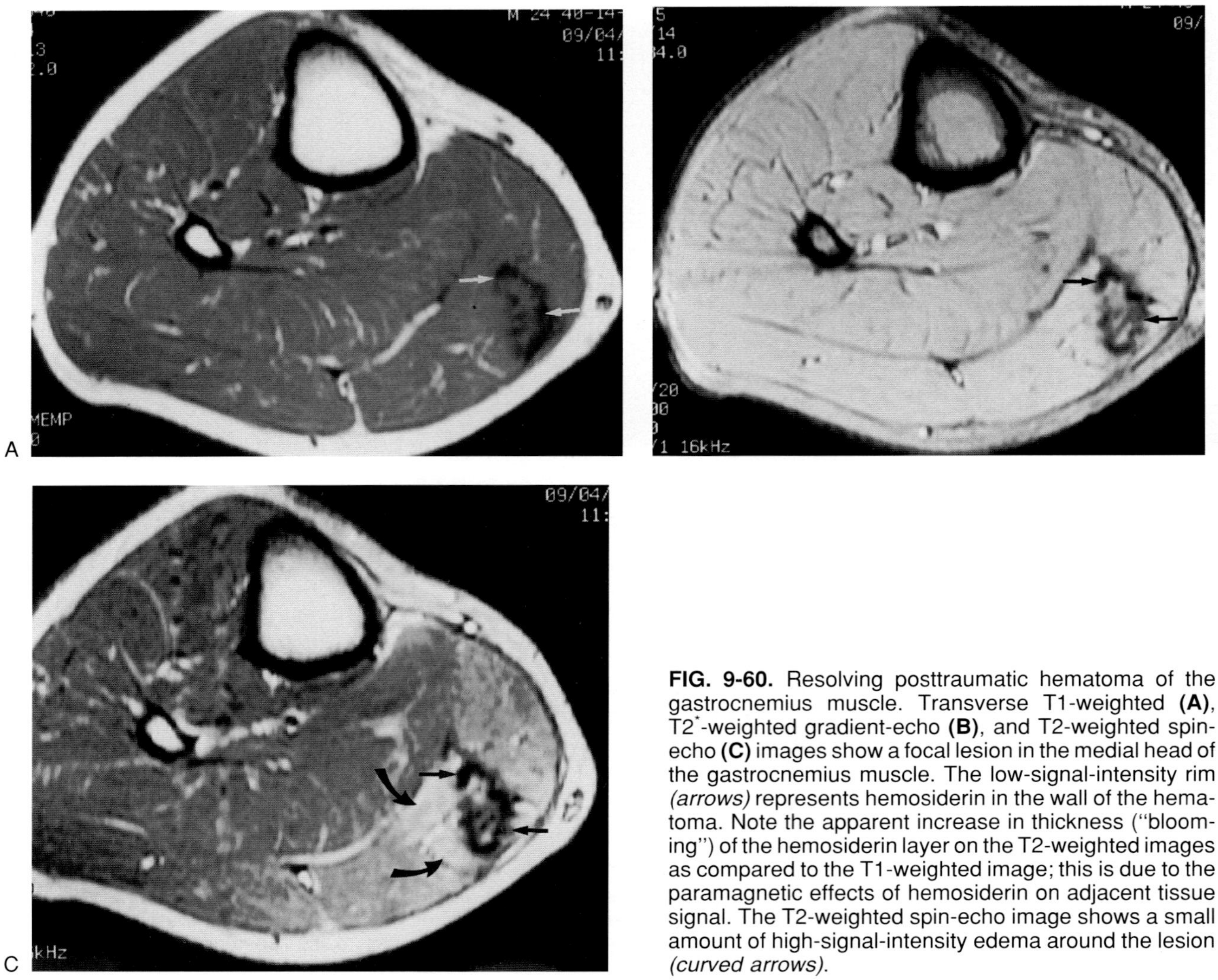

FIG. 9-60. Resolving posttraumatic hematoma of the gastrocnemius muscle. Transverse T1-weighted **(A)**, T2*-weighted gradient-echo **(B)**, and T2-weighted spin-echo **(C)** images show a focal lesion in the medial head of the gastrocnemius muscle. The low-signal-intensity rim *(arrows)* represents hemosiderin in the wall of the hematoma. Note the apparent increase in thickness ("blooming") of the hemosiderin layer on the T2-weighted images as compared to the T1-weighted image; this is due to the paramagnetic effects of hemosiderin on adjacent tissue signal. The T2-weighted spin-echo image shows a small amount of high-signal-intensity edema around the lesion *(curved arrows)*.

On imaging, lipomas typically appear as well-marginated lesions composed almost entirely of mature fat. A few fibrous septations are frequently seen in benign lipomas; the amount of septation is equal to or less than that of the subcutaneous fat. Intramuscular lipomas occasionally have infiltrative margins, producing a misleading appearance of an aggressive lesion (286). MR imaging shows the signal characteristics of a lipoma to be identical to those of subcutaneous fat on all pulse sequences (Fig. 9-61). In our experience and in the literature, MR imaging allows a confident and accurate diagnosis of lipoma to be made in the vast majority of cases, thus obviating the need for further investigation or biopsy (26,272,273,287,288). Fat-suppressed images, using STIR techniques or frequency-selective fat saturation, are very useful in assessment of fatty tumors. Simple lipomas will show complete suppression of signal, with no residual high-signal-intensity cellular regions (see Fig. 9-61). The presence of thick septations is typical of well-differentiated liposarcoma; the finding of a soft-tissue component within a fatty tumor is typical of dedifferentiation (280,289). Parosteal lipomas originate adjacent to the periosteum, resulting in the typical appearance of a fatty mass associated with a bony excrescence of reactive periosteal ossification (156).

Other types of benign fatty tumors include lipoblastomas, hibernomas, and various types of lipomatosis; all these conditions are rare. Lipoblastomas are well-defined tumors containing immature lipoblasts and a variable amount of mature lipocytes. Lipoblastomas are most common in children and may occur in focal or diffuse (lipoblastomatosis) forms (286,290,291). Hibernomas are rare tumors composed of brown fat. These tumors tend to occur in the mediastinal, retroperitoneal, and intercapsular regions and are most common in middle-aged women (292). We have imaged two cases of hibernoma on MRI; in both cases the hibernoma had an appearance indistinguishable from a lipoma. Lipomatoses are rare conditions in which fat extensively infiltrates an anatomic region, often in a bilateral and symmetric fashion (286). No discrete mass is present; rather, the infiltrating fat is intermixed with muscles, nerves, vessels, and connective tissues. A wide variety of lipomatoses have been described,

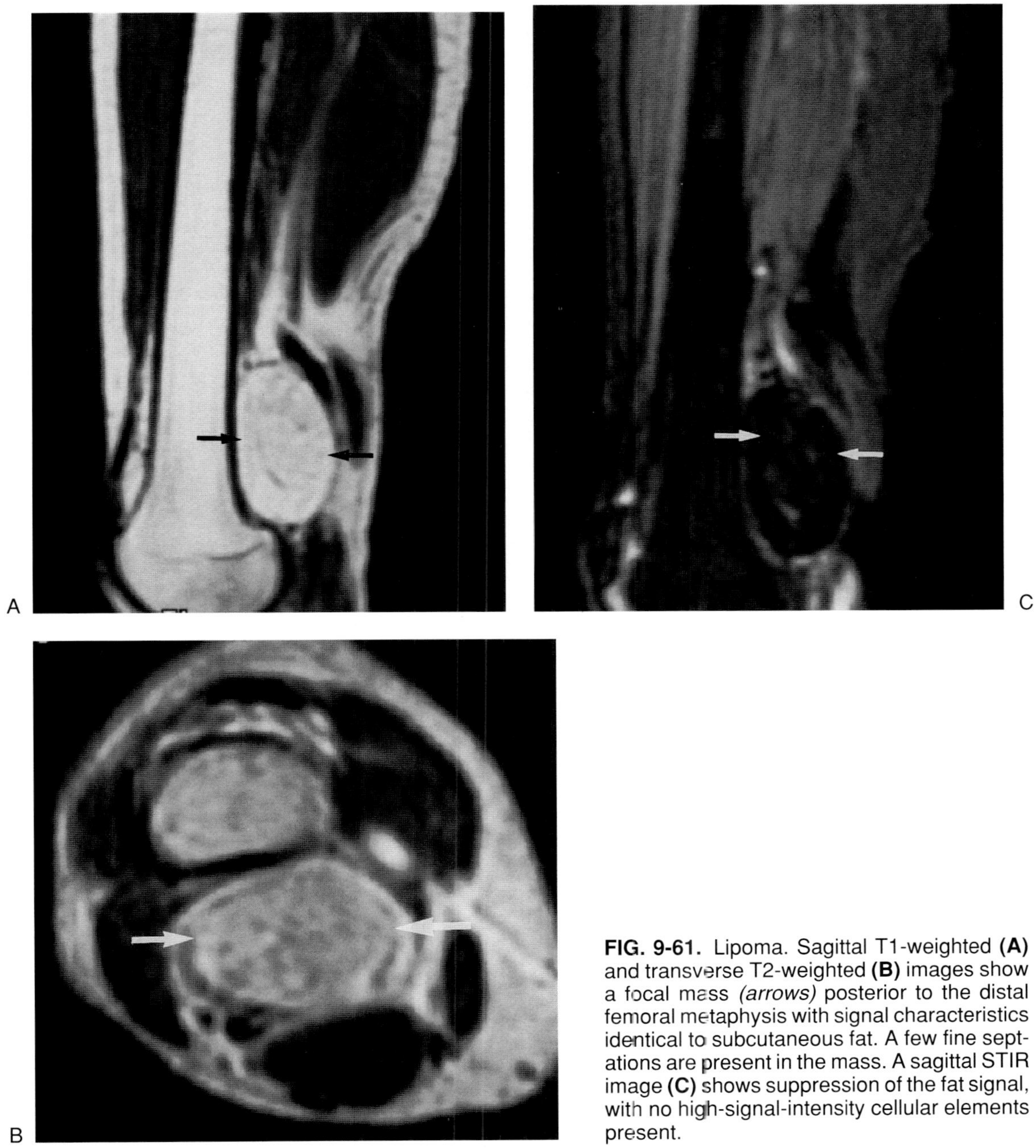

FIG. 9-61. Lipoma. Sagittal T1-weighted **(A)** and transverse T2-weighted **(B)** images show a focal mass *(arrows)* posterior to the distal femoral metaphysis with signal characteristics identical to subcutaneous fat. A few fine septations are present in the mass. A sagittal STIR image **(C)** shows suppression of the fat signal, with no high-signal-intensity cellular elements present.

many of which are associated with abnormalities in glucose and lipid metabolism (293–296).

Of note, other benign tumors may contain visible fat on MR images, including hemangiomas, arteriovenous malformations, and hamartomas (i.e., chondrolipoma, fibrolipoma, angiolipoma) (297–300).

Malignant Fatty Tumors

Liposarcomas are malignant mesenchymal tumors that histologically have features of adipose differentiation. As in the nomenclature of all sarcomas, the prefix (e.g., *lipo, fibro, chondro*) does not indicate that the tumor arose from a known precursor tissue; instead, it indicates that the tumor has differentiated toward a specific tissue type. Liposarcomas are the second-most-common soft-tissue sarcoma in adults, after malignant fibrous histiocytoma (280,301,302). The biological behavior of liposarcomas covers a spectrum from low-grade tumors with no metastatic potential to high-grade malignancies producing significant mortality (303).

Low-grade liposarcomas are variously described as *well-differentiated liposarcomas*, *atypical lipomas*, or *lipoma-like liposarcomas*. All these terms describe histologically identical tumors composed predominantly of mature fat, with thick or numerous septations. Some authors reserve the term *well-differentiated liposarcoma* for retroperitoneal lesions and use *atypical lipoma* for an identical lesion in the extremities (304). These tumors have essentially no risk of distant metastasis but will recur locally if incompletely excised. On MR images, a low-grade liposarcoma appears as a predominantly fatty mass with thick or nodular septations (280). T2-weighted or fat-suppressed images are very helpful to highlight the presence of high-signal-intensity soft-tissue components within the fatty mass.

The intermediate-grade liposarcomas consist largely of the myxoid subtype. These common tumors often do not contain macroscopic amounts of fat on CT or MR images (Fig. 9-62). In a study by Jelinek and colleagues, only two of 19 myxoid liposarcomas contained more than 25% fat (by volume), and 11 contained no visible fat (280). If macroscopic fat is visible within the tumor, it is often distributed in lacy or linear strands (Fig. 9-63) (305). Myxoid liposarcomas often have an appearance suggestive of a cyst, with well-defined margins, homogeneous low signal intensity on T1-weighted images, and high signal intensity on T2-weighted images (280). The CT appearance can also resemble a cyst, because the myxoid material produces attenuation values similar to those of fluid. Sonography is occasionally useful to assess definitively the cystic versus solid nature of a soft-tissue mass.

High-grade liposarcomas generally contain minimal or no visible fat and are often indistinguishable from other soft-tissue sarcomas on MR imaging. These tumors have low signal intensity on T1-weighted images and high signal intensity on T2-weighted images, often with heterogeneous signal characteristics. The most common histologic subtypes of high-grade liposarcoma are pleomorphic and round-cell.

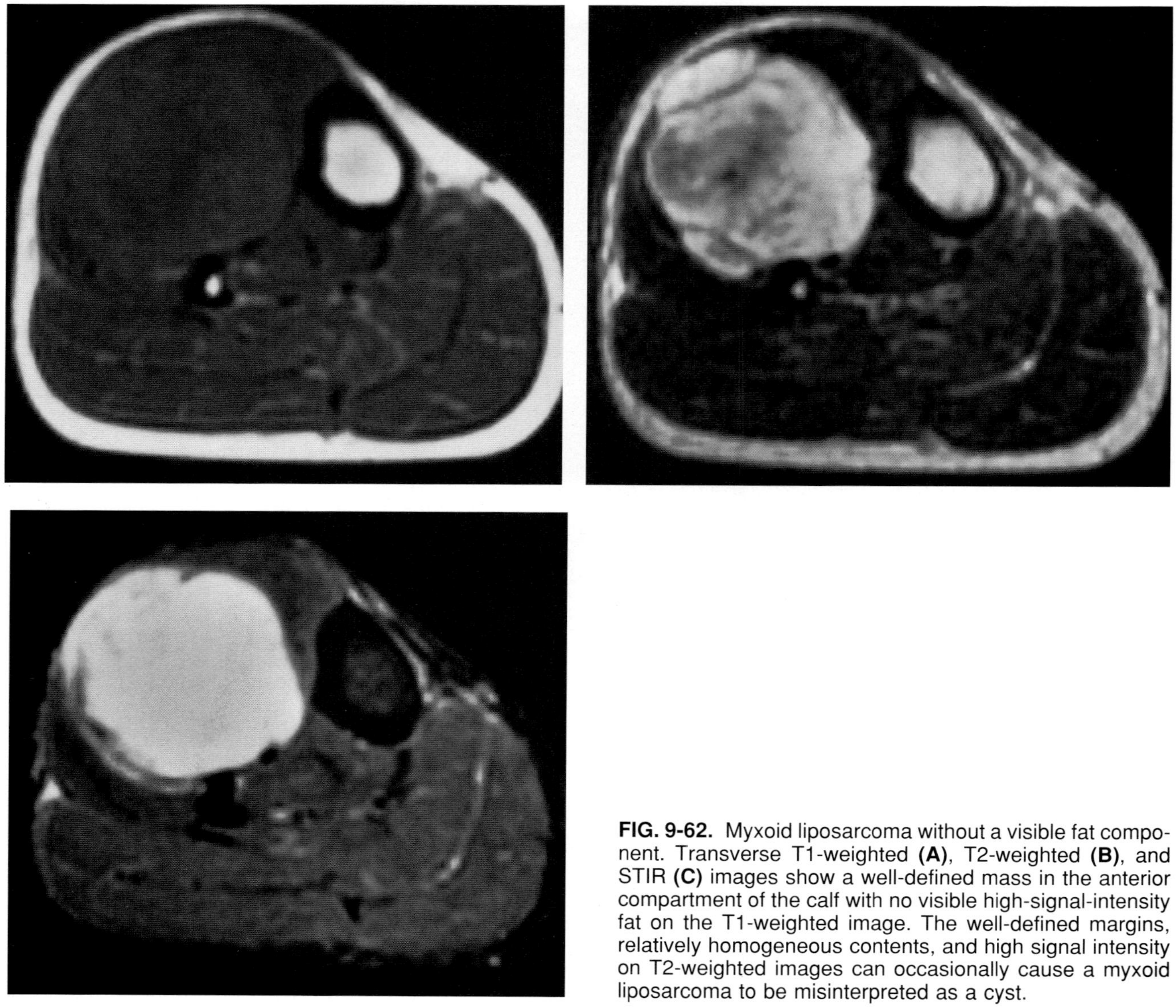

A B C

FIG. 9-62. Myxoid liposarcoma without a visible fat component. Transverse T1-weighted **(A)**, T2-weighted **(B)**, and STIR **(C)** images show a well-defined mass in the anterior compartment of the calf with no visible high-signal-intensity fat on the T1-weighted image. The well-defined margins, relatively homogeneous contents, and high signal intensity on T2-weighted images can occasionally cause a myxoid liposarcoma to be misinterpreted as a cyst.

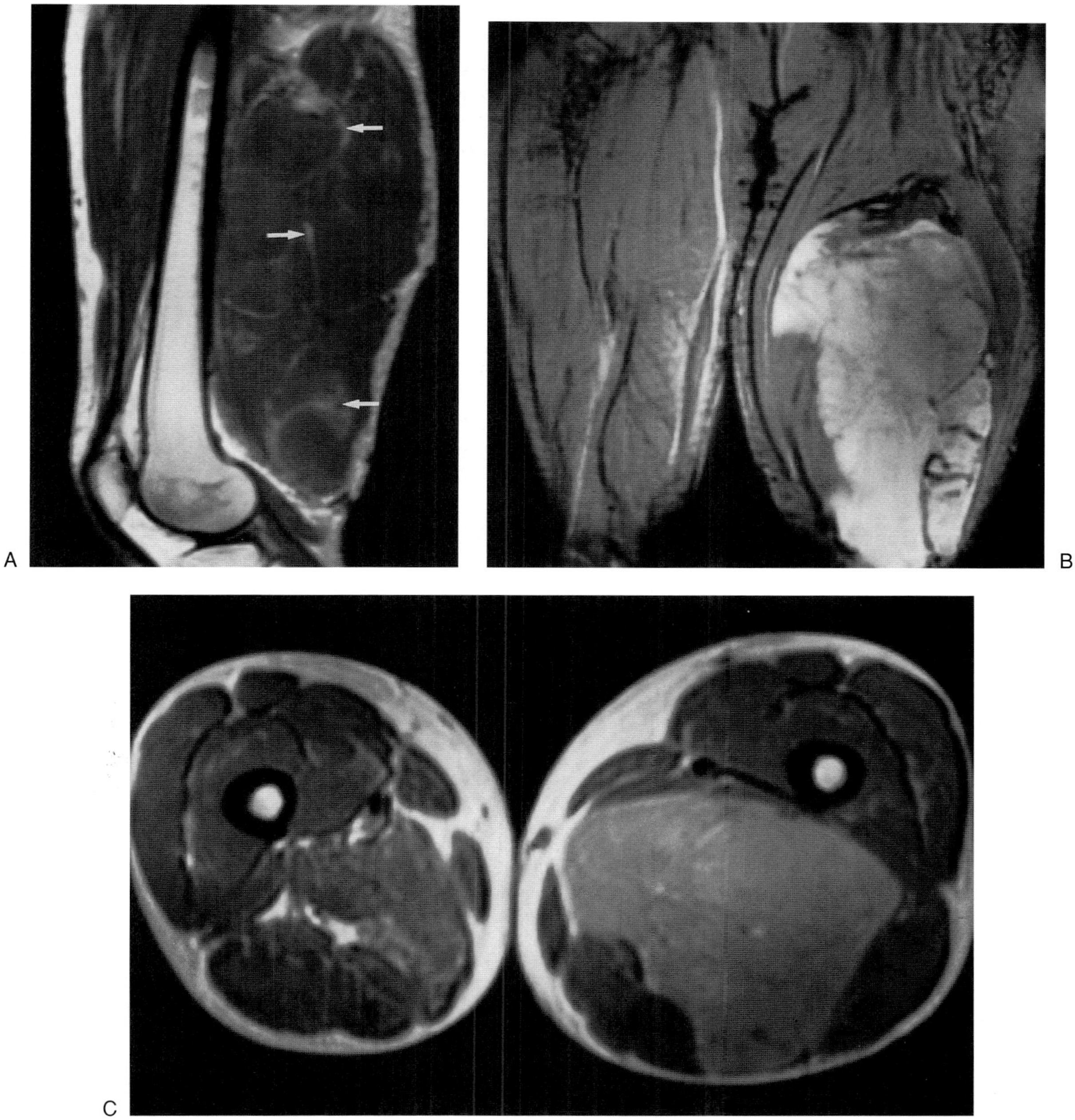

FIG. 9-63. Myxoid liposarcoma with visible fatty components. **A:** A sagittal T1-weighted image shows a huge mass in the posterior compartment of the thigh, which contains linear lacy strands of high-signal-intensity fat *(arrows).* Coronal T2*-weighted **(B)** and transverse T2-weighted **(C)** images show displacement and effacement of the hamstring and adductor muscles by the huge lobulated inhomogeneous tumor.

These aggressive tumors have a high rate of metastasis and cause significant morbidity and mortality.

Vascular Tumors

Hemangiomas

Hemangiomas are common benign vascular tumors, comprising approximately 8% of benign soft-tissue tumors (285). Hemangiomas are composed of variable proportions of fat, fibrous septae, thrombus, and vascular spaces filled with stagnant blood. Hemangiomas are further classified as capillary or cavernous types, depending on the size of the vascular spaces.

Hemangiomas have a characteristic MRI appearance that, in most cases, allows a confident and accurate diagnosis to be made (Fig. 9-64) (306). In most cases, T1-weighted images show strands of high-signal-intensity fat interspersed

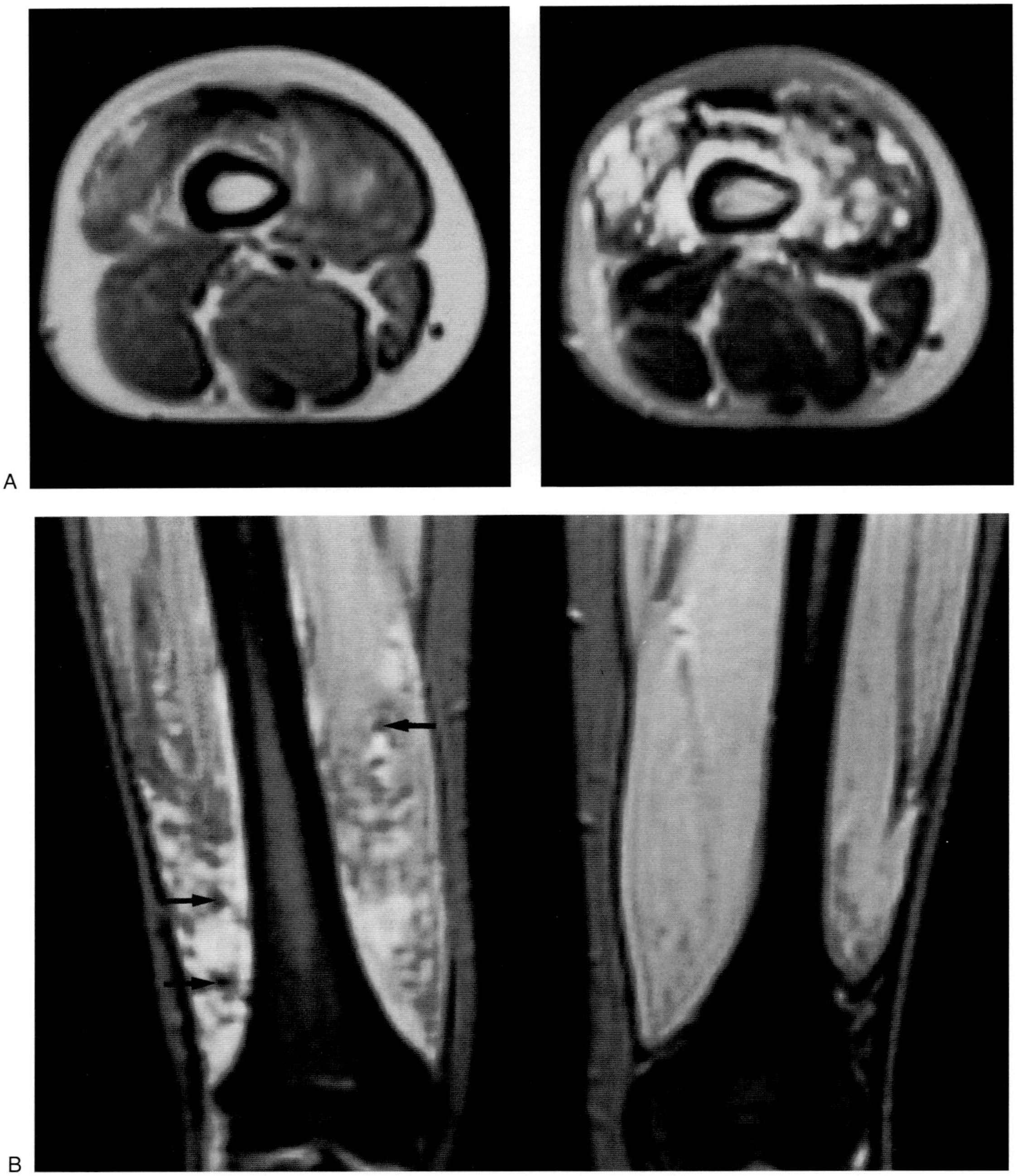

FIG. 9-64. Infiltrating hemangioma. **A:** Transverse T1-weighted *(left)* and T2-weighted images *(right)* show a hemangioma infiltrating the quadriceps muscle and prefemoral fat. Strands of high-signal-intensity fat are visible on the T1-weighted image. The T2-weighted image shows many high-signal-intensity locules of the fluid within the vascular spaces of the hemangioma. A coronal STIR image **(B)** shows a few low-signal-intensity foci *(arrows)* consistent with phleboliths or thrombi within the hemangioma. Intramuscular hemangiomas are often extensively infiltrating, as shown in this case.

with low-signal-intensity blood-filled spaces and fibrous septations. T2-weighted images show locules of high signal intensity, representing the blood-filled spaces (306). Fluid–fluid levels may be found in the larger cavernous spaces, because of stagnation and sedimentation of the blood into cellular and serum components (307). Focal signal voids may also be present, representing phleboliths or hemosiderin-laden thrombus (1,274,287,308). Hemangiomas may be well defined or may involve multiple contiguous structures (hemangiomatosis). MR is more accurate than CT or angiography for determining the extent of these lesions and is thus the preferred modality for preoperative planning (309,310).

Vascular Malformations

A variety of high-flow and low-flow vascular malformations have been described, including venous malformations, arteriovenous malformations, arteriovenous fistulae, and mixed lesions. Venous malformations are abnormal dilatations of the postcapillary vessels, with slow (venous) flow. Arteriovenous malformations are high-flow lesions consisting of multiple connections between the arterial and venous circulation without an interposed capillary bed. Arteriovenous fistulae consist of a single connection between an artery and a vein (311). These lesions are usually congenital; however, arteriovenous fistulae can also arise from penetrating trauma to adjacent arteries and veins.

MR imaging can characterize vascular malformations as high-flow or low-flow lesions. In slow-flow lesions such as venous malformations, T2-weighted images show high signal intensity arising from the vascular spaces. In high-flow lesions, T2-weighted images show signal voids representing the vascular spaces (311–313). Flow-related phase-encoding artifacts may also be seen arising from high-flow vessels. Venous malformations often extend along the long axis of a limb, following neurovascular structures, and may be associated with muscle atrophy and hypertrophy of the subcutaneous fat. Arteriovenous malformations and fistulae usually have the additional findings of enlarged feeding and draining vessels proximal to the lesion (311). Of note, some sarcomas are markedly vascular and can look like a vascular malformation. Particular attention must be paid to the presence or absence of a soft-tissue mass in association with the abnormal vessels, because this finding suggests a vascular neoplasm. Sarcomas that contain multiple enlarged vessels suggestive of a vascular malformation include angiosarcomas, hemangiopericytomas, and alveolar-cell sarcomas (314,315).

Vascular malformations may be treated by surgical excision, angiographic embolization, or percutaneous embolization (316). MR imaging is the preferred modality for determining the extent of the lesion, often showing areas of involvement not appreciated on clinical examination or angiography.

Neurogenic Tumors

Benign Neurogenic Tumors

The common benign tumors of peripheral nerves are schwannomas (also known as neurilemoma or neurinoma) and neurofibromas (285). Schwannomas are encapsulated tumors that arise from the nerve sheaths of peripheral nerves; thus, these tumors are eccentrically positioned within the nerve bundle and usually can be resected without sacrificing the nerve. Neurofibromas, on the other hand, arise from the nerve sheath and fibroblasts of peripheral nerves, and infiltrate and intermix with nerve fibers (317). Neurofibromas occasionally cannot be fully resected without neurologic damage (318,319). Schwannomas usually occur in 20–40-year-old patients and are more common in women than in men. Schwannomas and neurofibromas most commonly occur in patients without neurofibromatosis. However, schwannomas are associated with neurofibromatosis types I and II, and neurofibromas are associated with neurofibromatosis type I. The presence of multiple neurofibromas is strongly suggestive of neurofibromatosis; the finding of a plexiform neurofibroma is diagnostic of neurofibromatosis type I in essentially all cases (320,321). Malignant transformation is occasionally seen in neurofibromas but is rare in schwannomas (322). Patients with solitary benign peripheral nerve tumors present with a mass lesion, muscle atrophy, pain, and weakness or dysesthesia in the distribution of the involved nerve (323).

Solitary neurofibromas and schwannomas typically present as small, well-defined masses of low signal intensity on T1-weighted images and of high signal intensity on T2-weighted images. These tumors enhance markedly after intravenous gadolinium chelate administration (Fig. 9-65). In the extremities, neurogenic tumors are frequently located along the course of a major nerve trunk; thus, the location of the lesion can suggest the correct diagnosis. Fatty atrophy of muscle in the distribution of the involved nerve is occasionally found on MR imaging and is strongly suggestive of a neurogenic tumor (324).

Schwannomas and neurofibromas can often be differentiated on T2-weighted MR images. Schwannomas typically have an inhomogeneous mottled appearance on T2-weighted images; the relatively high-signal-intensity areas correspond histologically to hypocellular myxoid areas (Antoni type B tissue), the lower-signal-intensity areas represent cellular regions (Antoni type A tissue) (see Fig. 9-65) (325–327). Long-standing schwannomas may contain areas of amorphous calcification, cystic degeneration, and prominent vascularity, mimicking a malignant mass (328).

Neurofibromas often have a ''target'' appearance on T2-weighted images. The central low-signal-intensity area histologically represents dense collagen and fibrillary tissue, whereas the high-signal-intensity periphery represents cellular and stromal tissue with a high water content. This ''target'' appearance was found in seven of 10 neurofibromas and in none of four schwannomas in a series reported by Suh and colleagues (326). Plexiform neurofibromas appear as diffuse thickening and beading along a major nerve trunk, often in a bilaterally symmetric fashion. Plexiform neurofibromas may have an infiltrative appearance, because the tumor extends along many small branches of a nerve trunk (329). Asymmetry or rapid enlargement of any region of a plexiform neurofibroma is suggestive of malignant degeneration; however, malignant degeneration cannot be reliably diagnosed by MR imaging, and biopsy is required (317,330).

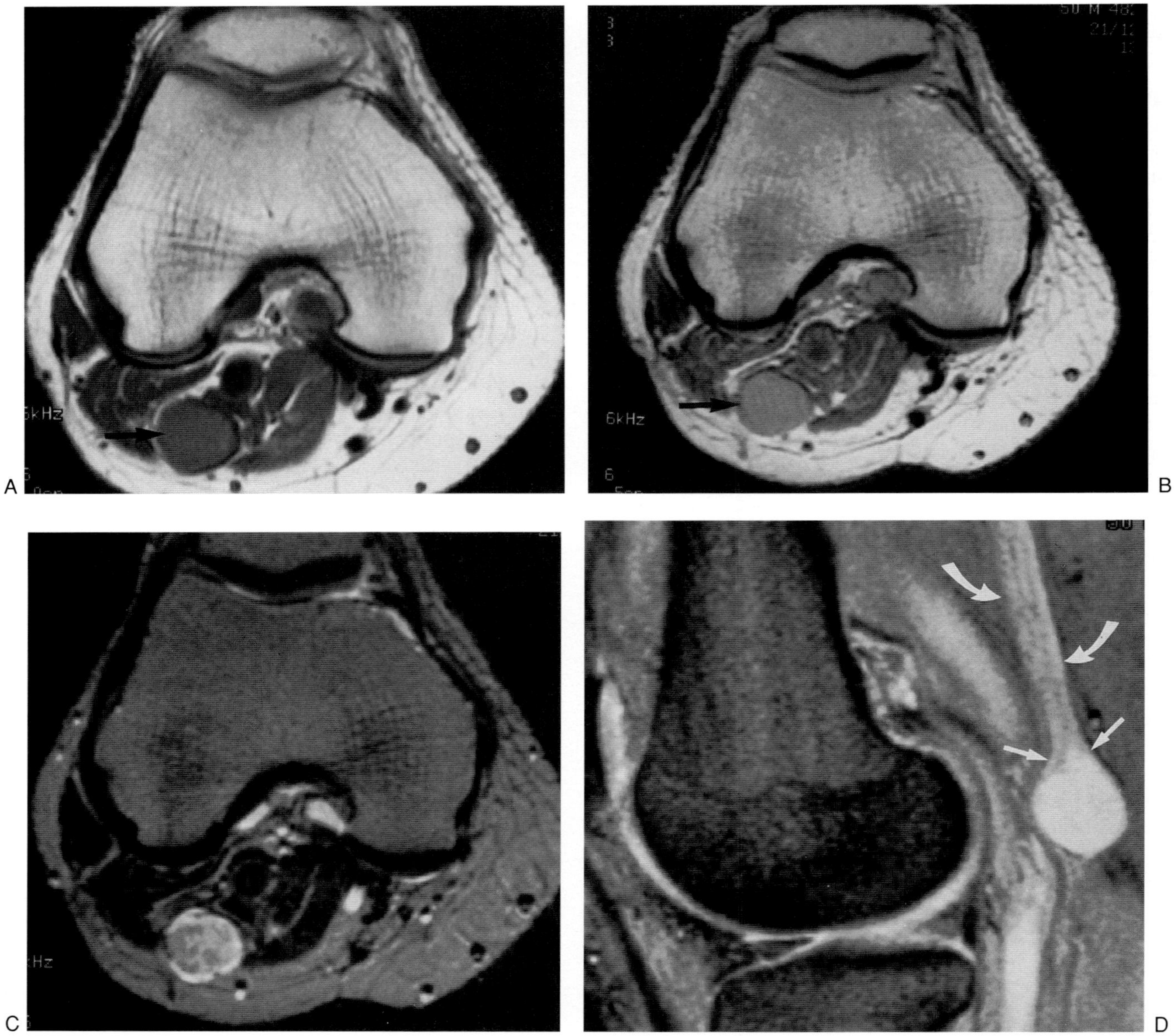

FIG. 9-65. Schwannoma of the posterior tibial nerve. Transverse T1-weighted images obtained before **(A)** and after **(B)** intravenous gadolinium administration show a well-defined round enhancing mass *(arrow)* in the popliteal fossa. A transverse T2-weighted image **(C)** shows the typical mottled appearance of schwannomas, resulting from admixture of cellular and myxoid tissue within the lesion. A sagittal T2*-weighted image **(D)** shows prominent thickening of the posterior tibial nerve above the level of the tumor *(curved arrows)*, and flaring of the nerve around the mass *(arrow)*. These features strongly suggest the neurogenic origin of the tumor.

Malignant Neurogenic Tumors

Malignant degeneration occurs much more commonly in neurofibromas than in schwannomas and is most common in patients with extensive plexiform neurofibromas (331,332). In the limited reports available in the literature, these tumors had nonspecific MRI appearances, with low signal intensity on T1-weighted images and high signal intensity on T2-weighted images. The "target" appearance of neurofibromas has not been described in neurofibrosarcoma (326).

Fibrous Tumors

Benign Fibrous Tumors

Benign fibrous tumors range in biological activity from relatively quiescent fibromas to locally aggressive and destructive cases of fibromatosis. Tumors that contain a predominance of mature collagen will appear hypointense on T2-weighted images, whereas tumors with a predominantly cellular composition will be hyperintense on T2-weighted images (282). Fibromas frequently are well-defined masses with low signal intensity on T2-weighted images. Aggressive fibromatosis (extra-abdominal desmoid) is a very infiltrative and locally destructive tumor; however, it does not produce distant metastases. These tumors have a high rate of local recurrence after attempted resection and may require major resection or limb amputation for control (333,334). Aggressive fibromatosis appears as infiltrative, inhomogeneous tumors that readily invade adjacent structures; these features mimic a malignant neoplasm (Fig. 9-66). On T2-weighted images, the tumor is predominantly of high signal intensity because of the cellularity of the tissue. However, in a series by Hartman and colleagues, focal low-signal-intensity fibrous areas were present on T2-weighted images in 88% of primary cases, and in 90% of recurrent cases (335). Thus, the finding of focal low-signal-intensity areas within an otherwise high-signal-intensity infiltrative mass is suggestive of aggressive fibromatosis.

Other benign fibrous mass lesions may be encountered, including hypertrophic scars and granulomatous reactions around foreign bodies (Fig. 9-67). The MR imaging characteristics of these lesions have not been described in the literature, to our knowledge.

Malignant Fibrous Tumors

Malignant fibrous histiocytoma is the most common soft-tissue sarcoma in adults, accounting for 24% of cases in a large series (302,336). These tumors tend to occur in older adults, with a mean age of 59 years. The most common sites of origin are the thigh, pelvis, retroperitoneum, and shoulder (302). Malignant fibrous histiocytomas are histologically described by grade and subtype. The grading system assesses the degree of dedifferentiation; the subtypes describe the tumor as myxoid, storiform-pleomorphic, giant cell, inflammatory, or angiomatoid (336). These tumors have significant metastatic potential and require wide local resection for local control.

On MR imaging, high-grade malignant fibrous histiocytomas often have the typical malignant features of ill-defined margins and internal heterogeneity. Internal septations and hemorrhage are not uncommon in high-grade malignant fibrous histiocytomas (Fig. 9-68). The low-grade or myxoid subtypes may show well-defined margins and more homogeneous internal signal characteristics (Fig. 9-69). Metaplastic ossification occasionally occurs in malignant fibrous histiocytomas, producing focal signal voids on MR images (336). Necrosis within a malignant fibrous histiocytoma may occur, producing an MR appearance that resembles abscess or hematoma (Fig. 9-70).

Dermatofibrosarcoma protuberans is a malignant fibrous sarcoma closely related to malignant fibrous histiocytoma that accounts for approximately 6% of all soft-tissue sarcomas (302,337) These tumors are composed histologically of fibroblasts, often in a storiform pattern. Although dermatofibrosarcoma protuberans is usually a low-grade sarcoma, regions of high-grade fibrosarcoma are not uncommonly found within the lesion (338). A characteristic clinical and imaging feature of dermatofibrosarcoma protuberans is that this tumor typically arises in the subcutaneous tissues, with infiltration and thickening of the overlying skin. The MR signal characteristics are nonspecific, with low signal intensity on T1-weighted images and high signal intensity on T2-weighted images; however, the finding of a soft-tissue mass in a superficial location with thickening or infiltration of the skin should suggest the diagnosis of dermatofibrosarcoma protuberans.

Other Soft-Tissue Tumors

An extensive variety of soft-tissue tumors have been described, many of which can produce mass lesions in the knee region. A few of these have unique or unusual clinical and imaging features and thus warrant mention in this discussion.

Alveolar Soft-Part Sarcoma

Alveolar soft-part sarcoma is uncommon, comprising only 0.5% of all soft-tissue sarcomas (302). This tumor has the unusual clinical feature of occurring in relatively young patients (10–30 years old). The thigh is the most common site of origin. Histologically, alveolar soft-part sarcomas are composed of nests of large tumor cells separated by highly vascular septations. The tissue of origin is unknown. On imaging, the hypervascularity of these tumors produces the unusual findings of large vascular channels within that lesion, prominent draining veins, and marked contrast enhancement (314). The degree of vascular enlargement may mimic that of an arteriovenous malformation in extreme cases and may produce a pulsatile mass with an audible bruit (315). Alveolar soft-part sarcomas are highly malignant, and hematogenous and lymphatic metastases are commonly present at the time of diagnosis.

Synovial Sarcoma

Synovial sarcoma is a relatively common soft-tissue malignancy that tends to affect younger patients (20–50 years old) and has a propensity to affect the distal extremities (302,339). Some authors state that synovial sarcoma is the most common type of soft-tissue sarcoma in the foot and ankle region; occurrence in the knee region and thigh is also common (274,302). Histologically, synovial sarcomas are often biphasic, with pseudoglandular epithelioid regions and spindle-cell regions (340,341). Monophasic tumors, consist-

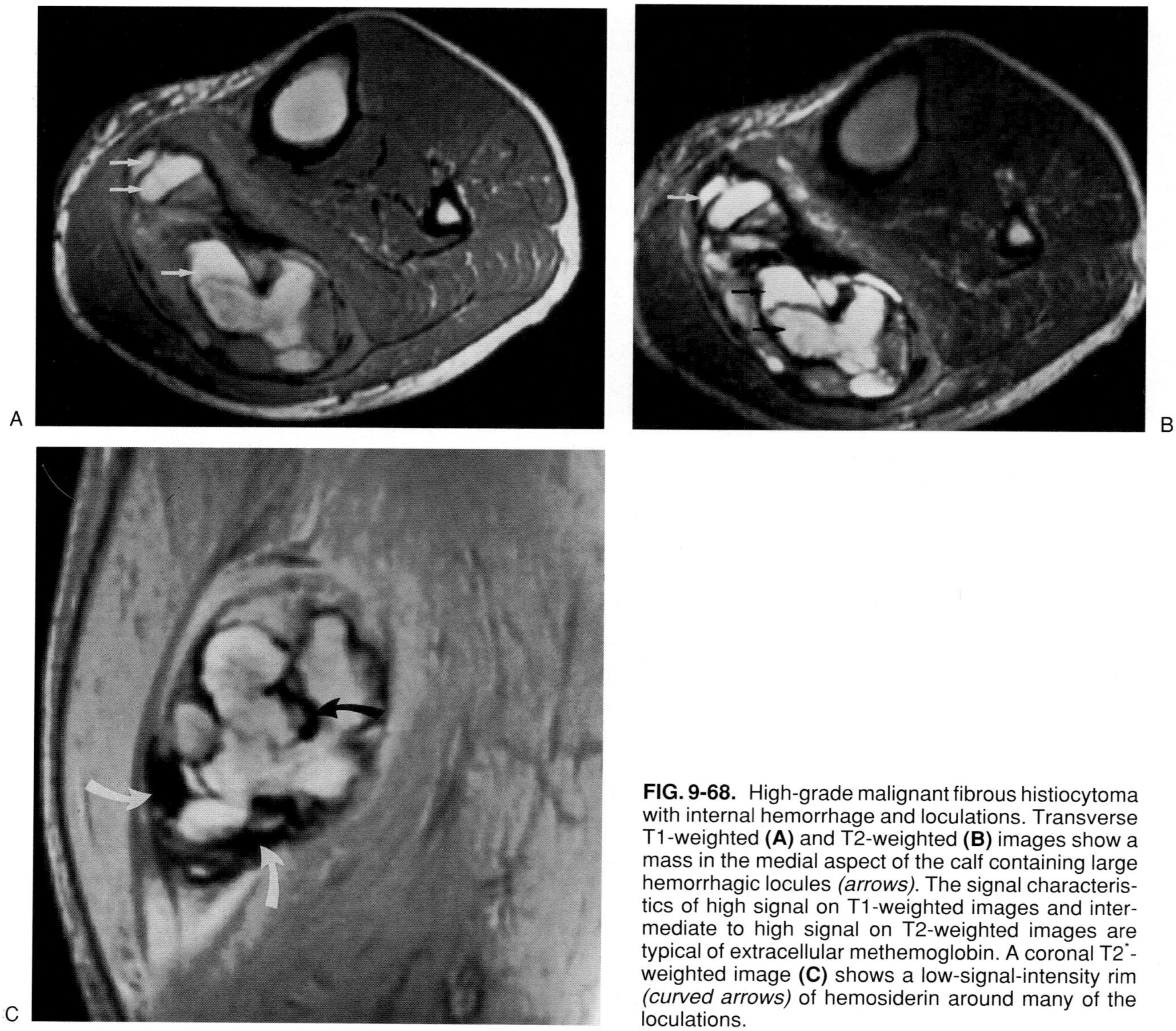

FIG. 9-68. High-grade malignant fibrous histiocytoma with internal hemorrhage and loculations. Transverse T1-weighted **(A)** and T2-weighted **(B)** images show a mass in the medial aspect of the calf containing large hemorrhagic locules *(arrows)*. The signal characteristics of high signal on T1-weighted images and intermediate to high signal on T2-weighted images are typical of extracellular methemoglobin. A coronal T2*-weighted image **(C)** shows a low-signal-intensity rim *(curved arrows)* of hemosiderin around many of the loculations.

free intervals (5,36,37,347,348). Noninvasive assessment of tumor response to neoadjuvant therapy is clinically valuable because this information affects treatment type, duration, dosage, and patient prognosis (19). Considerable information is available regarding the use of MRI, with and without gadolinium enhancement, for this purpose (4,5,16,19,36,37). The goals of MRI in this setting are to evaluate changes in tumor size, tumor necrosis, tumor vascularity, and peritumoral edema in response to adjuvant treatment (349–351).

Unenhanced MRI imaging allows assessment of changes in tumor volume, peritumoral edema volume, and tumor signal intensity (4). Increased tumor volume or edema volume indicates a poor response to chemotherapy (36). Minimal or no reduction in tumor volume after chemotherapy, with residual soft-tissue mass visible, is predictive of poor response in Ewing's sarcoma (352). The findings of decreased tumor volume and edema volume, and improved demarcation of the tumor are suggestive of a good histopathologic response (3,5,353). On T2-weighted images, a decrease in signal intensity has been correlated with histopathologic evidence of tumor response to chemotherapy (5,37). However, the extent of tumor necrosis is difficult to determine on unenhanced MRI images, because the signal intensities of necrotic tumor tissue and edematous tumor tissue overlap considerably.

The presence and degree of tumor enhancement on dynamic MRI after intravenous contrast administration have been shown to correlate with tumor response and necrosis (33,353). Necrotic areas appear as nonenhancing regions that can be easily distinguished from viable tumor and can be

A B C

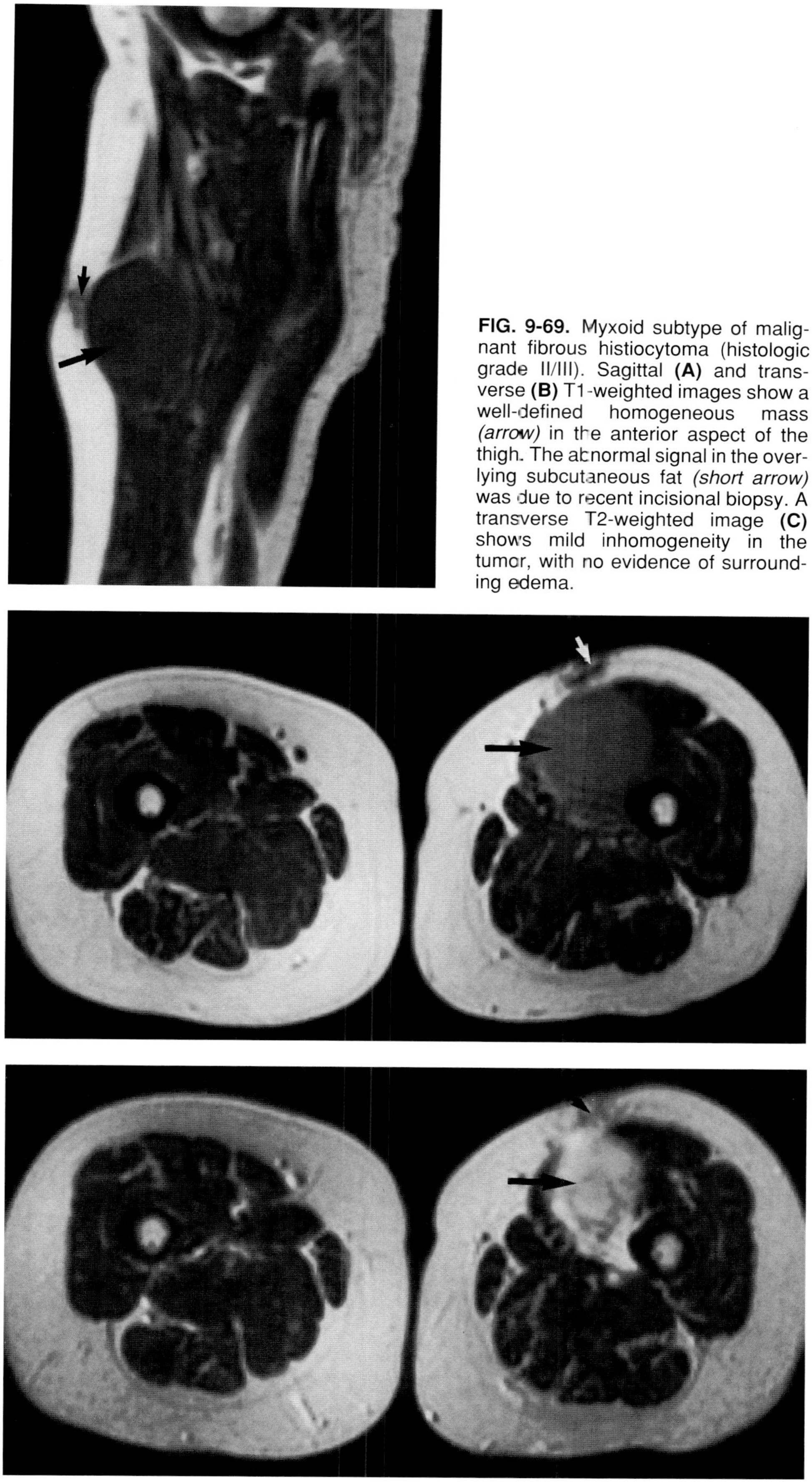

FIG. 9-69. Myxoid subtype of malignant fibrous histiocytoma (histologic grade II/III). Sagittal **(A)** and transverse **(B)** T1-weighted images show a well-defined homogeneous mass *(arrow)* in the anterior aspect of the thigh. The abnormal signal in the overlying subcutaneous fat *(short arrow)* was due to recent incisional biopsy. A transverse T2-weighted image **(C)** shows mild inhomogeneity in the tumor, with no evidence of surrounding edema.

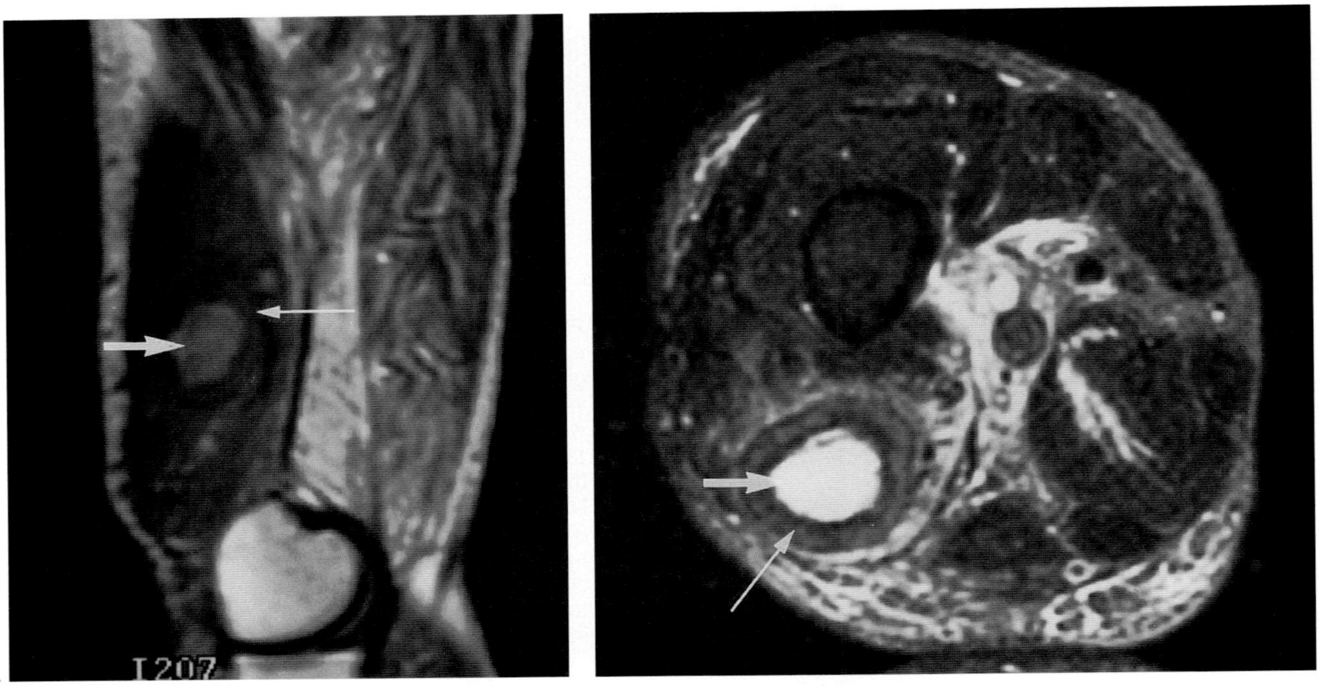

A B

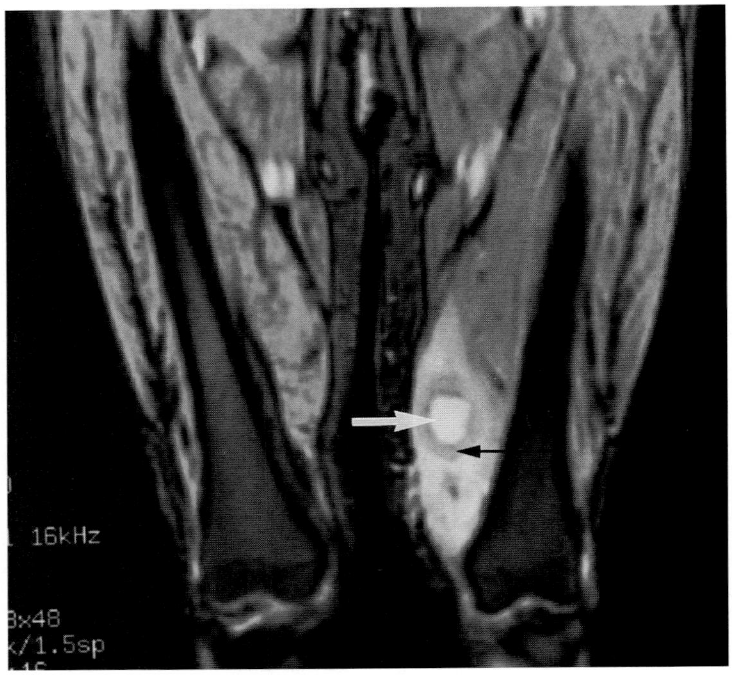

C

FIG. 9-70. Malignant fibrous histiocytoma with central necrosis. Sagittal T1-weighted **(A)**, transverse fat-suppressed T2-weighted **(B)**, and coronal STIR **(C)** images show a mass in the vastus medialis with extensive surrounding edema. The center of the mass *(large arrow)* is of intermediate signal intensity on T1-weighted images and high signal intensity on T2-weighted images; aspiration showed thick proteinaceous fluid in the necrotic center of the tumor. The rind of soft tissue around the periphery of the lesion *(long arrow)* was viable tumor at histology. The extensive perilesional edema visible on the T2-weighted and STIR images is typical of a high-grade sarcoma.

quantified by volume. Serial measurement of the volume of necrosis within a tumor is a useful index of response to chemotherapy. Dynamic contrast-enhancement techniques can been used to assess the perfusion and vascularization of tumors before and after neoadjuvant treatment. Untreated sarcomas and some vascular benign tumors typically show very rapid enhancement; normal tissue, reactive tissue, and necrotic tumor have much slower enhancement (16,18,19,33,353–355).

MR spectroscopy may be useful in the assessment of tumor response to neoadjuvant therapy. Measurement of phosphorus metabolites within the tumor provides information on tumor oxygenation, pH, and viability (278,348). Successful chemotherapy produces an increase in inorganic phosphorus and a decrease in phosphomonoesters and phosphodiesters; these changes are indicative of disruption of normal tissue energetics. MR spectroscopy is a particularly promising technique for evaluation of tumor response be-

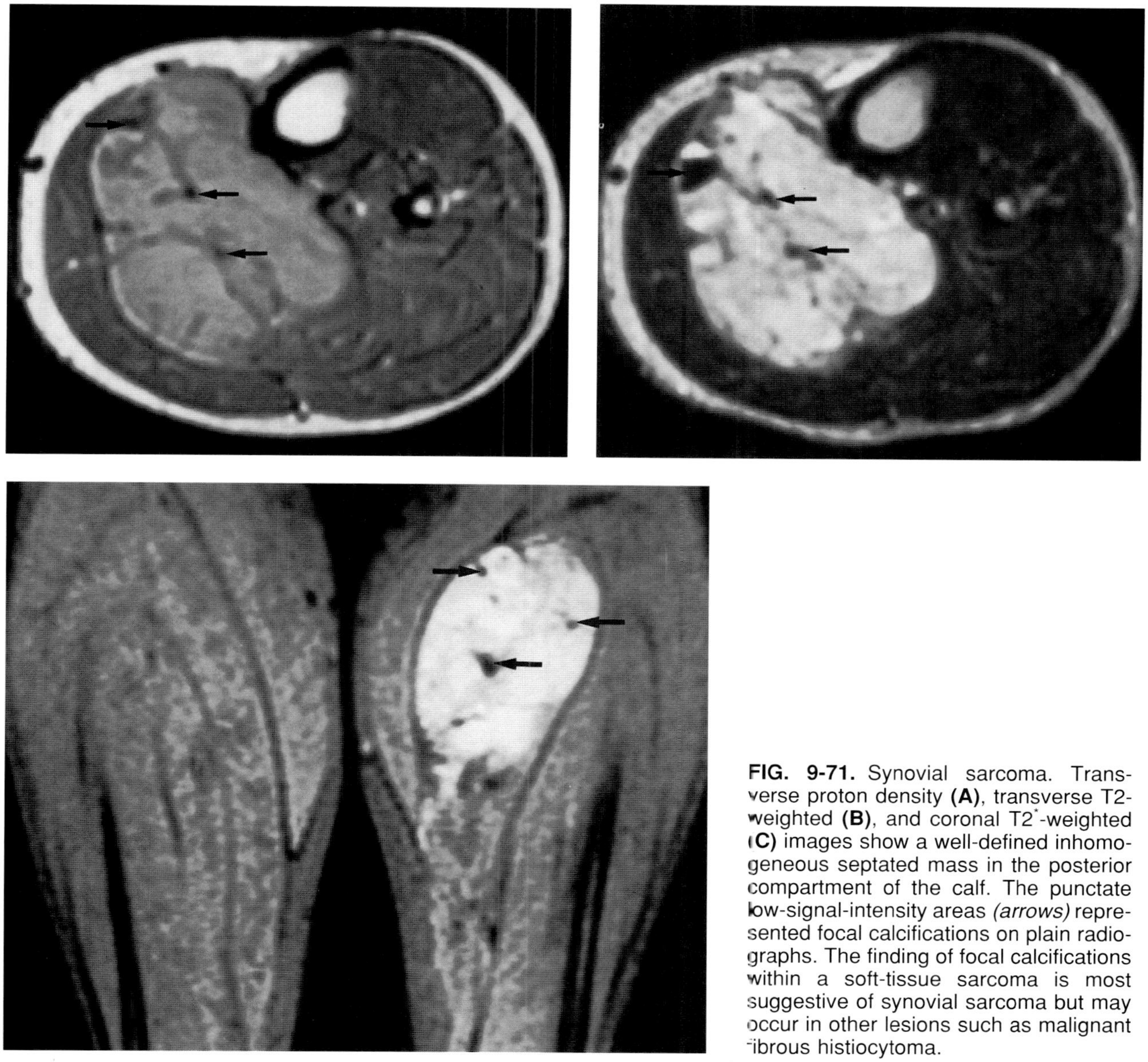

FIG. 9-71. Synovial sarcoma. Transverse proton density **(A)**, transverse T2-weighted **(B)**, and coronal T2*-weighted **(C)** images show a well-defined inhomogeneous septated mass in the posterior compartment of the calf. The punctate low-signal-intensity areas *(arrows)* represented focal calcifications on plain radiographs. The finding of focal calcifications within a soft-tissue sarcoma is most suggestive of synovial sarcoma but may occur in other lesions such as malignant fibrous histiocytoma.

cause it provides quantifiable measurements that can be obtained soon after treatment (3,356,357).

REFERENCES

1. Kransdorf MJ, Jelinek JS, Moser RP Jr. Imaging of soft tissue tumors. *Radiol Clin North Am* 1993;31:359–372.
2. Richardson ML, Gillespy T. Magnetic resonance imaging. In: Kricun ME, ed. *Imaging of bone tumors.* Philadelphia: WB Saunders, 1993:358–446.
3. Berquist TH. Magnetic resonance imaging of primary skeletal neoplasms. *Radiol Clin North Am* 1993;31:411–424.
4. Sundaram M, McLeod RA. MR imaging of tumor and tumorlike lesions of bone and soft tissue. *AJR* 1990;155:817–824.
5. Holscher HC, Bloem JL, Nooy MA, Taminiau AH, Eulderink F, Hermans J. The value of MR imaging in monitoring the effect of chemotherapy on bone sarcomas. *AJR* 1990;154:763–769.
6. Dalinka MK, Zlatkin MB, Chao P, Kricun ME, Kressel HY. The use of magnetic resonance imaging in the evaluation of bone and soft-tissue tumors. *Radiol Clin North Am* 1990;28:461–470.
7. Council on Scientific Affairs. Musculoskeletal applications of magnetic resonance imaging. *JAMA* 1989;262:2420–2427.
8. Berquist TH. Magnetic resonance imaging of musculoskeletal neoplasms. *Clin Orthop* 1989;244:101–118.
9. Haggar AM, Freolich JW. MR imaging strategies in primary and metastatic malignancy. *Radiol Clin North Am* 1988;26:689–696.
10. Kalmar JA, Eick JJ, Merritt DR, et al. A review of applications of MRI in soft tissue and bone tumors. *Orthopedics* 1988;11:417–425.
11. Shuman WP, Patten RM, Baron RL, Liddle RM, Conrad EU, Richardson ML. Comparison of STIR and spin-echo imaging at 1.5 T in 45 suspected extremity tumors: lesion conspicuity and extent. *Radiology* 1991;179:247–251.
12. Golfieri R, Baddeley H, Pringle JS, Souhami R. The role of the STIR sequence in magnetic resonance imaging examination of bone tumors. *Br J Radiol* 1990;63:251–256.
13. Beltran J, Chandnani V, McGhee RJ, Kursonoglu-Brahme S. Gadopentetate dimeglumine-enhanced MR imaging of the musculoskeletal system. *AJR* 1991;156:457–466.

14. Seeger LL, Widoff BE, Bassett LW, Rosen G, Eckardt JJ. Preoperative evaluation of osteosarcoma: value of gadopentetate dimeglumine-enhanced MR imaging. *AJR* 1991;157:347–351.
15. Mirowitz SA, Totty WG, Lee JKT. Characterization of musculoskeletal masses using dynamic Gd-DTPA enhanced spin-echo MRI. *J Comput Assist Tomogr* 1992;16:120–125.
16. Verstraete KL, Deene YD, Roels H, Dierick A, Uyttendaele D, Kunnen M. Benign and malignant musculoskeletal lesions: dynamic contrast-enhanced MR imaging: parametric "first-pass" images depict tumor vascularization and perfusion. *Radiology* 1994;192:835–843.
17. Munk PL, Vellet AD. The musculoskeletal system. In: Higgins CB, Hricak H, Helms CA, ed. *Magnetic resonance imaging of the body*, 2nd ed. New York: Raven, 1992:1381–1389.
18. Erlemann R, Reiser M, Peters P, et al. Musculoskeletal neoplasms: static and dynamic Gd-DTPA-enhanced MR imaging. *Radiology* 1989;171:767–773.
19. Fletcher BD, Hanna SL, Fairclough DL, Gronemeyer SA. Pediatric musculoskeletal tumors: use of dynamic, contrast-enhanced MR imaging to monitor response to chemotherapy. *Radiology* 1992;184: 243–248.
20. Schima W, Amann G, Stiglbauer R, et al. Preoperative staging of osteosarcoma: efficacy of MR imaging in detecting joint involvement. *AJR* 1994;163:1171–1175.
21. Vanel D, Shapeero LG, De Baere T, et al. MR imaging in the follow-up of malignant and aggressive soft-tissue tumors: results of 511 examinations. *Radiology* 1994;190:263–268.
22. Dooms GC, Hricak H, Sollitto RA, Higgins CB. Lipomatous tumor and tumors with fatty component: MR imaging potential and comparison of MR and CT. *Radiology* 1985;157:479–483.
23. Aisen AM, Martel W, Braunstein EM, McMillin KI, Phillips WA, King TF. MRI and CT evaluation of primary bone and soft-tissue tumors. *AJR* 1986;146:749–756.
24. Reiser M, Rupp N, Heller HJ, et al. MR in the diagnosis of malignant soft tissue tumors. *Eur J Radiol* 1984;4:288–293.
25. Petterson H, Slone RM, Spanier S, Gillespy T III, Fitzsimmons JR, Scott KN. Musculoskeletal tumors: T1 and T2 relaxation times. *Radiology* 1988;167:783–785.
26. Berquist TH, Ehman RL, King RL, Hodgman CG, Ilstrup DM. Value of MR imaging in differentiating benign from malignant soft-tissue masses: study of 95 lesions. *AJR* 1990;155:1251–1255.
27. Kransdorf MJ, Jelinek JS, Moser RP Jr, et al. Soft-tissue masses: diagnosis using MR imaging. *AJR* 1989;153:541–547.
28. Resnick D, Nimayama G. *Diagnosis of bone and joint disorders*, 2nd ed. Philadelphia: WB Saunders, 1988.
29. Weatherall PT, Maale GE, Mendelsohn DB, Sherry CS, Erdman WE, Pascoe HR. Chondroblastoma: classic and confusing appearance at MR imaging. *Radiology* 1994;190:467–474.
30. Assoun J, Richardi G, Railhac JJ, et al. Osteoid osteoma: MR imaging versus CT. *Radiology* 1994;191:217–223.
31. Beltran J, Simon DC, Katz W, Weis LD. Increased MR signal in skeletal muscle adjacent to malignant tumors: pathological correlation and clinical relevance. *Radiology* 1987;162:251–255.
32. Kroon HM, Bloem JL, Holscher HC, van der Woede HJ, Reijnierse M, Taminiau AHM. MR imaging of edema accompanying benign and malignant bone tumors. *Skeletal Radiol* 1994;23:261–269.
33. Schoenberg NY, Beltran J. Contrast enhancement in musculoskeletal imaging: current status. *Radiol Clin North Am* 1994;32:337–352.
34. Bloem JL, Reiser MF, Vanel D. Magnetic resonance contrast agents in the evaluation of the musculoskeletal system. *Magn Reson Q* 1990; 6:136–163.
35. McDonald DJ. Limb-salvage surgery for treatment of sarcomas of the extremities. *AJR* 1994;163:509–513.
36. Holscher HC, Bloem JL, Vanel D, et al. Osteosarcoma: chemotherapy-induced changes at MR imaging. *Radiology* 1992;182:839–844.
37. Pan G, Raymond AK, Carrasco CH, et al. Osteosarcoma: MR imaging after preoperative chemotherapy. *Radiology* 1990;174:517–526.
38. Nolan DJ, Middlemiss H. Chondroblastoma of bone. *Clin Radiol* 1975;26:343–346.
39. McLeod RA, Beabout JW. The roentgenographic features of chondroblastoma. *AJR* 1973;118:464.
40. Huvos AG, Marcove RC. Chondroblastoma of bone. A critical review. *Clin Orthop Rel Res* 1973;95:300.
41. Dahlin DC, Ivins JC. Benign chondroblastoma. A study of 125 cases. *Cancer* 1972;30:401.
42. Aronsohn RS, Hart WR, Martel W. Metaphyseal chondroblastoma of bone. *AJR* 1976;127:686.
43. Springfield DS, Capanna R, Gherlinzoni F, et al. Chondroblastoma: a review of seventy cases. *J Bone Joint Surg* 1985:67A:748–755.
44. Kurt AM, Unni KK Sim FH, McLeod RA. Chondroblastoma of bone. *Hum Pathol* 1989;20:965–976.
45. Bloem JL, Mulder JD. Chondroblastoma: a clinical and radiological study of 104 cases. *Skeletal Radiol* 1985;14:1–9.
46. Fobben ES, Dalinka MK, Scheibler ML, et al. The magnetic resonance imaging appearance at 1.5 Tesla of cartilaginous tumors involving the epiphysis. *Skeletal Radiol* 1987;16:647–651.
47. Gravanis MB, Giansanti JS. Benign chondroblastoma. Report of four cases with a discussion of the presence of ossification. *Am J Clin Pathol* 1971;55:624.
48. Huvos AG, Higginbotham NL, Marcove RC, O'Leary P. Aggressive chondroblastoma. Review of the literature on aggressive behavior and metastases with report of one new case. *Clin Orthop Rel Res* 1977; 126:266.
49. Present D, Bacchini P, Pignatti G, Picci P, Bertoni F, Campanacci M. Clear cell chondrosarcoma of bone. *Skeletal Radiol* 1991;20:187–191.
50. Bjornsson J, Unni KK, Dahlin DC, et al. Clear-cell chondrosarcoma of bone: observations in 47 cases. *Am J Surg Pathol* 1984;8:223.
51. Kransdorf MJ, Sweet DE, Buetow PC, Giudici MA, Moser RP Jr. Giant cell tumor in skeletally immature patients. *Radiology* 1992;184: 233–237.
52. McInerney DP, Middlemiss JH. Giant cell tumor of bone. *Skeletal Radiol* 1978;2:195–204.
53. Dahlin DC. Giant cell tumor of bone: highlights of 407 cases. *AJR* 1985;144:955–960.
54. Moser RP Jr, Kransdorf MJ, Gilkey FW, Manaster BJ. Giant cell tumor of the upper extremity. *Radiographics* 1990;10:83–102.
55. Carrasco CH, Murray JA. Giant cell tumors. *Orthop Clin North Am* 1989;20:395–405.
56. Marcove RC, Miller TR, Cohen WC. The treatment of primary and metastatic bone tumors by repetitive freezing. *Bull NY Acad Med* 1968;44:532.
57. Manaster BJ, Doyle AJ. Giant cell tumors of bone. *Radiol Clin North Am* 1993;31:299–323.
58. Tubbs WS, Brown LR, Beabout JW, Rock MG, Unni KK. Benign giant-cell tumor of bone with pulmonary metastases: clinical findings and radiologic appearance of metastases in 13 cases. *AJR* 1992;158: 331–334.
59. Nojima T, Takeda N, Matsuno T, Inoue K, Nagashima K. Case report 869: benign metastasizing giant cell tumor of bone. *Skeletal Radiol* 1994;23:583–585.
60. Present D, Bertoni F, Hudson T, Enneking WF. The correlation between the radiologic staging studies and histopathologic findings in aggressive stage 3 giant cell tumor of bone. *Cancer* 1986;57:237–244.
61. Meis JM, Dorfman HD, Nathanson SD, et al. Primary malignant giant cell tumor of bone: "dedifferentiated" giant cell tumor. *Mod Pathol* 1989;2:541–546.
62. Dahlin DC, Cupp RE, Johnson EW Jr. Giant cell tumor: a study of 195 cases. *Cancer* 1970;25:1061–1070.
63. Tehranzadeh J, Murphy BJ, Mnaymneh W. Giant cell tumor of the proximal tibia: MR and CT appearance. *J Comput Assist Tomogr* 1989;13:282–286.
64. Herman SD, Mesgarzadeh M, Bonakdarpour A, et al. Role of magnetic resonance imaging in giant cell tumor of bone. *Skeletal Radiol* 1987; 16:635.
65. Abdelwahab IF, Kenan S, Hermann G, Klein MJ, Lewis MM. Case report 845: fluid-filling giant cell tumor with an aneurysmal bone cyst component. *Skeletal Radiol* 1994;23:317–319.
66. Welkerling H, Dreyer T, Delling G. Morphological typing of chondrosarcoma: a study of 94 cases. *Virchows Archiv A Pathol Anat* 1991; 418:419–425.
67. Ishida T, Kikuchi F, Machinami R. Histological grading and morphometric analysis of cartilaginous tumours. *Virchows Archiv A Pathol Anat* 1991;418:149–155.
68. Varma DGK, Ayala AG, Carrasco CH, Guo SQ, Kumar R, Edeiken J. Chondrosarcoma: MR imaging with pathologic correlation. *Radiographics* 1992;12:687–704.
69. Giudici NM, Moser RP Jr. Kransdorf MJ. Cartilaginous bone tumors. *Radiol Clin North Am* 1993;31:237–259.
70. Mirra JM, Gold R, Downs J, Eckardt JJ. A new histologic approach

to the differentiation of enchondroma and chondrosarcoma of the bones: a clinicopathologic analysis of 51 cases. *Clin Orthop* 1985; 201:214–237.
71. Rosenthal DI, Schiller AL, Mankin HJ. Chondrosarcoma: correlation of radiological and histological grade. *Radiology* 1984;150:21–26.
72. Cohen EK, Kressel HY, Frank TS, et al. Hyaline-cartilage origin bone and soft-tissue neoplasms: MR appearance and histologic correlation. *Radiology* 1988;167:477–481.
73. Golfieri R, Baddeley H, Pringle JS, et al. Primary bone tumors: MR morphologic appearance correlated with pathologic examinations. *Acta Radiol* 1991;32:290–298.
74. Meyers SP, Hirsch WL Jr, Curtin HD, Barnes L, Sekhar LN, Sen C. Chondrosarcomas of the skull base: MR imaging features. *Radiology* 1992;184:103–108.
75. Reinus WR, Kyriakos M, Gilula LA, Brower AC, Merkel K. Plasma cell tumors with calcified amyloid deposition mistaken for chondrosarcoma. *Radiology* 1993;189:505–509.
76. Reutner G, Mutschler W. Radiomorphologic classification of central chondrosarcomas. *ROFO* 1989;150:1–7.
77. Geirnaerdt MJA, Bloem JL, Eulderink F, Hogendoorn PCW, Taminiau AHM. Cartilaginous tumors: correlation of gadolinium-enhanced MR imaging and histopathologic findings. *Radiology* 1993;186: 813–817.
78. Aoki J, Sone S, Fujioka F, et al. MR of enchondroma and chondrosarcoma: rings and arcs of Gd-DTPA enhancement. *J Comput Assist Tomogr* 1991;15:1011–1016.
79. Wu KK, Collon DJ, Guise ER. Extra-osseous chondrosarcoma: report of five cases and review of literature. *J Bone Joint Surg* 1980;62A: 189.
80. Norman A, Sissons HA. Radiographic hallmarks of peripheral chondrosarcoma. *Radiology* 1984;151:589.
81. Garrison RC, Unni KK, McLeod RA, Pritchard DJ, Dahlin DC. Chondrosarcoma arising in osteochondroma. *Cancer* 1982;49:1890–1897.
82. Hudson TM, Springfield DS, Spanier SS, et al. Benign exostoses and exostotic chondrosarcomas: evaluation of cartilage thickness by CT. *Radiology* 1984;152:595–599.
83. Larsson SE, Lorentzon R, Boquist L. Fibrosarcoma of bone. *J Bone Joint Surg* 1976;58B:412.
84. Hudson TM, Stiles RG, Monson DK. Fibrous lesions of bones. *Radiol Clin North Am* 1993;31:279–297.
85. Huvos AG, Higinbotham NL. Primary fibrosarcoma of bone: a clinicopathologic study of 130 patients. *Cancer* 1975;35:837–847.
86. Lorigan JG, Libshitz HI, Peuchot M. Radiation-induced sarcoma of bone: CT findings in 19 cases. *AJR* 1989;153:791–794.
87. Kumar R, Madewell JE, Lindell MM, Swischuk LE. Fibrous lesions of bone. *Radiographics* 1990;10:237–256.
88. Lee J, Yao L, Phelps CT, Pilon VA, Wirth CR. Case report 459: fibrosarcomatous dedifferentiation of chondrosarcoma of bone. *Skeletal Radiol* 1988;17:60–65.
89. Taconis WK, Mulder JD. Fibrosarcoma and malignant fibrous histiocytoma of long bones: radiographic features and grading. *Skeletal Radiol* 1984;11:237–245.
90. Capanna R, Beroni F, Bacchini P, et al. Malignant fibrous histiocytoma of bone. *Cancer* 1984;54:177–187.
91. Huvos AG, Heilwell M, Bretsky SS. The pathology of malignant fibrous histiocytoma of bone. *Am J Surg Pathol* 1985;9:853–871.
92. Feldman F, Norman D. Intra- and extraosseous malignant fibrous histiocytoma. *Radiology* 1972;104:497–508.
93. Bertoni F, Calderoni P, Bacchini P, et al. Benign fibrous histiocytoma of bone. *J Bone Joint Surg Am* 1986;68:12225–1230.
94. Taconis WK, Schutte HE, van der Heul RO. Desmoplastic fibroma of bone: a report of 18 cases. *Skeletal Radiol* 1994;23:283–288.
95. Crim JR, Gold RH, Mirra JM, Eckardt JJ, Bassett LW. Desmoplastic fibroma of bone: radiographic analysis. *Radiology* 1989;172: 827–832.
96. Dahlin DC. Pathology of osteosarcoma. *Clin Orthop Rel Res* 1975; 111:23–36.
97. Enneking WF, Springfield DS. Osteosarcoma. *Orthop Clin North Am* 1977;8:875–885.
98. Bloem JL, Kroon HM. Osseous lesions. *Radiol Clin North Am* 1993; 31:261–278.
99. Huvos AG, Rosen G, Bretsky SS, et al. Telangiectatic osteogenic sarcoma. *Cancer* 1982;4:1679.
100. Unni KK, Dahlin DC, Beabout JW. Periosteal osteogenic osteosarcoma. *Cancer* 1976;37:2476.
101. Unni KK, Dahlin DC, Beabout JW, Ivins JC. Parosteal osteogenic sarcoma. *Cancer* 1976;37:2466.
102. Sundaram M, McGuire MH, Herbold DR. Magnetic resonance imaging of osteosarcoma. *Skeletal Radiol* 1987;16:23–27.
103. Gillespy T III, Manfrini M, Ruggieri P, et al. Staging of intraosseous extent of osteosarcoma: correlation of preoperative CT and MR imaging with pathologic macroslides. *Radiology* 1988;167:765–767.
104. Bloem JL, Taminiau AH, Eulderink F, Herman J, Pauwels EK. Radiologic staging of primary bone sarcoma: MR imaging, scintigraphy, angiography, and CT correlated with pathologic examination. *Radiology* 1988;169:805–810.
105. Seeger LL, Eckardt JJ, Bassett LW. Cross-sectional imaging in the evaluation of osteogenic sarcoma: MRI and CT. *Semin Roentgenol* 1989;24:174–184.
106. Boyko OB, Cory DA, Cohen MD, et al. MR imaging of osteogenic sarcoma and Ewing's sarcoma. *AJR* 1987;148:317.
107. Larsson SE, Lorentzon R, Boquist L. Telangiectatic osteosarcoma. *Acta Orthop Scand* 1978;49:589.
108. Dahlin DC. Case Report 27. *Skeletal Radiol* 1977;1:249.
109. De Santos LA, Murray JA, Finklestein JB, Spjut HJ, Ayala AG. The radiographic spectrum of periosteal osteosarcoma. *Radiology* 1978; 127:123.
110. Edeiken J, Farrel C, Ackerman LV, Spjut HJ. Parosteal sarcoma. *AJR* 1971;111:579.
111. Smith J, Ahuja SC, Huvos AG, Bullough PG. Parosteal (juxtacortical) osteogenic sarcoma. *J Can Assoc Radiol* 1978;29:167.
112. Farr GH, Huvos AG. Juxtacortical osteogenic sarcoma: an analysis of fourteen cases. *J Bone Joint Surg Am* 1972;54:1205–1210.
113. Ahuja SC, Villacin AB, Smith JS, Bullough PG, Huvos AG, Marcove RC. Juxtacortical (parosteal) osteogenic sarcoma: histologic grading and prognosis. *J Bone Joint Surg Am* 1977;59:632.
114. Wold LE, Unni KK, Beabout JW, et al. Dedifferentiated parosteal osteosarcoma. *J Bone Joint Surg Am* 1984;66:53–59.
115. Rabhan WN, Rosai J. Desmoplastic fibroma: report of ten cases and review of the literature. *J Bone Joint Surg Am* 1968;50:487.
116. Sugiura I. Desmoplastic fibroma: case report and review of the literature. *J Bone Joint Surg Am* 1976;58:126.
117. Gebhardt MC, Campbell CJ, Schiller AL, Mankin HJ. Desmoplastic fibroma of bone: a report of eight cases and review of the literature. *J Bone Joint Surg Am* 1985;67:732–747.
118. Inwards CY, Unni KK, Beabout JW, Sim FH. Desmoplastic fibroma of bone. *Cancer* 1991,68:1978–1983.
119. McFarland GB Jr, Morden ML. Benign cartilaginous lesions. *Orthop Clin North Am* 1977;8:737.
120. Jaffe HL, Lichtenstein L. Solitary benign enchondroma of bone. *Arch Surg* 1943;46:480.
121. Crim JR, Seeger LL. Diagnosis of low-grade chondrosarcoma. *Radiology* 1993;189:503–504.
122. Lewis RJ, Ketcham AS. Maffucci's syndrome: functional and neoplastic significance: a case report and review of the literature. *J Bone Joint Surg Am* 1973;44:1564.
123. Schwartz H, Zimmerman NB, Simon MA, et al. The malignant potential of enchondromatosis. *J Bone Joint Surg* 1987;69:267–274.
124. Liu J, Hudkins PG, Swee RG, et al. Bone sarcomas associated with Ollier's disease. *Cancer* 1987;59:1376–1385.
125. Sun TC, Swee RG, Shives TC, et al. Chondrosarcoma in Maffucci's syndrome. *J Bone Joint Surg Am* 1985;67:1214–1219.
126. Unger EC, Kessler HB, Kowalyshyn MJ, Lackman RD, Morea GT. MR imaging of Maffucci syndrome. *AJR* 1988;150:351–353.
127. Phelan JT. Fibrous cortical defect and non-ossifying fibroma of bone. *Surg Gynecol Obstet* 1964;119:807–810.
128. Caffey J. On fibrous defects in cortical walls of growing tubular bones: their radiologic appearance, structure, prevalence, natural course and diagnostic significance. *Adv Pediatr* 1955;7:13–24.
129. Moser RP, Sweet DE, Haseman DB, et al. Multiple skeletal fibroxanthomas: radiologic-pathologic correlation of 72 cases. *Skeletal Radiol* 1987;16:353–359.
130. Marks KE, Bauer TW. Fibrous tumors of bone. *Orthop Clin North Am* 1989;20:377–393.
131. Ritschl P, Karnel F, Hajek P. Fibrous metaphyseal defects: determination of their origin and natural history using a radiomorphological study. *Skeletal Radiol* 1988;17:8–15.

248. Burk DL Jr, Dalinka MK, Kanal E, et al. Meniscal and ganglion cysts of the knee: MR evaluation. *AJR* 1988;150:331–336.
249. Fielding JR, Franklin PD, Kustan J. Popliteal cysts: a reassessment using magnetic resonance imaging. *Skeletal Radiol* 1991;20:433–435.
250. Munk PL, Helms CA. The knee. In: Higgins CB, Hricak H, Helms CA, eds. *Magnetic resonance imaging of the body*, 2nd ed. New York: Raven Press, 1992;1097–1119.
251. Schuldt DR, Wolfe RD. Clinical and radiographic findings in meniscal cysts. *Radiology* 1980;134:49–52.
252. Ferrer-Roca O, Vilalta C. Lesions of the meniscus. Part II: horizontal cleavages and lateral cysts. *Clin Orthop* 1980;146:301–307.
253. Becton JL, Young HH. Cysts of semilunar cartilage of the knee. *Arch Surg* 1965;90:708–712.
254. Haller J, Resnick D, Greenway G, et al. Juxtaacetabular ganglionic (or synovial) cysts: CT and MR features. *J Comp Assist Tomogr* 1989; 13:976–983.
255. Bauer TW, Dorfman HD. Intraosseous ganglion. A clinicopathological study of 11 cases. *Am J Surg Pathol* 1982;6:207–210.
256. Pope TJ Jr, Fechner RE, Keats TE. Intra-osseous ganglion: report of four cases and review of the literature. *Skeletal Radiol* 1989;18: 185–187.
257. Brown MF, Dandy DJ. Intra-articular ganglia of the knee. *Arthroscopy* 1990;6:322–323.
258. Recht MP, Applegate G, Kaplan P, et al. The MR appearance of cruciate ganglion cysts: a report of 16 cases. *Skeletal Radiol* 1995; 23:597–600.
259. McLaren DB, Buckwalter KA, Vahey TN. The prevalence and significance of cyst-like changes at the cruciate ligament attachments in the knee. *Skeletal Radiol* 1992;21:365–369.
260. Schajowicz F, Sainz MC, Slullitel JA. Juxta-articular bone cysts (intraosseous ganglia). *J Bone Joint Surg* 1979;61:107–111.
261. Munk PL, Poon PY, Chhem RK, Janzen DL. Imaging of soft-tissue sarcomas. *Can Assoc Radiol J* 1994;45:438–446.
262. Kransdorf MJ, Jelinek JS, Moser RP. Imaging of soft tissue tumors. *Radiol Clin North Am* 1993;31:359–372.
263. Taylor GA, Perlman EJ, Scherer LR, et al. Vascularity of tumors in children: evaluation with color Doppler imaging. *AJR* 1991;157: 1267–1271.
264. Mankin HJ, Lange T, Spanier S. The hazards of the biopsy in patients with malignant primary bone and soft tissue tumors. *J Bone Joint Surg Am* 1982;64:1121–1127.
265. Simon MA, Finn HA. Diagnostic strategy for bone and soft-tissue tumors. *J Bone Joint Surg Am* 1993;75:622–631.
266. Gustafson P, Dreinhofer KE, Rydholm A. Soft tissue sarcoma should be treated at a tumor center: a comparison of quality of surgery in 375 patients. *Acta Orthop Scand* 1994;65:47–50.
267. Arlen M, Marcove R. Sarcoma management based on a standardized TMN classification. *Semin Surg Oncol* 1992;8:98–103.
268. Musumeci M, Balzarini L, Ceglia E, Petrillo R, Reyner Y, Tesoro-Tess JD. Soft-tissue sarcomas. Imaging: an integrated approach. *Annals Oncology* 1992;3(suppl 2):555–556.
269. Tanabe KK, Pollock RE, Ellis LM, Murphy A, Sherman N, Romsdahl MM. Influence of surgical margins on outcome in patients with preoperatively irradiated extremity soft tissue sarcomas. *Cancer* 1994;73: 1652–1659.
270. Yu JS, Resnick D. MR imaging of accessory soleus muscle appearance in six patients and a review of the literature. *Skeletal Radiol* 1994; 23:525–528.
271. Kransdorf MJ. Magnetic resonance imaging of musculoskeletal tumors. *Orthopedics* 1994;17:1003–1016.
272. Crim JR, Seeger LL, Yao L, et al. Diagnosis of soft-tissue masses with MR imaging: can benign masses be differentiated from malignant ones? *Radiology* 1992;185:581–586.
273. Binkovitz LA, Berquist TH, McLeod RA. Masses of the hand and wrist: detection and characterization with MR imaging. *AJR* 1990; 154:323–326.
274. Wetzel LH, Levine E. Soft-tissue tumors of the foot: value of MR imaging for specific diagnosis. *AJR* 1990;155:1025–1030.
275. Hermann G, Abdelwahab IF, Miller TT, et al. Tumor and tumor-like conditions of the soft-tissues: magnetic resonance imaging features differentiating benign from malignant masses. *Br J Radiol* 1992;65: 14–20.
276. Dewhirst MW, Sostman HD, Leopold KA, et al. Soft-tissue sarcomas: MR imaging and MR spectroscopy for prognosis and therapy monitoring. *Radiology* 1990;174:847–853.
277. Sostman HD, Charles HC, Rockwell S, et al. Soft-tissue sarcomas: detection of metabolic heterogeneity with P-31 spectroscopy. *Radiology* 1990;176:837–843.
278. Negendank WG, Crowley MG, Ryan JR, Keller NA, Evelhoch JL. Bone and soft-tissue lesions: diagnosis with combined H-1 MR imaging and P-31 MR spectroscopy. *Radiology* 1989;173:181–188.
279. Sostman HD, Charles HC. Bone and soft-tissue lesions: diagnosis with combone H-1 MR imaging and P-31 MR spectroscopy. *Invest Radiol* 1991;26:769–770.
280. Jelinek JS, Kransdorf MJ, Shmookler BM, et al. Liposarcoma of the extremities: MR and CT findings in the histologic subtypes. *Radiology* 1993;186:455–459.
281. Jones BC, Sundaram M, Kransdorf MJ. Synovial sarcoma: MR imaging findings in 34 patients. *AJR* 1993;161:827–830.
282. Sundaram M, McGuire MH. Soft-tissue masses: histologic basis for decreased signal (short T2) on T2-weighted MR images. *AJR* 1987; 148:1247–1250.
283. Sundaram M, Chalk D, Merenda J, et al. Case report 563: pigmented villonodular synovitis of the knee. *Skeletal Radiol* 1989;18:463–465.
284. Jelinek JS, Kransdorf MJ, Schmookler BM, Aboulafia AA, Malawer MM. Giant cell tumor of the tendon sheath: MR findings in nine cases. *AJR* 1994;162:919–922.
285. Kransdorf MJ. Benign soft-tissue tumors in a large referral population: distribution of specific diagnoses by age, sex, and location. *AJR* 1995; 164:395–402.
286. Ha TV, Kleinman PK, Fraire A, et al. MR imaging of benign fatty tumors in children: report of four cases and review of the literature. *Skeletal Radiol* 1994;23:361–367.
287. Miller TT, Potter HG, McCormack RR Jr. Benign soft tissue masses of the wrist and hand: MRI appearances. *Skeletal Radiol* 1994;23: 327–332.
288. Fortier M, Mayo JR, Swensen SJ, Munk PL, Vellet AD, Muller NM. MR imaging of chest wall lesions. *Radiographics* 1994;14:597–606.
289. Kransdorf MJ, Meis JM, Jelinek JS. Dedifferentiated liposarcoma of the extremities: imaging findings in four patients. *AJR* 1993;161: 127–130.
290. Kaufman SL, Stout AP. Lipoblastic tumors of childhood. *Cancer* 1959;12:912–917.
291. Jimenez JF. Lipoblastoma in infancy and childhood. *J Surg Oncol* 1986;32:238–241.
292. Seynaeve P, Mortelmans L, Kockx M, Van Hoye M, Mathijs R. Case report 813: hibernoma of the left thigh. *Skeletal Radiol* 1994;23: 137–138.
293. Enzi G, Biondetti PR, Fiore D, Mazzoleni F. Computed tomography of deep fat masses in multiple symmetrical lipomatosis. *Radiology* 1982;144:121–124.
294. Enzi G, Carrari R, Alfieri P, et al. Shoulder girdle lipomatosis. *Ann Intern Med* 1992;117:749–750.
295. Enzi G, Digito M, Enzi GB, Fiore D. Asymmetrical lipomatosis: report of two cases. *Postgrad Med J* 1985;61:797–800.
296. Enzi G. Multiple symmetric lipomatosis: an updated clinical report. *Medicine* 1984;63:56–64.
297. Cavallero MC, Taylor JAM, Gorman JD, Haghighi P, Resnick D. Imaging findings in a patient with fibrolipomatous hamartoma of the median nerve. *AJR* 1993;161:837–838.
298. Chew FS, Hudson TM, Hawkins IF. Radiology of infiltrating angiolipoma. *AJR* 1989;135:781–787.
299. Nigrisoli M, Ruggieri P, Picci P, Pignatti G. Hibernoma. *Skeletal Radiol* 1988;17:432–435.
300. Sundaram M, McGuire MH, Herbold DR, Beshany S, Fletcher J. High signal intensity soft tissue masses on T1-weighted pulsing sequences. *Skeletal Radiol* 1987;16:30–35.
301. Enzinger FM, Weiss SW. *Soft tissue tumors*, 2nd ed. St. Louis: Mosby-Year Book, 1988.
302. Kransdorf MJ. Malignant soft-tissue tumors in a large referral population: distribution of diagnoses by age, sex, and location. *AJR* 1995; 164:129–134.
303. London J, Kim EE, Wallace C, Shirkhoda A, Coan J, Evans H. MR imaging of liposarcomas: correlation of MR features and histology. *J Comput Assist Tomogr* 1989;13:832–835.
304. Azumi N, Curtis J, Kempson RL, et al. Atypical and malignant neo-

plasms showing lipomatous differentiation. *Am J Surg Pathol* 1987; 11:161–183.
305. Sundaram M, Baran G, Merenda G, McDonald DJ. Myxoid liposarcoma: magnetic resonance imaging with clinical and histological correlation. *Skeletal Radiol* 1990;19:359–362.
306. Suh JS, Hwang G, Hahn SB. Soft tissue hemangiomas: MR manifestations in 23 patients. *Skeletal Radiol* 1995;23:621–625.
307. Ehara S, Sone M, Tamakawa Y, Nishida J, Abe M, Hachiya J. Fluid-fluid levels in cavernous hemangioma of soft tissue. *Skeletal Radiol* 1994;23:107–109.
308. Buetow PC, Kransdorf MJ, Moser RP Jr, Jelinek JS, Berrey JH. Radiologic appearance of intramuscular hemangioma with emphasis on MR imaging. *AJR* 1990;154:563–567.
309. Levine E, Wetzel HL, Neff JR. MR imaging and CT of extrahepatic cavernous hemangiomas. *AJR* 1986;147:1299–1304.
310. Kaplan PA, Williams SM. Mucocutaneous and peripheral soft-tissue hemangiomas: MR imaging. *AJR* 1987;163:163–166.
311. Rak KM, Yakes WF, Ray RL, et al. MR imaging of symptomatic peripheral vascular malformations. *AJR* 1992;159:107–112.
312. Cohen JM, Weinreb JC, Redman HC. Arteriovenous malformations of the extremities: MR imaging. *Radiology* 1986;158:475–479.
313. Meyer JS, Hoffer FA, Barnes PD, Mulliken JB. Biologic classification of soft-tissue vascular anomalies: MR correlation. *AJR* 1991;157: 559–564.
314. Lorigan JG, O'Keeffe FN, Evans HL, Wallace S. The radiologic manifestations of alveolar soft-part sarcoma. *AJR* 1989;153:335–339.
315. Temple HT, Scully SP, O'Keefe RJ, Rosenthal DI, Mankin HJ. Clinical presentation of alveolar soft-part sarcoma. *Clin Orthop* 1994;300: 213–218.
316. Yakes WF, Parker SH. Diagnosis and management of vascular anomalies. In: Castaneda-Zuniga WR, ed. *Interventional Radiology,* 2nd ed. Philadelphia: Williams & Wilkins, 1991;152–189.
317. Bass JC, Korobkin M, Francis IR, Ellis JH, Cohan RH. Retroperitoneal plexiform neurofibromas: CT findings. *AJR* 1994;163:617–620.
318. Berlin O, Stener B, Lindahl S, Irstam L, Lodding P. Vascularization of peripheral neurilemomas: angiographic, computed tomographic, and histologic studies. *Skeletal Radiol* 1986;15:275–283.
319. Harkin JC, Reed RJ. Tumors of the peripheral nervous system. *Atlas of tumor pathology.* Washington, DC: Armed Forces Institute of Pathology, 1969;67–69.
320. NIH consensus development group. Neurofibromatosis. *Arch Neurol* 1988;45:575–578.
321. Aoki S, Barkovich AJ, Nishimura K, et al. Neurofibromatosis types 1 and 2: cranial MR findings. *Radiology* 1989;172:527–534.
322. Ducatman BS, Scheithauer BW, Peipgras DG, Reiman HM, Ilstrup DM. Malignant peripheral nerve sheath tumors: a clinicopathologic study of 120 cases. *Cancer* 1986;57:2006–2021.
323. Donner TR, Voorhies RM, Kline DG. Neural sheath tumors of major nerves. *J Neurosurg* 1994;81:362–373.
324. Stull MA, Moser RP, Kransdorf MJ, et al. MR appearance of peripheral nerve sheath tumors. *Skeletal Radiol* 1991;20:9–14.
325. Kim SH, Choi BI, Han MC, Kim YI. Retroperitoneal neurilemoma: CT and MR findings. *AJR* 1992;159:1023–1026.
326. Suh JS, Abenoza P, Galloway HR, Everson LI, Griffiths HJ. Peripheral (extracranial) nerve tumors: correlation of MR imaging and histologic findings. *Radiology* 1992;183:341–346.
327. Getachew MM, Whitman GJ, Chew FS. Retroperitoneal schwannoma. *AJR* 1994;163:1356.
328. Schultz E, Sapan MR, McHeffey-Atkinson B, Naidich J, Arlen M. Case report 872: "ancient" schwannoma (degenerated neurilemoma). *Skeletal Radiol* 1994;23:593–595.
329. Sullivan TP, Seeger LL, Doberneck SA, Eckardt JJ. Case report 828: plexiform neurofibroma of the tibial nerve invading the medial and lateral gastrocnemius muscles and plantaris muscle. *Skeletal Radiol* 1994;23:149–152.
330. Ros PR, Eshaghi N. Plexiform neurofibroma of the pelvis: CT and MRI findings. *Magn Reson Imaging* 1991;9:463–465.
331. Morris JH, Schoene WC. The nervous system. In: Robbins SL Cotran R, Kumar V, eds. *Pathologic basis of disease,* 3rd ed. Philadelphia: WB Saunders, 1984;1370–1436.
332. Coleman BG, Arger PH, Dalinka MK, Oblinger AC, Raney BR, Meadow AT. CT of sarcomatous degeneration of neurofibromatosis. *AJR* 1983;141:383–387.
333. Wara WM, Phillips TL, Hill DR, et al. Desmoid tumors: treatment and prognosis. *Radiology* 1977;124:225–226.
334. Rock MG, Pritchard DJ, Reiman HM, et al. Extraabdominal desmoid tumors. *J Bone Joint Surg Am* 1984;66A:1369–1374.
335. Hartman TE, Berquist TE, Fetsch JF. MR imaging of extraabdominal desmoids: differentiation from other neoplasms. *AJR* 1992;158: 581–585.
336. Miller TT, Hermann G, Abdelwahab IF, Klein MJ, Kenan S, Lewis MM. MRI of malignant fibrous histiocytoma of soft tissue: analysis of 13 cases with pathologic correlation. *Skeletal Radiol* 1994;23: 271–275.
337. Kransdorf MJ, Meis-Kindblom JM. Dermatofibrosarcoma protuberans: radiologic appearance. *AJR* 1994;163:391–394.
338. Connelly JH, Evans HL. Dermatofibrosarcoma protuberans: a clinicopathologic review with emphasis on fibrosarcomatous areas. *Am J Surg Pathol* 1992;16:921–925.
339. Hajdu SI, Shiu MH, Fortner JG. Tendosynovial sarcoma: a clinicopathological study of 136 cases. *Cancer* 1977;39:1207–1207.
340. Evans HL. Synovial sarcoma: a study of 23 biphasic and 17 probable monophasic examples. *Pathol Annu* 1980;15:309–331.
341. Enterline HT. Histopathology of sarcomas. *Semin Oncol* 1981;8: 133–155.
342. Blacksin M, Acekosan A, Benevenia J. Case report 871: synovial sarcoma, monophasic type. *Skeletal Radiol* 1994;23:589–591.
343. Reeves BR, Smith S, Fisher C, et al. Characterization of the translocation between chromosomes x and 18 in human synovial sarcomas. *Oncogene* 1989;4:373–378.
344. Mahajan H, Lorigan JG, Shirkhoda A. Synovial sarcoma: MR imaging. *Magn Reson Imaging* 1989;7:211–216.
345. Morton MJ, Berquist TH, McLeod RA, Unni KK, Sim FH. MR imaging of synovial sarcoma. *AJR* 1991;156:337–340.
346. Maxwell JR, Yao L, Eckardt JJ, Doberneck SA. Case report 878: densely calcifying synovial sarcoma of the hip metastatic to the lungs. *Skeletal Radiol* 1995;23:673–675.
347. Link MP, Goorin AM, Miser AW, et al. The effect of adjuvant chemotherapy on relapse-free survival in patients with osteosarcoma of the extremities. *New Engl J Med* 1986;314:1600–1606.
348. Sostman HD, Prescott DM, Dewhirst MW, et al. MR imaging and spectroscopy for prognostic evaluation of soft-tissue sarcomas. *Radiology* 1994;190:269–275.
349. Rosen G, Caarros B, Huvos AG, et al. Preoperative chemotherapy for osteogenic sarcoma: selection of post-operative adjuvant chemotherapy based on the response of the primary tumor to preoperative chemotherapy. *Cancer* 1982;49:1221–1230.
350. Eilber FR, Morton DL, Eckardt J, Grant T, Weisenburger T. Limb salvage for skeletal and soft tissue sarcomas. *Cancer* 1984;53: 2579–2584.
351. Jaffe N, Robertson R, Takaue T, et al. Control of primary osteosarcoma with chemotherapy. *Cancer* 1985;56:461–466.
352. van der Woude HJ, Bloem JL, Holscher HC, et al. Monitoring the effect of chemotherapy in Ewing's sarcoma of bone with MR imaging. *Skeletal Radiol* 1994;23:493–500.
353. Vanel D, Lacombe MJ, Couanet D, Kalifa C, Speilmann M, Genin J. Musculoskeletal tumors: follow-up with MR imaging after treatment with surgery and radiation treatment. *Radiology* 1987;164: 243–244.
354. Petterson H, Eliasson J, Egund N, et al. Gadolinium-DTPA enhancement of soft tissue tumors in magnetic resonance imaging: preliminary clinical experience in five patients. *Skeletal Radiol* 1987;17:319–323.
355. Erlemann R, Reiser M, Peters PE, et al. Time-dependent changes in signal intensity in neoplastic and inflammatory lesions of the musculoskeletal system following intravenous administration of Gd-DTPA. *Radiology* 1988;28:269–276.
356. Redmond OM, Stack JP, Dervan PA, Hurson BJ, Carney DN, Ennis JT. Osteosarcoma: use of MR imaging and MR spectroscopy in clinical decision making. *Radiology* 1989;172:811–815.
357. Ross B, Helsper J, Cox I, et al. Osteosarcoma and other neoplasms of bone: magnetic resonance spectroscopy to monitor therapy. *Arch Surg* 1987;122:1464–1469.

MRI of the Knee, Second Edition,
edited by P. L. Munk and C. A. Helms.
Lippincott-Raven Publishers, Philadelphia © 1996.

CHAPTER 10

Magnetic Resonance Imaging of the Pediatric Knee

E. Michel Azouz, Paul Babyn, and Rethy K. Chhem

With its many advantages—including unrestricted multiplanar imaging capability, high-resolution and maximal soft-tissue contrast—magnetic resonance imaging (MRI) is now a well-recognized tool in the evaluation of pediatric musculoskeletal disorders, and it is particularly well suited for the evaluation of large joints such as the knee.

Plain radiographs should always be obtained first, but often these are normal, because most abnormalities of the adult and pediatric knee involve only or mainly the soft tissues, including the synovium, epiphyseal, articular or growth plate cartilage, menisci, ligaments, tendons, or muscles.

Plain films will usually suffice in dysplasias and other congenital anomalies and in most cases of fractures, arthritis, Osgood-Schlatter disease, bone and joint infection, osteochondritis dissecans, and Blount's disease. Most fractures are straightforward and do not need additional cross-sectional imaging. Bone scintigraphy, computed tomography, or MRI may be used for rapid diagnosis of an occult fracture not visible on plain films. Depending on the clinical context (and laboratory results), a knee effusion seen on plain films may be posttraumatic or secondary to inflammatory or septic arthritis and may require needle aspiration and fluid analysis rather than expensive imaging that could delay management.

In some conditions (e.g., popliteal or other cystic lesions, knee joint effusion, synovial thickening, tendinous and ligamentous injuries, and soft-tissue masses) ultrasound may be used for diagnosis. It is certainly noninvasive and less expensive than MRI, but it is operator dependent and may be difficult to reproduce.

Computed tomography (CT) is less expensive than MRI and may be very useful for the diagnosis of a large number of pathologic conditions involving bone and/or soft tissues around the knee (e.g., soft-tissue calcification, osteochondral fractures, osteomyelitis, osteoid osteoma, and other benign bone tumors). In most cases, however, MRI provides better contrast resolution and better delineates the full extent of soft-tissue masses and bone marrow involvement.

In the last few years, knee arthrography has been almost totally replaced by MRI and/or arthroscopy, where available, and MRI can effectively replace diagnostic arthroscopy of the knee (1).

TECHNIQUE

The child is usually examined supine, with the lower extremities straight, the knees extended, and the legs in a position of rest, in approximately 15° external rotation. This degree of external rotation is usually comfortable during imaging; moreover, it allows optimal visualization of the anterior cruciate ligament on the sagittal images. Selection of a small field of view (e.g., 12–16 cm) and the use of a knee or flexible coil are crucial to obtain good spatial resolution and perfect anatomic detail. We use a slice thickness of 3–5 mm with a 0–1 mm gap between the slices. A routine knee protocol for the evaluation of internal derangements should be available. For the evaluation of suspected or proven conditions other than internal derangements, the examination must be tailored to the individual patient. Most examinations should include sagittal and coronal T1-weighted and sagittal T2-weighted spin-echo (SE) sequences. Additional sequences may include a 15–30° sagittal gradient-echo sequence for the evaluation of cartilage, and axial imaging for evaluation of masses and for study of the patellofemoral joint. SE T2-weighted sequences require more time to obtain and have a low signal-to-noise ratio. In children, rapid scanning without sacrificing detail is essen-

E. M. Azouz and P. Babyn: Department of Diagnostic Imaging, The Hospital for Sick Children, University of Toronto, Toronto, Ontario, Canada M5G 1X8.

R. K. Chhem: Department of Daignostic Radiology, Montreal General Hospital, McGill University, Montreal, Quebec, Canada H3G 1A4.

tial, and fast SE T2-weighted sequences without or with fat suppression may be used. Short tau inversion recovery (STIR) and other T2-fat-suppression techniques are useful for the demonstration of inflammatory or posttraumatic soft-tissue or bone marrow edema, abscess formation, or venous malformations.

The protocol for tumor examination differs considerably from that for internal knee derangement and must be tailored to the individual child. Choosing appropriate pulse sequences and imaging planes requires consideration of the location, size, and radiographic appearance of the lesion and likely potential sites of local and distant spread. Important features affecting limb salvage surgery must be specifically assessed, including neurovascular bundle involvement and extent through the physis or into the joint. Determination of involved compartments and the status of the neurovascular bundle involvement are best provided by T2-weighted SE imaging, whereas intramedullary extent and overall tumor length are usually best shown on sagittal or coronal T1-weighted SE and inversion recovery (IR) imaging. Of course, imaging must be done before biopsy to avoid post-surgical inflammation and hemorrhage, which complicate the interpretation of the MR study.

Scanning after intravenous gadolinium chelate injection (Gd) is required for the evaluation of arthritis and other synovial lesions (2) and may be useful in musculoskeletal infection, osteochondritis dissecans, and avascular necrosis. Although controversial, Gd can be used to better characterize osseous and soft-tissue masses and may be helpful for differentiating tumor from peritumoral edema and recurrent tumor from fibrotic scarring.

Adequate sedation [e.g., with intravenous sodium pentobarbital (Nembutal) up to a maximum of 6 mg/kg (or rarely general anesthesia)] is usually required for children below 4 or 5 years. Infants under 6 months of age can be adequately sedated using oral chloral hydrate at doses between 50 and 100 mg/kg. Newborns often require no sedation at all (3). Nembutal should be given slowly intravenously or intramuscularly. The child must be adequately monitored with pulse oximetry for any transient fall of oxygen saturation during the whole time of sedation (4).

THE NORMAL PEDIATRIC KNEE

The child's knee reflects the development of the surrounding epiphyses, and its appearance on MR will depend upon the age and maturation of the individual. At birth, only the ossific centers of the distal femur and proximal tibia are present, with patellar ossification appearing at 3–4 years of age. Early on, the ossific centers are surrounded by an extensive amount of cartilage that is responsible for the formation of congruent articular surfaces and allows for future longitudinal growth of the bone (growth plate) and maturation of the ossific nucleus (epiphyseal cartilage).

The growth plate has a variable MR appearance, depending upon pulse sequences used and degree of resolution (5). Generally, for clinical imaging, the growth plate cartilage has similar imaging characteristics to articular cartilage (6). Epiphyseal cartilage may show subtle inhomogeneity in signal, especially on sagittal T2-weighted imaging posteriorly within the distal femoral epiphysis. Initially, the marrow signal within the ossific nucleus is hematopoietic, but fatty marrow is found very soon after the appearance of the ossific center. Irregularities in contour of the distal femoral ossification center are often seen in young children and should not be mistaken for osteochondritis dissecans. Uniform fatty signal will be seen with normal developmental contour irregularity. The marrow signal within the metaphyses depends on the patient's age and ratio of hematopoietic to fatty marrow. Young children typically have hematopoietic marrow, whereas older children and adolescents may show inhomogeneous or streaky metaphyseal marrow signal, before complete conversion to fatty marrow occurs (7). Hematopoietic marrow may show enhancement following Gd, as may the vessels contained within the epiphyseal cartilage surrounding the ossific nucleus.

Normally, minimal joint fluid, if any, is seen in the pediatric knee joint. The menisci appear to develop early on, with close to adult-sized menisci evident by 3–4 years of age. Similarly, the cruciate and collateral ligaments can all be identified from birth, but for their study thin sections need to be obtained with small fields of view.

Avulsive cortical irregularity of the distal femur is commonly seen in children and adolescents, particularly boys, as a cortical irregularity or defect on the posteromedial side of the distal femoral metaphysis (Fig. 10-1A). It is a developmental defect or the result of stress at tendinous attachment of the adductor magnus muscle or the medial head of the gastrocnemius muscle (8). It is very unlikely to be symptomatic. Plain radiographic diagnosis is usually definitive. The defect is sometimes seen as an incidental finding on CT or MRI of the knees (Fig. 10-1B). It is often bilateral. On MRI the defect is hypointense on T1 and shows areas of signal hyperintensity on T2 (9).

CONGENITAL LESIONS

The vast majority of congenital bone conditions and skeletal dysplasias involving the pediatric knee can be diagnosed on plain radiographs. Only rarely is CT or MRI needed for further assessment. MR can document the (congenital) absence of the anterior cruciate ligament, which is a common component of knee dysplasias (10), and the absent or hypoplastic patella (e.g., in the Fong's nail–patella syndrome). Isolated absence of the menisci and cruciate ligaments of the knee has been described (11). Children with congenital dislocation of the knee usually have menisci, but the ligaments are very lax or absent. Other congenital bony, cartilaginous, muscular, or vascular anomalies involving the thigh, knee, or leg may benefit from an MRI and/or MR angiogra-

A 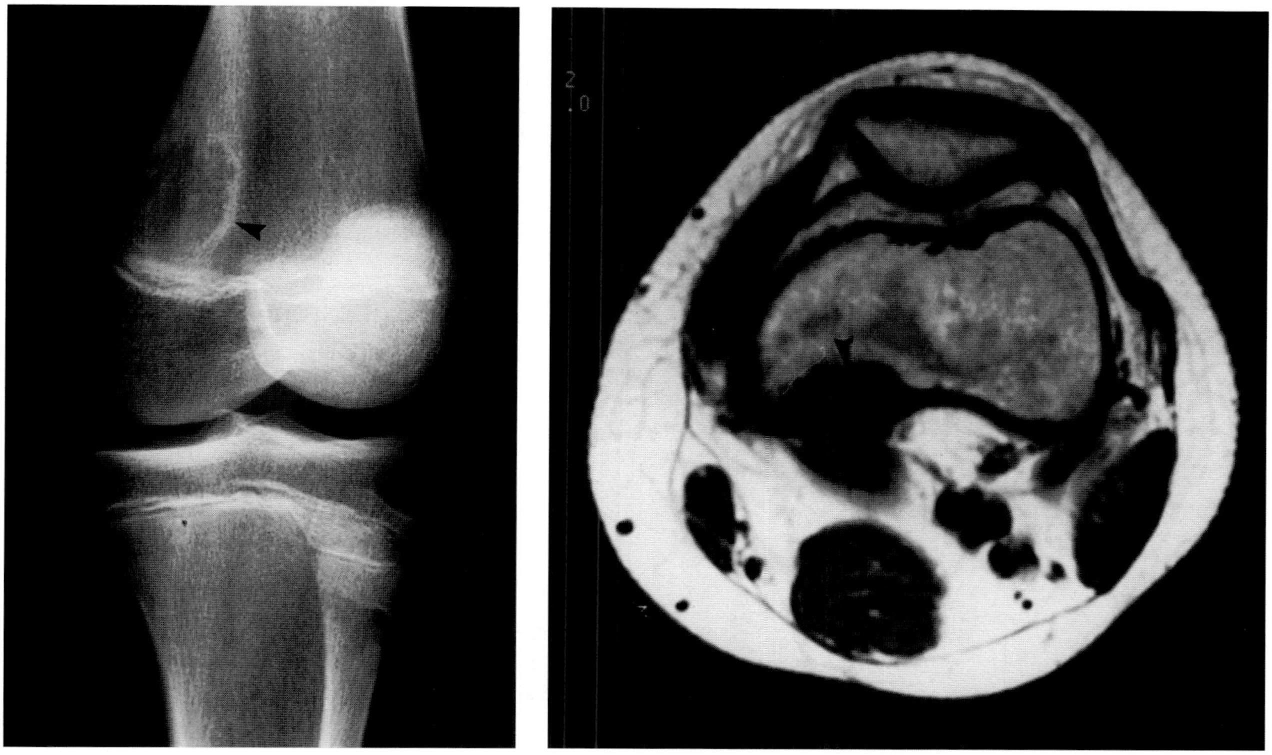 B

FIG. 10-1. Avulsive cortical irregularity of the left distal femur in an 1[illegible]-year-old girl. **A:** Oblique plain radiograph showing a well-defined irregular defect in the posteromedial cortex of the distal femoral metaphysis *(arrowhead)*. **B:** Axial T1-weighted SE image (TR 533, TE 16) showing the lesion *(arrowhead)* as an area of low signal intensity. Note its close proximity to the attachment of the adductor muscle. Irregular metaphyseal marrow signal is a normal finding for the patient's age before complete conversion to fatty marrow. The MRI study was requested for a possible meniscal tear.

phy (MRA) of the abnormal anatomy, particularly if corrective surgery is contemplated. Discoid lateral menisci are relatively common congenital abnormalities. When imaged, they often show tears and degeneration. They will be discussed with the traumatic soft-tissue lesions.

TRAUMATIC LESIONS

Traumatic Bony and Cartilaginous Lesions

MRI may reveal an undisplaced fracture, an osteochondral fracture, or a bone bruise (bone contusion) in children suffering from posttraumatic knee pain and with normal bone appearance on plain radiographs. In cases of occult cortical or trabecular bone fractures, bone scintigraphy will show an area of increased uptake (12). However, close proximity to the growth plate in children often renders interpretation of the bone scan difficult in these situations. In osteochondral fracture, MRI will demonstrate the bony and/or cartilaginous defect, the fragment—whether it is in situ, detached, or displaced—and any associated joint effusion (Fig. 10-2).

Bone contusions are probably occult subchondral trabecular microfractures. With lateral patellar dislocation, they are seen in the patella and in the lateral femoral condyle, often with a chondral or osteochondral fracture. With trauma to the knee involving anterior cruciate ligament tear, there is typically an area of bone contusion in the proximal tibia posteriorly and in the femoral condyle anteriorly, representing the sites of impaction in knee hyperextension (13–17). In children, a bone contusion may also be seen as an isolated finding following trauma. Bone contusion is shown as homogeneous or reticular low-signal-intensity areas on the T1-weighted images, with edema or hemorrhage demonstrated as high signal intensity on the long TR (repetition time) sequences without or with fat suppression and on IR technique (Fig. 10-3). Bone contusions and their significance, classification, and prognosis have been recently studied extensively by many investigators, including Lynch and colleagues (15), Mink and Deutsch (16), Newberg and Wetzner (18), and Vellet (19).

Osgood-Schlatter (OS) disease is seen predominantly in adolescent boys and is probably secondary to repetitive minor avulsive trauma exerted by the patellar tendon on the anterior tibial tuberosity. It is primarily clinical, and involvement may be bilateral or unilateral. Plain radiographs will show localized soft-tissue swelling (Fig. 10-4A). Eventually, there will be fragmentation of the tibial tuberosity. Bone

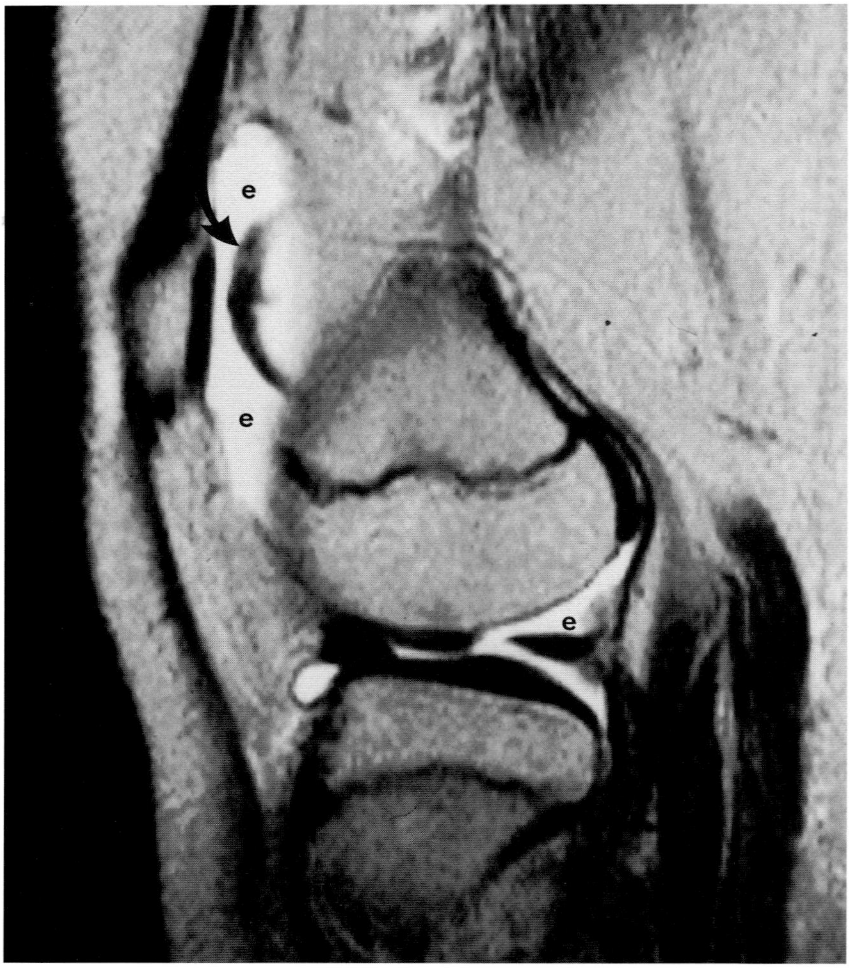

FIG. 10-2. Fracture of the articular cartilage of the lateral femoral condyle in a 14-year-old boy. Sagittal T2-weighted SE imaging (TR 5000, TE 120) showing the large crescent-shaped chondral fragment to be displaced superiorly and anteriorly *(curved arrow)*. Also seen are a moderately large effusion (e) showing high signal intensity, and the interrupted contour of the femoral condyle due to the missing (fractured and displaced) piece of articular cartilage.

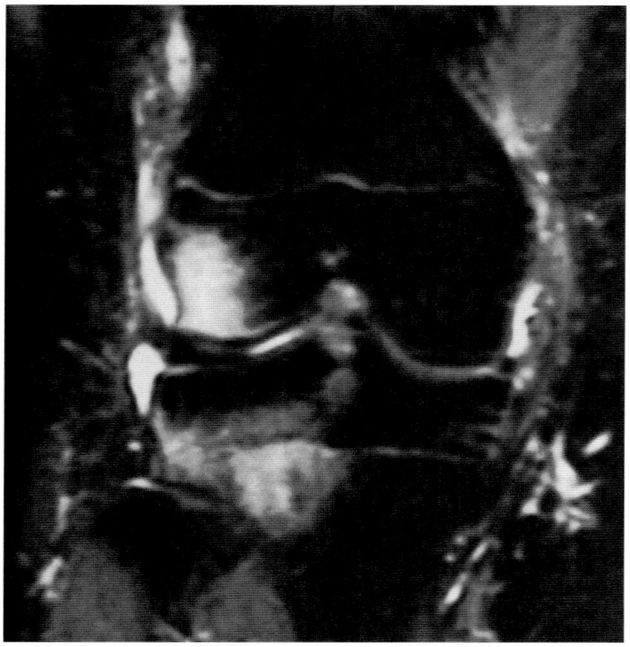

FIG. 10-3. Bone contusion seen after knee trauma (falling from a height) in a 17-year-old girl. Inversion recovery technique (TR 5000, TE 38, TI 160), coronal image shows high-signal-intensity areas in the lateral femoral condyle and in the lateral half of the proximal tibial epiphysis and metaphysis. The bone marrow is otherwise all dark on this sequence. There is an associated knee joint effusion.

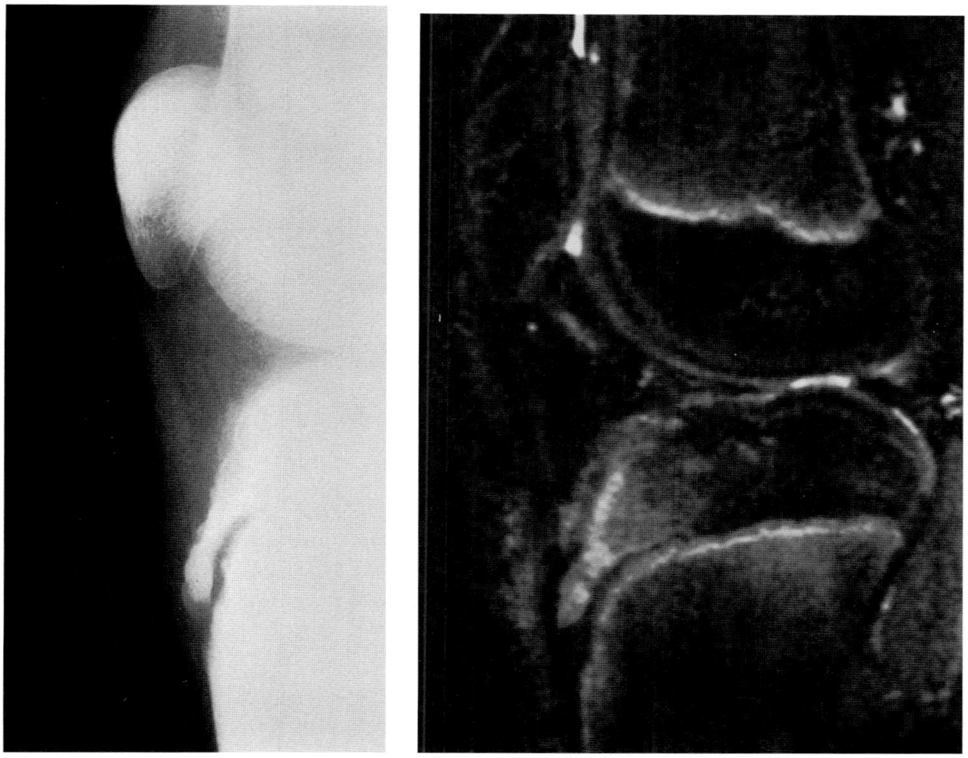

A B

FIG. 10-4. Osgood-Schlatter disease in a 13-year-old boy. **A:** Lateral plain radiograph showing irregularity of the tibial tuberosity—without fragmentation—and anterior soft-tissue swelling. **B:** Sagittal image, IR sequence (TR 4500, TE 40, TI 160) showing high-signal tibial tuberosity edema and, to a lesser degree, edema of the soft tissues anterior and posterior to the lower end of the patellar tendon.

scintigraphy will demonstrate a localized area of increased uptake in and immediately adjacent to the tibial tuberosity, and MRI will show edema of the tibial tuberosity, patellar tendon, and adjacent soft tissues (17) (Fig. 10-4B). This is best demonstrated with T2-weighted sequences, preferably with fat suppression, or with IR technique. On these sequences, edema will show high signal intensity. The appearance is less dramatic on the T1-weighted images, where edema of the tibial tuberosity will show as low signal intensity. A distended deep infrapatellar bursa may be seen in some cases (20). In the spondyloarthropathies, tibial tuberosity enthesitis shows plain-film, scintigraphic, and MRI findings that are identical to those of (traumatic) OS disease. Actually, the patient whose knee is shown in Fig. 10-4 also has nail pitting and a family history of psoriatic arthritis. In Sinding-Larsen-Johansson (SLJ) disease, a process similar to OS disease occurs in the lower pole of the patella. MRI is not essential for the study of the soft-tissue changes in OS and SLJ. The patellar tendon is successfully imaged using high-resolution ultrasound (21).

The articular surfaces of the patella are covered by a thick layer of hyaline cartilage. Chondromalacia of the patella is rare in childhood but may be encountered in adolescence and is likely posttraumatic. It is the most common overuse syndrome that afflicts athletes (22). The diagnosis is clinical with anterior knee pain, particularly when the knee is flexed (e.g., ascending or more often descending stairs or after prolonged sitting as in a theater). Plain films and even arthrography are often normal, unless CT-arthrography is used (23). Optimal MRI evaluation of the patellar (hyaline) cartilage should include axial and sagittal images. These will show initial focal cartilage swelling and edema, and later irregular cartilage ulceration and thinning. Eventually, subchondral patellar (bony) cysts may develop. Gradient-echo images (23–27) or T2-weighted images with fat suppression (28) can be used to achieve high contrast between articular cartilage and adjacent structures (fluid, marrow fat, and muscle) and to assess the patellar cartilage.

A fatigue-type stress fracture resulting from prolonged and repetitive muscular action on a normal bone may be seen in the proximal tibia or rarely in the proximal fibula or distal femur (29). Initially negative or showing only soft-tissue swelling, plain films may later reveal periosteal reaction and/or a fracture line (Fig. 10-5A). The bone scan will reveal a nonspecific increased tracer uptake (Fig. 10-5B). A transverse or oblique linear low-signal area representing the fracture line, with surrounding edema of the medullary fat and soft tissues, is seen on MRI (Fig. 10-5C). Runners may suffer a longitudinal stress fracture of the proximal tibia. In these cases, CT with sagittal reformatting will demonstrate

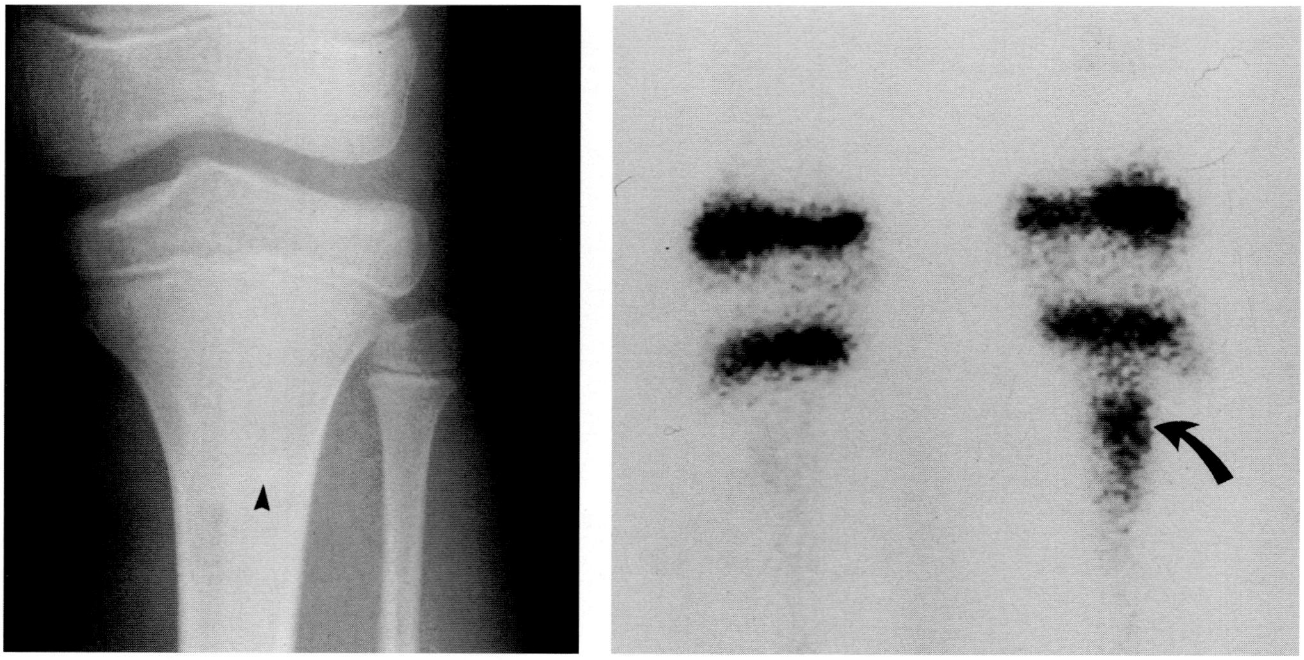

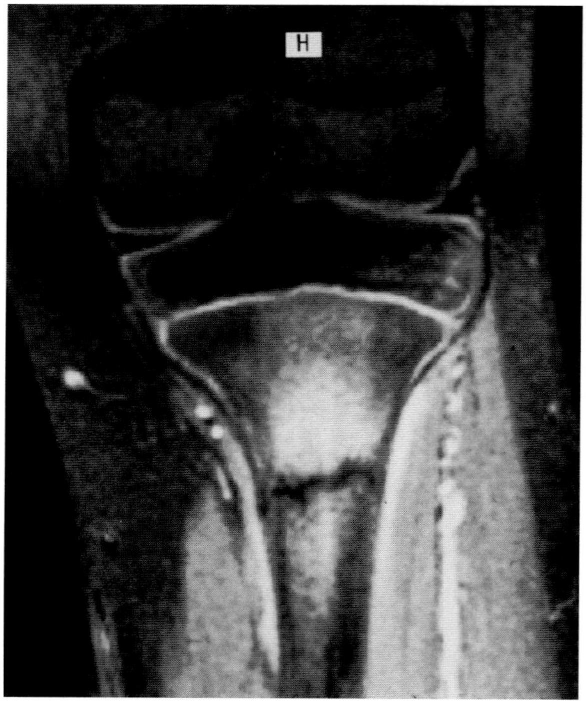

FIG. 10-5. Stress fracture of the proximal tibia in a 9-year-old girl with localized pain following intensive ballet lessons. **A:** Anteroposterior radiograph of the left knee showing only a faint transverse sclerotic line *(arrowhead)*. **B:** Bone scan, AP view, showing increased tracer uptake in the proximal left tibial metaphyseal region *(curved arrow)*. Normal physeal cartilage of the distal femora and proximal tibiae also shows increased uptake. **C:** Coronal, IR image (TR 1900, TE 20, TI 150) showing the fracture as an irregular transverse line of low signal intensity surrounded by intense high-signal edema of the bone marrow and adjacent soft tissues.

the longitudinal lucent fracture line to better advantage (30). An important role for MRI examination in stress fractures is to exclude bone infection and tumor (29,31).

Posttraumatic bone bridging and bars across the physis may be demonstrated using conventional tomography, CT with sagittal and coronal reformatting, or MRI (32,33). CT and MRI are used in the investigation of acute complex physeal and epiphyseal injuries, particularly prior to the appearance of the secondary ossification centers (34). The ability of MRI to depict bone, cartilage, and other soft-tissue structures in any plane is most helpful (35).

Traumatic Soft-Tissue Lesions

Imaging of menisci, ligaments, and tendons in the pediatric age group is similar to that in adults. The detailed anatomy, pathology, and signal abnormalities of the menisci can-

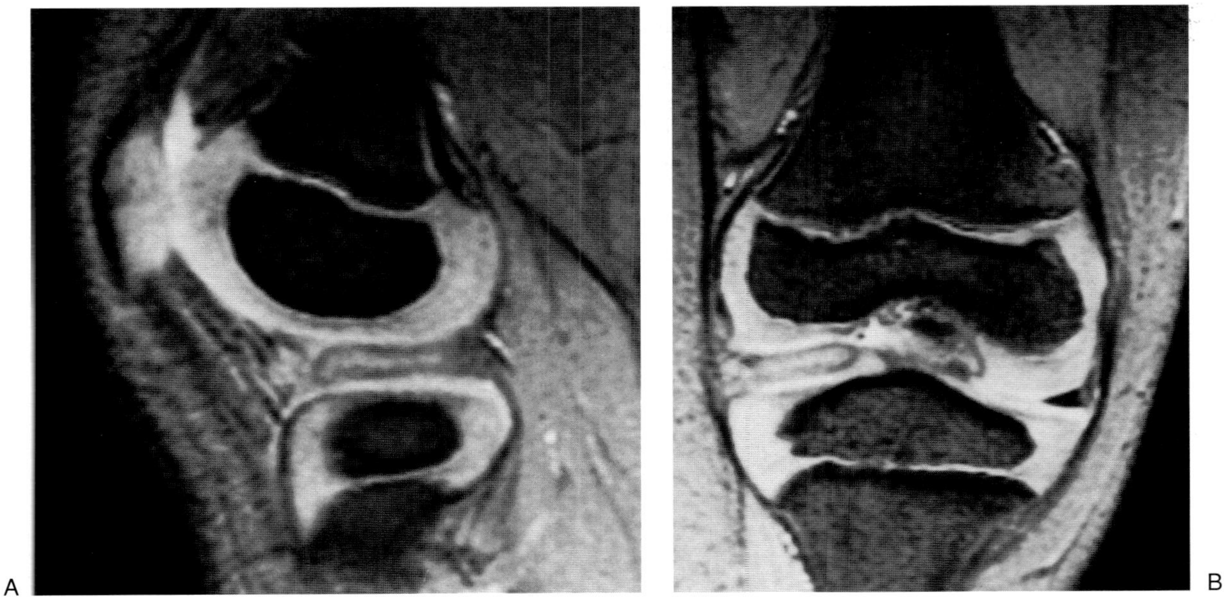

FIG. 10-6. Symptomatic discoid lateral meniscus in a 4-year-old girl. **A:** Sagittal and **B:** coronal gradient-echo images (TR 500, TE 14, flip angle 30°) showing the abnormally large, somewhat rectangular, high-signal-intensity lateral meniscus. The normal, triangular-shaped, low-signal-intensity medial meniscus is also seen on the coronal view.

not be given in this short chapter on MRI of the pediatric knee. The use of rapid gradient-echo sequences has proved to be very useful in the study of the menisci and ligaments of children and adolescents.

A common meniscal abnormality is the discoid lateral meniscus, which may be asymptomatic or may present with a snapping sound when the child walks (on knee flexion and/or extension). It may be unilateral or, more frequently, bilateral. MRI gives a direct view of the abnormally large meniscus, which may not demonstrate the typical "bow-tie" configuration on sagittal MRI (Fig. 10-6A). The diagnosis should be confirmed on coronal images, where it is often easier to detect (13) (Fig. 10-6B). The discoid meniscus usually lacks the normal triangular configuration, not tapering toward its free edge, or it may show a triangular configuration with increased thickness (height). It is thick, is elongated, and extends to the intercondylar region. It is prone to degeneration and tears at an early age and, after trauma, may become more symptomatic with pain and intermittent locking. On MRI, single or often multiple high-signal-intensity tears are seen in addition to the abnormal meniscal size and configuration.

In adolescents, traumatic lesions often include a combination of posterior horn of medial meniscus and anterior cruciate ligament tears together with a medial collateral ligament injury, the so-called O'Donoghue's triad (36). In the pediatric age group, bone contusions may be isolated or associated with anterior cruciate ligament tears (13–17).

The quadriceps or the patellar tendon may be injured and show contusion or tear. Spontaneous rupture of these tendons does occur in patients with renal failure or hyperparathyroidism (37). In adolescents, patellar tendon injuries (and tibial tubercle avulsions) are much more common than quadriceps tendon injuries (38). MRI has greatly improved our ability to detect and characterize these injuries (39). They are seen on MRI as focal or diffuse enlargement of the tendon with intrasubstance increased signal intensity. They are best evaluated on sagittal MRI. Caution has to be exercised when interpreting these studies, as Reiff and colleagues found that the normal patellar tendon is of uniform thickness but displays a focal expansion at its proximal and distal ends, which may show high signal intensity on gradient-echo sequences (40). Osgood-Schlatter's disease is associated with abnormalities of the distal patellar tendon (20). In "jumper's knee" or patellar tendinitis, abnormal findings are seen just distal to the inferior pole of the patella (17,41). They are secondary to repetitive stress. Pain and tenderness occur after jumping, running, or climbing (38). Pathologically, microruptures and areas of focal degeneration are seen in the tendon. Acute traumatic complete rupture of either tendon is unusual, and MRI will demonstrate the site of discontinuity as well as hemorrhage between the two fragments of the ruptured tendon (13). With the rare event of a complete tear of the quadriceps musculotendinous unit (e.g., in runners), the patella is displaced inferiorly and the patellar tendon demonstrates an undulating (wrinkled or wavy) appearance caused by quadriceps muscle retraction and an abnormal extensor mechanism (39,42). Tendons are successfully examined by high-resolution ultrasound but sonography is operator dependent, displays a small field of view, and has limited soft-tissue contrast. CT achieves a much better soft-

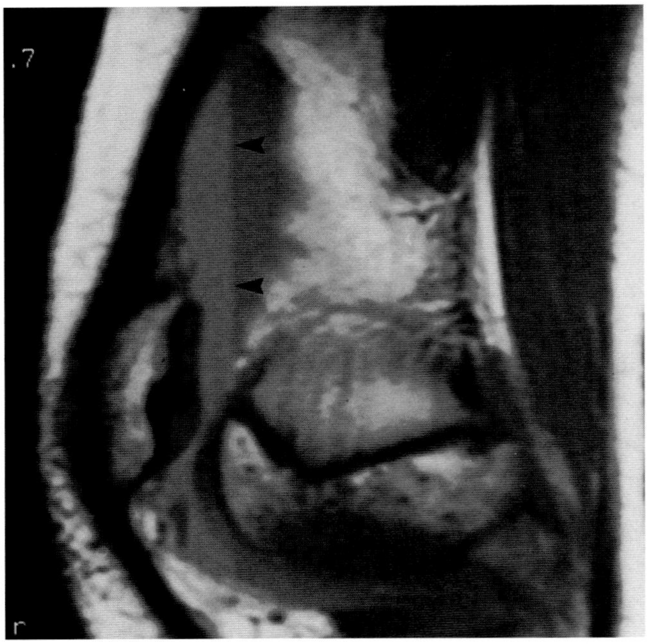

FIG. 10-7. Layered, posttraumatic large effusion (hemarthrosis) in a 10-year-old girl. This sagittal T1-weighted image (TR 400, TE 11) shows a fluid–fluid level *(arrowheads)*. There was no fat signal seen in the knee effusion and no associated fracture.

tissue contrast, but transverse imaging is not appropriate for the study of tendons around the knee.

Hemarthrosis

Hemarthrosis is encountered after acute knee injury and in hemophilia and other bleeding disorders. The condition is diagnosed as knee effusion on plain radiographs. Posttraumatic effusion does not always show a fat–fluid level or lipohemarthrosis on MRI. Unless fat signal is revealed, layered effusion should be more properly described as a fluid–fluid level (Fig. 10-7). In the instance of a true lipohemarthrosis, an associated fracture is invariably present, allowing escape of the bone marrow fat into the knee joint (43). Fresh hemorrhage will appear as low signal intensity on T1-weighted sequences and as high signal on the T2-weighted images, with possible settling of debris and the production of a fluid–fluid. A traumatic synovitis may also be seen, with foci of irregular synovial proliferation (44) and enhancement post-Gd (Fig. 10-8).

ARTHRITIS AND ENTHESITIS

Arthritis

Chronic arthritides of childhood include juvenile rheumatoid arthritis (JRA) and the spondyloarthropathies. Clinical and radiographic findings in these entities have been previously described (45–47). They all include a chronic synovial inflammation, often with joint effusion. On plain films, knee joint swelling is seen, but it is impossible to differentiate between fluid and proliferative synovitis (pannus). MRI is valuable in the assessment of early changes of the synovium and cartilage. Synovial proliferation (pannus) will show as thickening and irregularity of the synovium, which may be distinguished from effusion using standard SE sequences. The thickened synovium is of intermediate signal intensity on T1- and T2-weighted MRIs, compared with the low signal intensity of the effusion on T1 and the high signal intensity of the effusion on T2 (48,49).

Pannus is hypervascular, and after Gd it exhibits a rapid and marked increase of signal intensity, whereas adjacent fatty tissue, muscle, bone marrow, and synovial effusion demonstrate only minor changes, causing increased contrast between the thickened synovium and the joint effusion (50,51) (Fig. 10-9). This may be seen on many sequences, including T1-weighted spin-echo and gradient-echo techniques post-Gd injection (50,52). Normal synovium (and joint fluid) shows no visually apparent enhancement after Gd. Enhancement of the abnormal synovium is time dependent, and optimal imaging should be performed within minutes (e.g., 5 minutes) following Gd administration (2,53). Eventually, joint fluid also enhances, and this may cause

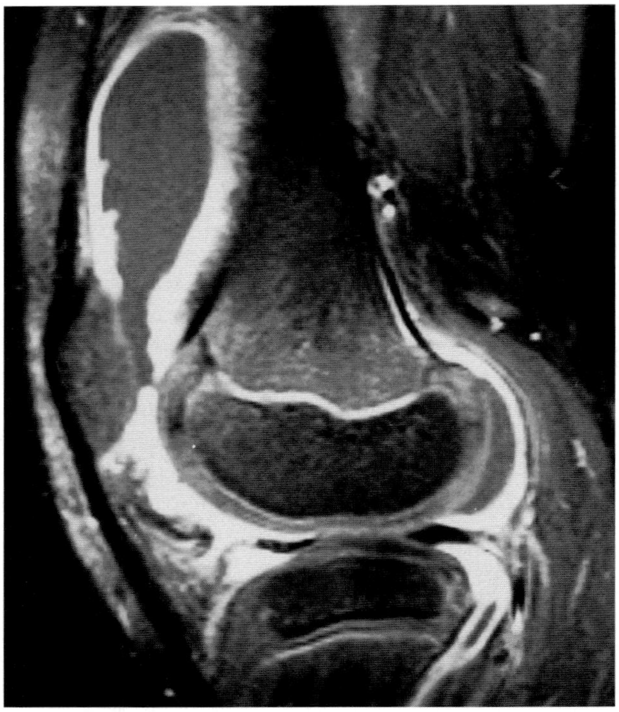

FIG. 10-8. Post-Gd sagittal proton-density image (TR 1155, TE 22) with fat suppression in a 17-year-old boy with traumatic synovitis, shows an intermediate-signal-intensity joint effusion and an intense enhancement of the synovium (post-Gd). The synovium is very thickened and irregular.

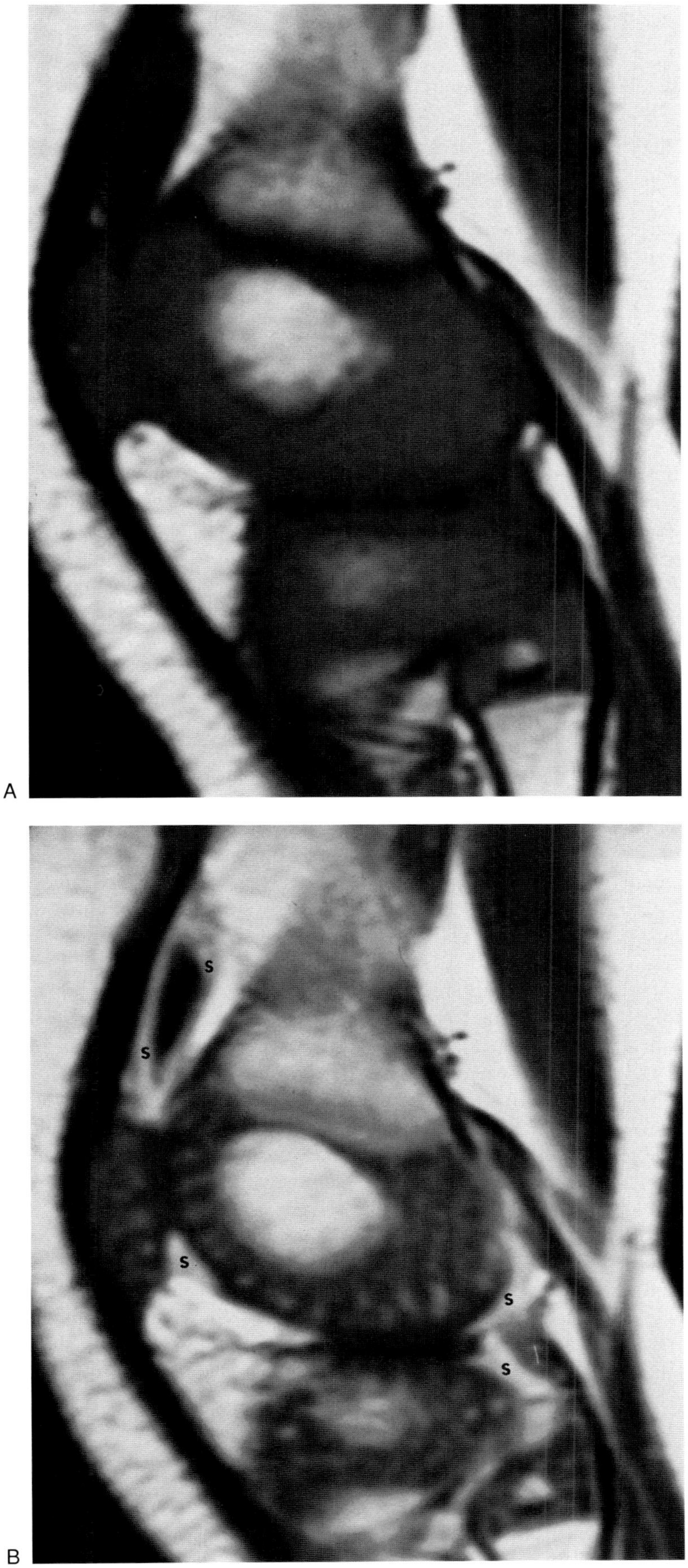

FIG. 10-9. Pauci-articular JRA with clinical involvement of the left knee for 6 months in a 19-month-old girl. **A:** Sagittal T1-weighted sequence (TR 650, TE 11) showing an intermediate signal suprapatellar effusion isointense with cartilage and muscle. The inflamed synovium is not well seen. **B:** Sagittal T1-weighted sequence post-Gd using the same imaging parameters as in Fig. 10-9A; shows the enhancing thickened synovium(s). The suprapatellar effusion is actually small. There is also some enhancement of the bone marrow and a reticulated appearance of the blood vessels seen in the cartilaginous structures (patella, femoral condyle, tibial plateau, and fibular head) post-Gd.

confusion in the interpretation of the MRIs (54). Herve-Somma and colleagues found that MRIs repeated 15 minutes after Gd injection in six patients with JRA show an increase in the signal intensity of the effusion, with blurring of the synovial outline caused by diffusion of contrast into the joint fluid (51).

In addition, MRI allows direct cartilage imaging and visualization of early articular cartilage erosion, irregularity, and thinning by the destructive pannus (55). At this stage, plain films will show joint space narrowing, and cartilage destruction is only inferred (56). In young patients the epiphyseal cartilage is very thick, and in chronic inflammatory arthritides a long time will elapse before it is gradually destroyed by pannus and actual bone erosions appear. Multiple new sequences are now being tried for optimal cartilage visualization and improved discrimination among it, the synovium, and joint fluid (57). Other changes that may be present in arthritis and seen on MRI include meniscal and cruciate ligaments atrophy or hypotrophy, a popliteal synovial cyst (which is a distended gastrocnemius–semimembranosus bursa), epiphyseal overgrowth, or posterior subluxation of the tibia at the knee secondary to quadriceps atrophy (3). Bone erosions are a late finding and are seen on both plain radiographs and MRI, but the latter detects a greater number of erosions compared to conventional radiography (58).

MRI may be indicated in the diagnosis, staging, follow-up, or planning of treatment of the knee involved with inflammatory arthritis (3). It has been used in the assessment of intra-articular steroid injection in the management of JRA (55). It cannot differentiate between the types of JRA (systemic onset, pauciarticular, or polyarticular) or between knee involvement in JRA and in the spondyloarthropathies.

In neuroarthropathy, MRI will show effusion with synovial debris, loose bodies, bone fragmentation, and joint disorganization, as well as synovial enhancement after Gd.

Hemophilic arthropathy is secondary to repeated bleeding into the joint (hemarthrosis), which leads to progressive joint destruction. MRI is capable of showing the synovial abnormalities, which are often marked (thickening and inflammation); erosions and thinning of cartilage; joint space narrowing; bone erosions; subchondral cysts; and epiphyseal overgrowth (59,60). Hemosiderin may deposit in the synovial lining (44,54). Bleeding in a large muscle (e.g., the quadriceps) may also be seen in hemophilia. Rarely, the hematoma fails to resolve. It becomes encapsulated and is called pseudotumor of hemophilia. It contains coagulated blood and is surrounded by a thick fibrous wall but may slowly expand if new bleeding occurs. The MRI signal characteristics of soft-tissue hemorrhage are variable, depending on the "age" of the hemorrhage (59,61).

Enthesitis

Enthesitis is the most specific clinical and radiological feature of the spondyloarthropathies and occurs more frequently in children than in adults. It represents inflammation at the site of attachment of ligament or tendon to bone and, in the knee region, may be present at the insertion of the patellar or quadriceps tendons and causes localized pain and swelling. Because of long-standing hyperemia, there may be localized bony overgrowth (Fig. 10-10). MRI demonstrates early inflammatory bone marrow edema, cortical erosion, and/or bone apposition as well as increased signal intensity within the tendon substance. The patellar and quadriceps tendons have no synovial sheath; therefore, tendinous and peritendinous inflammation directly involves the surrounding tissues (52).

INFECTION

Awareness of clinical symptoms and signs, laboratory confirmation, and tailored imaging are required for early diagnosis of osteomyelitis, septic arthritis, and soft-tissue infection. Aspiration and culture should be tried, to diagnose acute bone, joint, and soft-tissue infection (62). Prompt treatment is required to avoid permanent damage to bone and to articular, epiphyseal, and physeal cartilage of the distal femur and proximal tibia.

Knee infection may be hematogenous (e.g., in the child with sepsis) or may follow an open injury or surgery. Blood-borne microorganisms (usually *Staphylococcus aureus*) tend to settle in the metaphyses, where blood flow is relatively sluggish. Other specific infections include tuberculosis as well as viral and fungal infections.

Since metaphyseal capillaries penetrate the growth plate in infants, there may be concurrent metaphyseal and epiphyseal osteomyelitis and septic arthritis (63). Unless treated rapidly and efficiently, this will result in significant morbidity and long-lasting deformity with leg-length discrepancy and early and severe degenerative arthritis of the affected knee.

In the child more than 1 year of age, the vascular supplies to the metaphysis and epiphysis are separate and the growth plate acts, at least temporarily, as a barrier to infection. Epiphyseal osteomyelitis is rarely primary (63). It usually follows a metaphyseal infection or septic arthritis.

The knee joint is a site of predilection for septic arthritis, with the commonest microorganism being *Staphylococcus aureus*. Gonococcal or gram-negative joint sepsis is also relatively frequent. Drug abusers often develop infection in smaller joints. Prior joint trauma or surgery, juvenile rheumatoid arthritis, immunosuppressive agents, and systemic or local steroids predispose to septic arthritis during episodes of bacteremia. Subacute and chronic osteomyelitis are usually diagnosed on plain films, which may show periosteal reaction, bone destruction, metaphyseal channels and cavities, sequestra, or heavy sclerosis.

The plain-film finding of joint "space" narrowing is late and is the result of cartilage destruction. Plain radiographs do not show the early damages of bone, joint, or soft-tissue infection. Scintigraphy and MRI (and to a lesser extent CT) will show early bone marrow and soft-tissue changes (64).

Bone and joint scintiscans are highly sensitive for the di-

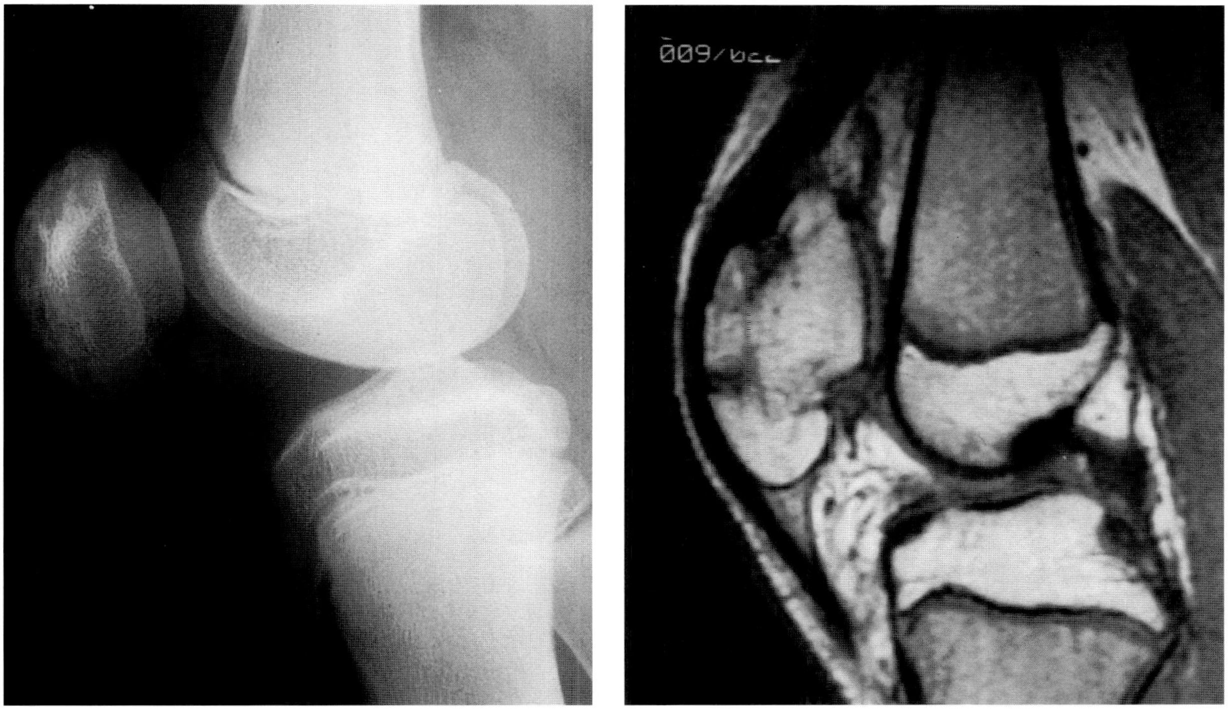

A B

FIG. 10-10. Sequel of patellar enthesitis in a 13-year-old boy with juvenile ankylosing spondylitis. **A:** Lateral plain radiograph of the knee showing patellar enlargement with irregular outline. **B:** Sagittal T1-weighted image (TR 666, TE 20) showing the same findings as in Fig. 10-10A. Fat signal is seen in the patella with no sign of marrow edema (also verified on other sequences). The cortical (and cartilaginous) outline of the patella is very irregular and notched.

agnosis of acute infection, but at times it is difficult to separate a bone marrow process from soft-tissue infection. Also, invasion of the growth plate is difficult to detect. These difficulties are not encountered with MRI. CT is the best imaging modality for the detection and localization of sequestra. Sonography may detect early changes in the soft tissues and synovium, subperiosteal abscess, and joint effusion.

Together with scintigraphy, MRI is very sensitive to early changes of infection in bone, joint, and soft tissues (65). In osteomyelitis, MRI will show bone marrow abnormality with low signal on T1 and high signal on T2 caused by edema, hyperemia, and exudate. Bone marrow changes are often extensive (66). In children the periosteum is only loosely adherent to the cortex and is easily lifted away, allowing large and sometimes diffuse subperiosteal abscesses to form (67,68). Linear periosteal new bone formation shows as low-signal-intensity lines separated from the adjacent cortex by fluid or granulation tissue (Fig. 10-11). Later, cortical bone thickening and remodeling are present. Adjacent soft tissues (fat, fascial planes, and muscles) may demonstrate variable degrees of edema, with irregular areas of increased signal intensity on long TR and on IR sequences. Using MRI one can detect foci of acute infection in chronic osteomyelitis or exclude active osteomyelitis, which is also important information in the patient's management (65,69).

A soft-tissue abscess may be present. It is not rare in the pediatric age group, where the cortex is easily permeated. It shows as a round, triangular, or oval mass of fluid accumulation, giving a bright signal on T2 and IR sequences and showing thick rim enhancement after Gd (64). The abscess margins are often irregular and serrated (68). MRI is highly sensitive in identifying these foci of soft-tissue infection and localized fluid collections. Abscess identification and localization are very useful prior to percutaneous or open surgical drainage A Brodie's abscess may be present in the distal femoral or proximal tibial or fibular metaphysis. It will show as a round or oval intraosseous low signal intensity on T1 and high signal intensity on T2 with a surrounding rim of hypointensity. Between the rim (of reactive bone sclerosis) and the abscess fluid there may be intermediate layers of vascular granulation tissue, of intermediate signal on T1 and of high signal on T2, which show marked enhancement after Gd injection (70). Rarely, a primary epiphyseal bone abscess may be seen, often in a femoral condyle (63,67) (Fig. 10-12). A sequestrum may be identified as an amorphous fragment of low signal intensity that does not enhance if Gd is given.

In septic arthritis of the knee, MRI will demonstrate synovial thickening and irregularity due to congestion, edema, and hypertrophy secondary to infection. Gd injection clearly delineates the abnormal synovium (2). Joint effusion, often with internal debris, follows invariably. Changes in signal

A 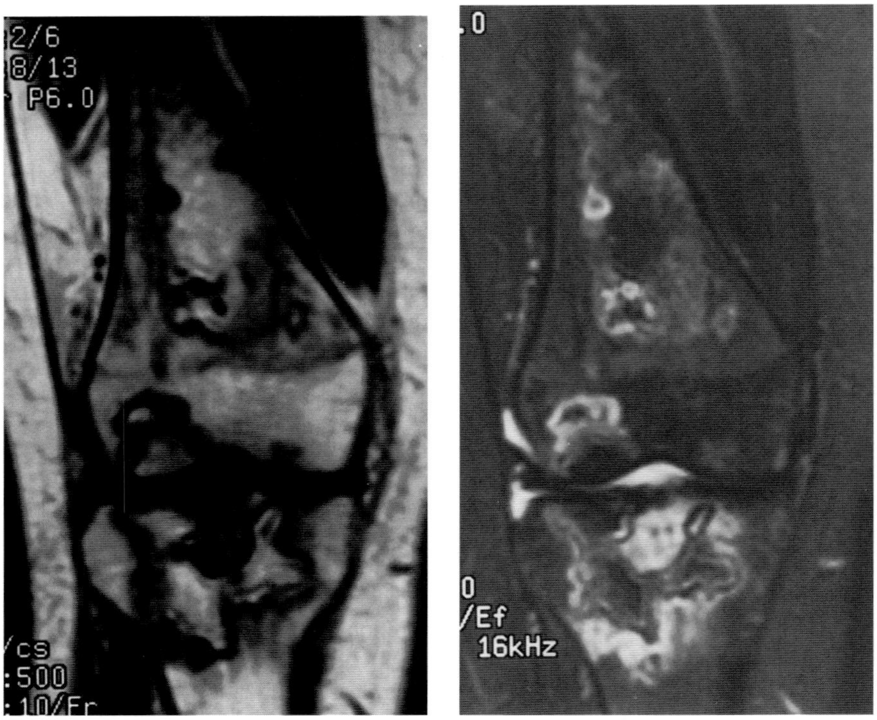 B

FIG. 10-16. Advanced changes of ischemic bone necrosis in a 16-year-old girl with leukemia, on long-standing steroid medication. **A:** Coronal T1-weighted sequence (TR 500, TE 10) and **(B)** coronal T2-weighted sequence (TR 2800, TE 102), with fat suppression showing multiple metaphyseal and epiphyseal geographic areas of abnormal signal intensity due to a mixture of bone marrow edema, fibrosis, and sclerosis. High-signal-intensity edema is well seen in **B** in the proximal tibia. Fibrosis and sclerosis show low-signal intensities on both T1- and T2-weighted sequences.

common in the West Indies and Scandinavia. Familial cases have been reported.

On plain radiographs there is an abrupt angulation of the tibia into varus deformity below the knee. Langenskiold described six radiographic stages (93), with the earliest changes seen between 1 and 3.5 years of age. The higher the stage (from 1 to 5), the more medial deformity is present, whereas stage 6 is characterized by a bony bridge across the physis (i.e., between the metaphysis and epiphysis).

Radiographic differential diagnosis includes physiologic bowing of the legs and the deformity seen in rickets, hypophosphatasia, and focal fibrocartilagenous dysplasia of the proximal tibia (94).

The rare adolescent type is usually unilateral, with narrowing of part of the medial growth plate and shortening of the tibia. There is premature irregular fusion of the medial aspect of the growth plate producing the Blount's deformity. There is no steplike deformity of the growth plate, and the etiology is usually posttraumatic, but may in rare cases be postinfectious. The age at presentation is usually between 8 and 13 years.

Magnetic resonance imaging is not part of the routine investigation of a classic case of Blount's disease. It certainly helps our understanding of the plain radiographic appearances by showing the cartilaginous component of the epiphysis, which is usually relatively large. It also demonstrates depression of the medial tibial metaphysis and epiphysis. A metaphyseal beak is formed, and this shows a variable signal intensity (95). The rest of the metaphysis shows normal signal on MRI. The tibial articular surface may be normal and horizontal if the cartilaginous component of the epiphysis compensates for the bony deformity (95). More often the joint line is depressed medially or posteromedially and compensation by the epiphyseal cartilage is only partial. The medial aspect of the epiphysis shows delay in ossification, and the adjacent physis is narrowed and irregular but shows normal signal intensity. The medial aspect of the epiphysis gradually ossifies and the epiphysis appears triangular or wedge-shaped and may be fragmented. It also shows normal signal intensity.

As a further step, early bridging of the physis medially will accentuate the deformity. The medial meniscus may be enlarged and its signal increased but the cruciates are normal.

TUMORS AND TUMORLIKE CONDITIONS

Commonly indicated for tumors arising from the knee joint or surrounding soft tissues in childhood, MRI is used primarily to delineate tumor anatomy. It provides better tu-

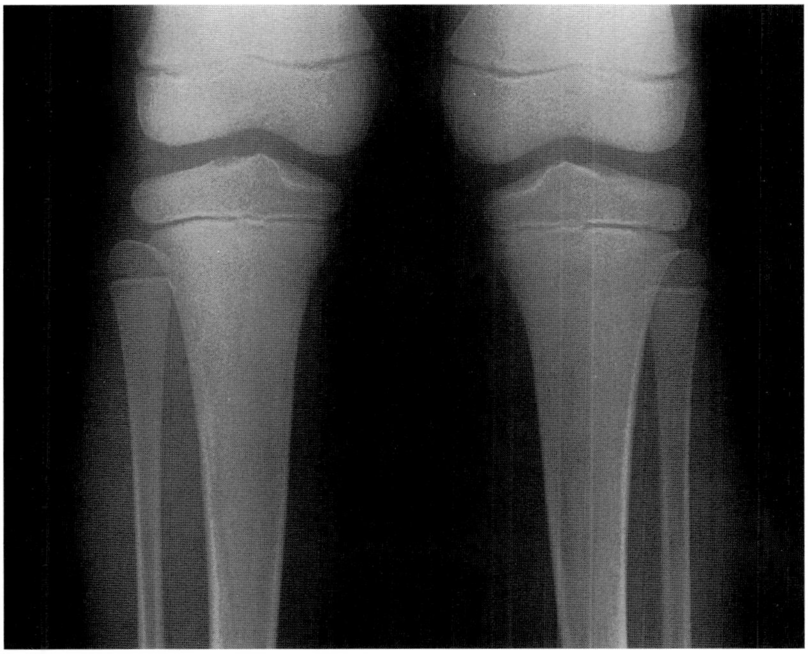

A

FIG. 10-17. Gaucher's disease in an 8-year-old girl. **A:** AP plain radiograph of both knees and proximal legs showing diffuse sclerosis with an indistinct bone trabecular pattern. **B:** Coronal, T1-weighted image (TR 500, TE 10) showing significant replacement of the bone marrow with a dramatic reduction of the normal marrow signal in the metaphyses but also—to a lesser extent—in the epiphyses and tibial diaphyses. **C:** Coronal T1-weighted image of the upper abdomen showing mild hepatomegaly and severe splenomegaly (S). The spleen measured 19 cm in its craniocaudal length.

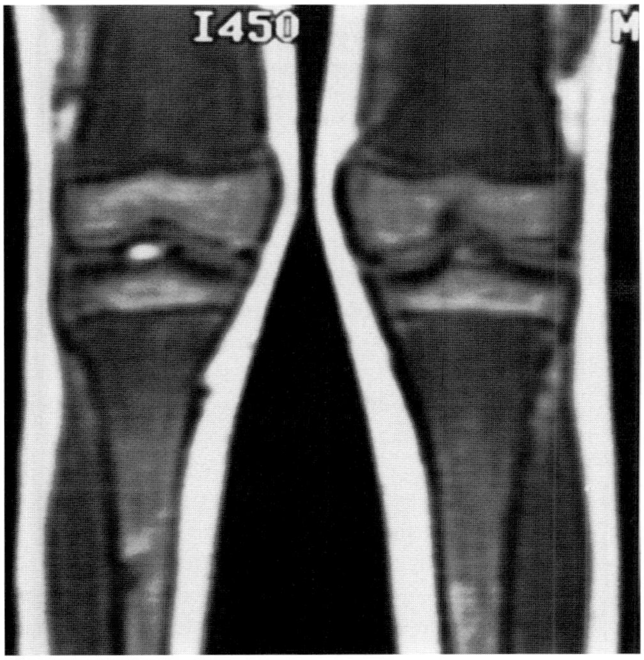

B

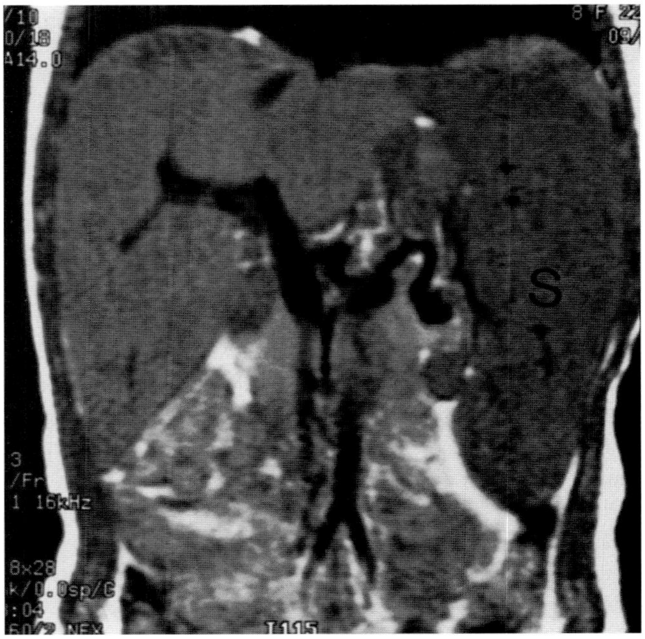

C

mor–tissue contrast than CT and improved definition of intramedullary tumor, extension into surrounding musculature and fascial planes, or involvement of neurovascular bundles (96,97). This section will highlight some of the more common entities encountered during childhood and the value of MRI in their investigation.

Bone Lesions

Characterization of pediatric bone tumors is usually best done by plain radiography based upon conventional strategies that include consideration of age of the child, site of origin (i.e., epiphysis, metaphysis, or diaphysis) and tumor appearance. Occasionally, however, MRI can add important information helpful in recognizing malignant lesions, especially with prior irradiation (Fig. 10-18).

Clearly, benign lesions on radiography such as osteochondromas do not require MRI investigation if surgery is not contemplated. When necessary, MRI may be used to define local anatomy, especially if articular or soft-tissue extent is suspected. Generally well recognized on plain films, osteoid osteomas may require CT or MRI for confirmation or exact

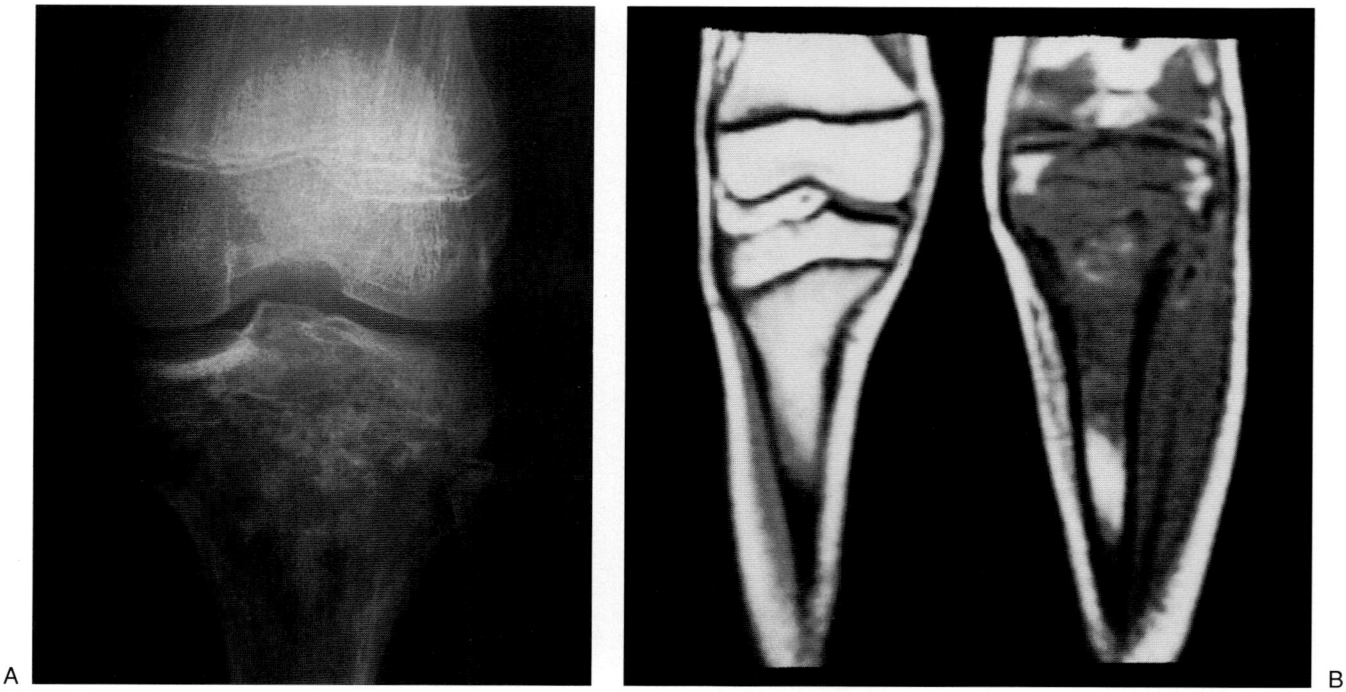

FIG. 10-18. Malignant fibrous histiocytoma. Thirteen-year-old boy developed knee pain and pathologic fracture 6 years following radiation therapy of lower extremity for rhabdomyosarcoma. **A:** Frontal radiograph shows mixed lytic sclerotic process within proximal tibial epiphysis and metaphysis, earlier thought to be radiation necrosis. **B:** Coronal T1-weighted image (TR 567, TE 10) with extensive marrow replacement from malignant fibrous histiocytoma.

localization prior to image-guided ablation (98). On MRI, the nidus of the osteoid osteoma is usually of low to intermediate signal intensity on T1-weighted SE imaging and of moderate to increased signal intensity on T2-weighted images. Extensive marrow edema or low signal on both T1 and T2 from reactive sclerosis are occasionally present along its periphery (98). Rarely encountered around the knee, osteoblastomas may show more heterogeneous signal intensity and diffuse inflammatory response (96).

Fibrous cortical defects and nonossifying fibromas arising particularly from the posteromedial aspect of the distal femoral metaphysis and proximal tibia are often encountered incidentally. These lesions usually show nonspecific low signal intensity on T1-weighted and high signal intensity on T2-weighted images and can be recognized from their characteristic plain-film appearance (8). Fibrous dysplasia may have similar signal intensity often bordered by a thick, low-signal-intensity sclerotic band (96).

Unicameral and aneurysmal bone cysts are common, usually appearing as well-defined metaphyseal lucencies often septated with bone expansion (99,100). Simple bone cysts have a typical fluid appearance on MRI with well-defined low signal intensity on T1 and uniform high signal intensity on T2, also often associated with a low-signal-intensity sclerotic rim (96). Internal hemorrhage (e.g., after fracture) may lead to a somewhat atypical MR appearance that may resemble an aneurysmal bone cyst (99) (Fig. 10-19). Often containing acute or chronic hemorrhage, fluid, and fibrous tissue, aneurysmal bone cysts may have high-signal-intensity regions on both T1 and T2 and characteristically multiple fluid–fluid levels (100) (Fig. 10-20). Fluid–fluid levels are not pathognomonic, as they occur in other benign or malignant bone and soft-tissue lesions in childhood, including osteosarcoma and synovial sarcoma (101). Transphyseal extent of aneurysmal bone cysts is more frequently recognized with MRI than with plain films alone.

Although Langerhans cell histiocytosis most often occurs in the diaphysis, occasionally localized involvement around the knee may be seen. In the incipient phase of Langerhans cell histiocytosis, Ewing sarcoma may be simulated on plain films with a poorly defined lytic lesion and lamellated periosteal reaction (102). On MRI striking peritumoral edema, periosteal new bone formation, and a soft-tissue component can suggest more aggressive malignant lesions (103). A low-signal-intensity periphery and enhancement following Gd may be seen (104).

Chondroblastomas, one of the commonest epiphyseal-based lesions, are often found at the knee in the distal femur and proximal tibia (105–107). They may extend through the physis or cortex into the surrounding metaphysis or soft tissues and have associated joint effusion or diametaphyseal periosteal reaction (105). Chondroblastomas usually have

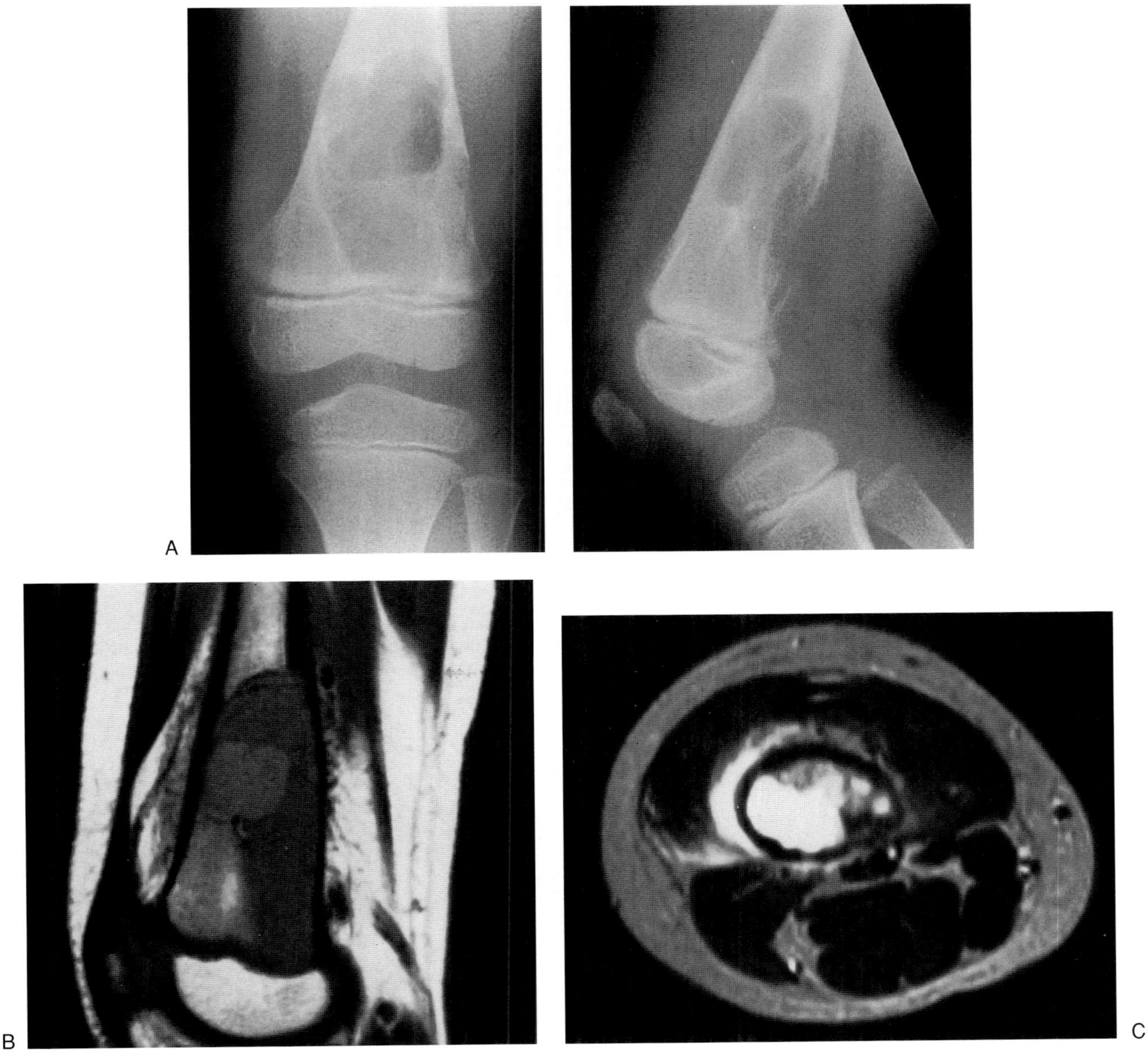

FIG. 10-19. Unicameral bone cyst of distal femoral metaphysis in an 8-year-old girl. **A:** AP and lateral radiographs showing septated distal femoral metaphyseal lesion with loss of cortex posteriorly and abutting physis inferiorly. **B:** Sagittal T1-weighted image (TR 700, TE 20) showing inhomogeneous signal intensity of the contained fluid in keeping with prior hemorrhage. **C:** Axial T2-weighted image (TR 2500, TE 80) with high signal of contained fluid and high signal within surrounding soft tissues, likely from small pathologic fracture.

A 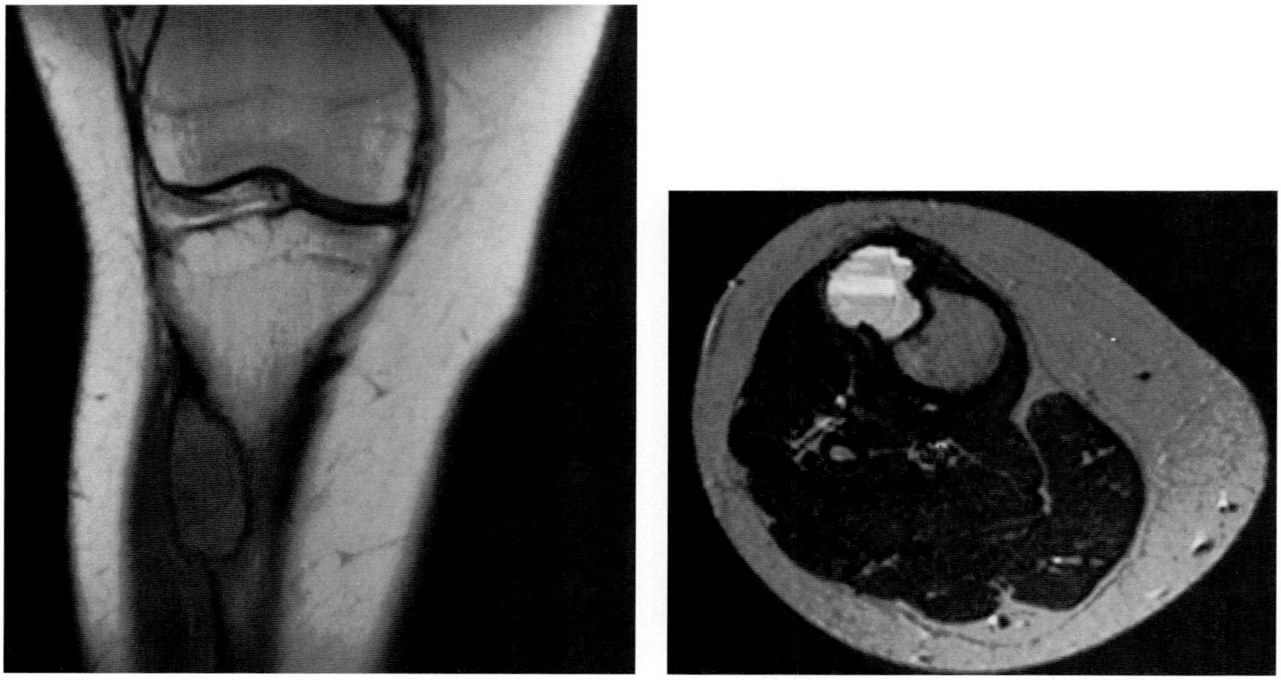 B

FIG. 10-20. Aneurysmal bone cyst presenting with expansile cortical-based lesion of proximal tibia. **A:** Coronal T1-weighted image (TR 600, TE 20) showing slightly heterogeneous lesion with intermediate signal, marginated by low signal intensity. **B:** Axial T2-weighted image (TR 2500, TE 80) with multiple fluid–fluid levels.

A 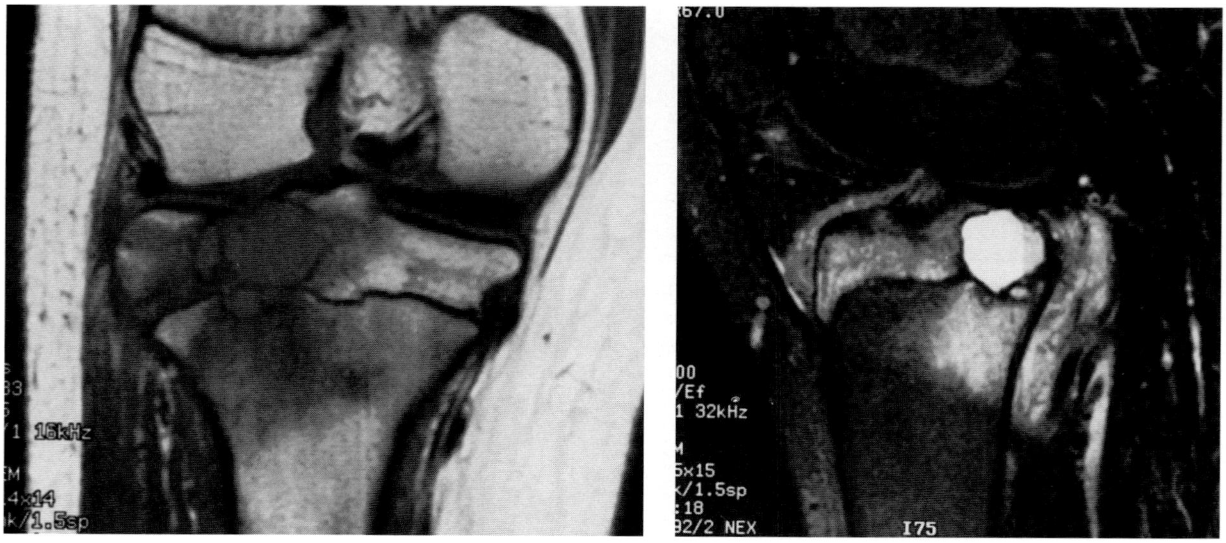 B

FIG. 10-21. Chondroblastoma presenting with knee pain in a 12-year-old boy. **A:** Coronal T1-weighted image (TR 633, TE 15) with low signal intensity periphery corresponding to sclerotic rim and diffuse, ill-defined low signal extending within epiphysis and metaphysis. **B:** Sagittal fast T2-weighted image (TR 3800, TE 84). Extensive high signal with fluid–fluid level in chondroblastoma and extensive bone and soft-tissue edema.

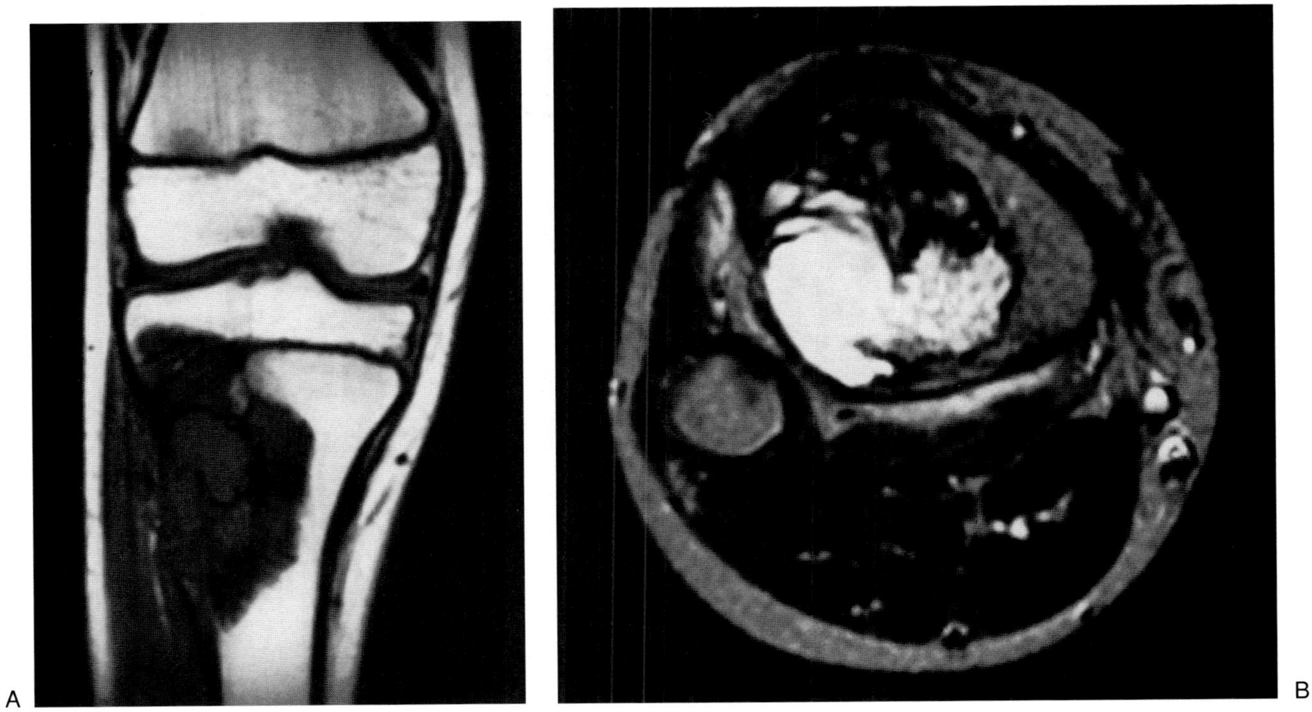

FIG. 10-22. Osteosarcoma presenting with knee pain in a 12-year-old boy. **A:** Coronal T1-weighted image (TR 500, TE 15) showing epiphyseal involvement and heterogeneous tumor signal within the metaphysis. **B:** Axial T2-weighted image (TR 2500, TE 80) showing heterogeneous tumor signal with low signal anteriorly from osteosclerosis and more extensive high signal within posterior aspect of the tibia.

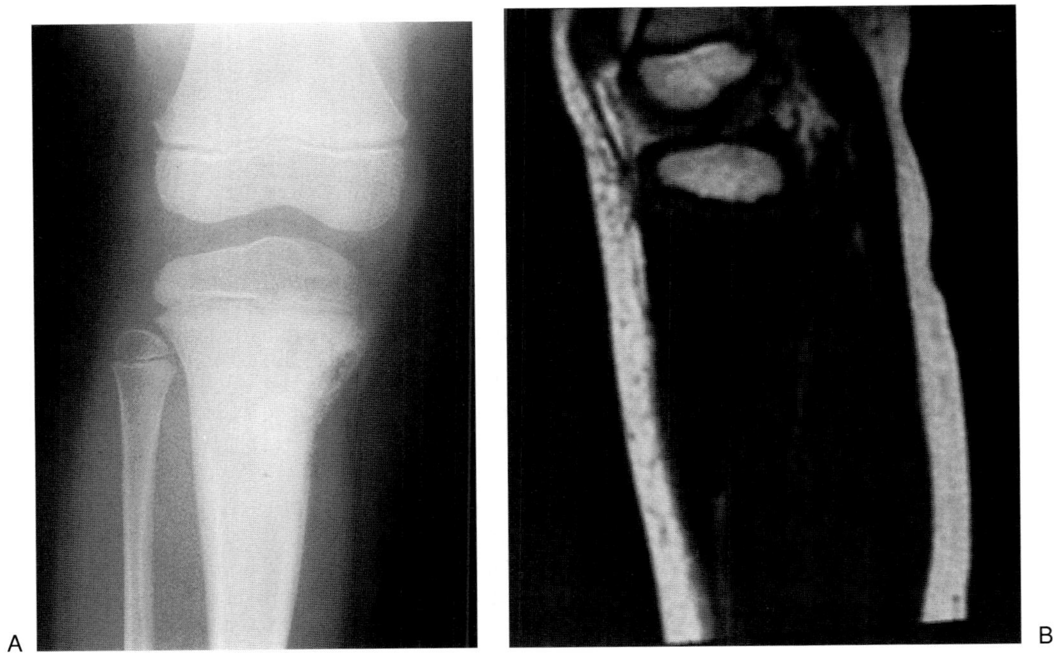

FIG. 10-23. Ewing's sarcoma presenting in an 8-year-old boy with acute onset of knee pain. **A:** Frontal radiograph showing an aggressive lesion of the proximal tibia with loss of cortex medially, periosteal reaction, and sclerosis. **B:** Sagittal T1-weighted image (TR 566, TE 11) with extensive replacement by tumor that abuts the physis proximally.

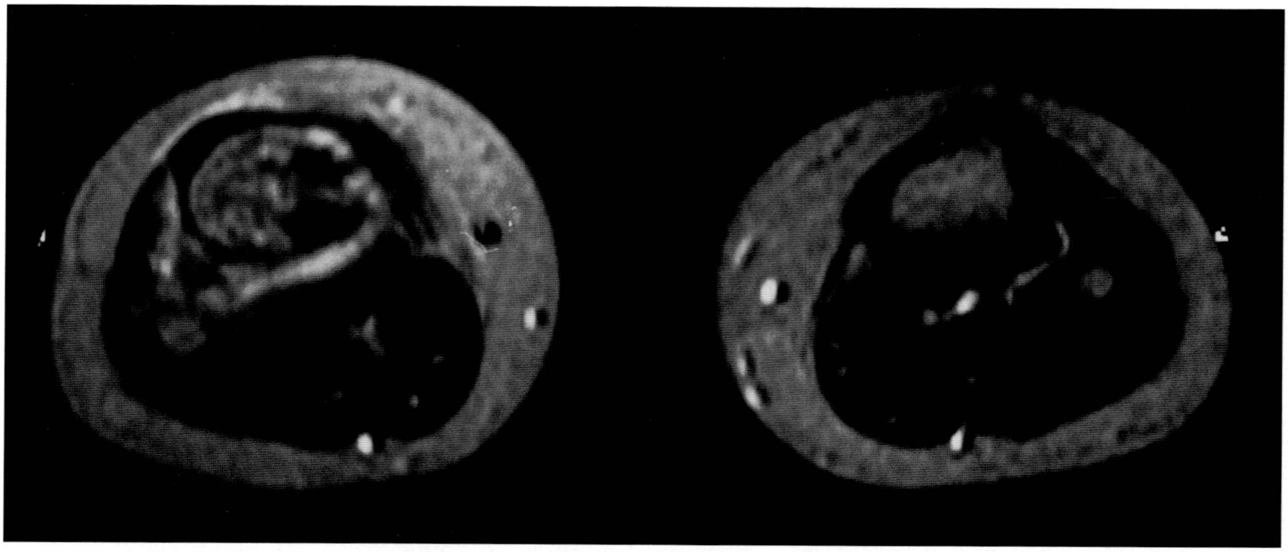

C

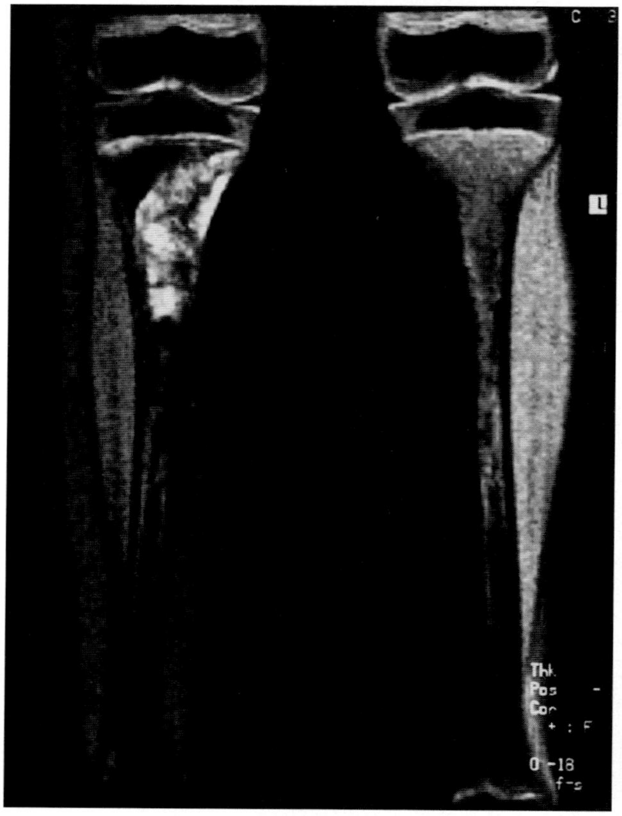

D

FIG. 10-23 *Continued.* **C:** Axial T2-weighted image (TR 2500, TE 80) showing minimal surrounding soft-tissue mass or edema. **D:** Follow-up at 3 months postchemotherapy IR image (TR 1800, TE 20, TI 150) showing reduction in extent of tumor but persistent high signal, compatible with necrosis and/or viable tumor.

well-defined low signal intensity on T1-weighted SE imaging with heterogeneous or high signal intensity on T2-weighted images, often associated with a low-signal-intensity sclerotic rim (105) and moderate surrounding epiphyseal marrow edema (Fig. 10-21). Chondroblastomas must be distinguished from other epiphyseal abnormalities, including osteomyelitis, Langerhans cell histiocytosis, fibrous defects, and erosions from juvenile chronic arthritis.

Osteosarcoma, the most common primary bone malignancy encountered in late childhood and adolescence, commonly arises from the distal femoral or proximal tibial metaphysis (97). Accurate preoperative assessment is essential before oncologic treatment and/or limb-sparing surgery can be planned. Formerly thought to be a barrier to tumor spread, conventional plain films cannot accurately exclude physeal involvement (108). Epiphyseal extent is now commonly noted, with 70–80% of cases of osteosarcomas showing direct transgression of the physis on MRI (108,109) (Fig. 10-

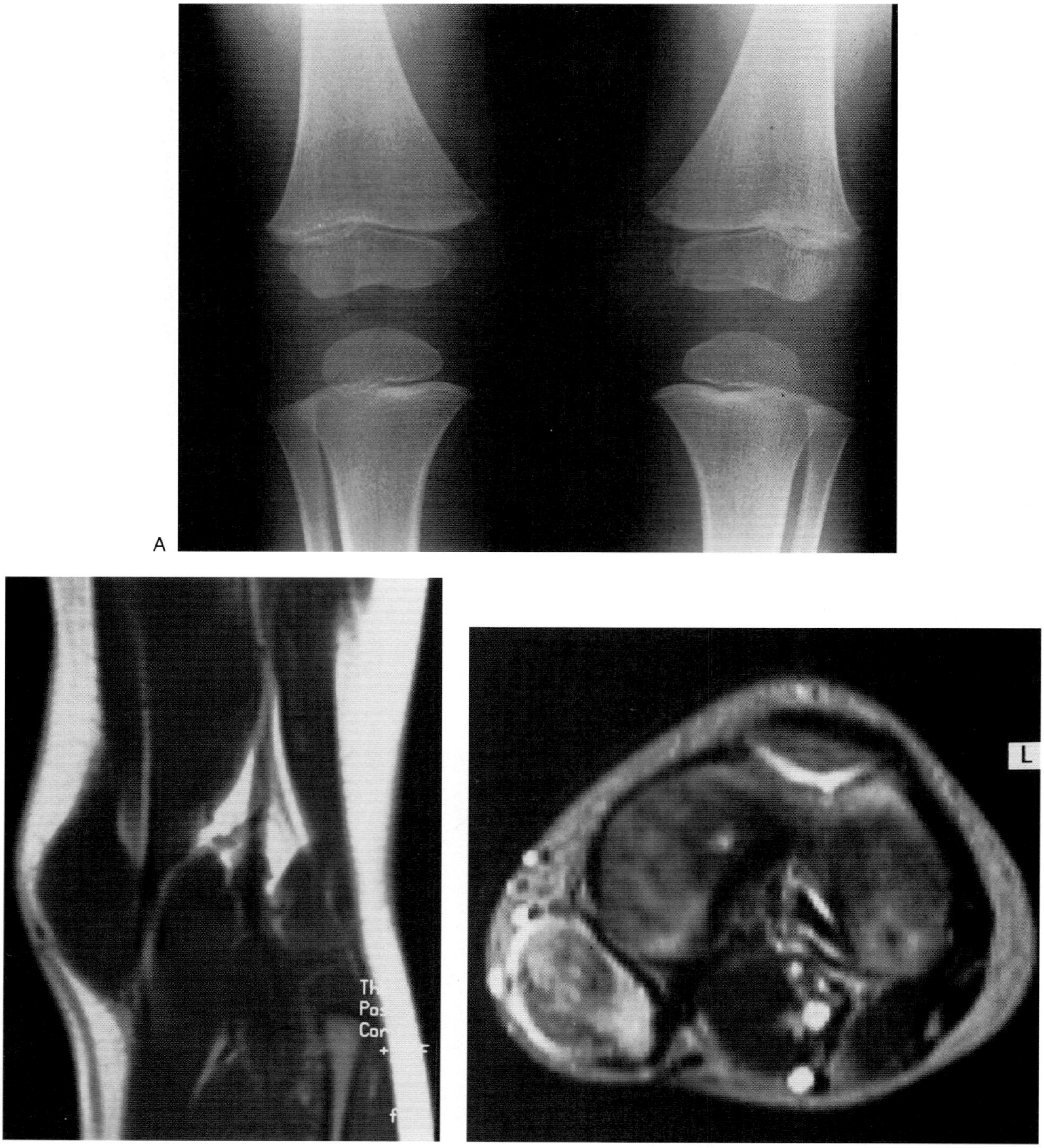

FIG. 10-24. Extra-osseous Ewing's presenting with a juxta-articular mass in a 2.5-year-old boy. **A:** Radiograph of left knee vaguely defines medial soft-tissue mass on left. **B:** Coronal T1-weighted image (TR 450, TE 10) with elongated homogeneous mass isointense to muscle. **C:** Axial T2-weighted image (TR 2500, TE 80) with well-defined mass extending into subcutaneous fat with heterogeneous increased signal.

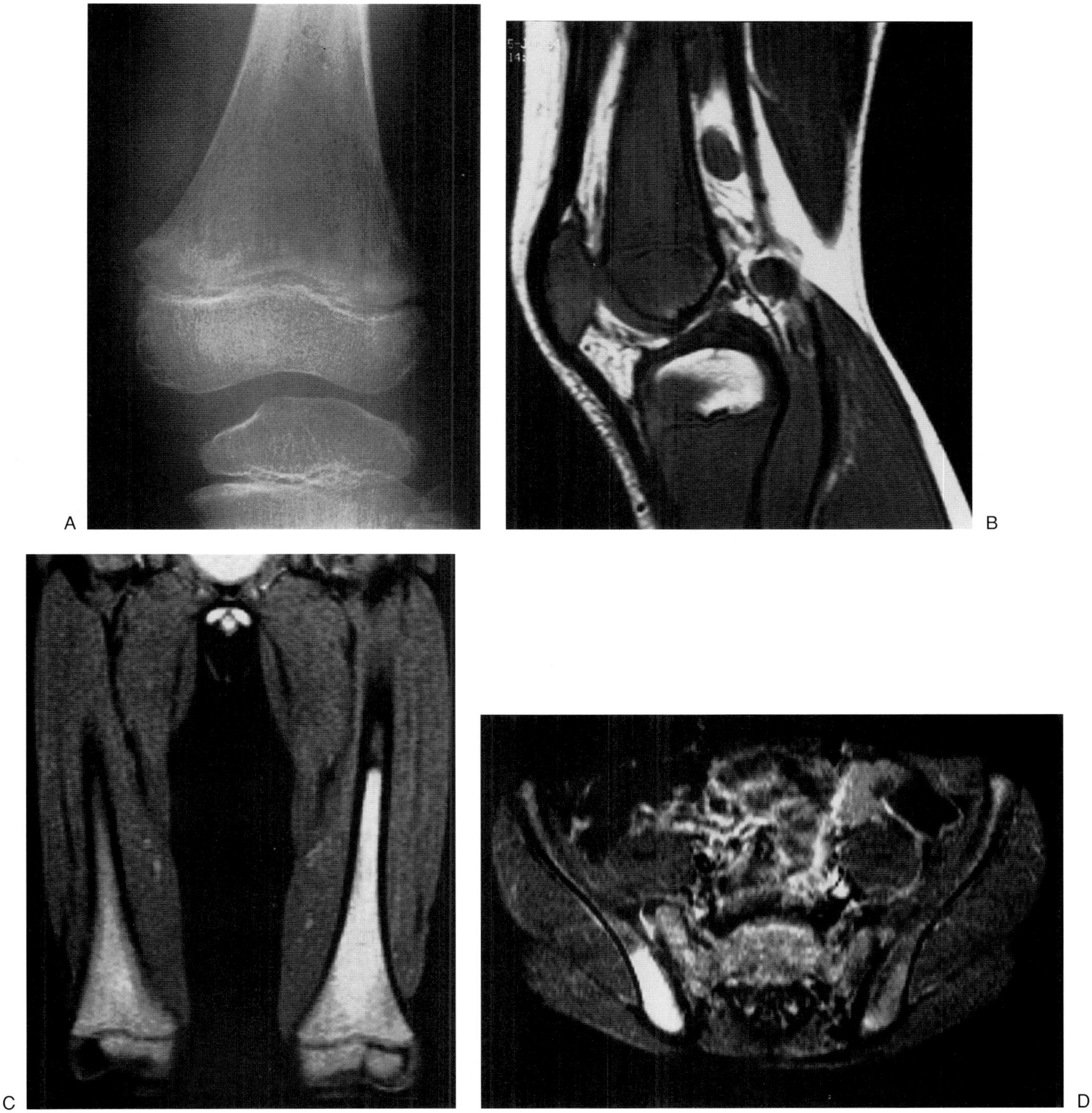

FIG. 10-25. Multifocal acute lymphatic leukemia presenting with knee pain in a 5-year-old boy. **A:** Radiograph of left knee showing typical features of leukemia with metaphyseal rarefaction, including linear juxtaphyseal band. MRI obtained after initial bone marrow aspiration was reported negative. **B:** Sagittal T1-weighted image (TR 630, TE 15) with diffuse marrow replacement, particularly within epiphyses of fatty marrow by leukemic cells. Note enlarged lymph nodes posterior to distal femur. **C:** Coronal IR image (TR 1800, TE 20, TI 150) showing more widespread abnormality. **D:** Axial IR image (TR 1980, TE 30, TI 145) showing relative sparing on left posterior iliac crest explaining initial negative marrow aspiration.

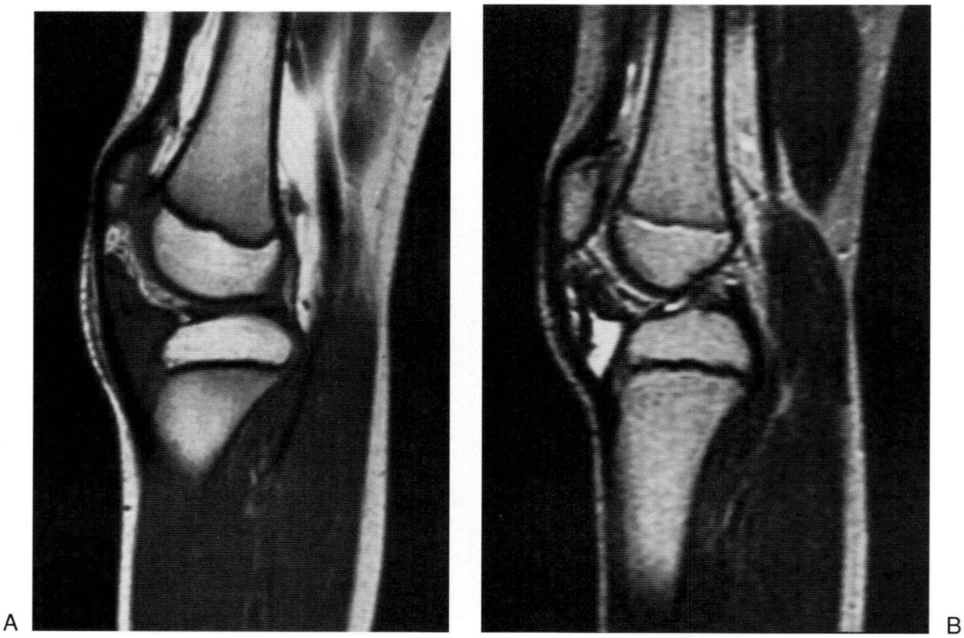

FIG. 10-26. Venous malformation in a 12-year-old boy presenting with intermittent knee pain and swelling. **A:** Sagittal T1-weighted image (TR 600, TE 20) with replacement of infrapatellar fat pad by venous malformation, isointense to muscle. **B:** Slightly more medial T2-weighted image (TR 2500, TE 80) with overall high-signal and low-signal voids present in the lesion.

22). Skip metastases are not infrequently seen, and imaging of the entire bone with MRI or bone scintigraphy is recommended (110). We prefer MRI evaluation as scintigraphy may not reveal small skip lesions. Transarticular spread across the joint should also be assessed and frequently can be seen. The MRI appearance of osteosarcoma is variable, depending upon the histologic constituents of the tumor and extent of hemorrhage and necrosis. Regions of osteosclerosis are typically low signal intensity on T1- and T2-weighted SE images, whereas foci of hemorrhage can show high signal on both T1- and T2-weighted images. With MRI, one can recognize cortical transgression with replacement of the normal low-signal-intensity cortical bone with intermediate signal. Periosteal reaction can also be recognized, especially when simple, layered, or lamellated. Sunburst periosteal reactions are more complex and less readily appreciated on MRI. Care should be taken not to confuse stress fractures or other traumatic injury for osteosarcoma.

Second in frequency to osteosarcoma, Ewing sarcoma is highly malignant and often spreads to bone marrow, bone, and lungs (97,111). Most often diametaphyseal in location rather than the classically thought diaphyseal lesion, it shows a variable aggressive appearance on plain films (111). Extensive lamellated periosteal reaction and a soft-tissue mass are usually present, and reactive bone sclerosis may be noted (111). On MRI, Ewing sarcoma is hyperintense compared with muscle on T2 and of intermediate to low signal on T1-weighted images (111) (Fig. 10-23). Uncommonly, extraosseous soft-tissue Ewing sarcoma can occur (Fig. 10-24).

Accurate monitoring of the effect of chemotherapy may have an impact on neoadjuvant treatment protocols and selection and timing of limb salvage surgery (112). MRI has been used to assess tumor response following chemotherapy. Tumor volume and signal-intensity changes have been evaluated, including both intra- and extramedullary edema and enhancement of residual areas of tumor post-Gd administration (109,112). One must recognize that residual high-signal-intensity regions following therapy for Ewing sarcoma may not reflect viable tumor, as can be seen with complete or incomplete tumor necrosis (112). Increase in tumor volume generally correlates with poor response in both osteosarcoma and Ewing sarcoma, whereas decrease in tumor volume is not necessarily an indicator of good tumor response (109).

Following limb salvage with use of cadaveric allograft placement in the absence of tumor recurrence, the graft may show heterogeneous low signal isointense to muscle on T1 and high signal intensity on T2, possibly related to persistent marrow necrosis within the marrow cavity of the graft (113).

MRI is rarely needed to examine children with leukemia, lymphoma, or metastatic tumor spread (Fig. 10-25). Marrow involvement in the epiphysis or metaphysis, with replacement of normal fatty or hematopoietic marrow can be exquisitely seen with MRI, occasionally suggesting more widespread disease than previously thought from the plain films alone.

Soft-Tissue Masses

MRI can be used to define the extent of childhood soft-tissue masses, but accurate determination of the benign or

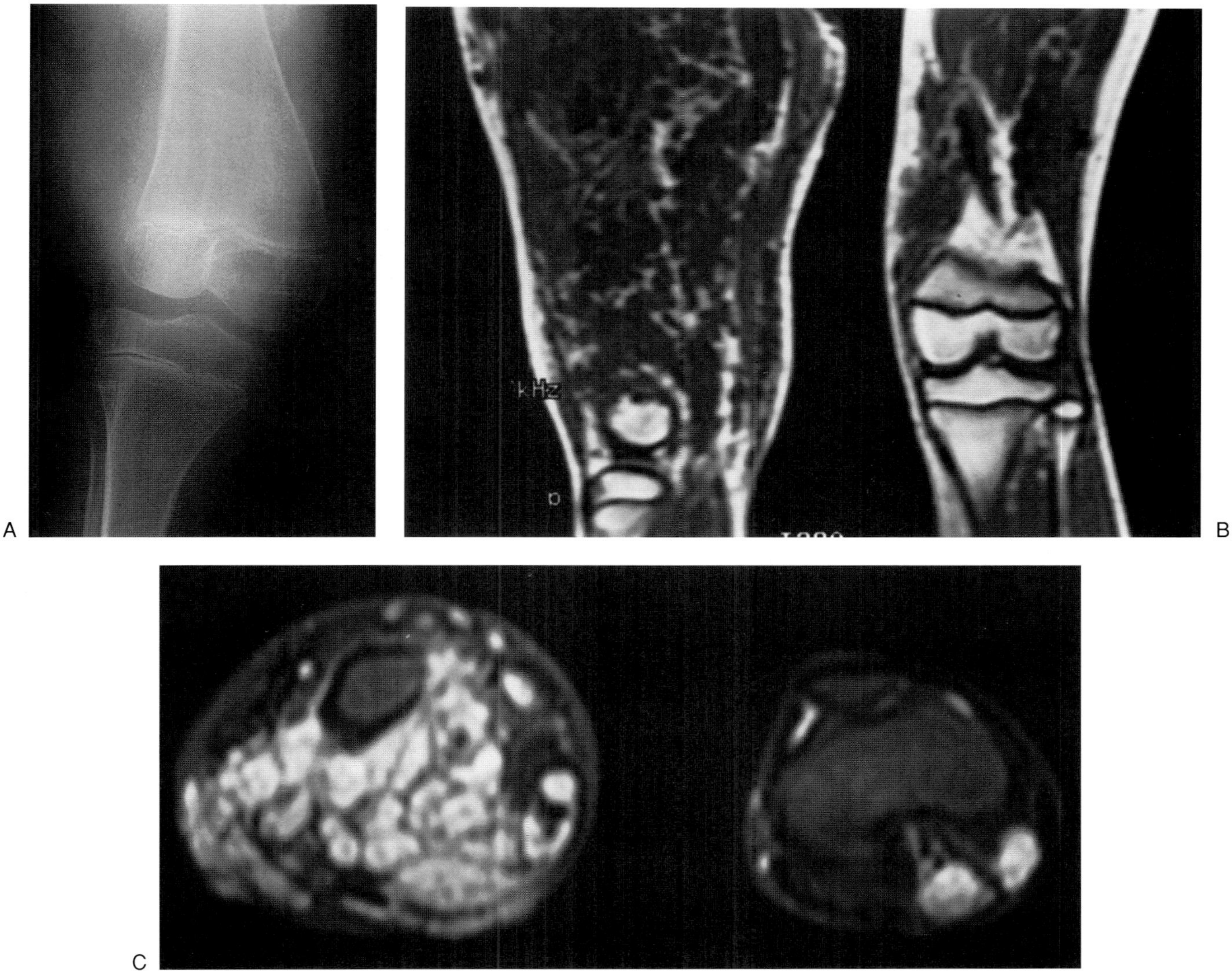

FIG. 10-27. Neurofibromatosis in an 11-year-old boy. **A:** Frontal radiograph with bone and soft-tissue abnormality secondary to neurofibromatosis. **B:** Coronal T1-weighted image (TR 600, TE 20) of thigh showing extensive soft-tissue enlargement with diffuse involvement. **C:** Axial T2-weighted image (TR 2500, TE 80) with overall high signal intermixed with low-signal septations. Note also contralateral limb involvement.

malignant nature of the majority of soft-tissue masses and their specific underlying histology is not always possible (114,115). The majority of benign childhood masses do have characteristic MRI features suggesting a specific diagnosis (114–116). These include lipomas, hemangiomas, hematomas, abscesses, and giant cell tumors of the tendon sheath. However, once those benign lesions with typical characteristics are excluded, MRI cannot accurately distinguish malignant from benign conditions, warranting biopsy in many cases (114,115).

Hemangiomas and vascular malformations are the commonest childhood benign soft-tissue masses that may be found anywhere in the body. Synovial "hemangiomas" are rare lesions occurring predominantly in children and young adults that frequently involve the knee. The nomenclature of these vascular lesions can be confusing. The term *hemangioma* should be restricted to vascular tumors that grow by rapid cellular proliferation, as typically seen in neonates. Vascular malformations, which in our experience are the usual lesions encountered, are structural abnormalities due to errors in morphogenesis with normal cell turnover rates. These malformations can mimic monoarticular juvenile rheumatoid arthritis with commonly reported symptoms of intermittent pain and swelling. Recurrent hemarthrosis, limited range of motion, and a soft, doughy mass are also often described. Plain-film findings of vascular malformations about the knee include phleboliths, soft-tissue swelling, osteopenia, epiphyseal overgrowth, and erosions. On T1-

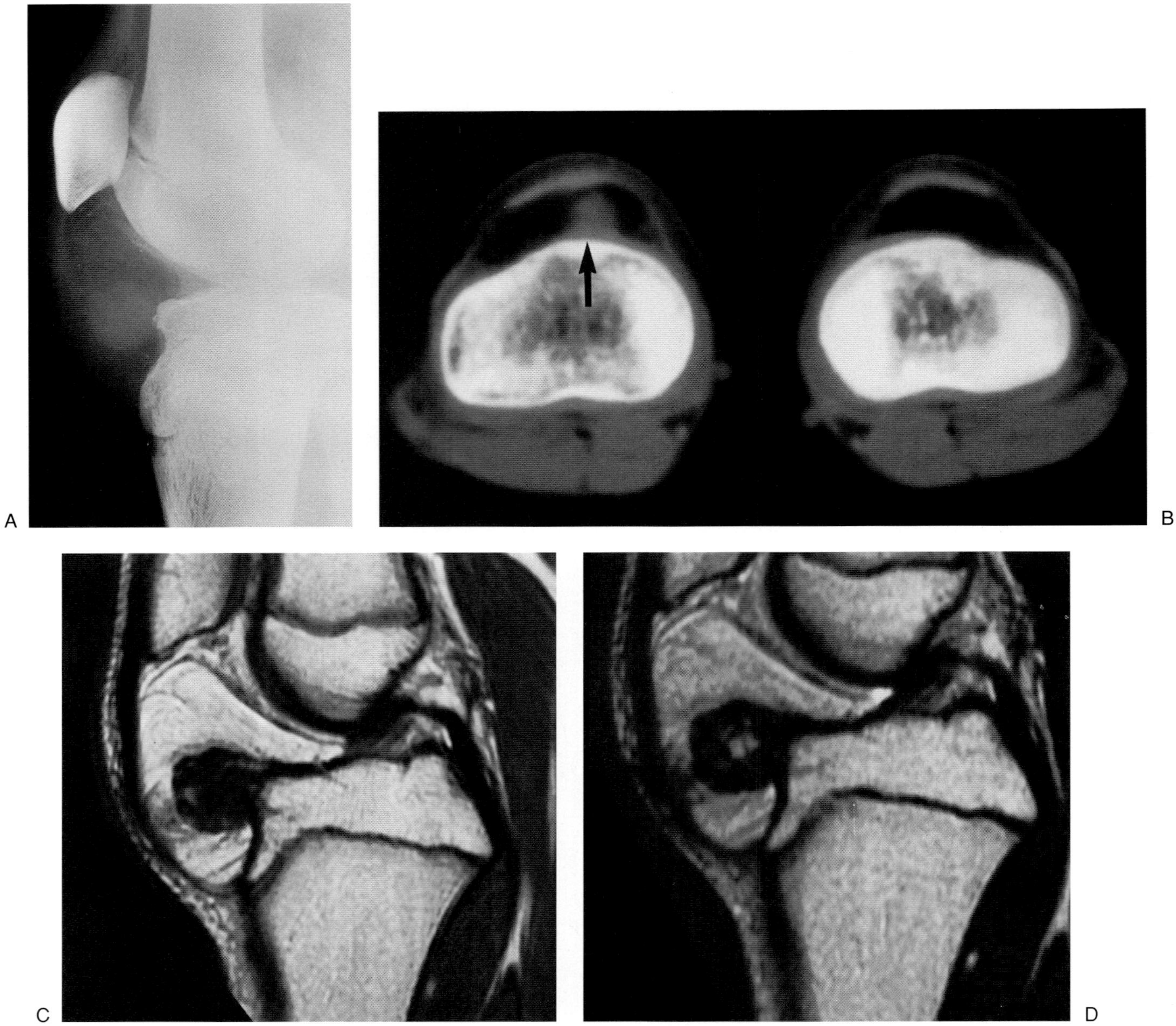

FIG. 10-28. Chondroma contained within infrapatellar fat pad in an 8-year-old girl. **A:** Radiograph showing soft-tissue rounded mass anterior to tibial plateau. **B:** Soft-tissue broad-based lesion on axial CT (*arrow*). **C:** Heterogeneous predominantly low-signal intensity on sagittal T1-weighted image (TR 550, TE 12). **D:** Corresponding T2-weighted fast spin-echo image with predominant low signal intensity (TR 2500, TE 102).

weighted SE imaging images, the mass may be lobulated in outline, isointense to muscle, or slightly heterogeneous in signal intensity. T2-weighted imaging best demonstrates the lesion, with overall high signal intensity interspersed with low-signal septations. Increased vascularity, central signal voids from calcifications, and hemosiderin deposits can also be seen. These lesions may involve the lower extremity and knee joint, but one can also see localized lesions limited to just the joint (Fig. 10-26).

Although they show no specific predilection for the knee, fatty lesions are not uncommon in the lower extremity and include not only simple lipomas but also infiltrating lipomas, diffuse lipomatosis, and rarely lipoblastomatosis (116). These lesions demonstrate typical MRI features of fat intermixed with other soft-tissue signal intensity, depending on the specific histopathology. The fibromatoses are a diverse group of soft-tissue lesions that may occur superficially or deeply (117). The MRI appearance is variable, depending

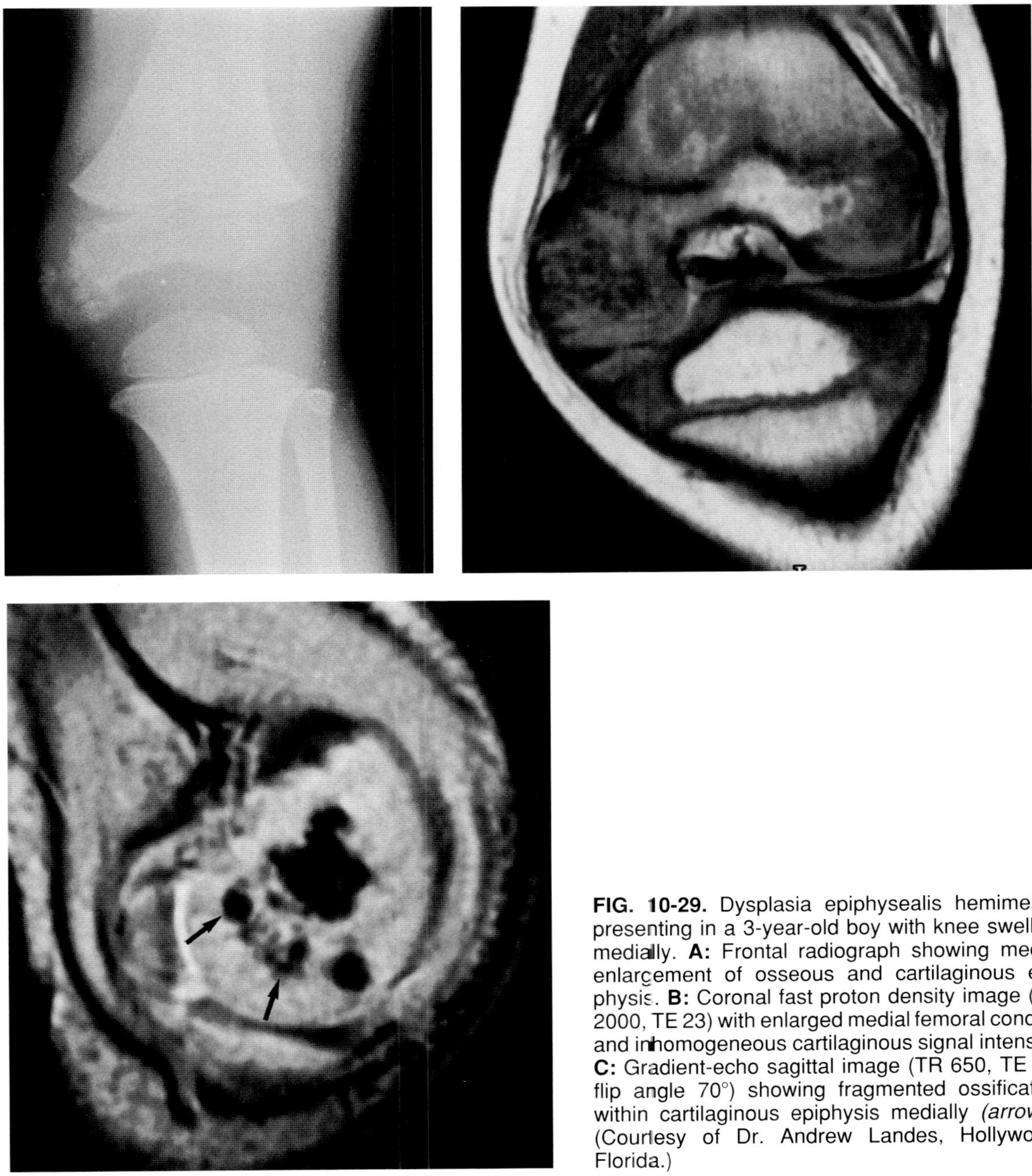

A B C

FIG. 10-29. Dysplasia epiphysealis hemimelica presenting in a 3-year-old boy with knee swelling medially. **A:** Frontal radiograph showing medial enlargement of osseous and cartilaginous epiphysis. **B:** Coronal fast proton density image (TR 2000, TE 23) with enlarged medial femoral condyle and inhomogeneous cartilaginous signal intensity. **C:** Gradient-echo sagittal image (TR 650, TE 11, flip angle 70°) showing fragmented ossification within cartilaginous epiphysis medially *(arrows)*. (Courtesy of Dr. Andrew Landes, Hollywood, Florida.)

on the degree of cellularity and collagen deposits, with most demonstrating decreased signal intensity on T1- and increased signal on T2-weighted imaging. Myxomatous fibrous lesions may have increased signal intensity on T1-weighted SE imaging, whereas hypocellular lesions with extensive collagen can show low signal on T1- and T2-weighted imaging (117). Microscopic tumor extensions are often present, despite margins being well defined on MRI, which mandates wide excisional biopsy (117).

Myositis ossificans of the soft tissues can mimic malignancy, with immature lesions presenting as soft-tissue masses with little in the way of calcification. Rapid growth may be evident without a history of trauma or neurologic compromise. High signal on T2 may be present (96). Diffuse soft tissue and bone abnormality may be seen in neurofibromatosis (Fig. 10-27) alone but rarely with superimposed malignancy.

The commonest soft-tissue malignancy encountered in childhood is rhabdomyosarcoma, often alveolar in type, with approximately one-third arising from the extremities (97). On MRI, the mass is usually large, is isointense to muscle on T1-weighted imaging, and shows increased signal on T2-

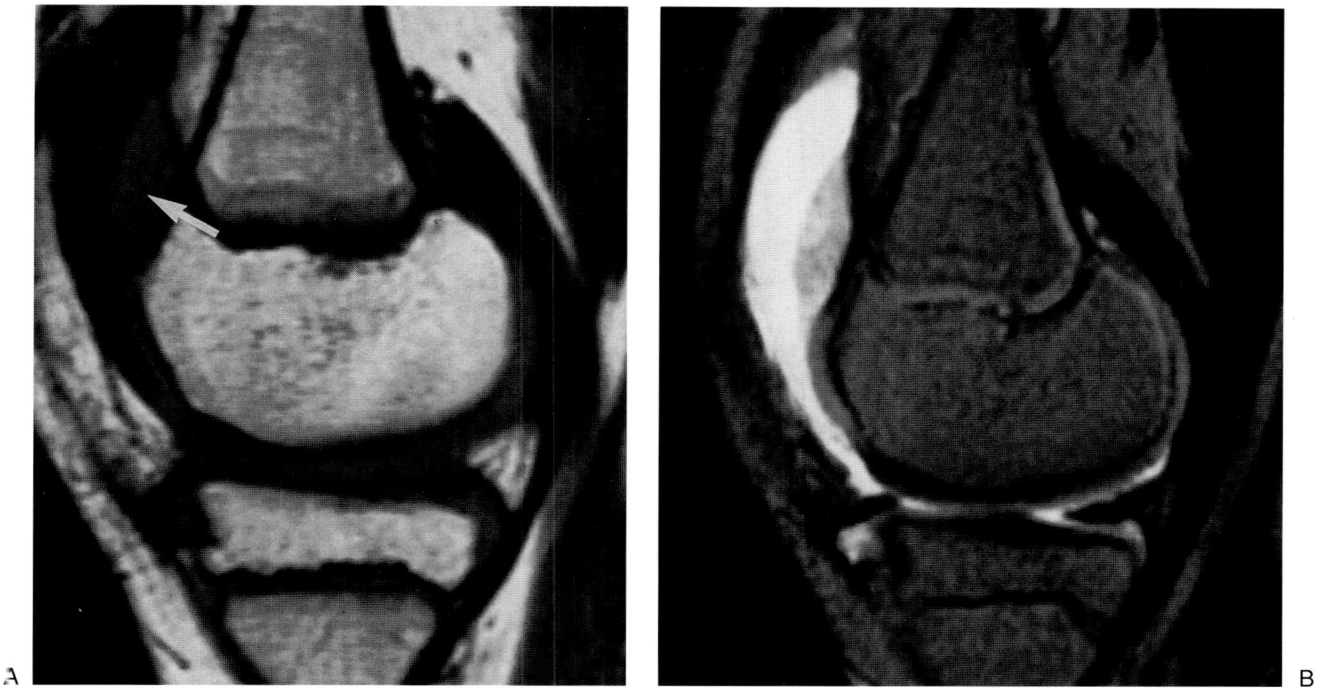

FIG. 10-30. Nodular synovitis in a 9-year-old girl with juvenile rheumatoid arthritis. **A:** Sagittal T1-weighted image (TR 666, TE 20) showing moderate joint effusion and nodular mass isointense to cartilage within suprapatellar bursa *(arrow)*. **B:** Corresponding T2-weighted image (TR 2500, TE 20) with high-signal fluid and intermediate signal from nodular synovitis. Note lack of low signal (as would be expected in PVNS) from absence of hemosiderin.

weighted imaging (97). Rhabdomyosarcomas are often heterogeneous in signal intensity and ill defined, but this is not always the case. Metastasis to regional lymph nodes in the popliteal or inguinal region frequently occurs, and these regions should be examined (96,97).

Second in frequency to rhabdomyosarcomas, synovial sarcomas account for approximately 10% of soft-tissue malignancies in childhood. Most occur in the lower extremity adjacent to the hip or knee joints. On MRI, synovial sarcoma usually shows as a large heterogeneous, multilocular mass with internal septations from hemorrhage occurring within regions of cyst formation or necrosis (118). Synovial sarcomas are most often isointense to muscle on T1-weighted images, but high signal foci can be seen on T1, likely from hemorrhage. On T2 imaging, synovial sarcomas typically show marked heterogeneity with fluid–fluid levels and foci of hyperintense, hypointense, or isointense signal intensity relative to fat. The margin may be poorly defined or infiltrative, but most often it is well defined, often in contiguity with adjacent bone (118). The presence of punctate calcification evident on plain film is a typical feature of synovial sarcoma that may not be appreciated on MRI.

Intra-articular Masses

Intra-articular mass lesions are uncommon but include synovial osteochondromatosis, chondromas, nodular synovitis, pigmented villonodular synovitis (PVNS), and lipoma arborescens (119). Synovial osteochondromatosis represents a chondroid metaplasia of the synovium with formation of cartilaginous masses that may eventually ossify. MRI may show multiple intermediate-signal-intensity masses on T1-weighted SE imaging that correspond to cartilage. The signal intensity can vary, depending on whether ossification and marrow are present within the lesions.

Soft-tissue chondromas are well-defined, solitary cartilage lesions separate from underlying bone that can occur within the knee joint, often in Hoffa's fat pad. They typically show signal characteristics similar to cartilage, with high signal on T2-weighted and intermediate signal intensity on T1-weighted SE imaging (107), but low signal lesions may be seen (Fig. 10-28). Chondromas should be distinguished from dysplasia epiphysealis hemimelica, a developmental overgrowth of epiphyseal cartilage. This may lead to unilateral swelling about the knee, often with a valgus or varus deformity from asymmetric growth of epiphyseal cartilage. Although usually readily recognized on plain films, MRI can clearly demonstrate its size and origin from epiphyseal cartilage (Fig. 10-29).

Pigmented villonodular synovitis (PVNS) is rare in children and exhibits a variable appearance on MRI. On T1 there may be evidence of a large joint effusion, hemosiderin deposition, and a lobulated intermediate-signal-intensity mass that may become high signal on T2. Its associated

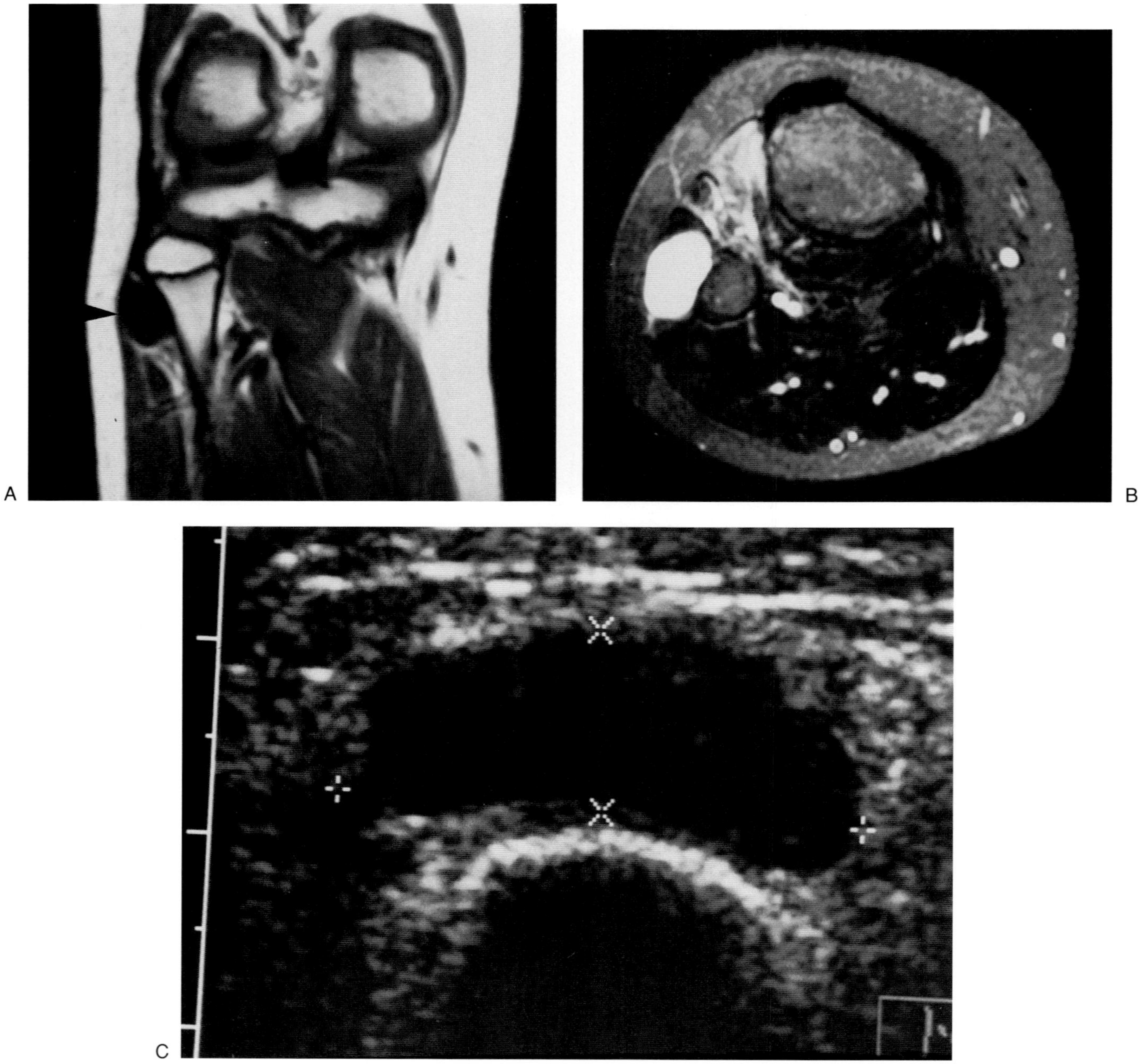

FIG. 10-31. Ganglion cyst with compressive neuropathy lateral to fibula in an 11-year-old boy presenting with knee pain and foot drop. **A:** Coronal T1-weighted image (TR 450, TE 16) with hypointense mass just subjacent to fibular head *(arrow)*. **B:** Axial fast T2-weighted image (TR 4000, TE 90) showing effect of compressive neuropathy within anterior tibialis and ganglion cyst. **C:** Cyst outlined on ultrasound.

hemosiderin can lead to low signal on T2. PVNS should be distinguished from nodular synovitis, which does not show evidence of hemosiderin either on MRI or on pathologic examination (Fig. 10-30).

Lipoma arborescens is a very rare lesion consistent with villous lipomatous proliferation of the synovium with a characteristic MR appearance (119). A frondlike mass, typically located within the suprapatellar bursa, lipoma arborescens has signal intensity similar to fat on all imaging sequences. Joint effusion may be present, but there is absence of magnetic susceptibility effects from hemosiderin (119).

Cystic Lesions

A wide variety of cystic lesions may be seen in the child's knee, similar to those in the adult (120), but overall they

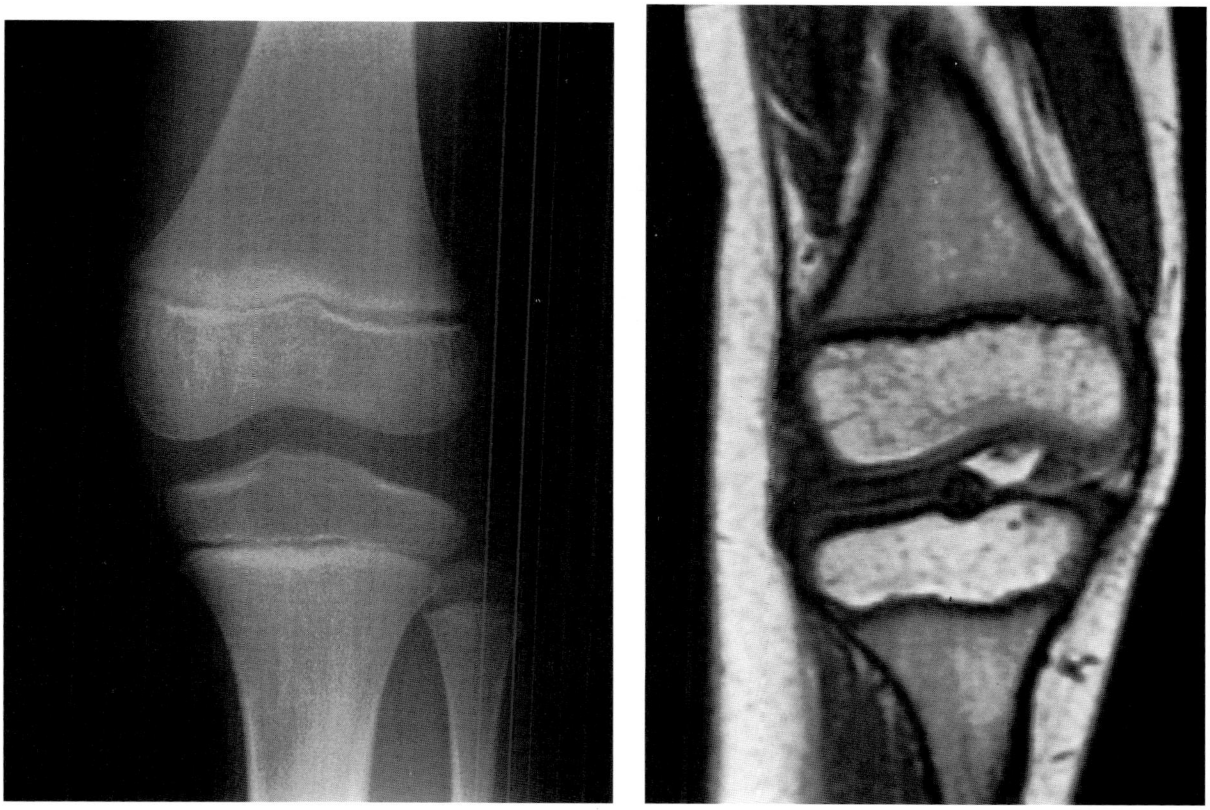

A B

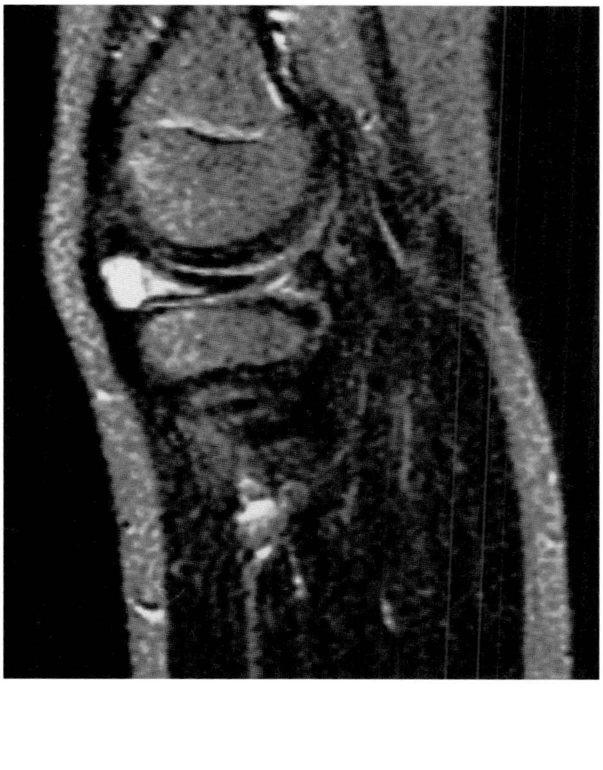

C

FIG. 10-32. Discoid meniscus with meniscal tear and cyst in a 7-year-old girl presenting with right knee pain and swelling. **A:** Frontal radiograph of right knee showing widened joint space laterally. **B:** Coronal T1-weighted (TR 600, TE 20) image with discoid pancake configuration of lateral meniscus. **C:** Sagittal T2-weighted image (TR 2500, TE 80) with high signal intensity of meniscal cyst compatible with fluid anteriorly.

are less common. Synovial cysts, representing herniations of synovium through the joint capsule, are the most common and are frequently bilateral in the popliteal region. These cysts are usually well-defined simple fluid collections on MRI that rarely contain debris. Other synovial cysts are less common but may be encountered in juvenile rheumatoid arthritis or in other patients with chronic knee effusions. We have seen one case of proximal tibiofibular cyst presenting with focal mass and compressive neuropathy of the common peroneal nerve (Fig. 10-31). Inflamed bursae around the knee may also appear as cysts, especially in the infrapatellar bursae. Intra-articular cysts include meniscal cysts likely arising from extruded joint fluid through horizontal tears of the menisci. In childhood these are usually associated with a torn discoid lateral meniscus. On MRI, these are usually small collections of fluid signal that may be simple or multi-loculated (Fig. 10-32). A similar MR appearance may be seen with intra-articular ganglia arising in association with cruciate ligaments or menisco-tibial attachments.

REFERENCES

1. Ruwe PA, Wright J, Randall RL, Lynch JK, Jokl P, McCarthy S. Can MR effectively replace diagnostic arthroscopy? *Radiology* 1992;183:335–339.
2. Whitten CG, Moore TE, Yuh WTC, Kathol MH, Renfrew DL, Walker CW. The use of intravenous gadopentetate dimeglumine in magnetic resonance imaging of synovial lesions. *Skeletal Radiol* 1992;21:215–218.
3. Kleinman PK, Spevak MR. Advanced pediatric joint imaging. *Radiol Clin North Am* 1990;28:1073–1109.
4. Strain JD, Campbell JB, Harvey LA, et al. IV Nembutal: safe sedation for children undergoing CT. *AJR* 1988;151:975–979.
5. Jaramillo D. Pediatric musculoskeletal MR imaging and CT: infection and trauma in syllabus. In: Seibert J, ed. *Current concepts: a categorical course in pediatric radiology.* RSNA Publications, 1994;125–134.
6. Hayes CW, Conway WF. Normal anatomy and magnetic resonance appearance of the knee. *Top Magn Reson Imaging* 1993;5:207–227.
7. Moore SG, Bisset GS, Siegel MJ, Donaldson JS. Pediatric musculoskeletal MR imaging. *Radiology* 1991;179:345–360.
8. Resnick D, Greenway G. Distal femoral cortical defects, irregularities, and excavations. *Radiology* 1982;143:345–354.
9. Yamazaki T, Maruoka S, Takahashi S, Saito H, Takase K, Nakamura M, Sakamoto K. MR findings of avulsive cortical irregularity of the distal femur. *Skeletal Radiol* 1995;24:43–46.
10. Thomas NP, Jackson AM, Aichroth PM. Congenital absence of the anterior cruciate ligament: a common component of knee dysplasia. *J Bone Joint Surg* 1985;67B:572–575.
11. Tolo VT. Congenital absence of the menisci and cruciate ligaments of the knee. *J Bone Joint Surg* 1981;63A:1022–1024.
12. Marks PH, Goldberg JA, Vezina WC, et al. Subchondral bone infractions in acute ligamentous knee injuries demonstrated on bone scintigraphy and magnetic resonance imaging. *J Nucl Med* 1992;33:516–520.
13. Kaplan PA, Dussault RG. Magnetic resonance imaging of the knee: menisci, ligaments, tendons. *Top Magn Reson Imaging* 1993;5:228–248.
14. Kaplan PA, Walker CW, Kilcoyne RF, Brown DE, Tusek D, Dussault RG. Occult fracture patterns of the knee associated with anterior cruciate ligament tears: assessment with MR imaging. *Radiology* 1992;183:835–838.
15. Lynch TCP, Crues JV III, Morgan FW, Sheehan WE, Harter LP, Ryu R. Bone abnormalities of the knee: prevalence and significance at MR imaging. *Radiology* 1989;171:761–766.
16. Mink JH, Deutsch AL. Occult cartilage and bone injuries of the knee: detection, classification, and assessment with MR imaging. *Radiology* 1989;170:823–829.
17. Munk PL, Vellet AD. Lesions of cartilage and bone around the knee. *Top Magn Reson Imaging* 1993;5:249–262.
18. Newberg AH, Wetzner SM. Bone bruises: their patterns and significance. *Semin Ultrasound CT MR* 1994;15:396–409.
19. Vellet D. Magnetic resonance imaging of bone marrow and osteochondral injury. *MRI Clin North Am* 1994;2:413–423.
20. Rosenberg ZS, Kawelblum M, Cheung YY, Beltran J, Lehman WB, Grant AD. Osgood-Schlatter lesion: fracture or tendinitis? Scintigraphic, CT and MR imaging features. *Radiology* 1992;185:853–858.
21. De Flaviis L, Nessi R, Scaglione P, Balconi G, Albisetti W, Derchi LE. Ultrasonic diagnosis of Osgood-Schlatter and Sinding-Larsen-Johansson diseases of the knee. *Skeletal Radiol* 1989;18:193–197.
22. Garrick JG. Anterior knee pain (chondromalacia patellae). *Phys Sports Med* 1989;17:75–84.
23. Conway WF, Hayes CW, Loughran T, et al. Cross-sectional imaging of the patello-femoral joint and surrounding structures. *Radiographics* 1991;11:195–217.
24. Disler DG, Peters TL, Muscoreil SJ, Ratner LM, Wagle WA, Cousins JP, Rifkin MD. Fat-suppressed spoiled GRASS imaging of knee hyaline cartilage: technique optimization and comparison with conventional MR imaging. *AJR* 1994;163:887–892.
25. Hodler J, Resnick D. Chondromalacia patellae. *AJR* 1992;158:106–107.
26. McCauley TR, Kier R, Lynch KJ, Jokl P. Chondromalacia patellae: diagnosis with MR imaging. *AJR* 1992;158:101–106.
27. Recht MP, Resnick D. MR imaging of articular cartilage: current status and future directions. *AJR* 1994;163:283–290.
28. Quinn SF, Rose PM, Brown TR, Demlow TA. MR imaging of the patellofemoral compartment. *MRI Clin North Am* 1994;2:425–440.
29. Tyrrell PNM, Davies AM. Magnetic resonance imaging appearances of fatigue fractures of the long bones of the lower limb. *Br J Radiol* 1994;67:332–338.
30. Saifuddin A, Chalmers AG, Butt WP. Longitudinal stress fractures of the tibia: MRI features in two cases. *Clin Radiol* 1994;49:490–495.
31. Stafford SA, Rosenthal DI, Gebhardt MC, Brady TJ, Scott JA. MRI in stress fracture. *AJR* 1986;147:553–556.
32. Bassett LW, Grover JS, Seeger LI. Magnetic resonance imaging of knee trauma. *Skeletal Radiol* 1990;19:401–405.
33. Jaramillo D, Shapiro F, Hoffer FA, et al. Post-traumatic growth plate abnormalities: MR imaging of bony-bridge formation in rabbits. *Radiology* 1990;175:767–773.
34. White PG, Mah JY, Friedman L. Magnetic resonance imaging in acute physeal injuries. *Skeletal Radiol* 1994;23:627–631.
35. Rogers LF, Poznanski AK. Imaging of epiphyseal injuries. *Radiology* 1994;191:297–308.
36. Staron RB, Haramati N, Feldman F, et al. O'Donoghue's triad: magnetic resonance imaging evidence. *Skeletal Radiol* 1994;23:633–636.
37. Munakata T, Nishida J, Shimamura T, Ichinohe S, Abe M, Ehara S. Simultaneous avulsion of patellar apexes bilaterally in a hemodialysis patient. *Skeletal Radiol* 1995;24:211–213.
38. Tehranzadeh J, Kerr R, Amster J. MRI of trauma and sports-related injuries of tendons and ligaments. Part II: pelvis and lower extremities. *Crit Rev Diagn Imaging* 1994;35:131–200.
39. Brandser EA, El-Khoury GY, Saltzman CL. Tendon injuries: application of magnetic resonance imaging. *Can Assoc Radiol J* 1995;46:9–18.
40. Reiff DB, Heenan SD, Heron CW. MRI appearances of the asymptomatic patellar tendon on gradient echo imaging. *Skeletal Radiol* 1995;24:123–126.
41. El Khoury GY, Wira RL, Berbaum KS, Pope TL, Monu JUV. MR imaging of patellar tendinitis. *Radiology* 1992;184:849–854.
42. Berlin RC, Levinsohn EM, Chrisman H. The wrinkled patellar tendon: an indication of abnormality in the extensor mechanism of the knee. *Skeletal Radiol* 1991;20:181–185.
43. Lee JH, Weissman BN, Nikpoor N, Aliabadi P, Sosman JL. Lipohemarthrosis of the knee: a review of recent experiences. *Radiology* 1989;173:189–191.
44. White EM. Magnetic resonance imaging in synovial disorders and arthropathy of the knee. *MRI Clin North Am* 1994;2:451–461.
45. Azouz EM, Levesque R-Y. Radiologic findings in children with seronegative spondyloarthropathies. *Can Fam Physician* 1992;38:1857–1867.
46. Petty RE, Malleson P. Spondyloarthropathies of childhood. *Pediatr Clin North Am* 1986;33:1079–1096.

47. Schaller JG. Arthritis in children. *Pediatr Clin North Am* 1986;33:1565–1580.
48. Singson RD, Zalduondo FM. Value of unenhanced spin-echo MR imaging in distinguishing between synovitis and effusion of the knee. *AJR* 1992;159:569–571.
49. Cardinal E, Dussault RG, Kaplan PA. Imaging and differential diagnosis of masses within a joint. *Can Assoc Radiol J* 1994;45:363–372.
50. Reiser MF, Bongartz GP, Erlemann R, et al. Gadolinium-DTPA in rheumatoid arthritis and related diseases: first results with dynamic magnetic resonance imaging. *Skeletal Radiol* 1989;18:591–597.
51. Herve-Somma CMP, Sebag GH, Prieur A-M, Bonnerot V, Lallemand DP. Juvenile rheumatoid arthritis of the knee: MR evaluation with Gd-DOTA. *Radiology* 1992;182:93–98.
52. Munk PL, Vellet AD, Romano C, Levin MF, Harth MF, Bell DA. The emerging role of magnetic resonance imaging in rheumatology. *Can Assoc Radiol J* 1994;45:270–276.
53. Yamato M, Tamai K, Yamaguchi T, Ohno W. MRI of the knee in rheumatoid arthritis: Gd-DTPA perfusion dynamics. *J Comput Assist Tomogr* 1993;17:781–785.
54. Weissman BN, Hussain S. Magnetic resonance imaging of the knee. *Rheum Dis Clin North Am* 1991;17:637–668.
55. Eich GF, Halle F, Hodler J, Seger R, Willi UV. Juvenile chronic arthritis: imaging of the knees and hips before and after intraarticular steroid injection. *Pediatr Radiol* 1991;24:558–563.
56. Yulish BS, Lieberman JM, Newman AJ, Bryan PJ, Mulopulos GP, Modic MT. Juvenile rheumatoid arthritis: assessment with MR imaging. *Radiology* 1987;165:149–152.
57. Peterfy CG, Majumdar S, Lang P, van Dijke CF, Sack K, Genant HK. MR imaging of the arthritic knee: improved discrimination of cartilage, synovium, and effusion with pulsed saturation transfer and fat-suppressed T1-weighted sequences. *Radiology* 1994;191:413–419.
58. Poleksic L, Zdravkovic D, Jablanovic D, Watt I, Bacic G. Magnetic resonance imaging of bone destruction in rheumatoid arthritis: comparison with radiography. *Skeletal Radiol* 1993;22:577–580.
59. Hermann G, Gilbert MS, Abdelwahab IF. Hemophilia: evaluation of musculoskeletal involvement with CT, sonography, and MR imaging. *AJR* 1992;158:119–123.
60. Nuss R, Kilcoyne RF, Geraghty S, Wiedel J, Manco-Johnson M. Utility of magnetic resonance imaging for management of hemophilic arthropathy in children. *J Pediatr* 1993;123:388–392.
61. Wilson DA, Prince JR. MR imaging of hemophilic pseudotumors. *AJR* 1988;150:349–350.
62. Morissy RT, Shore SL. Bone and joint sepsis. *Pediatr Clin North Am* 1986;33:1551–1564.
63. Azouz EM, Greenspan A, Marton D. CT evaluation of primary epiphyseal bone abscesses. *Skeletal Radiol* 1993;22:17–23.
64. Azouz EM, Chhem RK, Lambert R, Oudjhane K. Imaging for bone and joint infection in children and adults. *Curr Orthop* 1994;8:226–236.
65. Tehranzadeh J, Wang F, Mesgarzadeh M. Magnetic resonance imaging of osteomyelitis. *Crit Rev Diagn Imaging* 1992;33:495–534.
66. Munk PL, Vellet AD, Hilborn MD, Crues JV, Helms CA, Poon PY. Musculoskeletal infection: findings on magnetic resonance imaging. *Can Assoc Radiol J* 1994;45:355–362.
67. Dangman BC, Hoffer FA, Rand FF, O'Rourke EJ. Osteomyelitis in children: gadolinium-enhanced MR imaging. *Radiology* 1992;182:743–747.
68. Murphey MD, Gross TM, Rosenthal HG, Neff JR. Magnetic resonance imaging of soft tissue and cystic masses about the knee. *Top Magn Reson Imaging* 1993:5:263–282.
69. Tang JSH, Gold RH, Bassett LW, Seeger LL. Musculoskeletal infection of the extremities: evaluation with MR imaging. *Radiology* 1988;166:205–209.
70. Beltran J, Shankman S. Magnetic resonance imaging of bone marrow disorders of the knee. *MRI Clin North Am* 1994;2:463–473.
71. Tuite MJ, De Smet AA. MRI of selected sport injuries: muscle tears, groin pain, and osteochondritis dissecans. *Semin Ultrasound CT MR* 1994;15:318–340.
72. Milgram JW. Osteochondral fractures and loose bodies. In: *Radiologic and histologic pathology of nontumorous diseases of bones and joints.* IL: Northbook Publishing, 1990.
73. Shahabpour M, Osteaux M, Casteleyn P-P. The knee joint. In: Osteaux M, De Meirleir K, Shahabpour M, eds. *MRI and spectroscopy in sports medicine.* Berlin: Springer-Verlag, 1991.
74. Paille P, Quesnel C, Baunin C, et al. Computed arthrography: its role in the screening of joint diseases in pediatric radiology. *Pediatr Radiol* 1988;18:386–390.
75. Mesgarzadeh M, Sapega AA, Bonakdarpour A, Moyer RA, Maurer AH, Alburger PD. Osteochondritis dissecans: analysis of mechanical stability with radiography, scintigraphy, and MR imaging. *Radiology* 1987;165:775–780.
76. DeSmet AA. If a region of osteochondritis dissecans is identified on a radiographic examination of the knee, should an MR study be performed? *AJR* 1994;162:1495–1496.
77. DeSmet AA, Fisher DR, Graf BK, Langer RH. Osteochondritis dissecans of the knee: value of MR imaging in determining lesion stability and the presence of articular cartilage defects. *AJR* 1990;155:549–553.
78. Bureau NJ, Kaplan PA, Dussault RG. MRI of the knee: a simplified approach. *Curr Probl Diagn Radiol* 1995;24:1–49.
79. Kramer J, Stiglbauer R, Engel A, Prayer L, Imhof H. MR contrast arthrography (MRA) in osteochondritis dissecans. *J Comput Assist Tomogr* 1992;16:254–260.
80. Smith DS, Sharp DC, Resendes M. MRI of osteochondritis dissecans fragment with absorbable pins. *J Comput Assist Tomogr* 1994;18:832–833.
81. Weiner ES, Abeles M. Aseptic necrosis and glucocorticoids in systemic lupus erythematosus: a reevaluation. *J Rheumatol* 1989;16:604–608.
82. Haller J, Greenway G, Resnick KP, Kang HC. Intraosseous fat necrosis associated with acute pancreatitis. *Radiology* 1989;173:193–195.
83. Lanir A, Hadar H, Cohen I, Tal Y, Benmair J, Schreiber R, Clouse ME. Gaucher disease: assessment with MR imaging. *Radiology* 1986;161:239–244.
84. Rao VM, Fishman M, Mitchell DG, et al. Painful sickle cell crisis: bone marrow patterns observed with MR imaging. *Radiology* 1986;161:211–215.
85. Sanchez RB, Quinn SF, Walling A, Estrada J, Greenberg H. Musculoskeletal neoplasms after intraarterial chemotherapy: correlation of MR images with pathologic specimens. *Radiology* 1990;174:237–240.
86. Chang CC, Greenspan A, Gershwin ME. Osteonecrosis: current perspectives on pathogenesis and treatment. *Semin Arthritis Rheum* 1993;23:47–69.
87. Munk FL, Helms CA, Holt RG. Immature bone infarcts: findings on plain radiographs and MR scans. *AJR* 1989;152:547–549.
88. Rajah R, Young J, Conway WF. Acute hemorrhagic infarct with edema. *Skeletal Radiol* 1995;24:158–159.
89. Bonnerot V, Sebag G, de Montalembert M, et al. Gadolinium-DOTA enhanced MRI of painful osseous crises in children with sickle cell anemia. *Pediatr Radiol* 1994;24:92–95.
90. Vande Berg BZ, Malghem JJ, Labaisse MA, Michaux JL, Maldague BE. Apparent focal bone marrow ischemia in patients with marrow disorders: MR studies. *J Comput Assist Tomogr* 1993;17:792–795.
91. Vande Berg BZ, Malghem JJ, Labaisse MA, Noel HM, Maldague BE. Avascular necrosis of the hip: comparison of contrast-enhanced and non-enhanced MR imaging with histologic correlation. *Radiology* 1992;182:445–450.
92. Smith CF. Tibia vara (Blount's disease). *J Bone Joint Surg* 1982;64-A:630–632.
93. Langenskiold A. Tibia vara (osteochondrosis deformans tibiae): a survey of 23 cases. *Acta Chir Scand* 1952;103:1–22.
94. Reynolds RAK, Wedge JH, Babyn PS. Focal fibrocartilagenous dysplasia of the tibia: four cases of an unusual cause of tibia vara. *Iowa Orthop J* 1991;11:157–160.
95. Ducou le Pointe H, Mousselard H, Rudelli A, Montagne J-P, Filipe G. Blount's disease: magnetic resonance imaging. *Pediatr Radiol* 1995;25:12–14.
96. Richardson ML, Gillespy T III. Magnetic resonance imaging. in: Kricun ME, ed. *Imaging of bone tumors.* Philadelphia: WB Saunders, 1993;358–446.
97. Fletcher BD. Musculoskeletal tumor imaging in syllabus: current concepts. In: Seibert J, ed. *A categorical course in pediatric radiology.* RSNA Publications, 1994;245–252.
98. Baunin C, Puget C, Assoun J, et al. Percutaneous resection of osteoid osteoma under CT guidance in eight children. *Pediatr Radiol* 1994;24:185–188.

99. Burr BA, Resnick D, Syklawer R, Haghighi P. Fluid–fluid levels in a unicameral bone cyst: CT and MR findings. *J Comput Assist Tomogr* 1993;17:134–136.
100. Munk PL, Helms CA, Holt RG, Johnston J, Steinbach L, Neumann C. MR imaging of aneurysmal bone cysts. *AJR* 1989;153:99–101.
101. Tsai JC, Dalinka MK, Fallon MD, Zlatkin MB, Kressel HY. Fluid–fluid level: a nonspecific finding in tumors of bone and soft tissue. *Radiology* 1990;175:779–782.
102. George JC, Buckwalter KA, Cohen MD, Edwards MK, RR Smith. Langerhans cell histiocytosis of bone: MR imaging. *Pediatr Radiol* 1994;24:29–32.
103. Beltran J, Aparisi F, Bonmati LM, Rosenberg ZS, Present D, Steiner GC. Eosinophilic granuloma: MRI manifestations. *Skeletal Radiol* 1993;22:157–161.
104. Monroc M, Ducou le Pointe H, Haddad S, Josset P, Montagne J-P. Soft tissue signal abnormality associated with eosinophilic granuloma. Correlation of MR imaging with pathologic findings. *Pediatr Radiol* 1994;24:328–332.
105. De Boeck H, Aerts P, Casteleyn PP. Chondroblastoma of the upper end of the tibia, invading the attachment of the posterior cruciate ligament. *Acta Orthop Belg* 1989;55:129–134.
106. Fobben ES, Dalinka MK, Schiebler ML, et al. The magnetic resonance imaging appearance at 1.5 Tesla of cartilaginous tumors involving the epiphysis. *Skeletal Radiol* 1987;16:647–651.
107. Kransdorf MJ, Meis JM. Extraskeletal osseous and cartilaginous tumors of the extremities. *Radiographics* 1993;13:853–884.
108. Norton KI, Hermann G, Abdelwahab IF, Klein MJ, Granowetter LF, Rabinowitz JG. Epiphyseal involvement in osteosarcoma. *Radiology* 1991;180:813–816.
109. Lawrence JA, Babyn PS, Chan HSL, Thorner PS, Pron GE, Krajbich IJ. Extremity osteosarcoma in childhood: prognostic value of radiologic imaging. *Radiology* 1993;189:43–47.
110. Hopper KD, Moser RP Jr, Haseman DB, Sweet DE, Madewell JE, Kransdorf MJ. Osteosarcomatosis. *Radiology* 1990;175:233–239.
111. Eggli KD, Quiogue T, Moser RP Jr. Ewing's sarcoma. *Radiol Clin North Am* 1993;31:325–338.
112. van der Woude JH, Bloem JL, et al. Monitoring the effect of chemotherapy in Ewing's sarcoma of bone with MR imaging. *Skeletal Radiol* 1994;23:493–500.
113. Levin TL, Miller TT, Panicek DM, et al. MR signal characteristics of cadaveric bone allografts in three children with primary bone tumors treated with limb salvage therapy. *Pediatr Radiol* 1994;24:488–490.
114. Moulton JS, Blebea JS, Dunco DM, Braley SE, Bisset GS III, Emery KH. MR imaging of soft-tissue masses: diagnostic efficiency and value of distinguishing between benign and malignant lesions. *AJR* 1995;164:1191–1199.
115. Kransdorf MJ, Jelinek JS, Moser RP Jr. Imaging of soft tissue tumors. *Radiol Clin North Am* 1993;31:359–372.
116. Ha TV, Kleinman PK, Fraire A, et al. MR imaging of benign fatty tumors in children: report of four cases and review of the literature. *Skeletal Radiol* 1994;23:361–368.
117. Quinn SF, Erickson SJ, Dee PM, et al. MR imaging in fibromatosis: results in 26 patients with pathologic correlation. *AJR* 1991;156:539–542.
118. Jones BC, Sundaram M, Kransdorf MJ. Synovial sarcoma: MR imaging findings in 34 patients. *AJR* 1993;161:827–830.
119. Donnelly LF, Bisset GS III, Passo MH. MRI findings of lipoma arborescens of the knee in a child: case report. *Pediatr Radiol* 1994;24:258–259.
120. Janzen DL, Peterfy CG, Forbes JR, Tirman PFJ, Genant HK. Cystic lesions around the knee joint: MR imaging findings. *AJR* 1994;163:155–161.

MRI of the Knee, Second Edition,
edited by P. L. Munk and C. A. Helms.
Lippincott-Raven Publishers, Philadelphia © 1996.

CHAPTER 11

Postoperative Knee

Peter L. Munk, Dennis L. Janzen, Douglas G. Connell, and A. Dale Vellet

Until recently, most experience in magnetic resonance imaging (MRI) of the knee has been with the virgin knee—a knee that has not been previously operated on. Increasingly, with greater availability and widespread use of MRI, radiologists are being called upon to examine knees that have undergone a wide variety of procedures, ranging from diagnostic or therapeutic arthroscopies to complex ligament reconstructions and other surgical procedures. For this reason it is incumbent on the radiologist to be familiar with the appearance of the postoperative knee and the significance of the MRI findings in such patients.

The mere presence of metal in or near the knee joint does not necessarily preclude a diagnostically useful MRI, depending on the type of information being sought. This point is not well appreciated by many referring clinicians, or even by some radiologists. Should the area of interest be too near the metal—about one to one-and-a-half times the diameter of the metal implant—signal void will prevent adequate visualization. If the metal is ferrometallic, spectacular artifacts are produced, rendering the examination futile. Fortunately, most metal encountered will not be ferromagnetic (Fig. 11-1).

MRI of the postoperative knee may be an extremely difficult and challenging examination (1). Familiarity with the type of surgical procedure performed is extremely helpful. Previous MRI, CT, or arthrographic examinations as well as arthroscopic or surgical reports can be invaluable (1–4). At present, this is still an area of knee imaging that is in its early stages of development and is constantly undergoing refinement with greater experience.

P L. Munk: Department of Diagnostic Imaging, University of British Columbia, British Columbia Cancer Agency, Vancouver, British Columbia, Canada V5Z 4E6.

D. L. Janzen and D. G. Connell: Department of Radiology, Vancouver Hospital and Health Sciences Center, Vancouver, British Columbia, Canada V5Z 1M9.

A. D. Vellet: Department of Diagnostic Imaging, University of Calgary, Foothills Hospital, Alberta, Canada T2N 2T9.

ARTHROSCOPY

Arthroscopy is probably the single most common operative procedure performed by the orthopedic knee surgeon. As a diagnostic procedure it is certainly much more sensitive than clinical examination, especially in the evaluation of meniscal lesions, but unfortunately, it is invasive and expensive (5,6). With the increasing use of MRI, diagnostic arthroscopy is being used considerably less frequently than previously (7–9). Increasingly, arthroscopy is used selectively to perform therapeutic procedures that may be planned in advance based on imaging. Depending on the procedure performed, the number of arthroscopic ports that are made will vary, and both anterior and posterior ports may be required (10).

Like any other instrumentation elsewhere in the body, previous arthroscopy can often be recognized on MRI by the presence of numerous microscopic or small metallic fragments that are left behind along the instrumentation tract. With conventional spin-echo imaging as well as fast spin-echo imaging these will be seen as tiny areas of signal dropout (3). Gradient-echo imaging often accentuates these findings because of the blooming effect inherent with the magnetic susceptibility effect of these techniques, and arthroscopy tracts are therefore often much more obvious (Fig. 11-2). In addition, fibrotic scarring along the course of the tract may occur and can be followed as areas of relatively linear low signal on all sequences. This is often particularly striking in the area of Hoffa's fat pad, where the low-signal tract will be surrounded by higher-signal fat, particularly on T1-weighted sequences.

With extensive manipulation, particularly if the arthroscopy is difficult and if multiple instruments are utilized in the knee, tiny metallic fragments may also become embedded within the cartilage of the knee joint, particularly in the region of the femoral condyles (Fig. 11-3). We have also seen examples of metal within cartilage in patients who have not undergone arthroscopy but who have received joint injection.

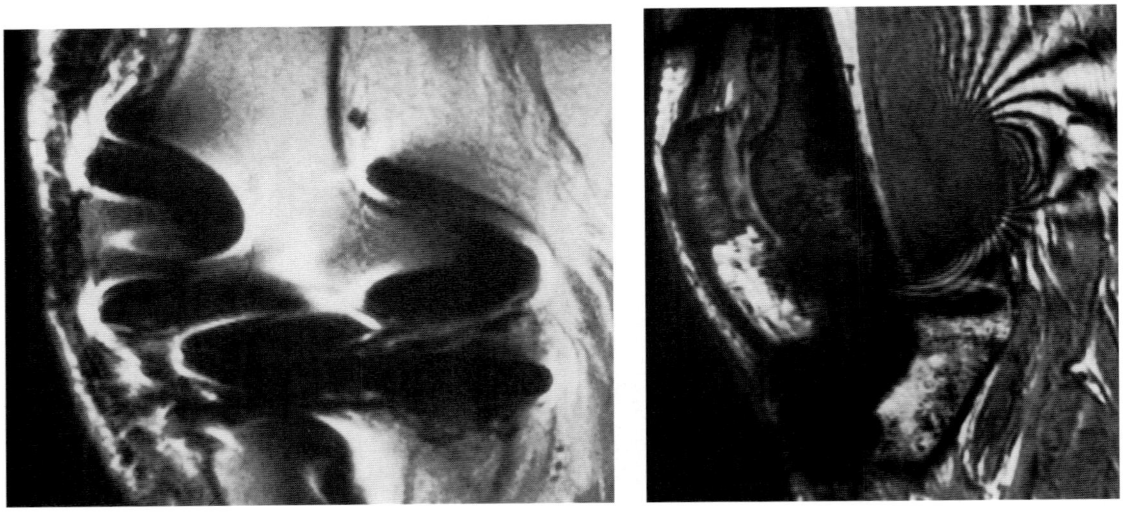

A B

FIG. 11-1. Examples of extensive artifact in patients with large metallic implants after surgery. **A:** Sagittal T1 spin echo (TR 600 msec, TE 20 msec). Large artifact following total knee arthroplasty, cruciate sparing variety. The extensive artifact precludes assessment of the cruciate ligament that had been preserved at the time of surgery. **B:** Sagittal T2* 3DFT gradient echo (TR 55 msec, TE 15 msec, flip angle 30°). Patellar tendon anterior cruciate neoligament with signal void adjacent to tibial bone plug due to interference screw. An additional screw had been placed in the distal femur at the time of revision surgery 2 years later.

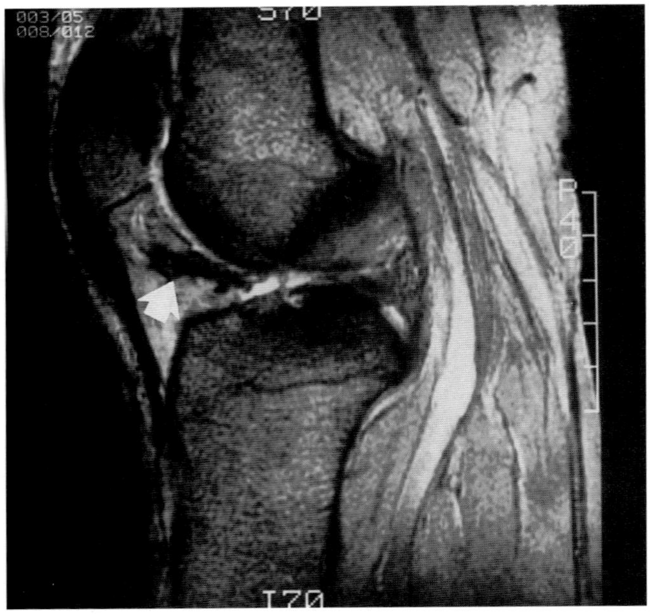

FIG. 11-2. Arthroscopy tract. Sagittal T2* gradient echo MPGR (TR 600 msec, TE 20 msec, flip angle 20°). An irregular linear band of low signal intensity *(arrow)* is present traversing Hoffa's fat pad representing the course of the instrument during the previous arthroscopy. The gradient-echo technique used makes the tract far more obvious than if spin-echo technique had been employed.

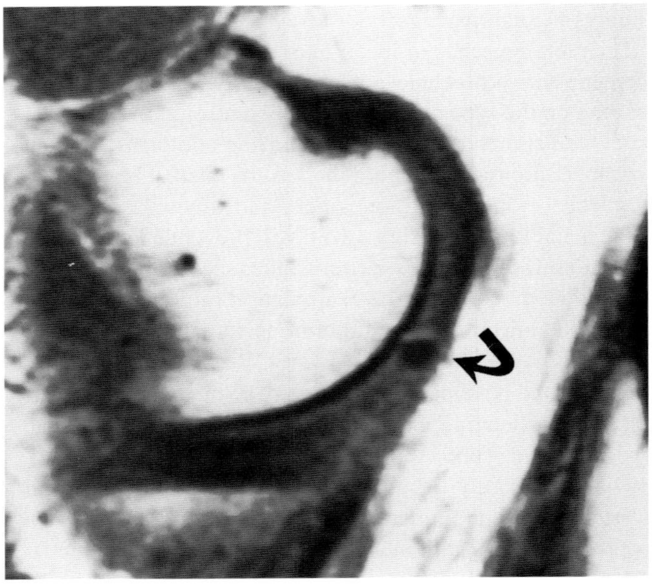

FIG. 11-3. Metal fragment. Sagittal T1 spin echo (TR 500 msec, TE 13 msec). Magnified image of the posterior aspect of the femoral condyle shows a tiny low signal area *(curved area)*. This is a fragment of metal left after a vigorous arthroscopy, not visible on radiographs. MRI is sufficiently sensitive to the presence of metal that plain film and CT often cannot show metal that is obvious on MRI. The presence of such tiny fragments is not usually of clinical significance.

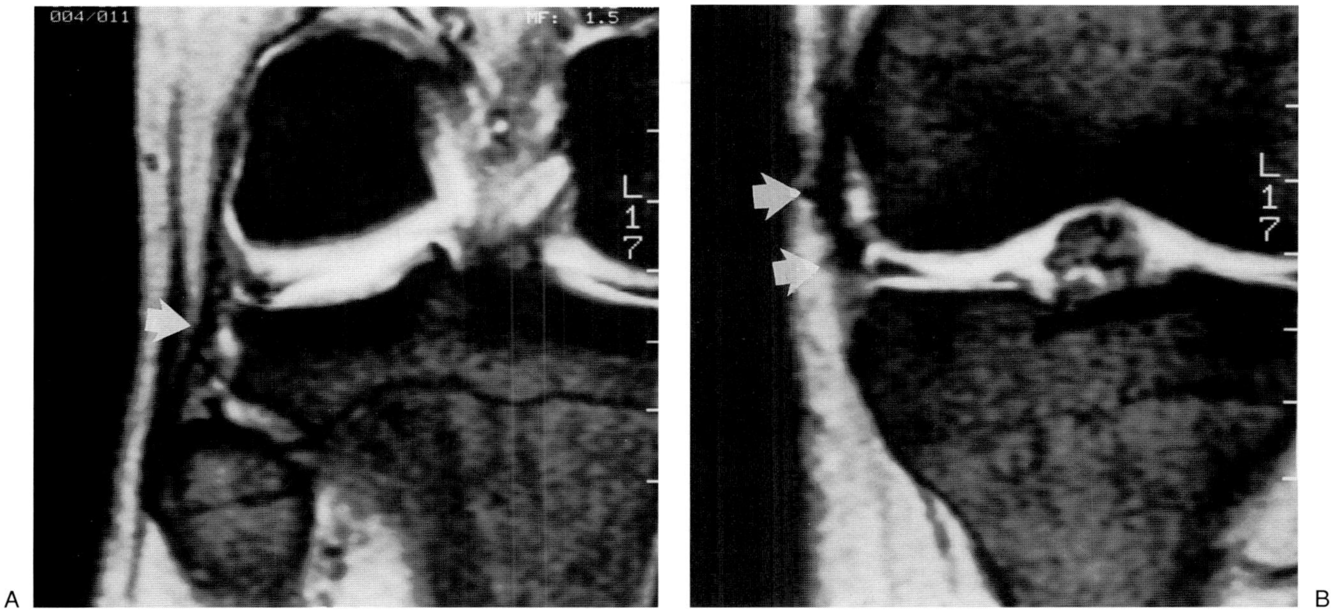

FIG. 11-4. Repaired peripheral tear of lateral meniscus. **A, B:** Adjacent coronal T2* gradient-echo MPGR (TR 400 msec, TE 20 msec, flip angle 20°) images. The periphery of the meniscus and adjacent capsular structures have a slightly bumpy contour [best seen in (B)—*arrows*], representing metal artifact at the site of the repair. The process of suturing is enough to leave behind tiny crystals of metal that produce this appearance.

MENISCAL SURGERY

In the past 40 years meniscal surgery has undergone revolutionary changes (11–16). The significance and importance of the meniscus in distribution of forces across the joint and maintaining stability have become increasingly well appreciated, and this has led to a tendency toward meniscal-sparing surgery and meniscal reconstruction (see Chapter 4). Preservation of even a partial meniscus has been shown to diminish peak loads markedly across the joint and to diminish significantly the degenerative changes that accompany meniscal resection (10,14,17–19).

Decisions regarding meniscal resection or repair are to a large degree based on location and morphology of the meniscal tear (Fig. 11-4). The peripheral portion of the meniscus is vascularized (''red zone''); therefore, tears through this region will usually heal with knee immobilization or placement of sutures. Surgeons can place sutures through these portions of the meniscus to give added stability, and this can be done either in an open procedure or arthroscopically. Tears at the junction of the vascularized and nonvascularized portion of the meniscus (''red–white junction'') also can undergo repair with a chance of healing. Methods to assess meniscal vascularity clinically, such as abrasion in the absence of a leg tourniquet, or laser Doppler have therefore been advocated (20). Tears that are in the central, poorly vascularized to nonvascularized portion of the meniscus (''white zone'') seldom undergo healing. For this reason the surgeon often elects to trim or recontour the meniscus. Recently, experimental procedures using synovial abrasion or application/injection of exogenous fibrin clot have been used to incite vascularization in these normally avascular portions of the meniscus and thereby promote healing (11,21–24). Some evidence suggests that this is less likely to be of value in chronic or complex tears. Supplementary fascia grafts have been advocated (23). The increasingly used vascularization procedures result in development of fibrovascular scar, which gradually remodels over a period of time to form ''regenerated'' meniscus. This process may take place more readily medially than laterally (25). Histologically, differences remain between these and areas of ''new'' meniscus and native fibrocartilage.

Depending upon the type of surgery performed, the appearance of the postoperative meniscus is extremely variable (Figs. 11-5 and 11-6). In an effort to categorize the expected appearance of these menisci Deutsch and colleagues, as well as other investigators, have divided menisci into three different groups, depending on the extent of resection (1,2). Group I consists of menisci that have been only minimally excised (25% or less). Group II is an intermediate group in which 25–75% of the meniscus has been resected. In group III, 75% or more of the meniscus has been excised.

In the first group, with only a minimal amount of meniscus removed, conventional diagnostic criteria for evaluation of meniscus are fairly accurate. In other words, grade III signal (a signal extending to the articulating surface of the meniscus) can generally be considered to indicate the presence of a meniscal tear with an accuracy similar to that of a meniscus

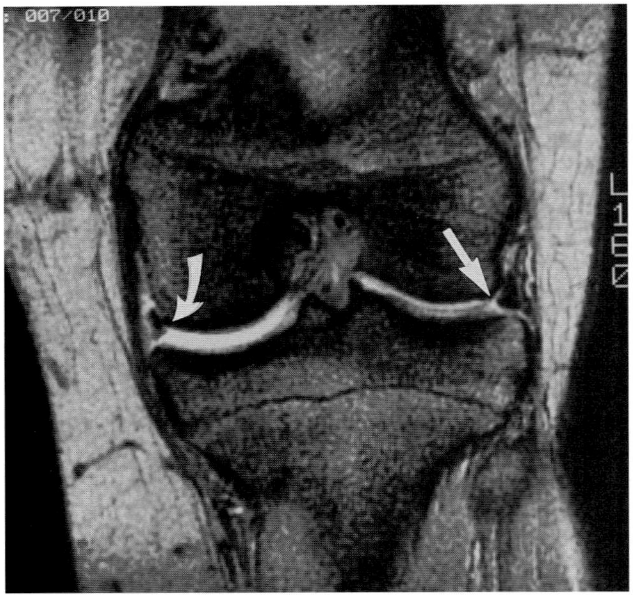

FIG. 11-5. Meniscal trimming. Coronal T2* gradient-echo MPGR (TR 500 msec, TE 20 msec, flip angle 20°). Both menisci had previously been trimmed at the time of arthroscopy over a year before. The medial meniscus had undergone more extensive resection *(curved arrow)*. Blunting of the lateral meniscal apex is also apparent (*arrow*), affecting the lateral meniscus.

that has not been operated on previously. With groups II and III these criteria cannot be employed to the same degree of accuracy, and indeed significant errors can be made if conventional criteria are employed. A meniscus that has a predominantly horizontal area of increased signal intensity within it may, after partial resection, have high-signal material extend to an articulating surface of the meniscus (4). In this way grade II signal intensity (linear signal intensity within the meniscus) will be converted into apparently grade III meniscus—a tear. Thus, mucoid degeneration may be misinterpreted as a tear.

With groups II and III careful evaluation of meniscal contour may be helpful. Generally speaking, surgeons attempt to restore an approximately triangular smooth contour to the meniscus following resection (3,26). Marked irregularity with step abnormalities or fragmentation are therefore very helpful signs. In this situation T2-weighted imaging may be helpful, particularly if there is a small amount of fluid within the joint, because a true tear may demonstrate extension of high signal into the substance of the meniscus (Figs. 11-7 and 11-8). Unfortunately, this will only be helpful in situations where a tear is not tightly coapted, thereby allowing fluid to enter the tear and be visualized. This sign is therefore highly specific and helpful when present; however, its absence is not as useful a finding. An additional problem is that menisci tend to adhere to damaged hyaline cartilage, preventing their morphology from being outlined by joint

A 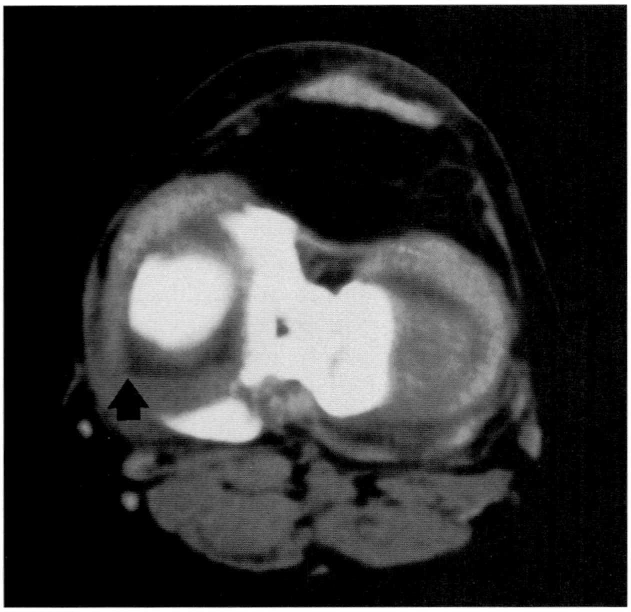 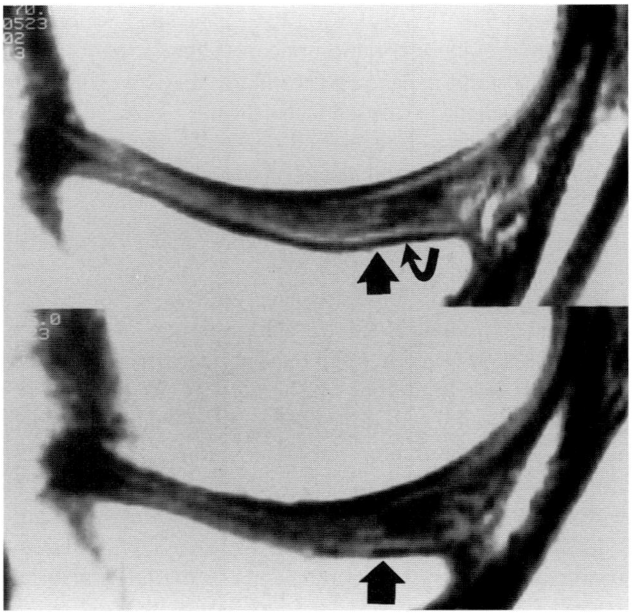 B

FIG. 11-6. Previous arthroscopic trimming of medical meniscal margin. **A:** Axial CT image 1.5 mm thick through the menisci. An angular configuration of the meniscal edge is present at junction of the posterior horn and body *(arrow)*. **B:** Magnified sagittal images T1-weighted spin echo (TR 800 msec, TR 20 msec) show an abrupt amputation of the meniscus *(arrows)* at the same site. On the top image some linear in-substance increased signal is also present as well as a small area of signal extending to the inferior surface of the posterior horn *(curved arrow)*, which at repeat arthroscopy was not a tear and presumably represents a healed tear.

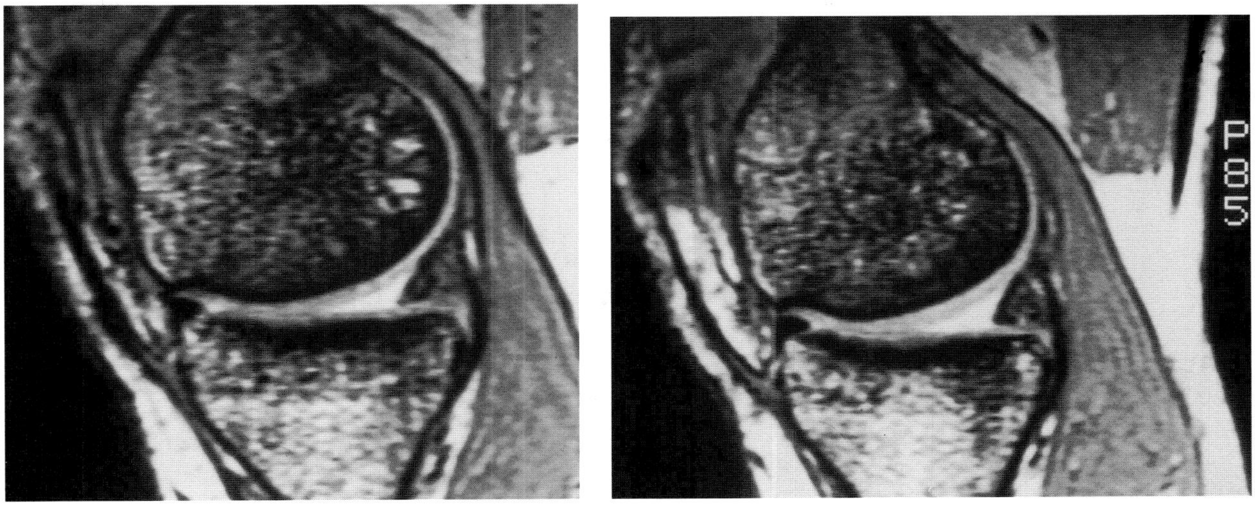

A B

FIG. 11-7. Previous meniscus resection and recontouring. **A, B:** Adjacent T2* gradient-echo 3DFT volumetric (TR 55 msec, TE 15 msec, flip angle 35°) images. Previous arthroscopic partial resection of the posterior meniscal horn has been performed. The remaining meniscus has a triangular configuration. The gap left following excision has been filled with bright joint fluid outlining both meniscus and hyaline cartilage. This arthrographic effect can be very helpful in evaluation of meniscal remnants and highlighting tears.

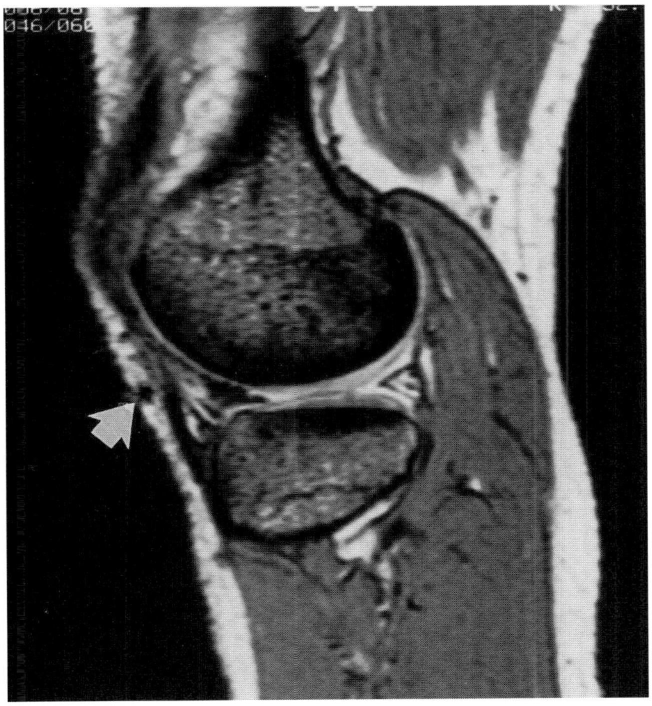

FIG. 11-8. Sagittal T2* gradient-echo 3DFT volumetric (TR 55 msec, TE 15 msec, flip angle 35°) through the lateral meniscus. A previous repair of a posterior horn tear had been performed as well as partial resection. High signal in-substance linear tears are seen in the posterior horn, which is outlined by high-signal-intensity joint fluid. Metal artifact is incidentally noted in the subcutaneous fat *(arrow)*.

fluid. For this reason it may be helpful to wrap the knee in a tension bandage in order to increase intra-articular pressure and encourage fluid to pass between coapted surfaces. T2- or T2*-weighted images can be helpful in this group in assessing meniscus morphology. We have also found that thin-section three-dimensional Fourier transform (3DFT) imaging can be helpful and aids in recognizing loose chondral or osteochondral bodies and/or meniscal fragments that are seen with greater frequency in this group of patients. Nodular synovitis as well as fibrin balls and degradation products from blood that contain hemosiderin can also be encountered.

Some authorities have suggested the use of MRI arthrography either by introduction of saline within the joint, in which case T2- or T2*-weighted sequences can be utilized, or by gadolinium arthrography using dilute gadolinium (approximately 1 in 200 volume ratio), which would allow T1-weighted images to be employed, with their superior signal-to-noise ratio (Fig. 11-9) (27). The presence of increased signal intensity extending to the meniscal surface has been found to be a very specific indicator of meniscal tear in the postoperative meniscus (4). It is likely that gadolinium arthrography will also prove highly specific and may be more sensitive than T2/T2*-weighted sequences, but it has the disadvantage of being slightly more invasive. Some authors have even suggested that conventional arthrography might be considered in the setting of a postoperative meniscus (4).

One feature of the healed meniscus that may produce considerable confusion and difficulty is that even healed tears often retain increased signal intensity relative to the sur-

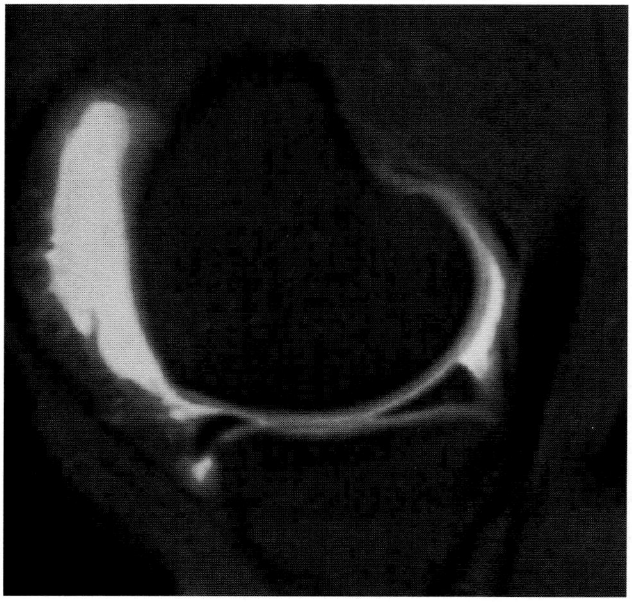

FIG. 11-9. Healed meniscal tear demonstrated by MRI arthrography. Sagittal T1-weighted image (TR 600 msec, TE 18 msec) with fat suppression following injection of a dilute solution of gadolinium–DTPA (1:250 dilution). The high-signal-intensity contrast outlines the meniscus and hyaline cartilage surfaces without penetrating into the meniscus. A faint high-signal-intensity linear region can be visualized (but having lower signal intensity than the intra-articular contrast) representing the healed tear, but no penetration of higher signal contrast is seen. This conclusively demonstrates that the zone of increased signal intensity within the meniscus is not a tear.

rounding original meniscus. For this reason, false-positives may be a problem. This problem could account for many of the false-positives mentioned in many studies that have assessed the accuracy of MRI in evaluating meniscal abnormalities (2). Whether these old meniscal tears serve as foci for new tears is not entirely clear. Also, regenerated menisci may be of increased signal intensity for a long time, or even permanently (Fig. 11-10).

Work is continuing in a few centers on the use of transplanted menisci harvested from cadavers that are cryopreserved before reimplantation (12,28). Very little has been written about their MRI appearance. Early results indicated that these menisci are of higher signal than native menisci and appear to be prone to tearing, particularly at the site of ligature. More recent reports have stated that short-term follow-up (months) shows that these menisci have an appearance similar to that of normal menisci, except that with T2-weighting high signal may be seen at the periphery (29). Definitive data await further follow-up and larger numbers of patients. Artificial collagen-based prostheses are currently being developed and may well appear in clinical trials in the near future. These prostheses are being developed with the idea of serving as a reabsorbable framework upon which fibrochondrocytes can develop a new meniscus (30). Experimental work on tendon autografts has also been reported (31).

ANTERIOR CRUCIATE LIGAMENT

The treatment of anterior cruciate ligament tears has been an area of significant controversy. In the past, many patients were treated conservatively, but increasingly a more aggressive approach has been adopted, with reconstructions being performed in the acute setting. This more aggressive approach has been due to a better understanding of the natural history of the untreated anterior cruciate ligament tear. It has become increasingly apparent that 80% or more of active patients will eventually develop some degree of progressive functional instability and/or degenerative joint disease if reconstruction is not performed (32–39). Although some patients may tolerate an anterior cruciate ligament tear with the use of exercises and braces and the elimination of certain physical activities, a significant number will develop gradually progressive symptoms. In this latter group, patients will often demonstrate joint effusions, thigh atrophy, and symptoms consistent with meniscal tears. Repair of meniscal tears has been proven to be more successful when the anterior cruciate is intact/reconstructed (40,41). More recent work has also shown that a large number of individuals with anterior cruciate tears will have evidence of subcortical bone infractions and that these changes may evolve into chondromalacia and eventually serve as the precursor lesions to osteoarthritis. Although conservative treatment may be well tolerated by sedentary individuals, particularly in the older age groups, those who are younger or active are being considered as candidates for anterior cruciate ligament reconstruction.

Tears of the anterior cruciate ligament are far more common than bone avulsions at the anterior cruciate attachments. If an avulsive injury occurs, a bone fragment is often carried off with the ligament, which permits reattachment surgically with good results (Fig. 11-11). In this setting postoperative MRI may only reveal some metal artifact (e.g., sutures/screws) at the site of reattachment. Primary anastomosis of in-substance tears is frequently impossible because of fraying, and even if this is not the case the strength of the repaired ligament is poor (Fig. 11-12) (42).

Once it has been determined that the anterior cruciate ligament is torn, various reconstructive procedures are available. Depending on a surgeon's preference and training, the type of reconstruction will vary considerably from one center to the next. Techniques that are entirely intra-articular, entirely extra-articular, or a combination of the two have been proposed and have their advocates and critics (34,35,43–55). Entirely extra-articular techniques have fallen into disfavor (56). At the present time it is unclear which type of reconstruction or reconstructions is preferable, and this undoubtedly will be a subject of clinical research for many years. Before attempting to interpret anterior cruciate ligament re-

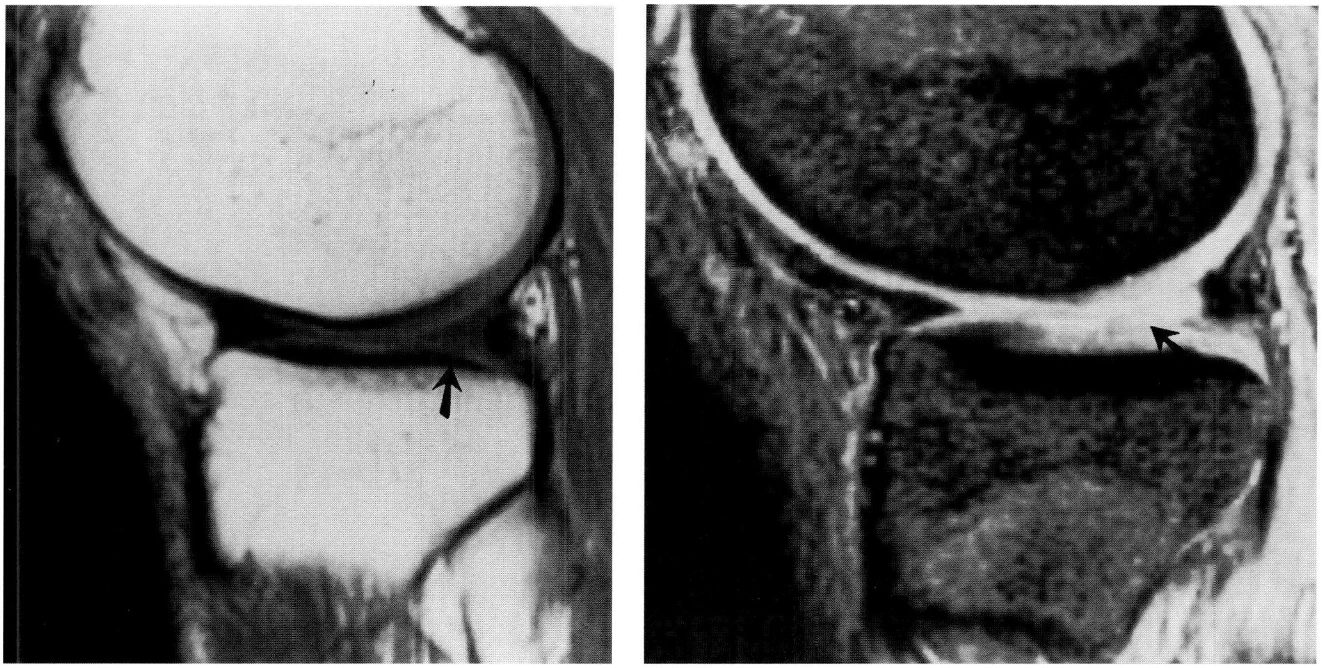
A B

FIG. 11-10. Regenerated meniscus. Resection of a large portion of the lateral meniscus had been performed more than 2 years previously, leaving behind a rim of vascularized peripheral meniscus. **A:** Sagittal T1-weighted spin echo (TR 600 msec, TE 20 msec). The apex and superior surface of the posterior horn *(arrow)* are of low signal intensity, less than that of adjacent hyaline cartilage. Fibrocartilage in regenerated menisci often has more signal than normal meniscus, and its appearance can easily mimic maceration. **B:** Sagittal T2* gradient echo MPGR (TR 400 msec, TE 20 msec, flip angle 30°) shows the regenerated meniscus *(arrow)* to be of high signal in this instance. Note the abrupt demarcation at the junction between original and regenerated meniscus.

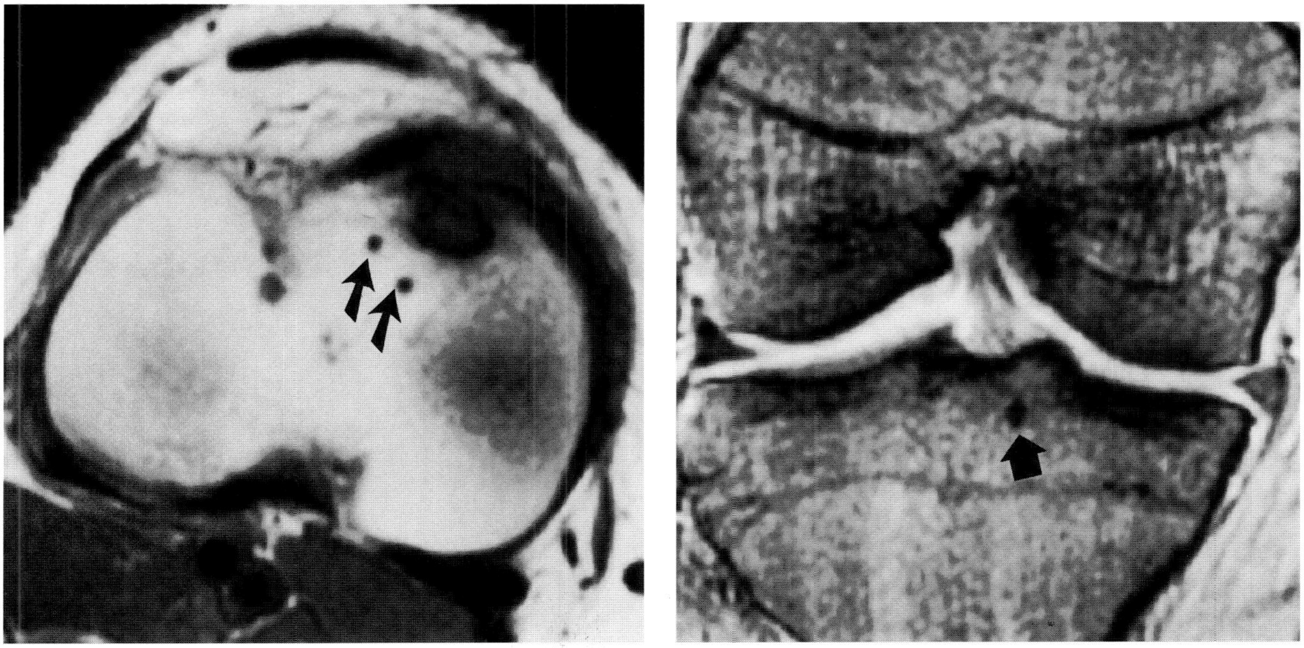
A B

FIG. 11-11. Distal anterior cruciate bone avulsion injury with repair by suturing bone fragment back into the donor site in the proximal tibia. **A:** Axial T1-weighted spin echo (TR 700 msec, TE 17 msec). Two low-signal dots *(arrows)* indicated the site of a metal suture used to transfix the avulsed fragment. **B:** Coronal T2* gradient echo MPGR (TR 550 msec, TR 19 msec, flip angle 20°) also shows the suture.

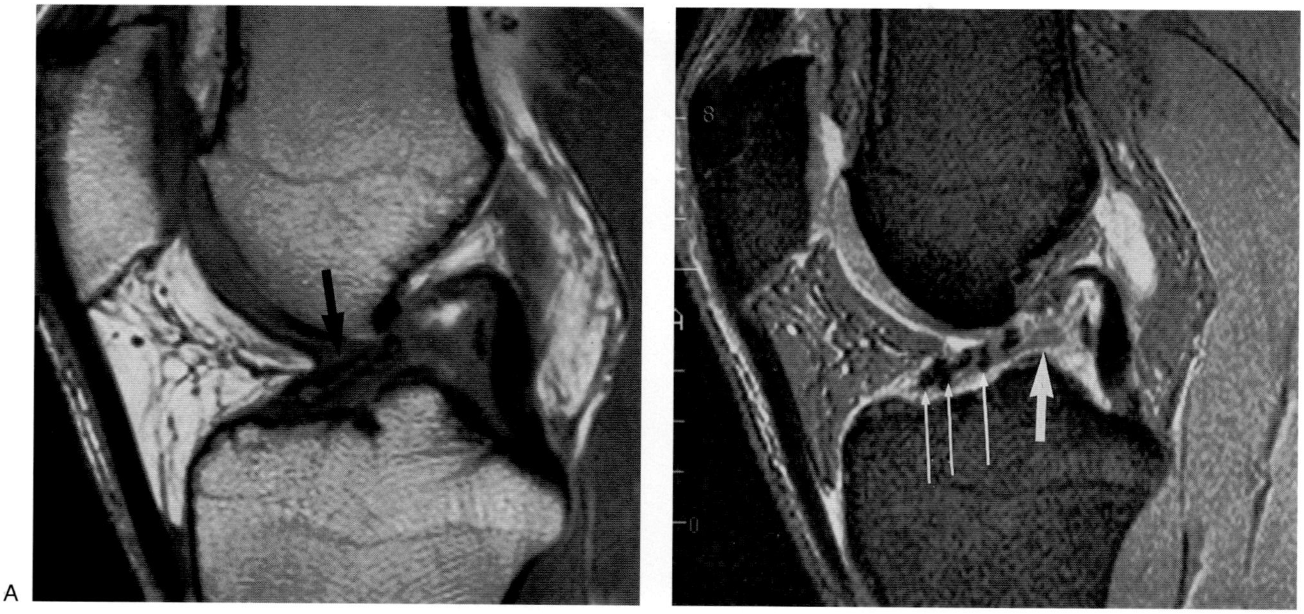

FIG. 11-12. Attempted primary repair of the anterior cruciate ligament. **A:** Sagittal T1-weighted spin echo (TR 800 msec, TE 20 msec). Nodular low-signal bands *(arrow)* are the anterior cruciate, which had been sutured in an attempted primary repair. **B:** Sagittal T2* gradient-echo MPGP (TR 400 msec TE 16 msec, flip angle 30°). The low-signal metal artifact is much more evident *(long, thin arrows)*. The fibers of the disrupted anterior cruciate can be seen as fine, wavy structures of low signal *(thick arrow)*.

construction MRIs it is extremely helpful to know what types of reconstruction are performed in patients being referred to your practice and, if possible, a specific type of reconstruction performed in any patient.

The reconstructions demonstrated in this text are principally of two types. Most of those shown here have been performed with a harvested semitendinosis graft reinforced by a polypropylene braid (a ligament augmentation device) (50,57–60) (Figs. 11-13 and 11-14). The other type has involved harvesting a segment of patellar tendon with segments of bone at its cranial and caudal ends from the patella and tibia (61). The bone plugs are either stapled/screwed into position or wedged into the tunnel alongside an interference screw (61,62) (Fig. 11-15). The intrinsic strength of patellar tendon grafts has been measured at 159–168% that of a normal anterior cruciate ligament. Hamstring tendons measure only 49–70%; therefore, augmentation, either with synthetic devices as noted earlier or with fascia, has been advised (57,63). Other materials—including gracilis tendon (usually sewn together with a concomitantly harvested semitendinosis tendon), quadriceps tendon, fascia lata, meniscus, bovine xenograft, and a number of different synthetic materials (especially Gortex)—have been used to construct neoligaments (34,35,64–75). Depending upon the type of material utilized as well as the technique employed, the appearance of grafts will vary (55,76–79).

Some techniques require construction of intra-osseous tunnels in both the tibia and femur (68,69,77,80) (Figs. 11-16–11-18). Many techniques, however, have dispensed with

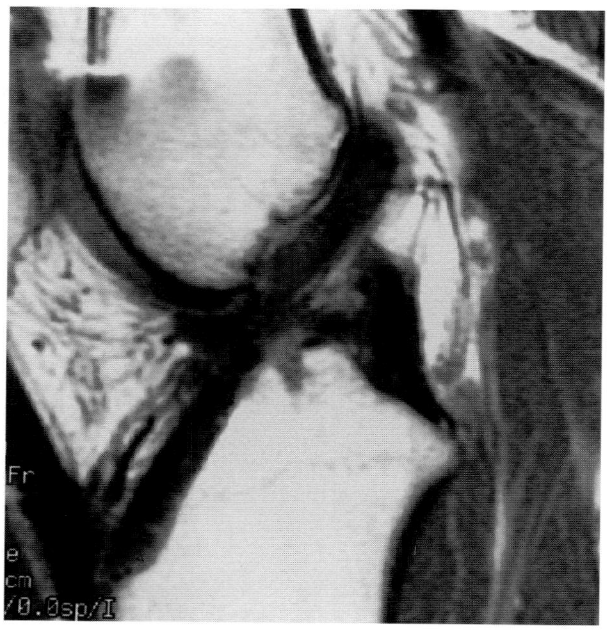

FIG. 11-13. Normal anterior cruciate neoligament. Sagittal T1-weighted spin echo (TR 800 msec, TE 20 msec). The thick low-signal band represents the harvested semitendinosis tendon running approximately along the expected course of a normal anterior cruciate ligament. The neoligament is uniformly of low signal, as would be expected in normal tendon.

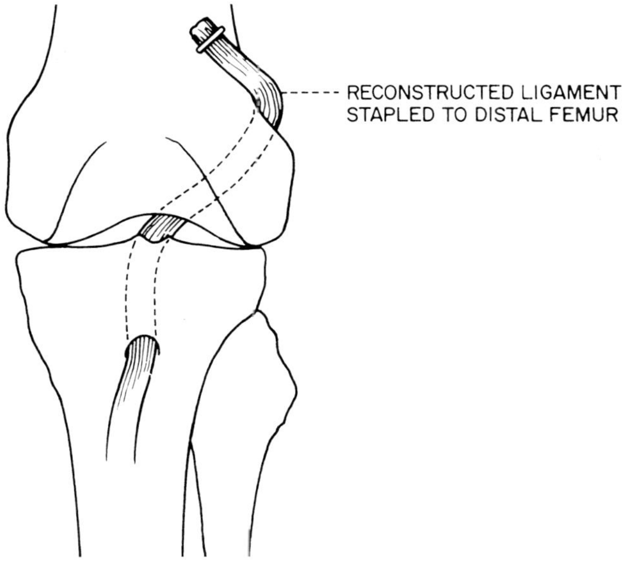

FIG. 11-14. Diagram anterior cruciate neoligament. The expected course of the neoligament is outlined. The distal portion is seen to enter a hole drilled in the anterior cortex of the proximal tibia and to enter the joint near the intercondylar spines; it then is brought superiorly and laterally behind the femur to be stapled to the femoral metaphysis.

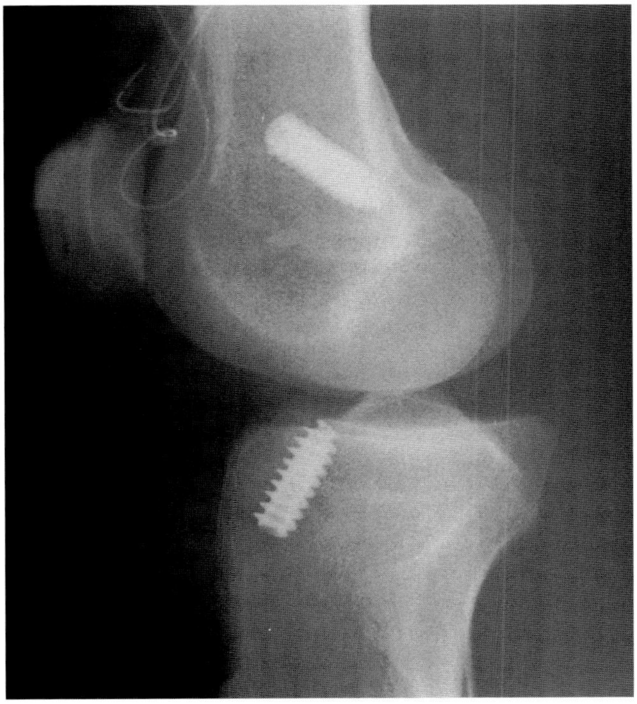

FIG. 11-15. Radiograph postoperative patellar tendon/bone plug graft. Lateral radiograph obtained the day after surgery. A bone–tendon–bone graft was obtained from the middle third of the patellar tendon and brought through a tibial tunnel. The distal bone plug was then wedged into position by placing the interference screw seen in the tibial. The femoral end of the graft was transfixed in a similar fashion.

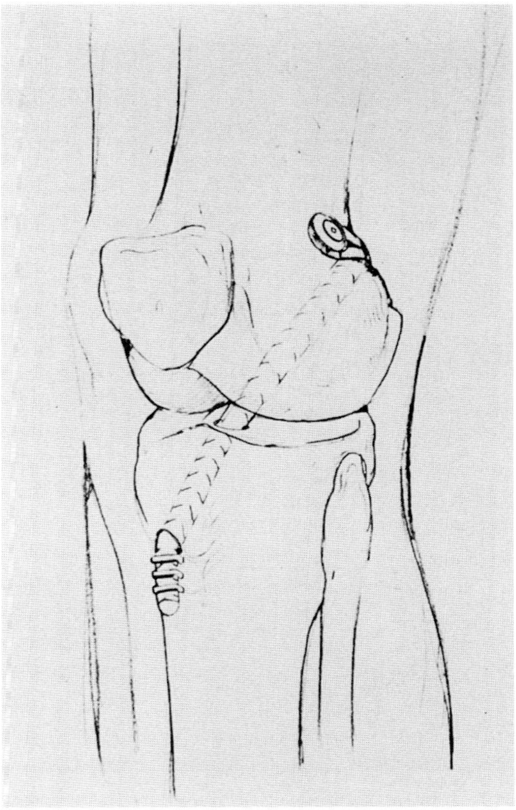

FIG. 11-16. Diagram anterior cruciate neoligament. Knee as seen from an oblique perspective, showing neoligament in situ traversing proximal femoral and distal tibial bone tunnels. In the extended position the course of the ligament should be straight.

the construction of a femoral tunnel and instead wrap the graft around the lateral femoral condyle and then staple it to the femoral metaphysis (''over-the-top'' technique) (45,55,81). Virtually all widely used technique use an intraosseous tibial tunnel, however.

With both the semitendinosis and patellar tendon techniques mentioned earlier as well as most other techniques, metallic fixation screws and/or staples are used to transfix the neoligament. These can sometimes produce significant metal artifact, making the portions of the graft immediately adjacent impossible to evaluate (Figs. 11-19 and 11-20). It has been reported that Perfix interference screws are ferromagnetic and therefore produce spectacular artifact on MRI (82). These patients cannot be adequately assessed with MRI, but fortunately are only a small population of patients with neoligaments. We have found, however, that spin-echo and fast spin-echo sequences usually produce images that allow the majority of neoligaments to be evaluated (55,61,62,77,78,83–85) (Fig. 11-21). Despite magnetic susceptibility effects, gradient-echo techniques utilizing 3DFT often produce exquisite images with great detail of the neoligaments (77) (Fig. 11-22). When using spin-echo or fast spin-echo sequences we attempt to angulate the plane of the

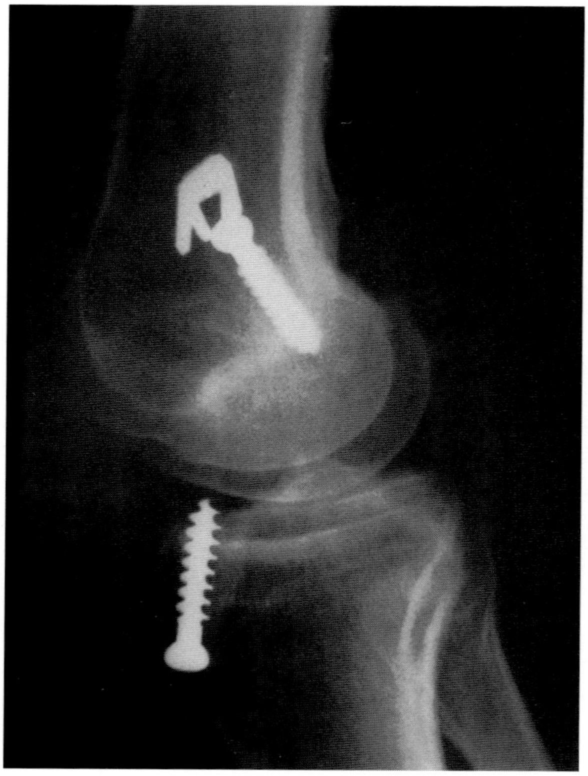

FIG. 11-17. Lateral radiograph showing bone screws and staples in a patient with dual bone tunnels from an anterior cruciate neoligament reconstruction.

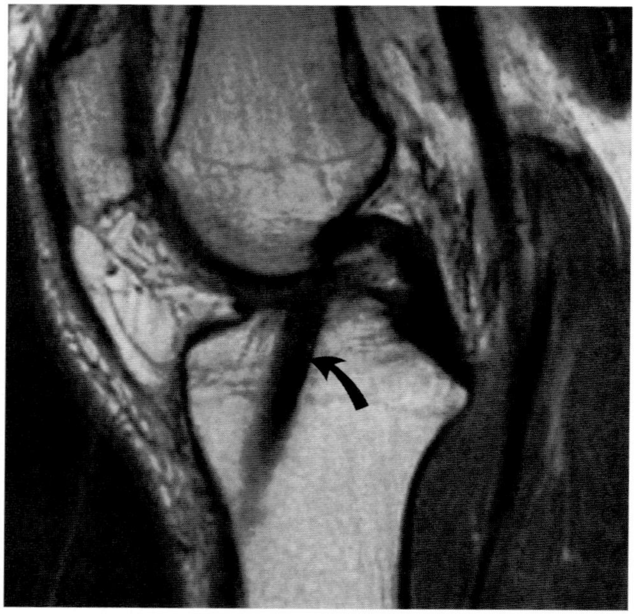

FIG. 11-19. Tibial bone tunnel. Sagittal T1-weighted spin echo (TR 600 msec, TE 18 msec). Tibial tunnel *(curved arrow)* is unobscured by any metal artifact in this semitendinosis reconstruction.

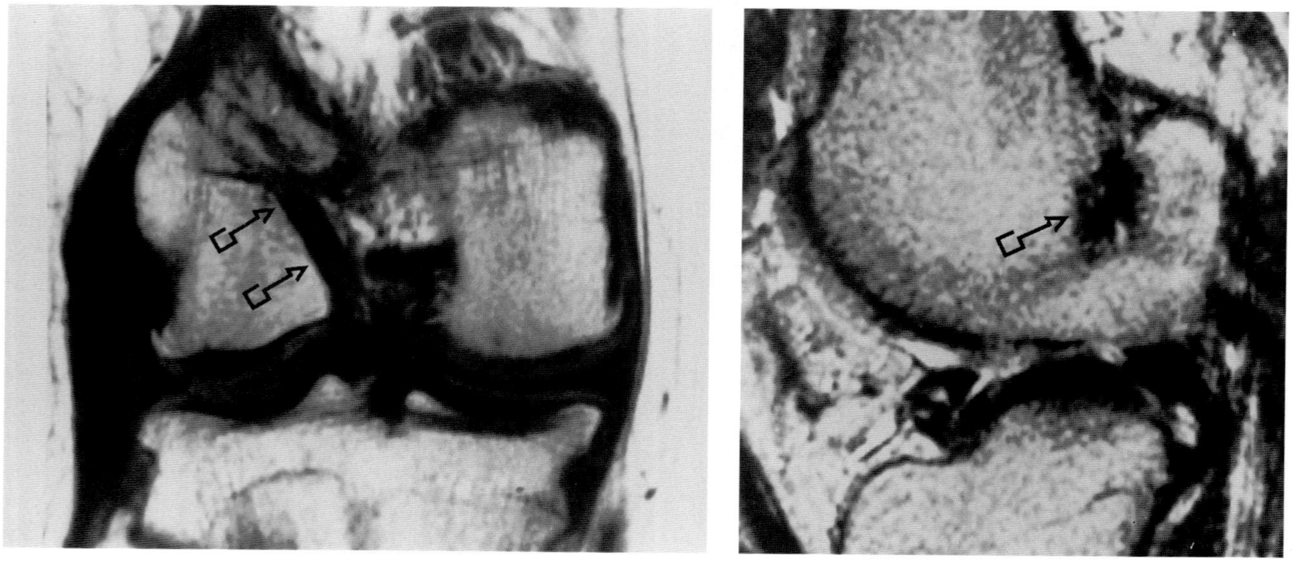

A B

FIG. 11-18. Dual tunnel anterior cruciate neoligament. **A:** Coronal T1-weighted spin echo (TR 600 msec, TE 20 msec) shows the femoral tunnel as an oblique band of low signal intensity running through the condyle *(arrows)*. **B:** Sagittal T2-weighted spin echo (TR 2102 msec, TE 80 msec) transects the tunnel in the femur so that it is seen end on *(arrow)*. (From Munk PL, et al. *Can Assoc Radiol J* 1992; 43:411–419. With permission.)

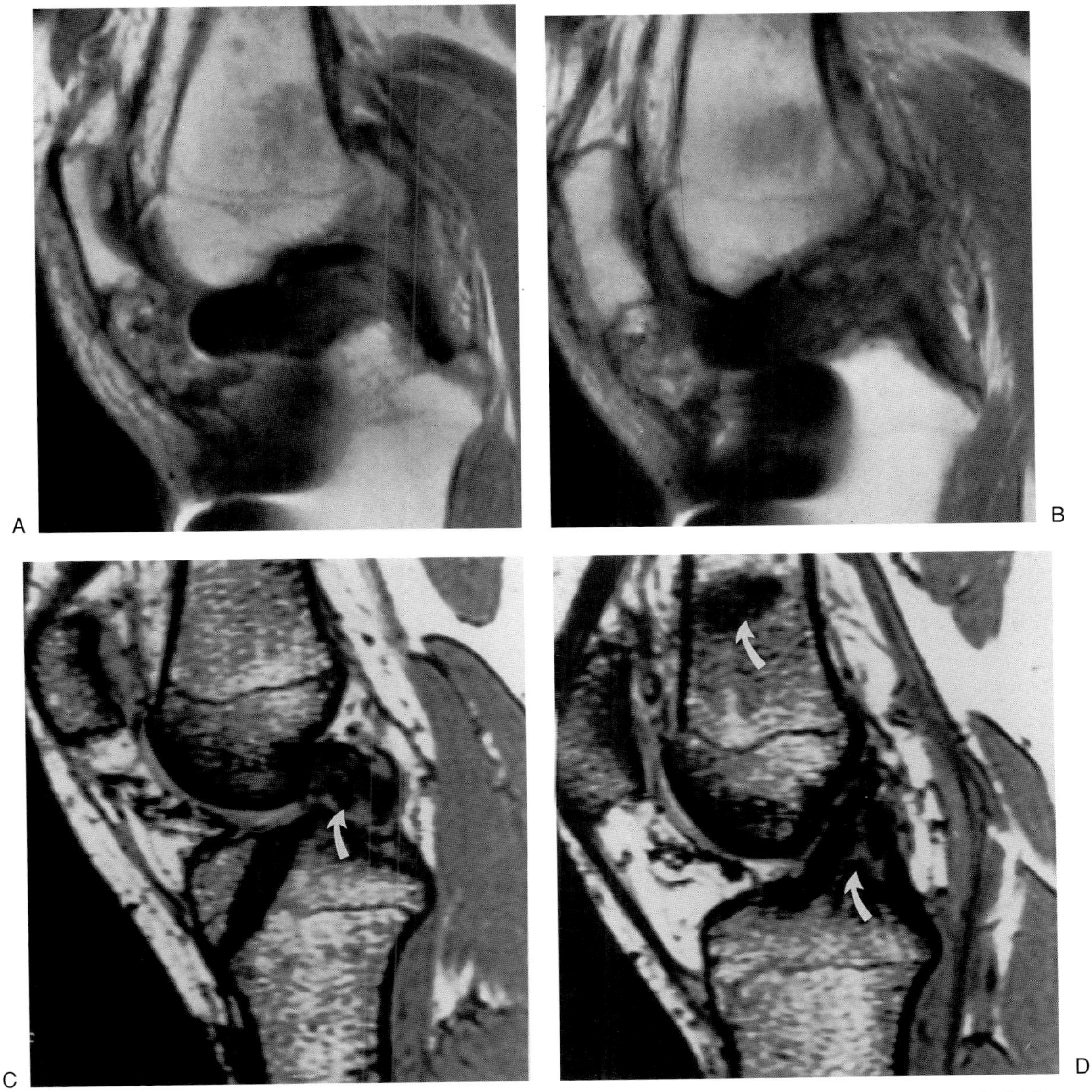

FIG. 11-20. Extensive artifact. **A,B:** Adjacent sagittal T1-weighted spin echo (TR 800 msec, TE 20 msec) from a patient with a patellar tendon graft has unusually marked metal artifact that completely obscures the portion of the neoligament running through the proximal tibia. **C,D:** Adjacent sagittal T2* 3DFT gradient echo (TR 55 msec, TE 15 msec, flip angle 35°) from a patient with a semitendinosis neoligament. The course of the neoligament is not significantly marred by metal artifact despite the use of gradient-echo technique allowing it to be adequately assessed. A few small metal artifacts can be seen *(arrows)*.

image along the course of the neoligament, which significantly facilitates interpretation (Figs. 11-23 and 11-24). Using T2 weighting is often very helpful in producing an arthrographic effect, allowing the fibers of the neoligament to be visualized to advantage (Figs. 11-25 and 11-26). When using 3DFT we have generally used a flip angle in the range of 30–50°, which allows the neoligament to be easily evaluated and differentiated from fluid and surrounding soft tissue or cartilage in most instances. If both femoral and tibial tunnels are present, it may be necessary to obtain several oblique sequences to visualize the whole course of the neoligament adequately.

Immediately after neoligament reconstruction, grafts will be of low signal intensity, as would be expected of normal patellar or hamstring tendons. When free tendon grafts are used the neoligament is avascular, because blood supply is completely disrupted during the process of transplantation and reconstruction. Some techniques have been developed

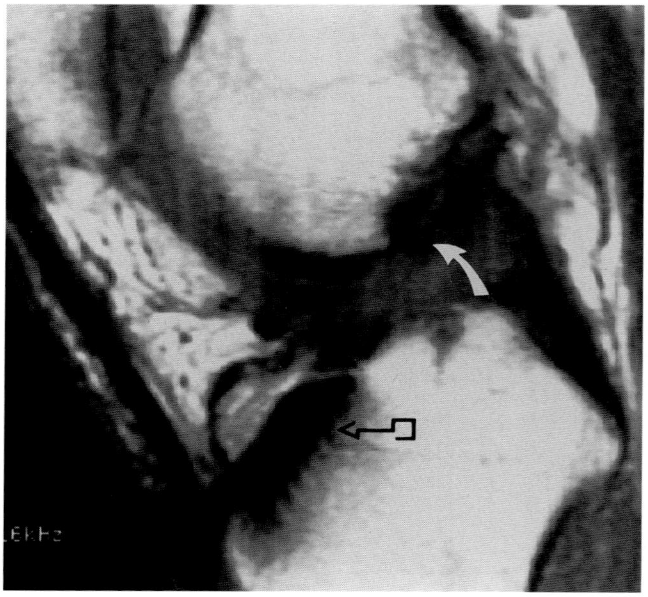

FIG. 11-21. Neoligament from patellar tendon graft. T1-weighted sagittal spin echo (TR 600 msec, TE 20 msec). Artifact from interference screw precludes visualization of distal portion of graft *(hollow arrow)*; note that the screw threads are visible. The intra-articular portion of the neoligament *(curved arrow)* is unaffected by artifact from the screw.

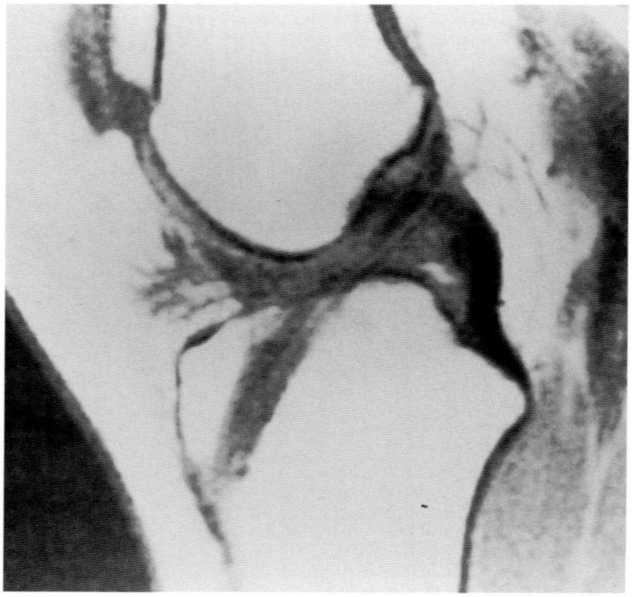

FIG. 11-23. Oblique sagittal image shows the whole neoligament (TR 600 msec, TR 20 msec).

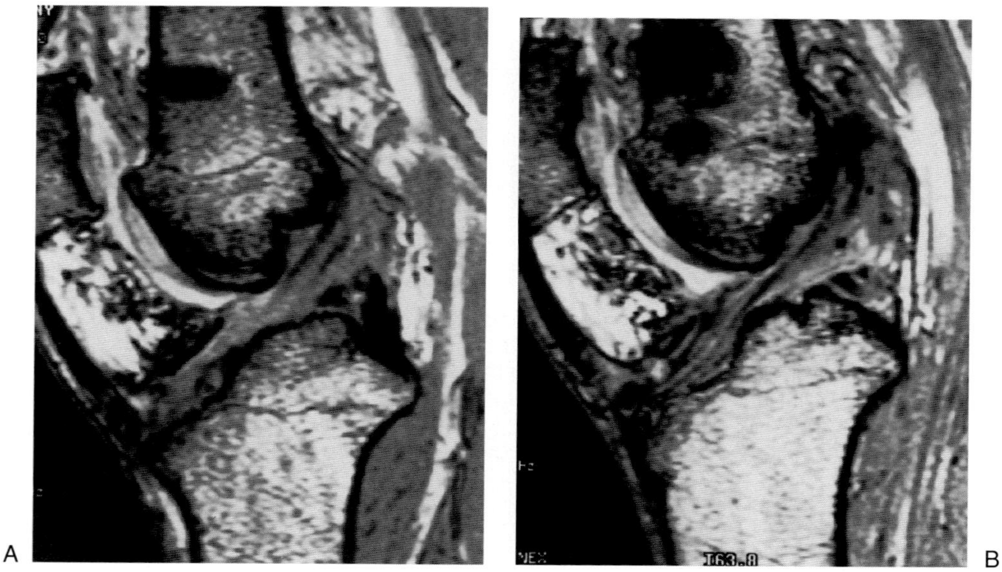

FIG. 11-22. Thin-section gradient-echo imaging. **A,B:** Nearly adjacent sagittal T2* 3DFT gradient echo (TR 55 msec, TR msec, flip angle 30°). The neoligament is of increased signal intensity, which is not unusual in grafts 2 years old like this one. A few low-signal fibers can clearly be appreciated and extend into the tibial tunnel. Incidentally noted is metal artifact. (From Munk PL, et al. *Can Assoc Radiol J* 1992; 43:411–419. Used with permission.)

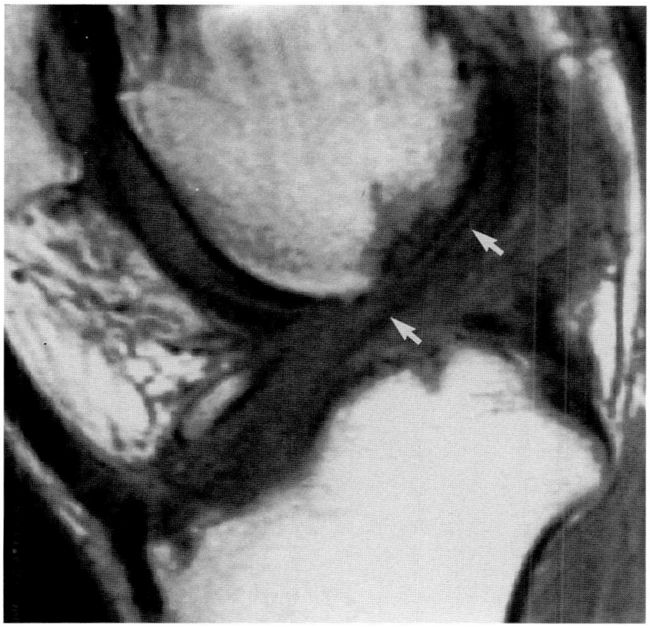

FIG. 11-24. Oblique sagittal spin-echo proton-density (TR 1800 msec, TE 20 msec) image of a ligament that had been reconstructed 2.5 years before. The whole length of the neoligament, except for the portion brought around the posterior femur proximally for stapling to metaphysis, can be seen. Note once again the low signal fibers *(arrows)*. (From Munk PL, et al. *Can Assoc Radiol J* 1992;43:411–419. Used with permission.)

in an effort to preserve the distal origin of the patellar tendon graft to maintain blood supply arising from the superior and inferior geniculate branches that supply the tendon (49,86–88).

Within a few weeks of implantation the neoligament is readily vascularized by the surrounding synovial membranes. The intraosseous portions of the graft also gradually become vascularized from endosteal vessels. It has been estimated that revascularization is complete within approximately 20 weeks, after which the vascularity of the graft surface gradually drops off. Once vascularized, the structure of the graft gradually becomes reorganized; given sufficient time, the tissue, if biopsied, will appear similar to that of a normal anterior cruciate ligament. Studies have shown that in the first several months water content and vascularity of the neoligament increase, which is accompanied by decreased strength. This decreased strength is only temporary and is more closely correlated with water content (63). This whole process has been termed *ligamentization*.

As this process of ligamentization occurs, a gradual increase in the signal intensity of the neoligament takes place. Grafts gradually become of intermediate signal intensity (within 6 months or even earlier), although it is not unusual for a few fibers of low signal intensity to persist (Figs. 11-27 and 11-28). This increase in signal intensity, therefore, does not necessarily indicate ligament failure or rerupture. Unfortunately, if impingement of the graft is present, this can also lead to increase in signal intensity with increased water content within the ligament and reduced strength. In

A

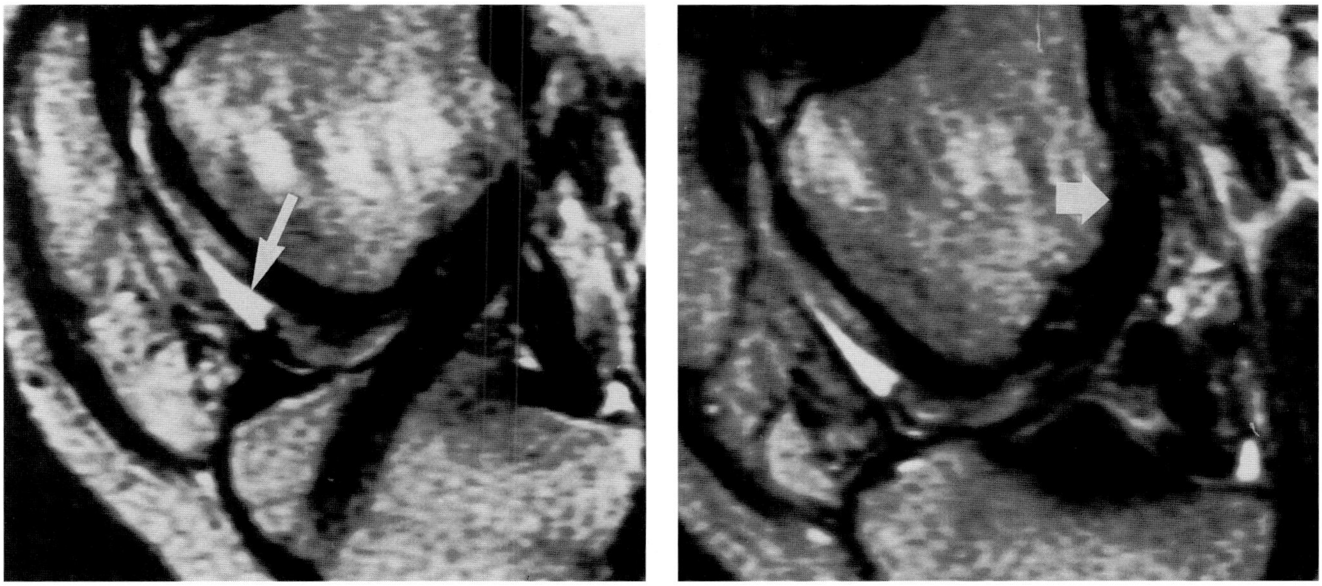

B

FIG. 11-25. A,B: Oblique sagittal images. T2-weighted spin echo (TR 2000 msec, TE 80 msec) shows most of the neoligament and can be seen ("over the top") curving over the posterior femoral metaphysis *(thick arrow)*. The small amount of fluid in the joint *(arrow)* is within normal limits. With larger effusions an arthrographic effect is produced.

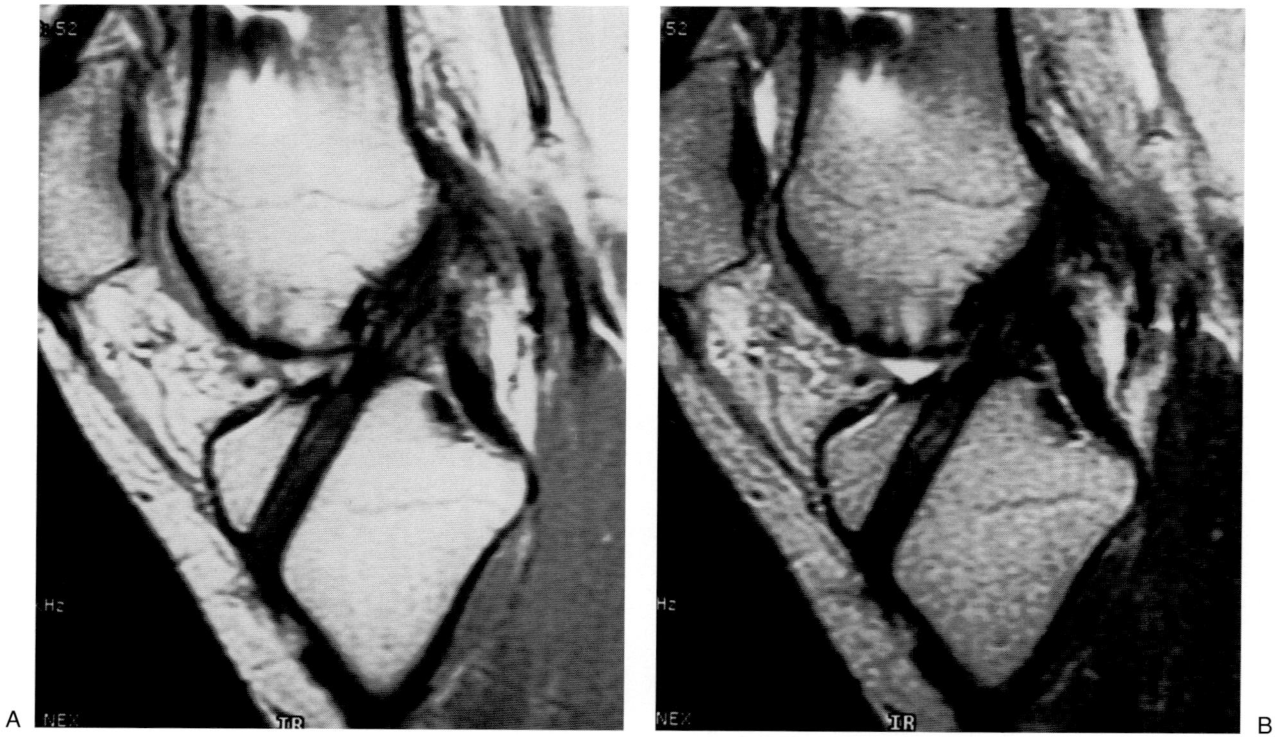

FIG. 11-26. Oblique sagittal proton density. **(A)** and **(B)** T2-weighted spin echo (TR 2000 msec, TE 20 & 80 msec) of a normal semitendinosis graft. The intra-articular and tibial portions are seen on a single image. It is not always possible to achieve this with oblique sagittals but usually fewer images need to be interpreted than with conventional sagittal imaging. Note the bright joint fluid in **B**.

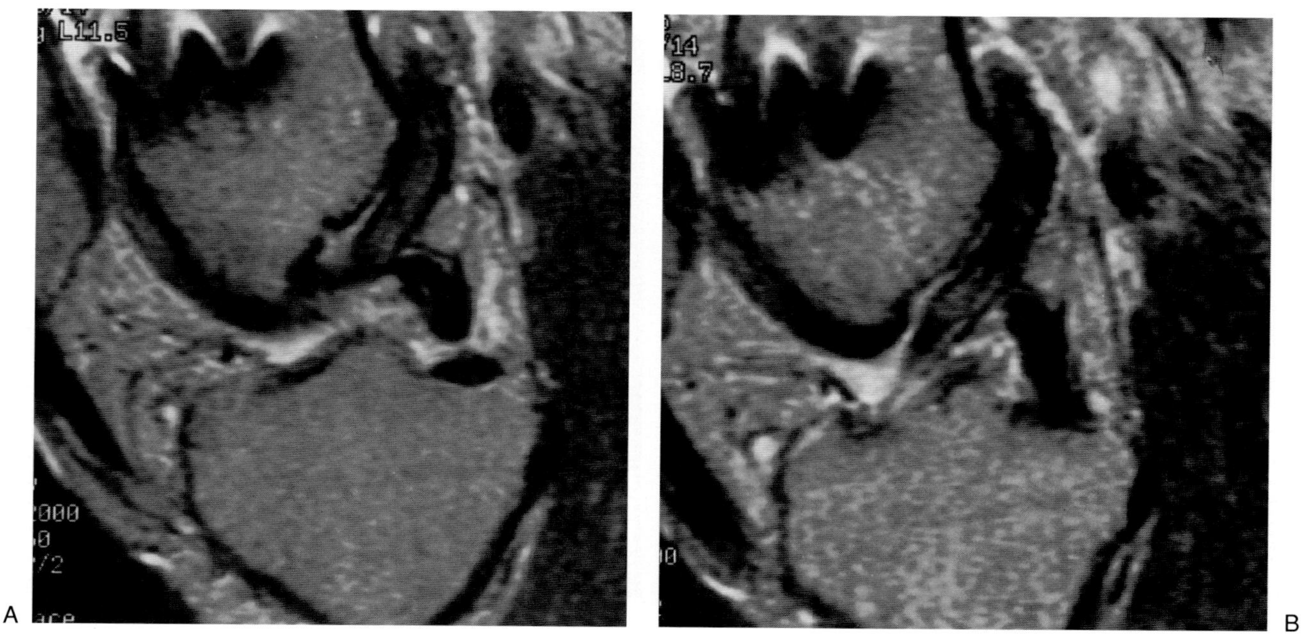

FIG. 11-27. Ligamentization. **A,B:** Adjacent oblique sagittal T2-weighted spin-echo images (TR 2400 msec, TE 80 msec) from a patient with a semitendinosis neoligament constructed more than 1 year previously. The intra-articular portion of the graft is well seen on these images. The periphery is of low-signal intensity but the core is of intermediate-signal intensity, as is normally the case in mature grafts, presumably because of microvascular ingrowth.

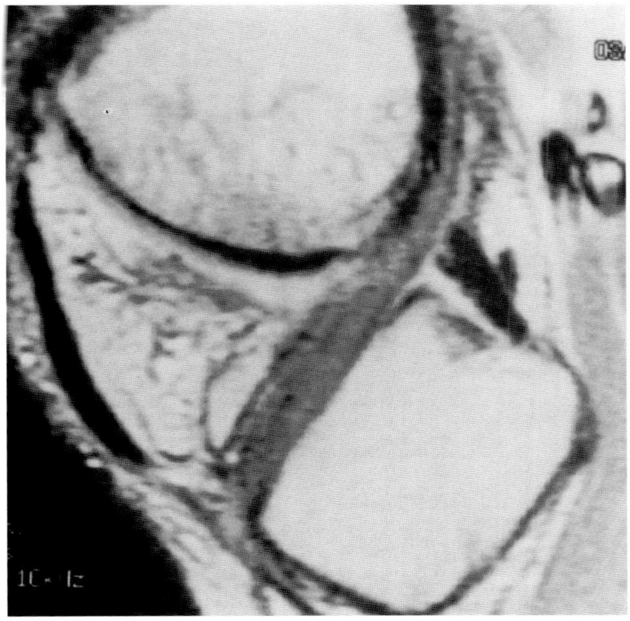

FIG. 11-28. The whole of the neoligament is of increased signal intensity on this oblique sagittal spin-echo image (TR 2500 msec, TR 90 msec) except for a few scattered fibers consistent with ligamentization in this 2-year-old neoligament.

this situation the graft is more likely to rupture, and some investigators have measured the change in signal intensity within the neoligament in impinged versus unimpinged grafts to support this hypothesis (79). In particular, this study suggests that presence of increased signal intensity on T1-weighted images of the distal portion of the graft may be a significant indication of impingement and a possible harbinger of impending failure. If impingement is relieved, signal intensity tends to diminish.

One of the most crucial aspects of neoligament reconstruction using these techniques has been accurate tibial tunnel placement (61,89) (Figs. 11-29 and 11-30). Should the tunnel be placed too anteriorly, when the knee is extended, the neoligament will bend around the anterior inferior edge of the intercondylar roof, thereby causing the neoligament to rasp over the bony surface (90). This predisposes the ligament to failure. For this reason enlargement of the intercondylar notch may be necessary (88,91). This diagnosis is extremely difficult to make clinically prior to neoligament failure. Plain-film findings on the lateral projection may sometimes suggest this if sclerosis of the osseous tibial tunnel can be visualized; however, tunnel position and the neoligament are more readily seen with MRI (92).

In patients with a normal reconstruction, the neoligaments and its fibers course straight through the intercondylar notch without any significant bending either anteriorly or posteriorly. The fibers are parallel to the tibial tunnel and the roof of the intercondylar notch. Marked bowing, frank discontinuity of fibers, or the absence of neoligament within the osseous tunnel indicates partial or complete failure of the neoligament (62,77,78) (Figs. 11-31 and 11-32). T2- and T2*-weighted images in particular are useful in this situation, because the osseous tunnel and neoligament remnants are often outlined by joint fluid (Figs. 11-33 and 11-34). If a patellar tendon reconstruction has been performed, the extensive metal artifact produced by the large interference screws (which are introduced into the osseous tunnel in an effort to wedge in the tendon bone block) can sometimes preclude visualization of most of the tibial tunnel and restrict the assessment of graft failure to the intra-articular portion of the graft.

Our experience indicates that failure of the graft is usually seen in the intra-articular portion or tibial tunnel portion and not more proximally. Some reports of visualization of a retracted portion of a graft toward the femoral insertion have appeared in the literature (1). An indirect sign of graft failure is anterior subluxation of the tibia in relation to the femur, which is best seen on sagittal images through the lateral compartment (Fig. 11-35).

Some work has been done with intravenous gadolinium in an effort to improve visualization of the neoligament (93). Enhancement of the synovial membrane surrounding the neoligament may allow the graft to be more readily identified. Preliminary studies indicate that relatively little enhancement of the neoligament itself is noted during the first 4 months following implantation, but by 7 months or more, a significant number of neoligaments demonstrate readily appreciable en-

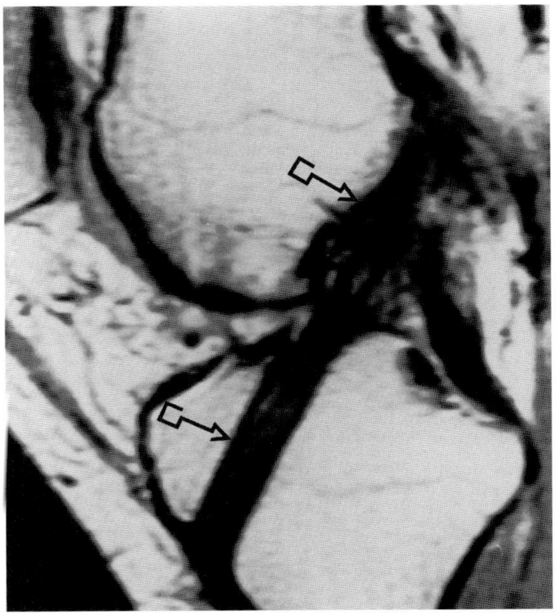

FIG. 11-29. Collinear tunnel. Oblique sagittal spin-echo proton density (TR 2000 msec, TE 30 msec) image from a 6-month-old neoligament of almost uniform low signal intensity. The intra-articular *(upper arrow)* and tibial *(lower arrow)* portions of the graft form a straight line when the knee is in the extended position, which is ideal. (From Munk PL, et al. *Can J Radiol* 1992;43:411–419. Used with permission.)

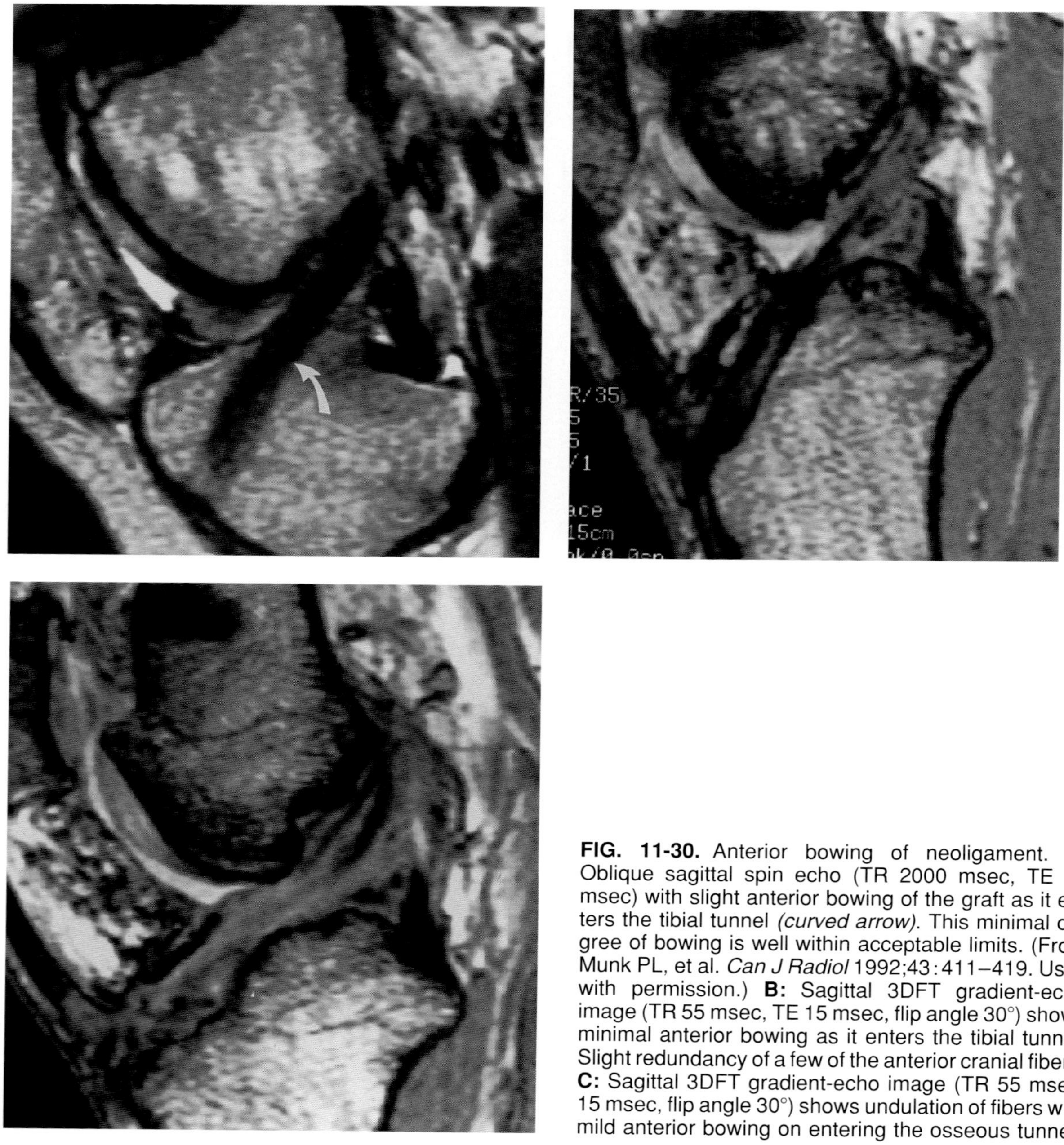

A B C

FIG. 11-30. Anterior bowing of neoligament. **A:** Oblique sagittal spin echo (TR 2000 msec, TE 60 msec) with slight anterior bowing of the graft as it enters the tibial tunnel *(curved arrow)*. This minimal degree of bowing is well within acceptable limits. (From Munk PL, et al. *Can J Radiol* 1992;43:411–419. Used with permission.) **B:** Sagittal 3DFT gradient-echo image (TR 55 msec, TE 15 msec, flip angle 30°) shows minimal anterior bowing as it enters the tibial tunnel. Slight redundancy of a few of the anterior cranial fibers. **C:** Sagittal 3DFT gradient-echo image (TR 55 msec, 15 msec, flip angle 30°) shows undulation of fibers with mild anterior bowing on entering the osseous tunnel.

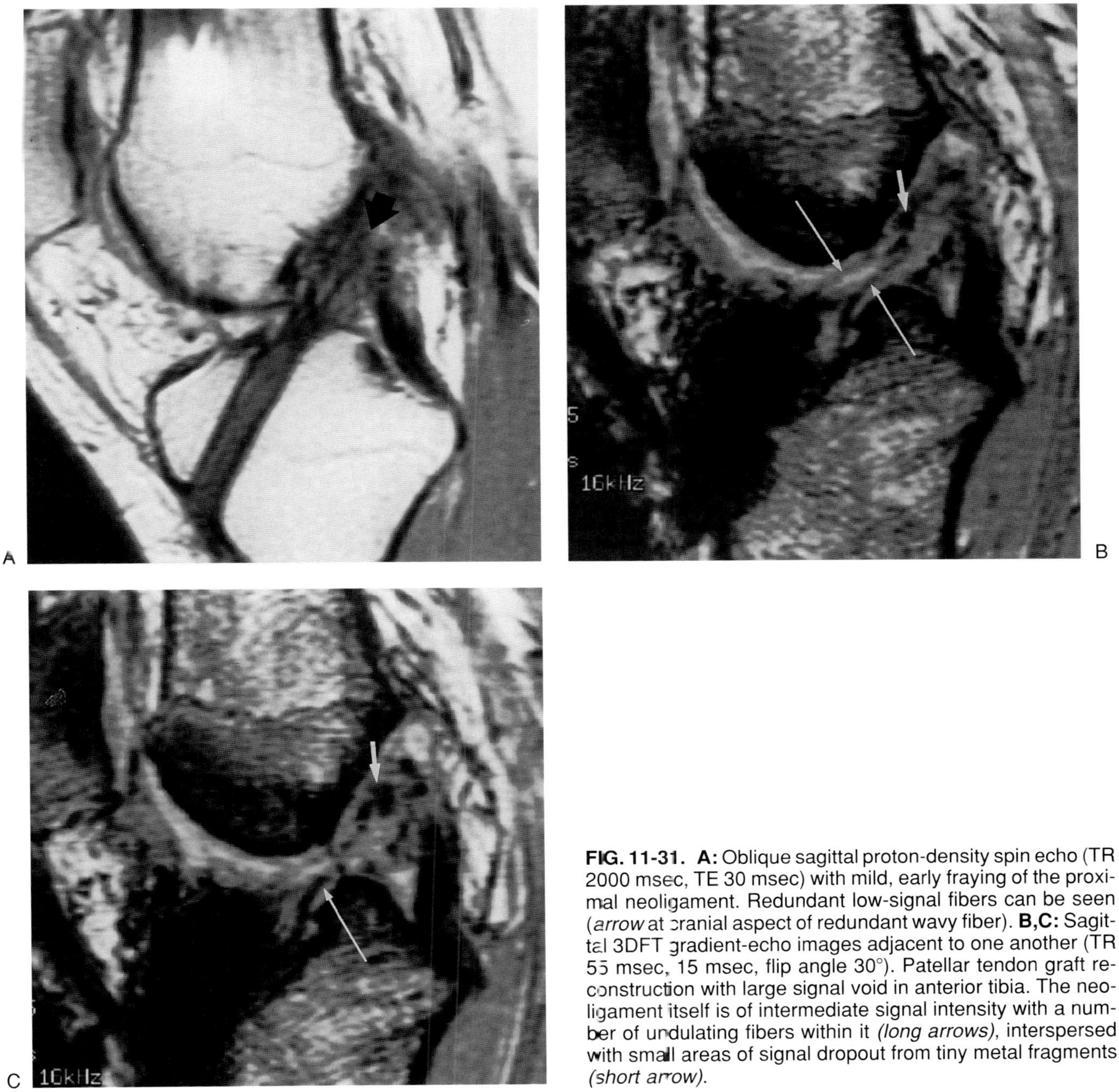

FIG. 11-31. A: Oblique sagittal proton-density spin echo (TR 2000 msec, TE 30 msec) with mild, early fraying of the proximal neoligament. Redundant low-signal fibers can be seen (*arrow* at cranial aspect of redundant wavy fiber). **B,C:** Sagittal 3DFT gradient-echo images adjacent to one another (TR 55 msec, 15 msec, flip angle 30°). Patellar tendon graft reconstruction with large signal void in anterior tibia. The neoligament itself is of intermediate signal intensity with a number of undulating fibers within it *(long arrows)*, interspersed with small areas of signal dropout from tiny metal fragments *(short arrow)*.

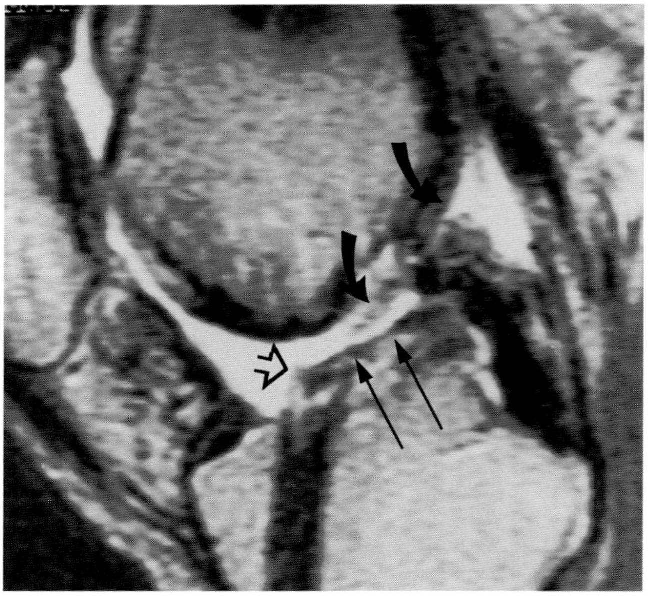

FIG. 11-32. Oblique sagittal T2-weighted spin-echo image (TR 2000 msec, TE 60 msec) of a high-grade tear of an anterior cruciate neoligament. A few cranial fibers remain in position *(curved arrow)*. Most of the fibers lie dependent in the posterior aspect of the joint space *(arrows)*. Marked angulation is present where the remnant of the neoligament enters the tibial tunnel *(hollow arrow)*. High-signal joint fluid helps outline these structures.

hancement. These changes parallel the ligamentization described earlier. Whether use of gadolinium routinely would provide more accurate evaluation of reconstructed anterior cruciate ligaments remains to be evaluated.

We have seen only a few examples of anterior cruciate reconstruction in the immature knee. This type of reconstruction requires that the proximal tibial epiphysis be violated—a situation normally best avoided. The appearance of the neoligament is similar to that in the mature knee (Fig. 11-36). Evidence of possible epiphysis plate fusion should be carefully searched for.

POSTERIOR CRUCIATE LIGAMENT

As discussed in the previous chapter on cruciate ligaments, tears of the posterior cruciate ligament are considerably less frequent than those of the anterior cruciate ligament, in large part because of its greater strength (94,95). Unfortunately, for many years the role of the posterior cruciate knee stabilization was not sufficiently appreciated (and still remains to some degree controversial); therefore, when the posterior cruciate ligament was damaged, limited interest in its reconstruction existed (94–97). For these reasons work on MRI assessment of posterior cruciate ligament reconstruction is not as extensive as that on anterior cruciate reconstruction.

Most disruptions of the posterior cruciate ligaments are actually avulsion injuries, usually accompanied by displacement of a bone fragment. Interstitial tears or femoral avulsions are far less common. If a tibial fragment has been avulsed, conservative therapy may be successful, with surgical union of the fragment or fixation of the bone (98,99). Primary repair is rarely possible because of fraying, and, if attempted, results in a significantly weaker ligament than normal (42) (Fig. 11-37).

Since considerable force is required to disrupt the posterior cruciate, associated injuries are very common, with isolated injury being in the 0–30% range. Proponents of reconstruction feel this ligament is crucial to knee stability and argue that all disruptions should be repaired, although whether this should be done acutely is unclear (97,100–103). Others propose reconstruction only if multidirectional instability exists (104). It has been established that deficiency of the posterior cruciate increases medial and patellofemoral compartment pressures, especially if posterolateral ligament/muscle insufficiency is present, which leads to multidirectional instability (105,106).

With increasing experience, promising results have been reported with neoligament construction, although these in general are still not as good as repair of avulsion injuries (103,107,108). Regardless of surgical technique used or whether conservative therapy is elected, patients who sustain their injury in athletic activities tend to do better than those involved in motor vehicle accidents (98,101).

Techniques have been developed for reconstruction of the posterior cruciate that have used a wide variety of different materials, including iliotibial band fascial grafts, patellar tendon, meniscus, popliteal tendon, Achilles tendon, semitendinosis tendon, and synthetics (77,94,95,100,102,104,109). Currently, the medial segment of the medial head of the gastrocnemius tendon is used by most surgeons. In this technique the tendon is directed in a trajectory similar to that of the posterior cruciate and passed through a femoral tunnel. Drill holes are also placed through the tibia most of the time through which sutures are passed. If possible, primary repair of the torn cruciate is also performed. Another method uses a patellar tendon–bone graft to construct a neoligament (99). As would be expected, the placement of the bone in the tunnels for the neoligament is different from that of the ante-

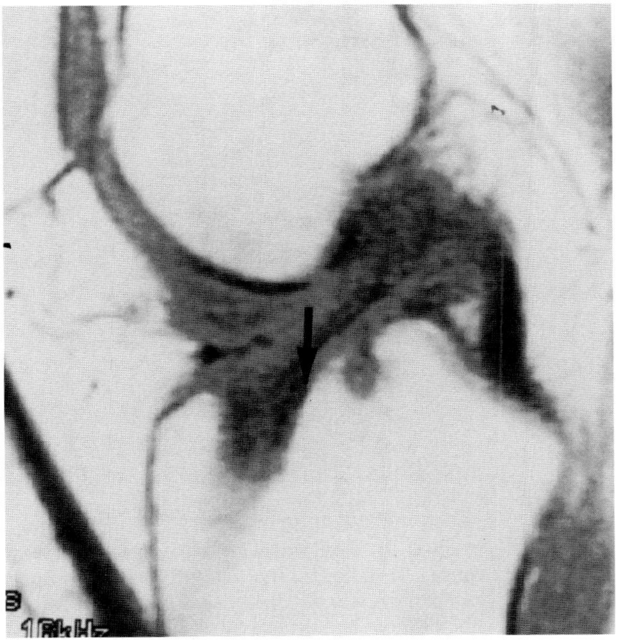

A

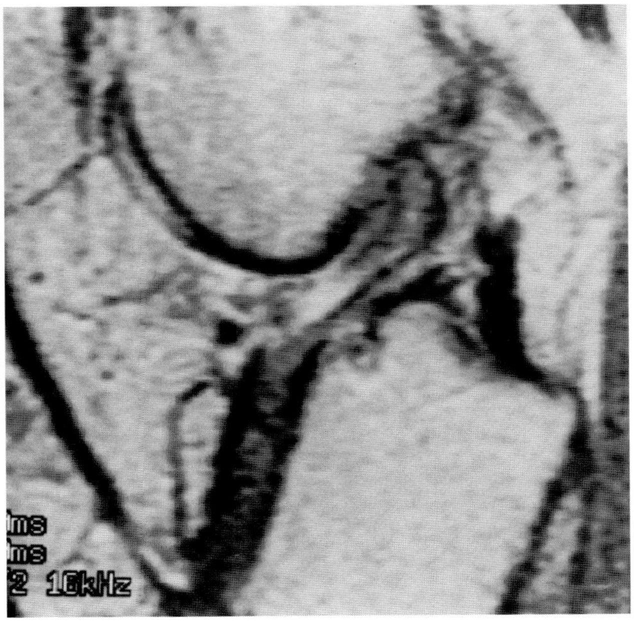

B

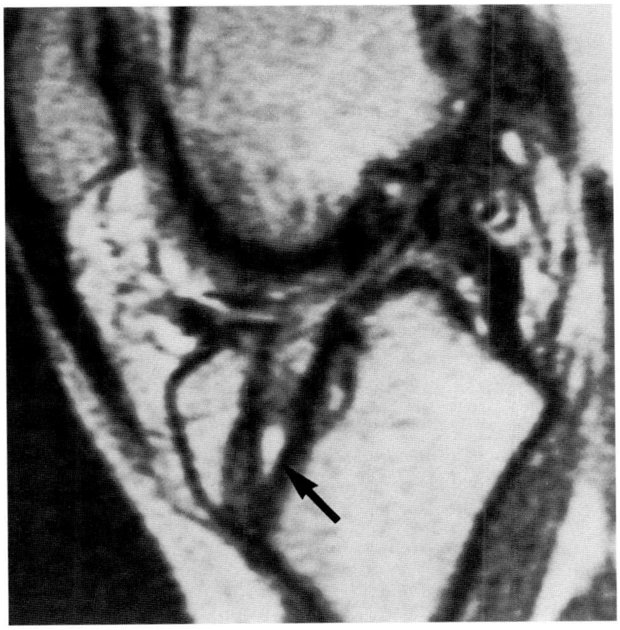

C

FIG. 11-33. High-grade, nearly complete tear. **A:** Sagittal T1-weighted spin echo (TR 600 msec, TE 18 msec) shows a thick-appearing neoligament of intermediate signal intensity, with low-signal fibers centrally. These low-signal fibers show abrupt angulation at the point of entry into the tibial tunnel *(arrow)*. The cranial portion of the neoligament has a mop-ended configuration. **B:** Oblique sagittal proton-density image (TR 2000 msec, TE 20 msec) from the same patient shows these findings more vividly. **C:** Similar features are seen from another patient on a oblique sagittal T2-weighted image (TR 2200 msec, TE 80 msec). In this instance a small amount of fluid is seen in the tibial tunnel *(arrow)*.

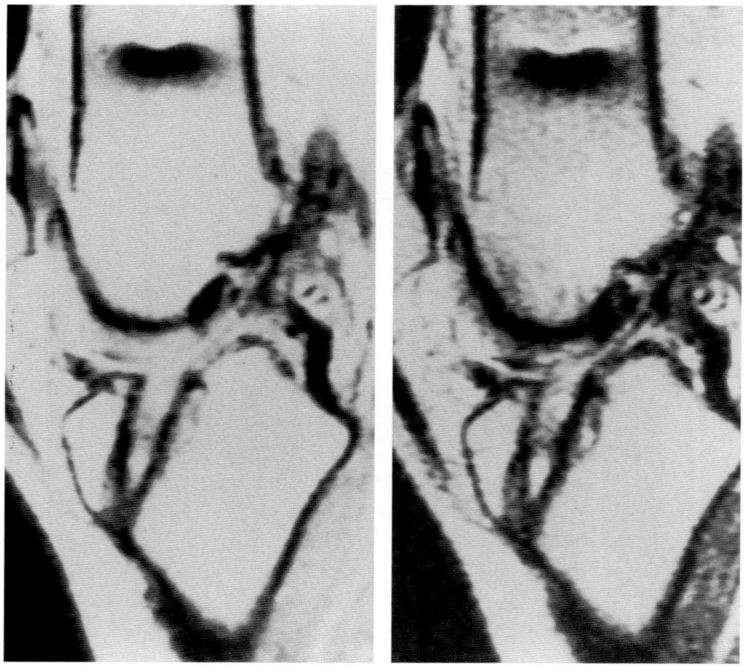

A B

FIG. 11-34. Complete neoligament tear. **A,B:** Oblique sagittal proton-density and T2-weighted (TR 2000 msec, TE 30 and 60 msec) images in a patient with a 2-year-old neoligament. The ligament is completely disrupted, with only a few wisplike cranial fibers seen. The tibial tunnel is completely filled with high-signal-intensity fluid.

rior cruciate (Fig. 11-38). The tibial tunnel is angulated to emerge more posteriorly in the region of the posterior lip of the tibia (Figs. 11-39 and 11-40). The femoral tunnel is angulated medially rather than laterally, as with the anterior cruciate reconstruction. This allows the intra-articular portion of the neoligament to run approximately in the same course as a normal posterior cruciate ligament. Because very extensive trauma is usually required to disrupt the posterior cruciate, the patient may undergo both anterior and posterior cruciate ligament repairs.

The literature on MRI of the posterior cruciate is very limited. Presumably, many of the same principles as imaging of the anterior cruciate neoligament would apply. We have found that the neoligament is of low signal intensity throughout, although a few ligaments that we have seen demonstrate slightly increased signal intensity, presumably reflecting the vascular ingrowth that has been documented with anterior cruciate neoligaments. Ideally, the ligament would be evaluated with images parallel to the plane in which it runs. For most reconstructions for the intra-articular portion of the neoligament, this would be close to the true sagittal plane. Evaluation of the intraosseous tunnel portion would require oblique sagittal images for the femoral and tibial components.

Considerably more experience will have to be accrued before criteria for evaluating the integrity of posterior cruciate neoligaments are available.

MEDIAL AND LATERAL COLLATERAL LIGAMENTS

The collateral ligaments are not frequently reconstructed in isolation. Isolated collateral ligament injuries probably do not require operative treatment and can be managed conservatively with good results, provided cruciate ligament damage and/or extensive meniscal injury are not present (110,111). Most patients who undergo reconstruction are also undergoing a cruciate ligament reconstruction, with collateral ligament augmentation being performed to give added stability to the joint. Repair of collateral ligaments may be important in preventing excessive loading of the cruciate ligaments (112).

In the vast majority of instances buttressing of the medial collateral ligaments (Figs. 11-41 and 11-42) is the procedure of choice; lateral reconstructions are done far less frequently (Fig. 11-43). In some cases, the torn medial collateral ligament may simply be sutured, and buttressing may be required if extensive disruption has occurred. In some cases, this may be accomplished by advancement of the pes anserine anteriorly. Laterally, reefing of the middle one-third of the capsule, tenodesis of the iliotibial band, and anterior transfer of the biceps tendon to the margin of Gerdy's tubercle are used, usually to treat anterolateral rotatory instability (111).

Extensive metal artifact is frequently present because of multiple sutures or staples used in the surgical repair. Since these staples may be relatively superficial, a small pseudobursa may be apparent adjacent to them, which is best appreciated with T2-weighted images (77) (Fig. 11-44). These reconstructions are best evaluated on coronal images. When these reconstructions are reviewed 6 months or more following reconstruction, they usually are uniformly of diminished signal intensity, reflecting the fact that the ligaments themselves are of low signal and the extensive scar that is coapted over the repaired area is of low signal inten-

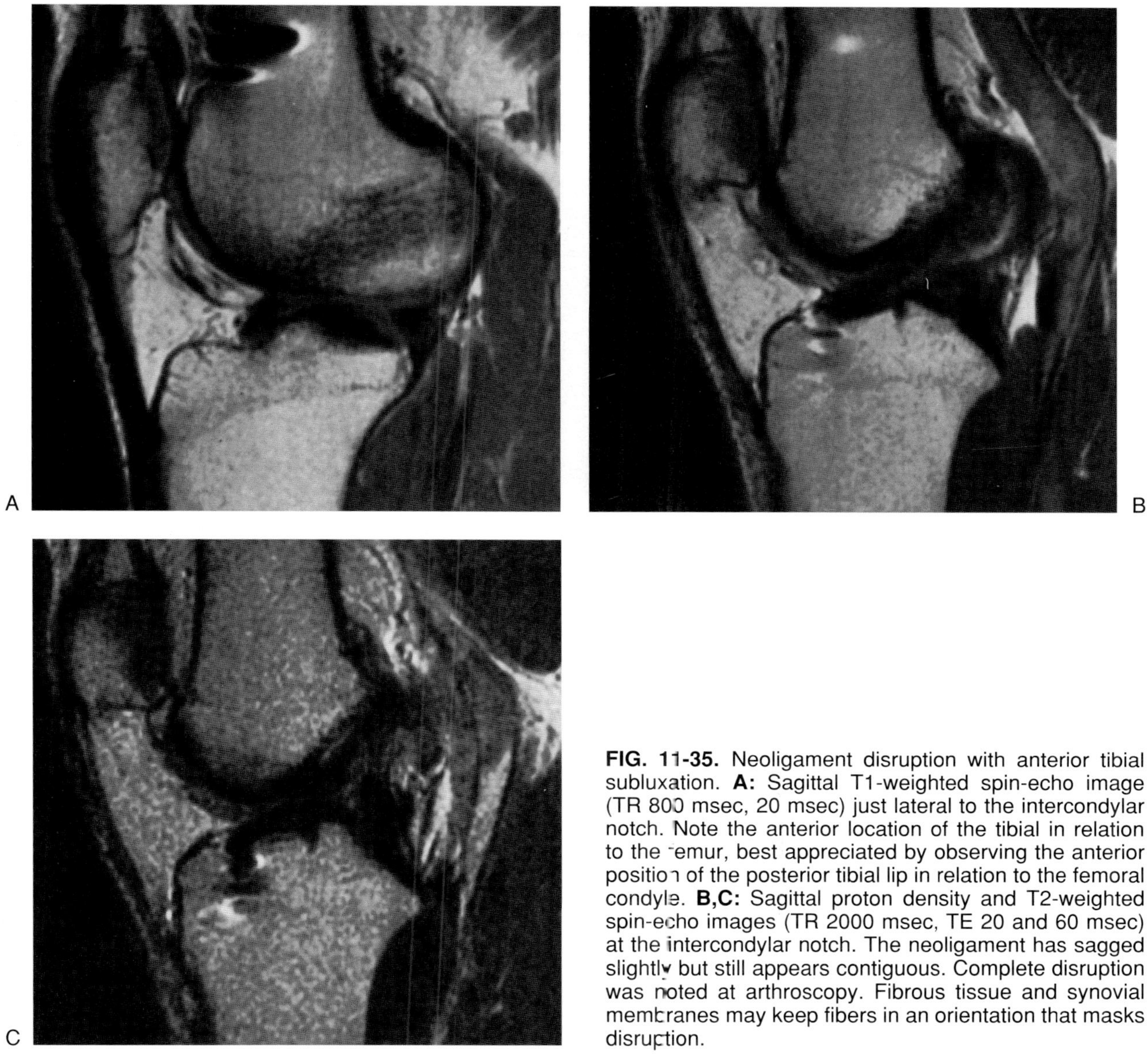

FIG. 11-35. Neoligament disruption with anterior tibial subluxation. **A:** Sagittal T1-weighted spin-echo image (TR 800 msec, 20 msec) just lateral to the intercondylar notch. Note the anterior location of the tibial in relation to the femur, best appreciated by observing the anterior position of the posterior tibial lip in relation to the femoral condyle. **B,C:** Sagittal proton density and T2-weighted spin-echo images (TR 2000 msec, TE 20 and 60 msec) at the intercondylar notch. The neoligament has sagged slightly but still appears contiguous. Complete disruption was noted at arthroscopy. Fibrous tissue and synovial membranes may keep fibers in an orientation that masks disruption.

sity. Linear areas of increased signal intensity are not unusual, however, and presumably reflect immature scar or areas of trapped fat or seroma and residual edema.

PATELLAR TENDON AND QUADRICEPS MECHANISM

The most frequent postoperative findings seen in this area relate to the patellar tendon. This is especially true in patients that have undergone anterior cruciate ligament reconstruction, because a large portion of these are reconstructed from harvested patellar tendon bone block grafts that are obtained either from the medial or central third of the patellar tendon. A small defect at the anterior, inferior portion of the patella can be seen. Immediately after harvesting, evidence of seroma and edema in the subcutaneous fat and Hoffa's fat pad is commonly encountered. These gradually recede, leaving a tendon that, with time, may actually be slightly thicker than normal due to the healing process. Small areas of increased signal intensity within the substance of the tendon are not unusual and are not necessarily significant. It has also been noted that the first-year postgraft harvesting, although a low patella (patella baja), is not unusual and may relate to weakness of the quadriceps muscles as well as to adhesions to the fat pad. As muscle strength returns with patient reconditioning following surgery, this usually disappears. An increased incidence of patellar fractures, patellar tracking abnormalities, and patellar rupture has been reported in these patients (1).

Patients who have undergone patellar tendon repairs following rupture usually have extensive metal artifact within the substance of the tendon and immediately adjacent to it.

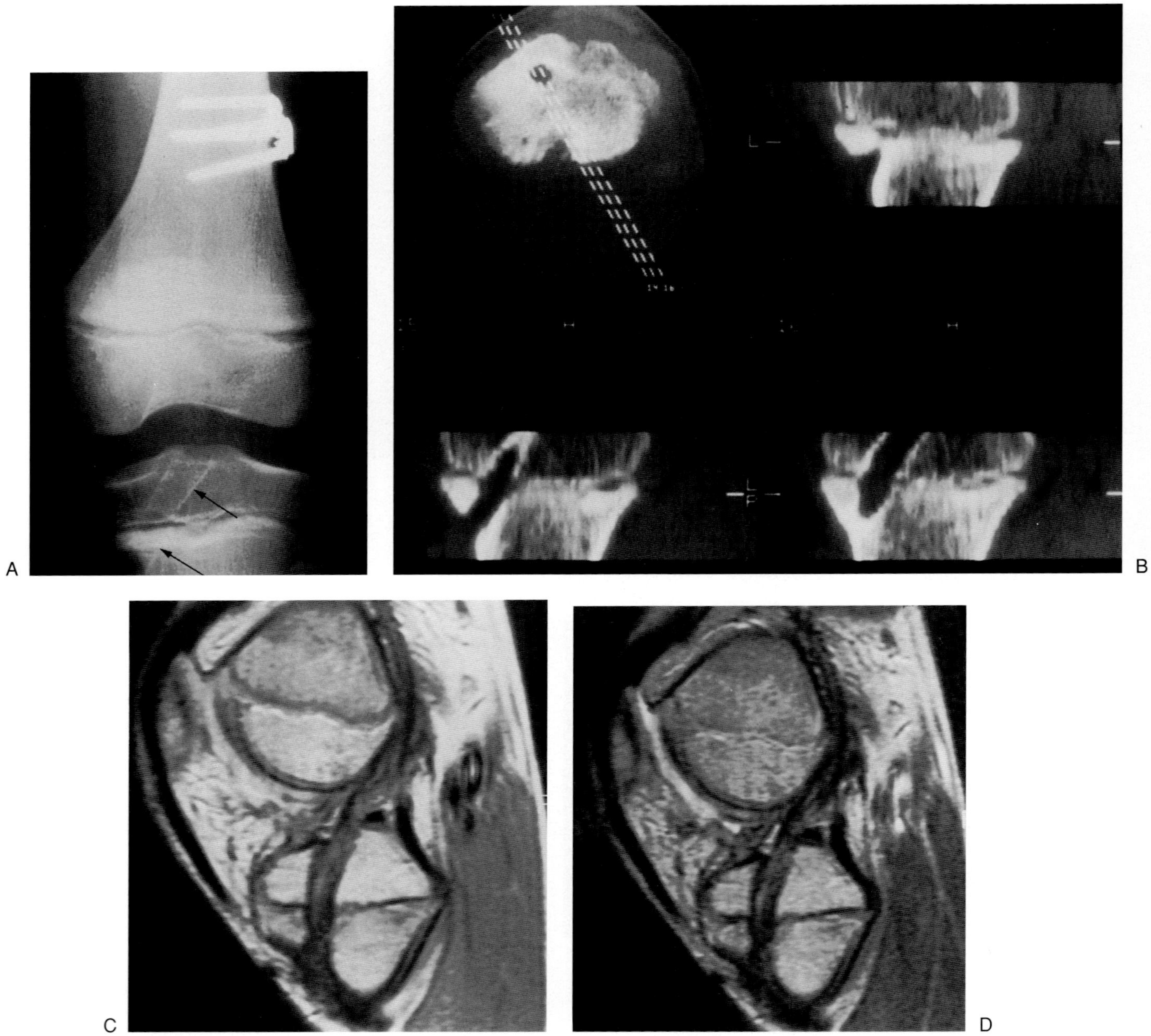

FIG. 11-36. Anterior cruciate neoligament in an immature knee. **A:** AP radiograph. Metal bone staples distal femur. Note the thin sclerotic lines in the proximal tibia, crossing the epiphyseal plate *(arrow)*. **B:** CT scan with thin sections and reformatting in an oblique plane show the epiphyseal plate and tibial tunnel. Since the plate is in the plane of section small areas of early fusion could easily be missed with this technique. In addition soft tissue is not optimal for displaying the neoligament. **C,D:** Oblique sagittal proton density and T2-weighted images (TR 2400 msec, TE 20 and 80 msec). The course of the neoligament is readily followed *(arrows)*. The epiphyseal plate is cut perpendicular to the slice, allowing any possible areas of fusion to be seen.

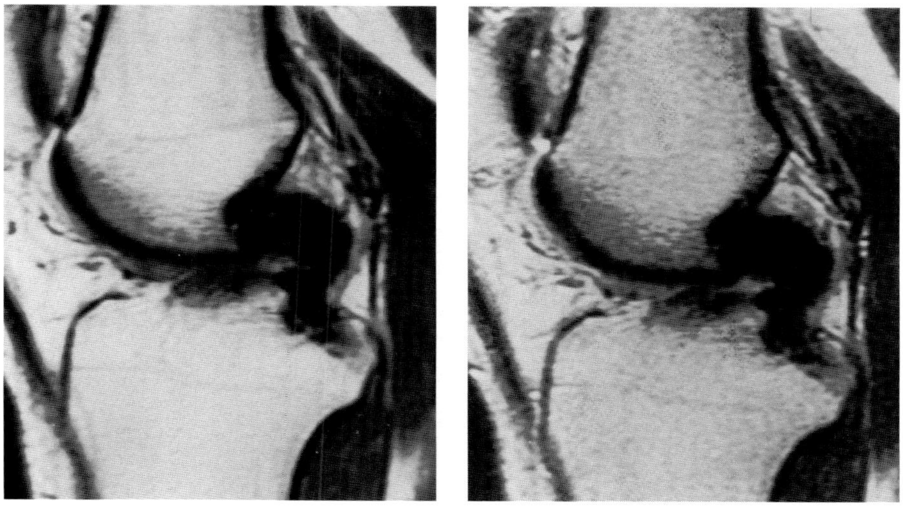

A B

FIG. 11-37. Sagittal T1-weighted **(A)** spin-echo (TR msec 800 msec, TR 20 msec) and T2-weighted **(B)** (TR 2000, TE 80) images from a patient who had a complete disruption of the posterior cruciate in its middle portion. The ligament was sutured together at this site and no neoligament was placed. The repaired ligament is of low signal intensity and appears thicker than normal, probably because of both scar tissue as well as signal dropout from numerous tiny metal fragments.

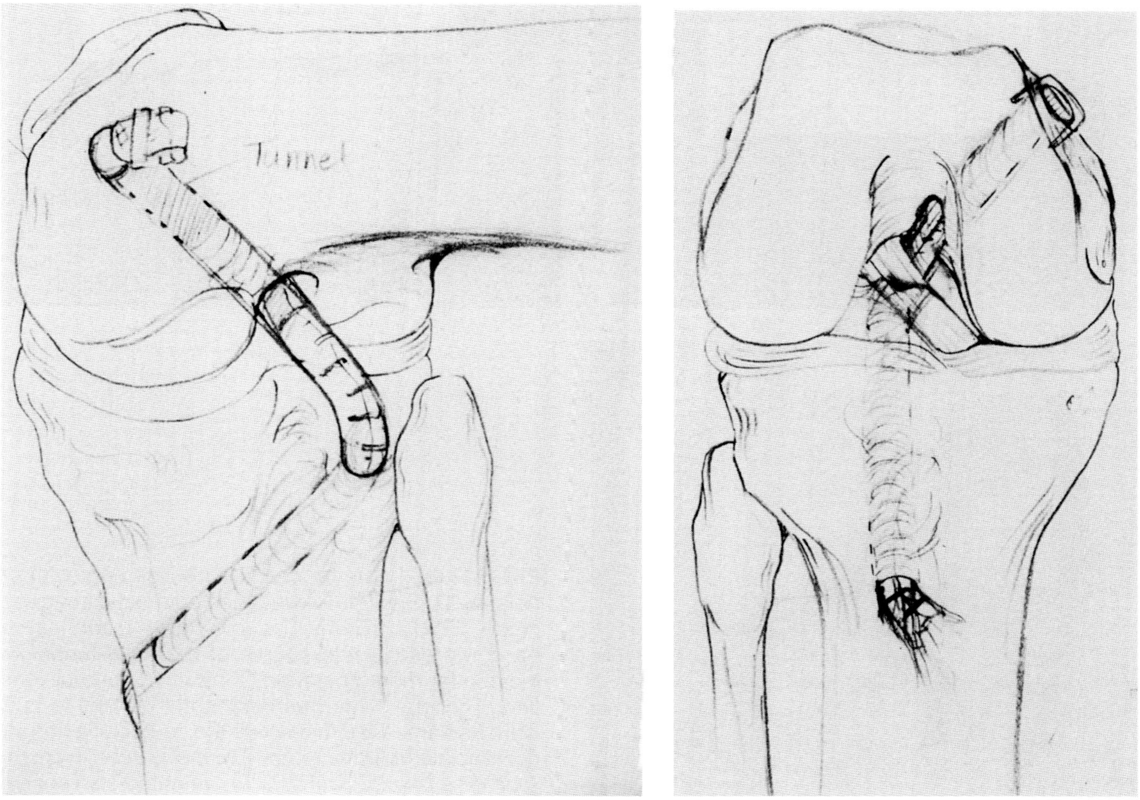

A B

FIG. 11-38. Posterior cruciate neoligament. **A,B:** Line diagrams showing a posterior cruciate neoligament in situ in a flexed knee as viewed from posterolaterally and AP.

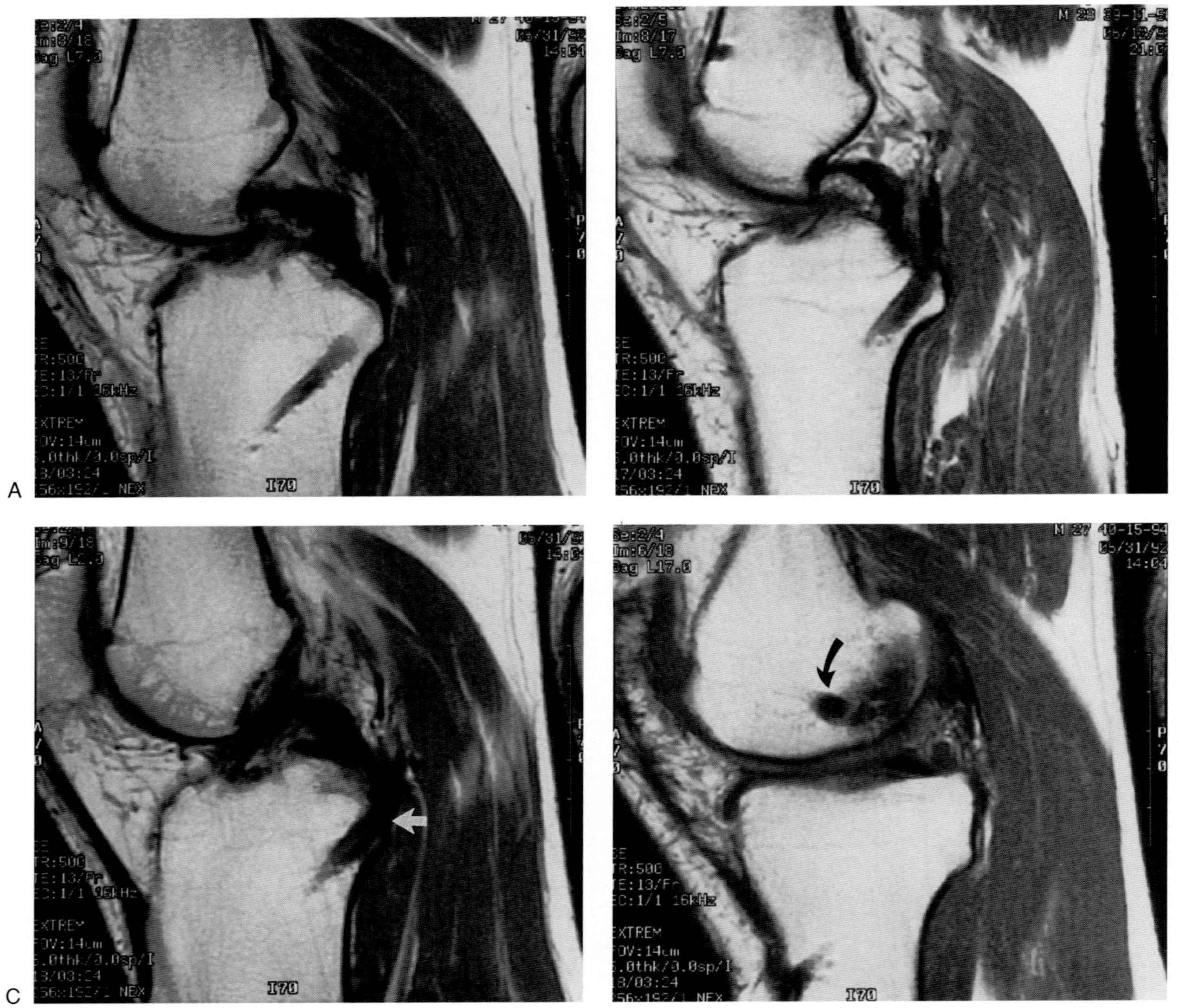

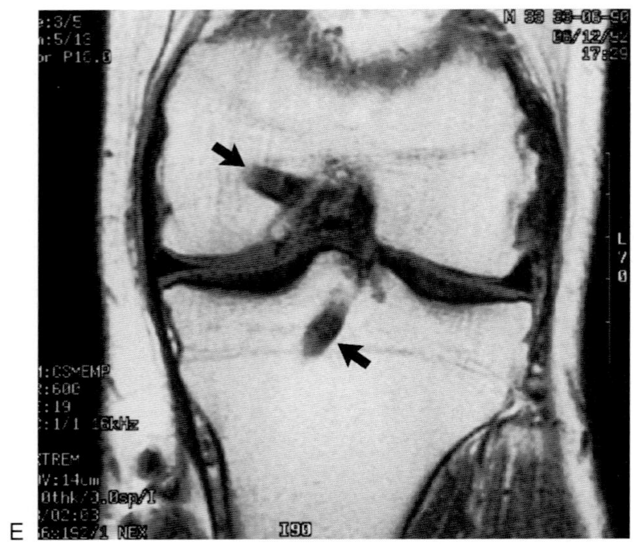

FIG. 11-39. Posterior cruciate neoligament with dual tunnels. **A–D:** Sagittal T1-weighted spin-echo images (TR 500 msec, TE 13 msec). The low-signal diagonally oriented band represents the course of the tibial tunnel, which is located far more posteriorly than in an anterior reconstruction. The graft emerges posteriorly *(arrow)* to curves upward and anteriorly mimicking the course of a normal posterior cruciate. In **D** the femoral tunnel is seen in cross section *(curved arrow)*. **E:** Coronal T1-weighted spin echo (TR 600 msec, TE 19 msec). Both femoral and tibial tunnels have been caught in tangent near the intercondylar notch and are seen as low-signal bands *(arrow)*.

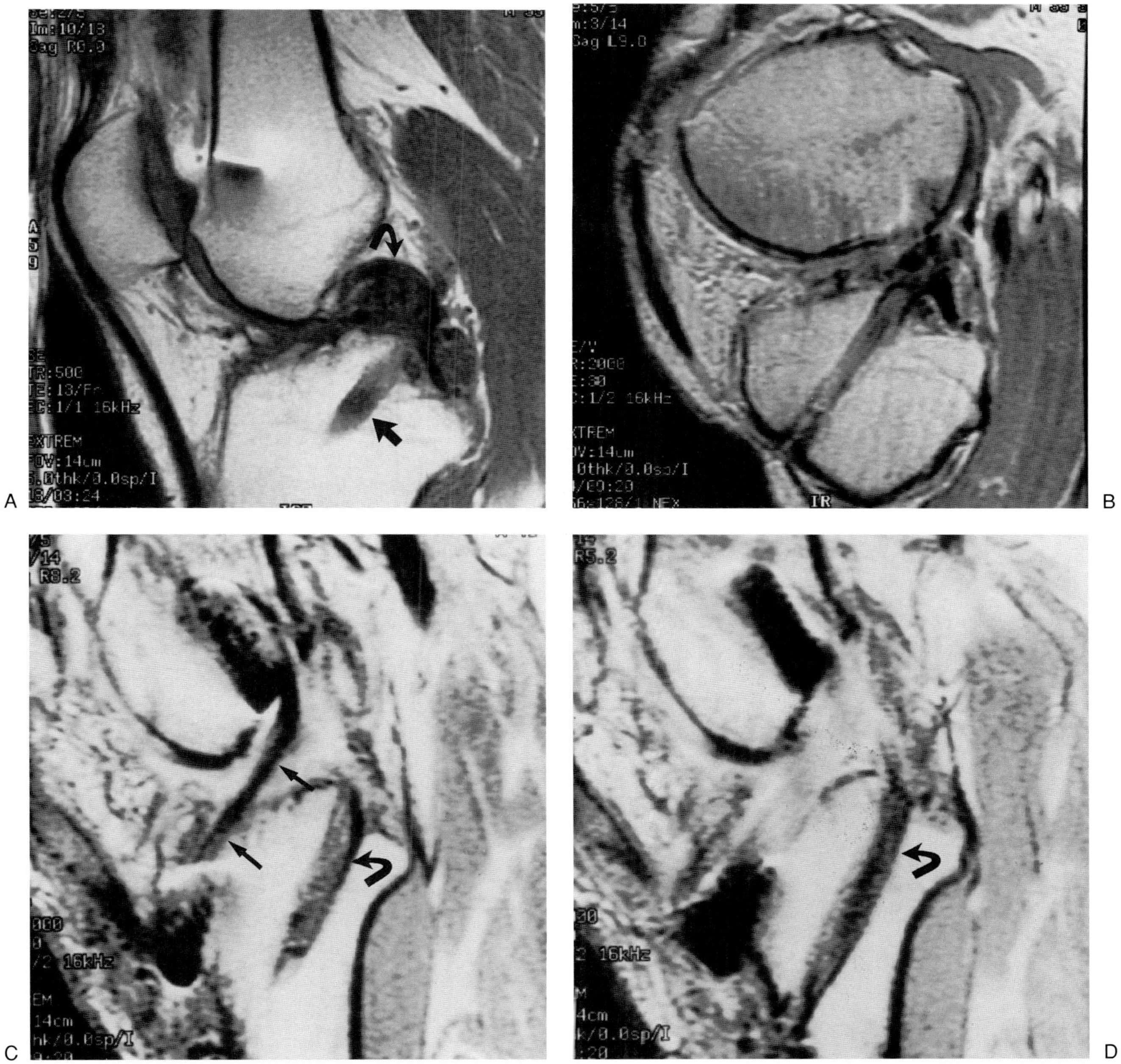

FIG. 11-40. Posterior cruciate reconstructions. **A:** Sagittal T1-weighted spin echo (TR 500 msec, TE 13 msec). The proximal tibial tunnel is located slightly more anteriorly than in the previous example shown *(arrow)*. The disrupted and slightly atrophic native posterior cruciate is seen below the intercondylar notch as a curled low-signal structure *(curved arrow)*. **B:** Oblique sagittal proton-density spin echo (TR 2000 msec, TE 30 msec). The neoligament is of intermediate signal intensity more than a year after surgery. **C,D:** Oblique sagittal T2-weighted spin echo (TR 2000 msec, TR 80 msec) in a patient who underwent reconstruction of both anterior and posterior cruciates. The anterior cruciate *(arrows)* is of lower signal intensity than the posterior *(curved arrow)*.

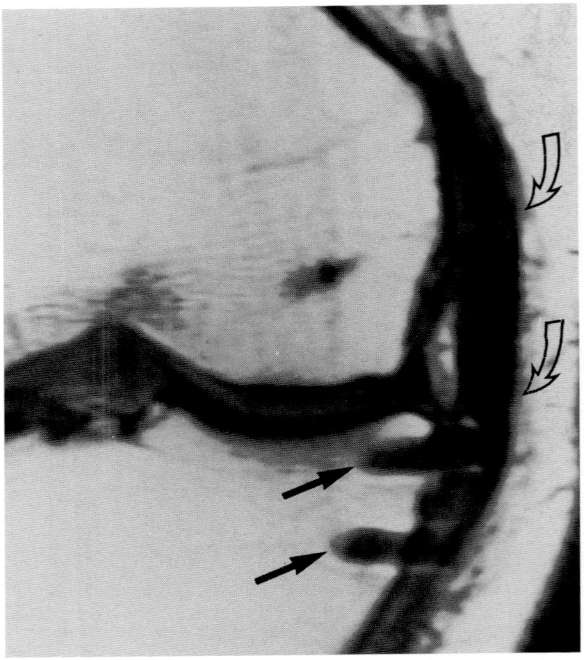

FIG. 11-41. Reconstructed medial collateral ligament. Coronal T1-weighted spin-echo image (TR 800 msec, TE 20 msec) shows the ligament as an irregular thick band of low signal intensity *(curved arrows)*. Two bone staples *(arrows)* used in transfixing the reconstructed ligament to the proximal tibia produce small linear areas of signal dropout. (From Munk PL, et al. *Can Assoc Radiol J* 1995; 43:411–419. With permission.)

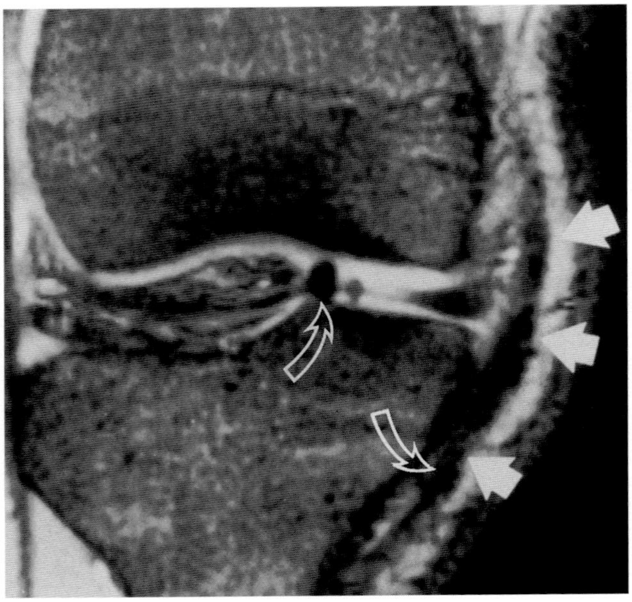

FIG. 11-42. Coronal gradient-echo MPRG (TR 400 msec, TE 20 msec, flip angle 30°). Buttressing of medial collateral ligament structures by advancing the pes anserine tendons. Marked thickening of the soft tissues at the medial aspect of the knee is present *(white arrows)*, which represents the pes anserine tendons that have been moved anteriorly and oversewn to improve support. *Curved arrows* indicate small areas of signal dropout caused by metal fragments.

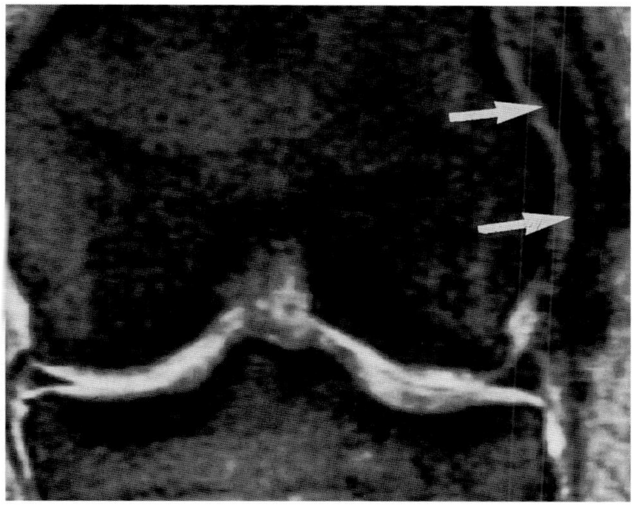

FIG. 11-43. Lateral ligament reconstruction. Coronal gradient-echo MPGR (TR 400 msec, TE 20 msec, flip angle 30°). Several thick bands of low-signal-intensity area seen at the lateral aspect of the knee, consistent with augmentation of the ligament *(arrows)*. Interspersed areas of low-signal "bloom" are due to tiny metal fragments that are more apparent with the gradient-echo technique used. (From Munk PL, et al. *Can Assoc Radiol J* 1995; 43:411–419. With permission.)

A 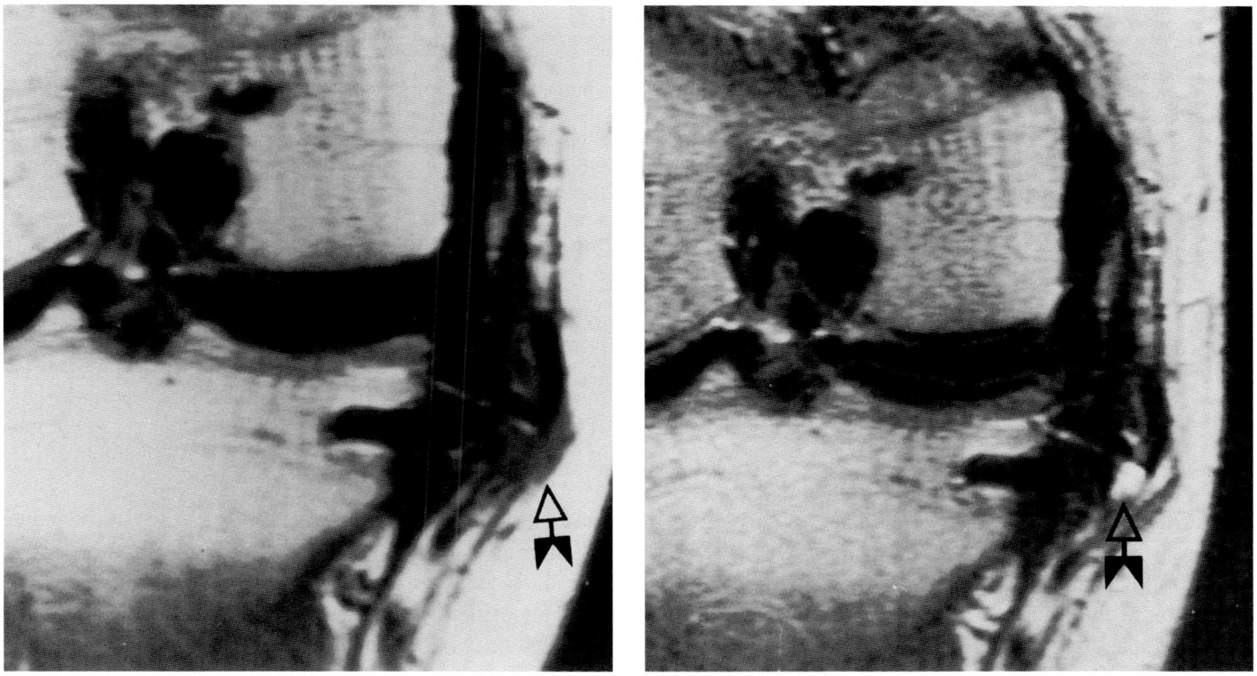 B

FIG. 11-44. Pseudo-bursae formation. **A,B:** Coronal proton-density and T2-weighted spin-echo (TR 2000 msec, TE 30 & 60 msec) images from a patient who underwent collateral ligament reconstruction 2 years previously and presented with pain adjacent to the joint line near the site of reconstruction, but no joint instability. Small fluid-filled structures may form overlying prominent pieces of hardware such as screws or staples as in this case. A small structure that brightens with T2 weighting *(arrow)* is a small pseudobursa at the surface of a protuberant staple. These may be treated by removal of the offending hardware or anti-inflammatory agents.

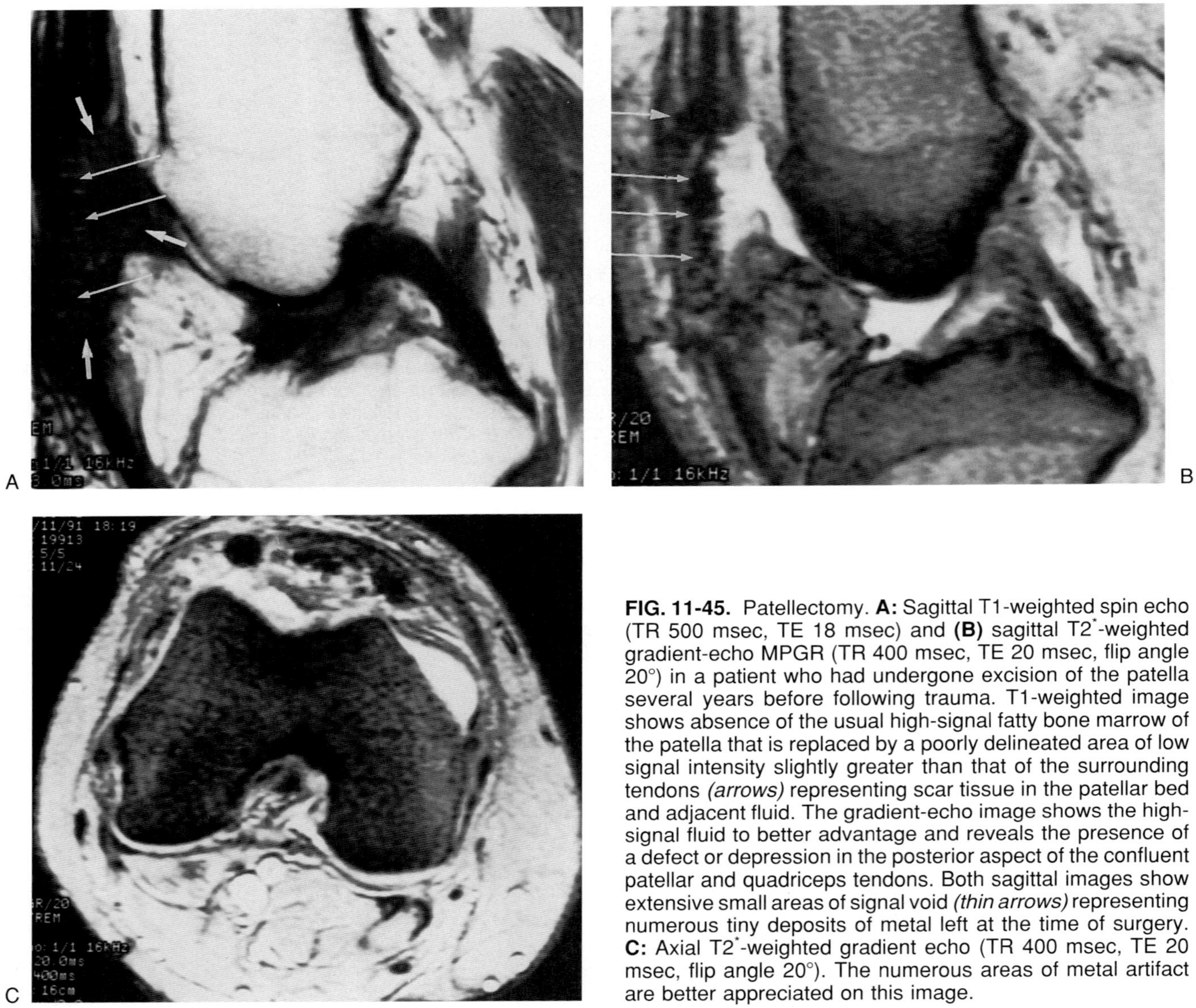

FIG. 11-45. Patellectomy. **A:** Sagittal T1-weighted spin echo (TR 500 msec, TE 18 msec) and **(B)** sagittal $T2^*$-weighted gradient-echo MPGR (TR 400 msec, TE 20 msec, flip angle 20°) in a patient who had undergone excision of the patella several years before following trauma. T1-weighted image shows absence of the usual high-signal fatty bone marrow of the patella that is replaced by a poorly delineated area of low signal intensity slightly greater than that of the surrounding tendons *(arrows)* representing scar tissue in the patellar bed and adjacent fluid. The gradient-echo image shows the high-signal fluid to better advantage and reveals the presence of a defect or depression in the posterior aspect of the confluent patellar and quadriceps tendons. Both sagittal images show extensive small areas of signal void *(thin arrows)* representing numerous tiny deposits of metal left at the time of surgery. **C:** Axial $T2^*$-weighted gradient echo (TR 400 msec, TE 20 msec, flip angle 20°). The numerous areas of metal artifact are better appreciated on this image.

The patellar tendon may also be thickened, and if early after surgery, may show increased signal intensity due to edema.

Excision of the patella, or patellectomy, is seldom performed, except in the treatment of complex fractures (113). These patients usually demonstrate a large amount of metal artifact at the site of the excision, and for this reason use of gradient-echo imaging is often unsatisfactory because of the marked degradation of the image (Fig. 11-45). The now confluent patellar and quadriceps tendons often have a markedly irregular contour, with islands of increased signal intensity representing immature scar, connective tissue, and residual islands of bone. Hoffa's fat pad is usually very irregular and distorted.

Patients who have been treated for unstable patellae and/or chondromalacia patella by elevation of the patella using such procedures as the Maquet or Trillat operations often display a relatively normal-appearing patella and quadriceps tendon; however, the anterior aspect of the tibia is elevated (114) (Fig. 11-46). The few examples of this that we have seen have been in patients long after their surgery, and the only abnormality visible is distortion of the anterior aspect of the tibia where a well-assimilated bone block has been placed.

BONE AND CARTILAGE

Probably the most common bone and cartilage abnormality encountered relates to previous meniscus surgery. With excision of the meniscus changes and stresses across the joint ensue that lead to accelerated osteoarthritis. Early in the evolution of this process subchondral cysts and islands of osteonecrosis may become apparent. Cartilage thinning and focal defects arise. The classic findings of osteonecrotic

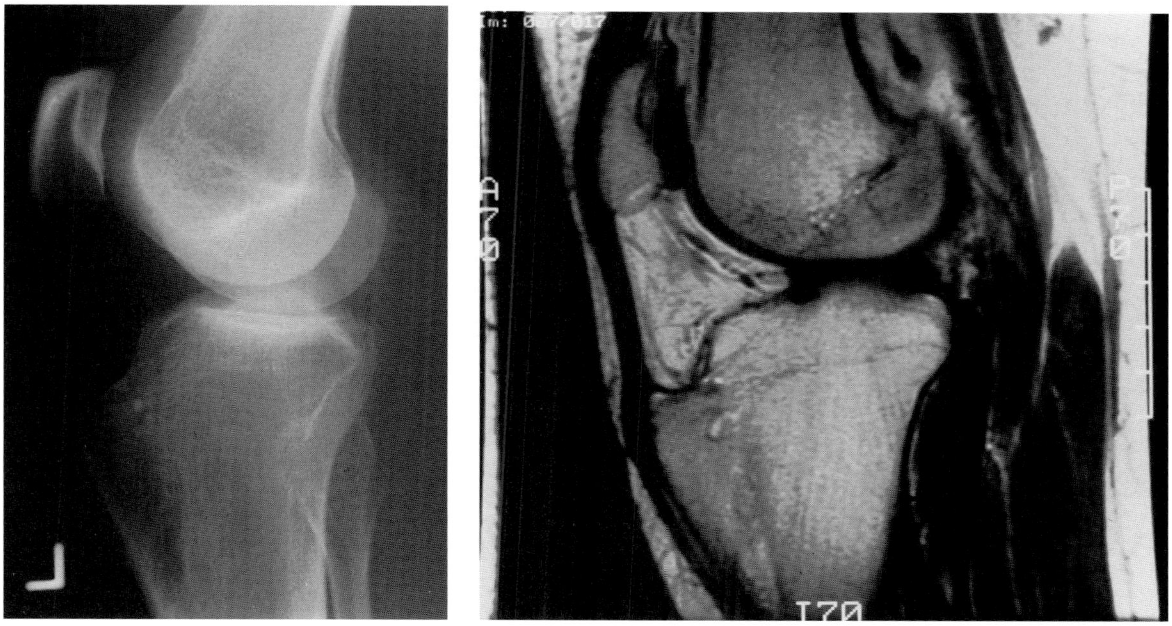

A B

FIG. 11-46. Patellar elevation. **A:** Lateral radiograph shows a very prominent tibial tuberosity. This patient had presented several years before with symptoms of chondromalacia patella unresponsive to conservative therapy and had undergone surgery with satisfactory results. **B:** Sagittal T1-weighted spin-echo image (TR 800 msec, TE 18 msec) from the same patient. The elevated tibial tuberosity shows good incorporation of the bone graft with confluence of the fatty marrow of the tibial shaft.

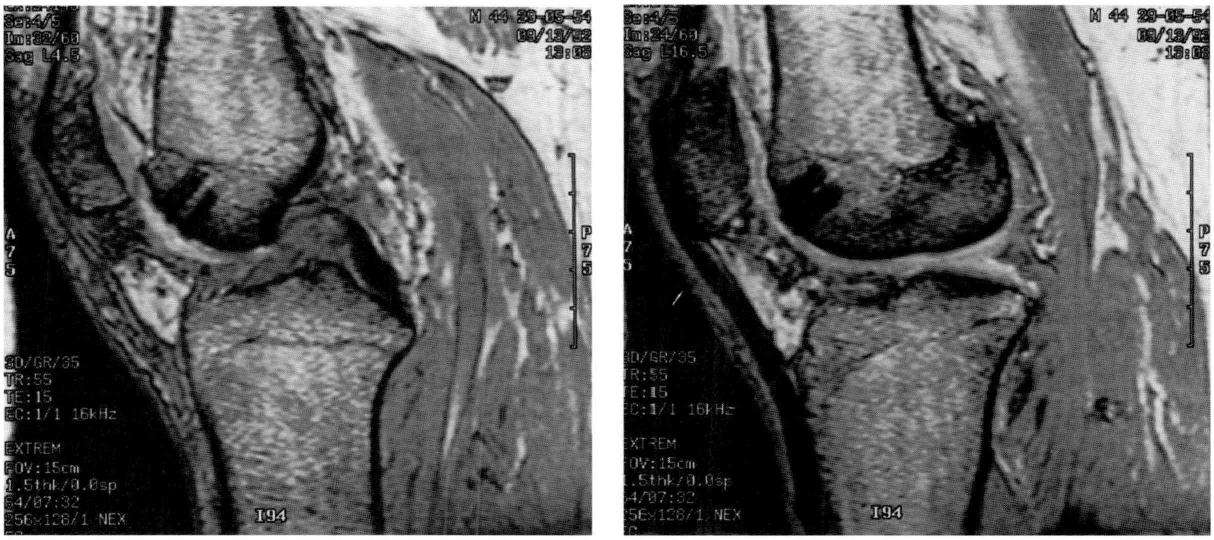

A B

FIG. 11-47. Carbon fiber implant patellofemoral compartment. **A,B:** Sagittal images 3DFT gradient-echo MPRG (TR 55 msec, TE 15 msec, flip angle 35°) noncontiguous. Two rectangular low-signal bands extend from the anterior femoral joint surface into the bone marrow, representing the arthroscopically placed carbon fiber plugs. These protrude very slightly above the level of the cortex, which is considered acceptable. The overlying cartilage has regenerated and appears intact.

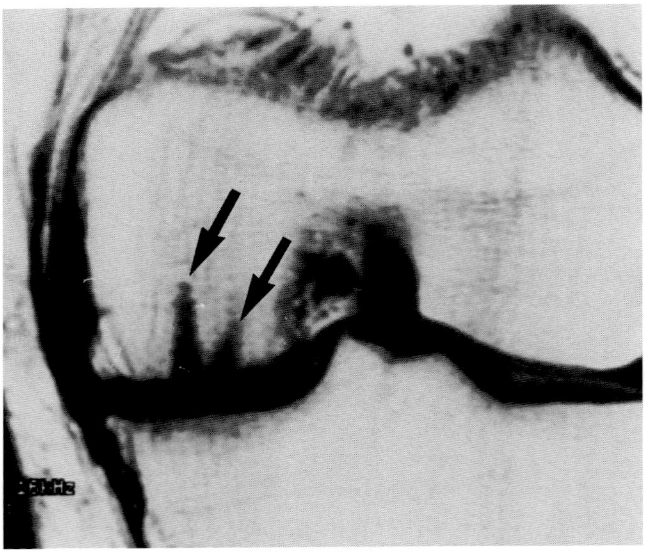

FIG. 11-48. Carbon fiber implant tibio-femoral compartment. Coronal T1-weighted spin echo (TR 600 msec, TE 20 msec). Rectangular areas of low signal intensity represent the sites where carbon fiber plugs have been inserted *(arrows)*.

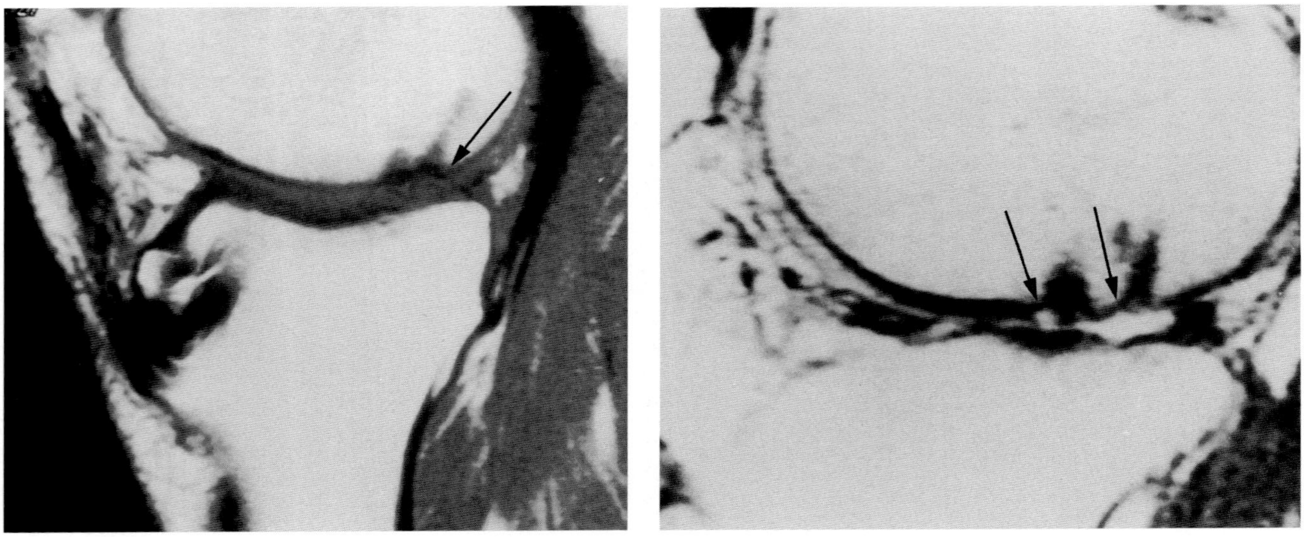

A B

FIG. 11-49. A: Sagittal T1-weighted spin echo (TR 800 msec, TE 18 msec). Obliquely oriented low-signal areas in the posterior aspect of the femoral condyle represent two carbon fiber plugs. The inferior aspect of the posterior plug is surrounded by intermediate signal fibrocartilage *(arrow)*. Metal artifact is seen in the anterior proximal tibia from previous ligament reconstructive surgery. **B:** Sagittal T2-weighted spin echo (TR 2000 msec, TE 60 msec). Low-signal areas in the posterior condyle represent well-incorporated carbon fiber plugs. High-signal fluid in the joint vividly demonstrates persistent defects in the cartilage *(arrows)*, which has not shown evidence of resurfacing more than a year after surgery.

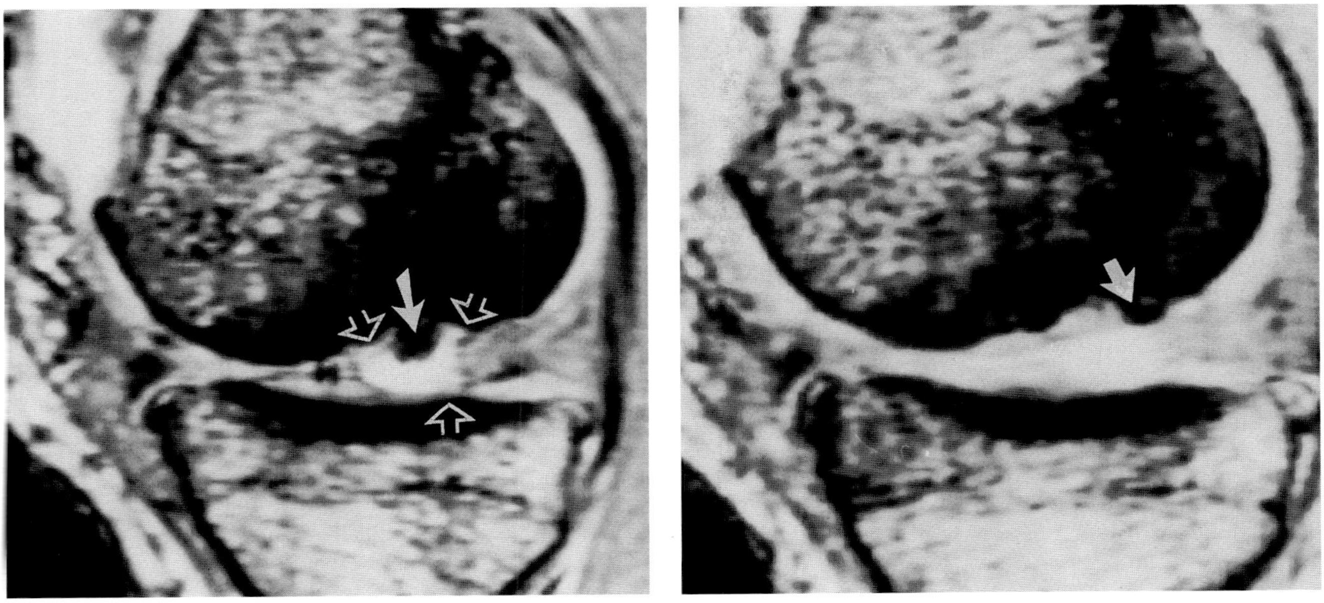

A B

FIG. 11-50. Failed carbon fiber implant. **A,B:** Adjacent sagittal T2* MPGR gradient echo (TR 55 msec, TE 15 msec, flip angle 35°). A large area of low signal intensity in the posterior femoral condyle. This represents the carbon fiber plug. A partially extruded segment of the plug is seen at the joint surface *(solid arrow)*. Defects in the surrounding cartilage both on the femoral condyle and tibial plateau *(hollow arrows)* are filled with high-signal-intensity joint fluid. Although a small amount of protrusion of the carbon fiber plug is acceptable and may even be helpful in promoting regeneration of fibrocartilage; marked protrusion, as in this case, signifies failure. The plug is likely to fragment and form loose bodies within the joint.

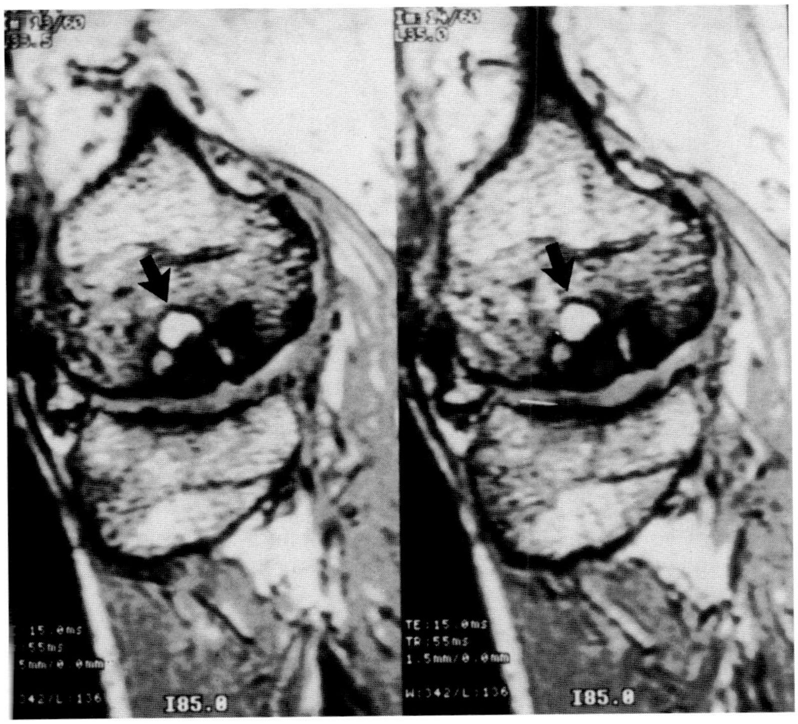

FIG. 11-51. Loose carbon fiber plug. Two adjacent 3DFT T2*-weighted MPGR gradient-echo images (TR 55 msec, TE 15 msec, flip angle 35°). A lobulated area of low signal intensity is present near the femoral condyle surface, representing the implanted carbon fiber plug. Well-demarcated high-signal-intensity areas are present at the margins of the plug *(arrow)*. These represent cysts that have formed around the plug and are indicative of loosening. Note the markedly irregular cortical surfaces of the joint.

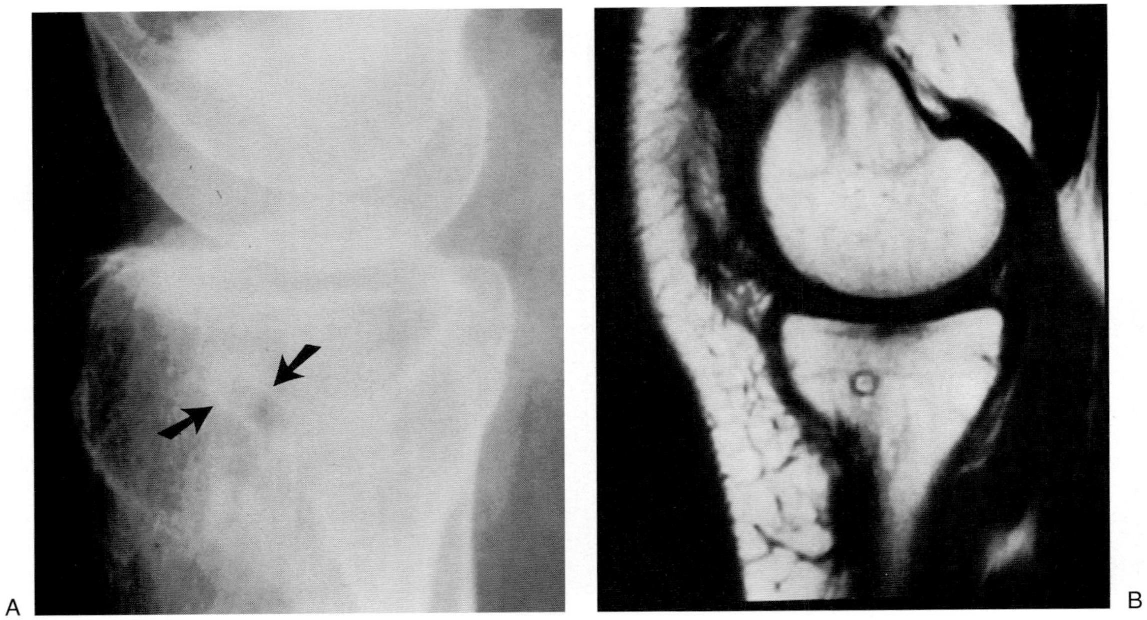

FIG. 11-52. Proximal tibial pin tract. **A:** Lateral radiograph of a patient who had previously treated with a complex fracture of the tibia with an Ilazarov external fixation device. The radiolucent pin tract surrounded by sclerosis is easily visualized *(arrow)*. **B:** Sagittal T1-weighted spin-echo image (TR 800 msec, TE 20 msec). The sclerotic margin of the pin tract is seen as a low-signal-intensity ring.

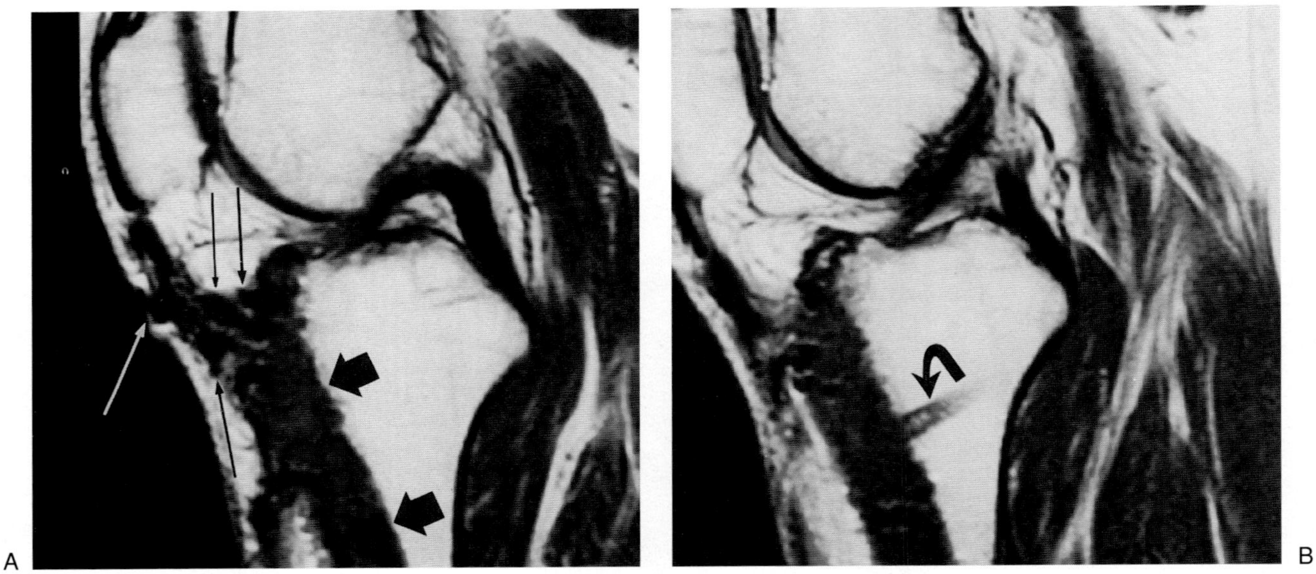

FIG. 11-53. Previous intramedullary rod fixation. **A,B:** Sagittal T1-weighted spin-echo images (TR 800 msec, TE 18 msec) from a patient who had undergone intramedullary rod placement for a fracture of a fracture of the mid-diaphysis of the tibia several years previously. The rod had been removed more than a year before. The path of the intramedullary rod can be seen in (A) and (B) as a broad, low-signal-intensity band nearly parallel to the cortex of the tibia *(thick arrows)*. Numerous tiny areas of signal dropout representing innumerable small metal fragments are present in the region of the patellar tendon and tibial tuberosity *(thin arrows)*. In addition, in (B) a small hatched low-signal area is noted perpendicular to the path of the intramedullary rod *(curved arrow)*. This represents the path of the proximal locking screw.

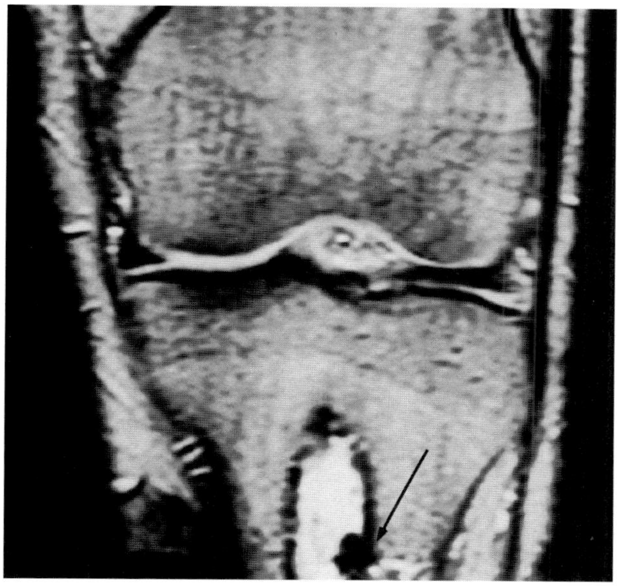

C

FIG. 11-53. *Continued.* **C:** Coronal T2*-weighted gradient-echo image (TR 400 msec, TE 16 msec, flip angle 30°). The path of the medullary rod that was seen as a low-signal-intensity band in (A) and (B) is seen to be of high signal intensity with this sequence. A low intensity, sclerotic/fibrotic rim is present with an embedded metal fragment seen due to its magnetic susceptibility artifact *(thin arrows)*. The path of the medullary rod has been filled in by granulation tissue.

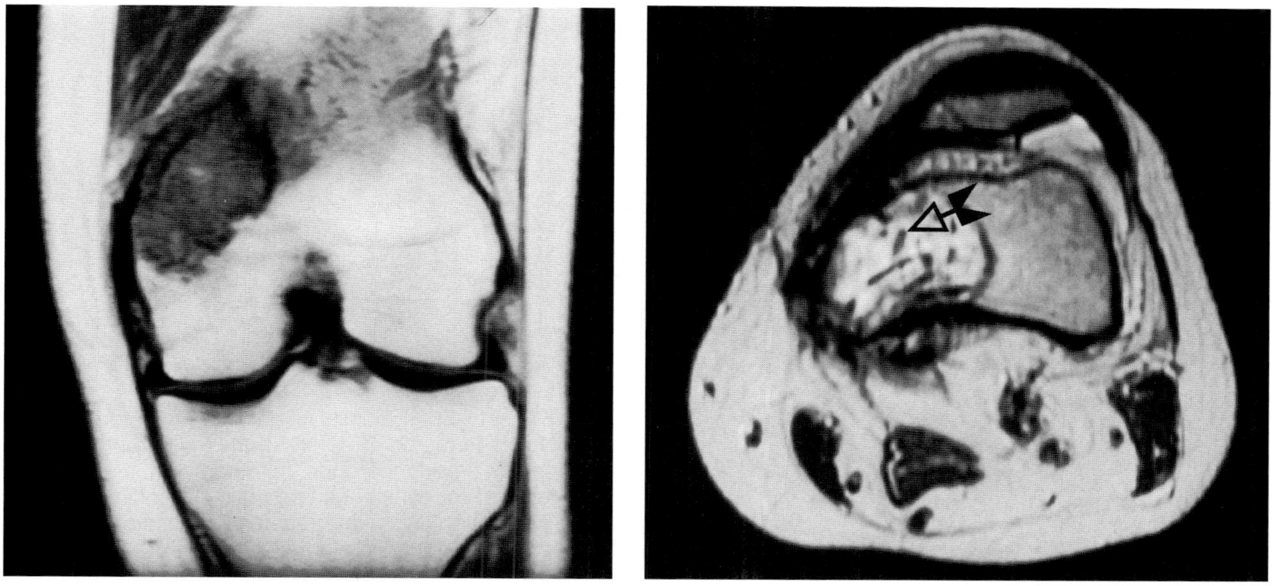

A B

FIG. 11-54. Bone tumor site post curettage. **A:** Coronal T1-weighted spin-echo image (TR 600 msec, TE 15 msec) from a patient with an osteogenic sarcoma that had inadvertently been curetted as a result of a mistaken preoperative diagnosis of giant cell tumor. Well-defined low-signal margins at the periphery represent fibrosis/sclerosis 2 months following surgery. **B:** Axial T2-weighted spin-echo image (TR 2800 msec, TE 80 msec). The curetted area had been filled in with bone chips. The linear low-signal densities within the area packed with chips represents individual bone fragments *(arrow)*. The surrounding high-signal-intensity material is thought to represent organizing granulation and scar tissue.

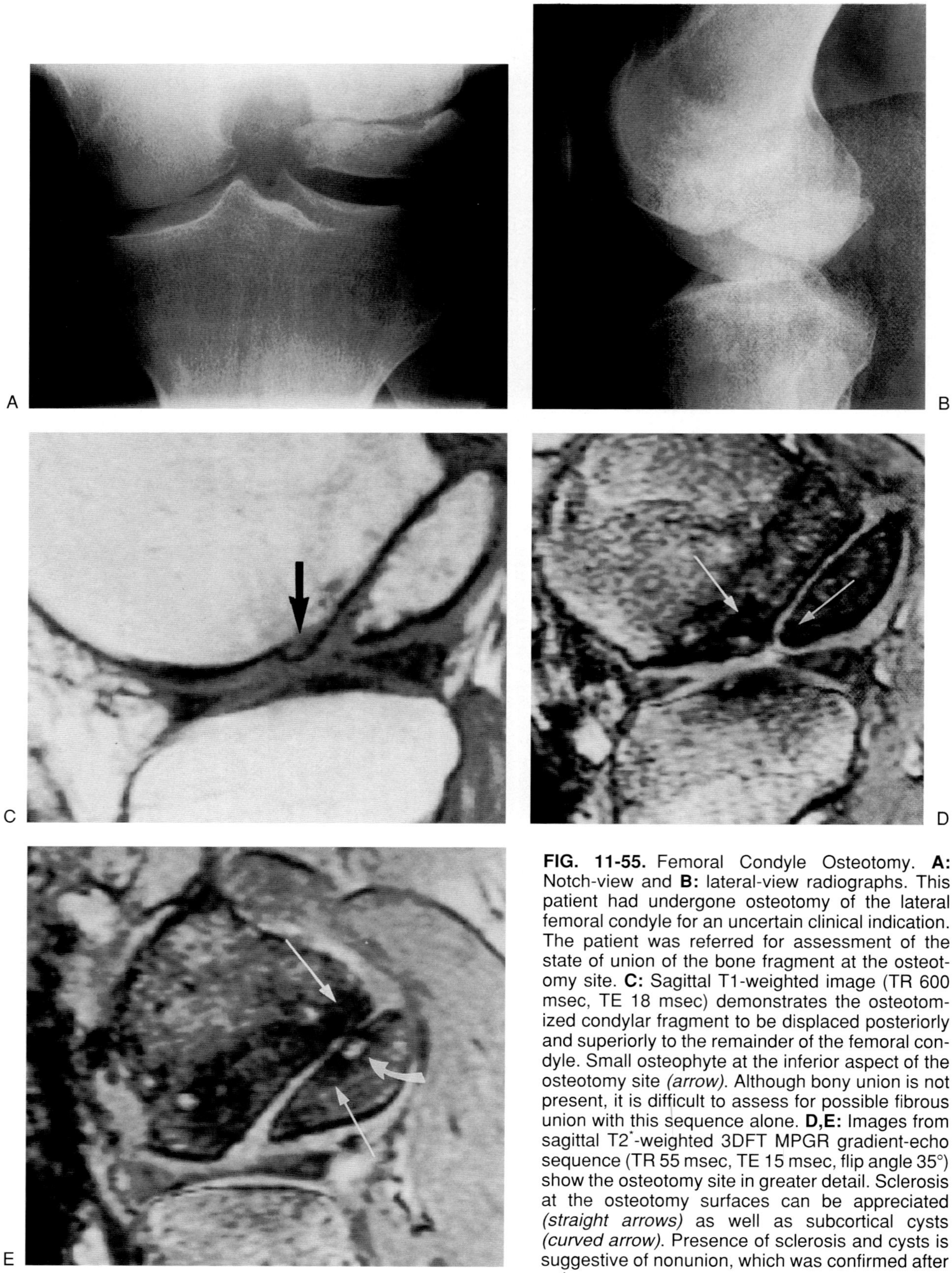

FIG. 11-55. Femoral Condyle Osteotomy. **A:** Notch-view and **B:** lateral-view radiographs. This patient had undergone osteotomy of the lateral femoral condyle for an uncertain clinical indication. The patient was referred for assessment of the state of union of the bone fragment at the osteotomy site. **C:** Sagittal T1-weighted image (TR 600 msec, TE 18 msec) demonstrates the osteotomized condylar fragment to be displaced posteriorly and superiorly to the remainder of the femoral condyle. Small osteophyte at the inferior aspect of the osteotomy site *(arrow)*. Although bony union is not present, it is difficult to assess for possible fibrous union with this sequence alone. **D,E:** Images from sagittal T2*-weighted 3DFT MPGR gradient-echo sequence (TR 55 msec, TE 15 msec, flip angle 35°) show the osteotomy site in greater detail. Sclerosis at the osteotomy surfaces can be appreciated *(straight arrows)* as well as subcortical cysts *(curved arrow)*. Presence of sclerosis and cysts is suggestive of nonunion, which was confirmed after arthroscopy.

bone described earlier become evident, and the presence of fluid within the joint is often helpful in demonstrating the overlying absence or thinning of the cartilage, especially if 3DFT is used. Loose osteochondral or chondral bodies within the joint should be searched for.

A few centers have embarked on investigation of carbon fiber implants to promote development of fibrocartilage resurfacing as treatment for early osteoarthritic changes. This method is still largely investigational.

On MRI, carbon fiber plugs appear as rectangular areas of diminished signal intensity on all sequences that are placed at right angles to the joint surface (Figs. 11-47–11-49). With successful incorporation of the carbon fiber into the bone the abrupt rectangular margins become less crisply delineated and thickening of the cartilage overlying the joint surface becomes apparent. Unfortunately, many of these carbon fiber plugs do not successfully incorporate; instead, they become loose and may break off and become loose bodies within the joint. Loosening of the plugs will be manifest as areas of increased signal intensity on T2- and T2*-weighted images, representing small cystic areas where fluid surrounds the plug (Fig. 11-50). With time gradual extrusion of the plug so that protrusion above the articular surface may be apparent (Fig. 11-51).

Recently, absorbable pins for bone fixation—particularly for small fragments and fractures—have been introduced. These are radiolucent and made of poly-L-lactic acid (115). Their appearance on MRIs is similar to that of carbon fiber, being of low signal intensity on all sequences (116).

Occasionally, other bony abnormalities may be encountered. Examples of this include pin tracks (Fig. 11-52) in patients being treated for fractures or other abnormalities may be placed to a distal femur or proximal tibia for traction purposes. These pin tracks usually demonstrate low-signal rims, representing cortication or fibrous material. After removal of such hardware as intramedullary rods (Fig. 11-53), the space fills with blood products, which gradually organize over time. The rims of the rod track are usually of low signal intensity, whereas the central portion is often of high signal intensity on T2- and T2*-weighted images until, with time, gradual filling in with fibrous tissue may be seen.

Occasionally after curettage or excision of bone tumors it may be necessary to evaluate the operative bed for residual and/or recurrent tumor. This is particularly common in patients who have have been treated for giant cell tumors or chondroblastomas, because these tumors can be treated with local excision and follow-up without significant risk of metastases. A baseline scan 6–10 weeks after surgery is very helpful in facilitating early detection of tumor on subsequent scans. Sclerosis at the edge of the curettage margins can often be appreciated once healing is well established, and low-signal areas from multiple bone chips can be appreciated for many years after surgery (Fig. 11-54).

Rarely, patients may undergo osteotomies that extend intra-articularly (Fig. 11-55). A normal osteotomy site is usually of low signal on all sequences. Nonunion is present when high-signal granulation tissue and/or fluid may be observed with T2 weighting. Fragment shifting is an even more obvious sign.

REFERENCES

1. Deutsch AL, Mink JH, Fox JM, Friedman MJ, Howell SM. The postoperative knee. *Magn Reson Q* 1992;8:23–54.
2. Deutsch AL, Mink JH, Fox JM, et al. Peripheral meniscal tears: MR findings after conservative treatment or arthroscopic repair. *Radiology* 1990;176:485–488.
3. Smith DK, Totty WG. The knee after partial meniscectomy: MR imaging features. *Radiology* 1990;176:141–144.
4. Farley TE, Howell SM, Love KF, Wolfe RD, Neumann CH. Meniscal tears: MR and arthrographic findings after arthroscopic repair. *Radiology* 1991;180:517–522.
5. Fowler PJ, Lubliner JA. The predictive values of five clinical signs in the evaluation of meniscal pathology. *Arthroscopy* 1989;5:184–186.
6. Johnson L. Impact of diagnostic arthroscopy on the clinical judgement of an experienced arthroscopist. *Clin Orthop Rel Res* 1982;167:75–83.
7. Spiers ASD, Meagher T, Ostlere SJ, Wilson DJ, Dodd CAF. Can MRI of the knee affect arthroscopic practice? *J Bone Joint Surg* 1993;75-B:49–52.
8. Ruwe PA, Wright J, Randall RL, Lynch JK, Jokl P, McCarthy S. Can MR imaging effectively replace diagnostic arthroscopy? *Radiology* 1992;183:335–339.
9. Boden SD, Labaopoulos PA, Vailas JL. MR scanning of the acutely injured knee: sensitive, but is it cost effective? *Arthroscopy* 1990;6:306–310.
10. Henning CH. Current status of meniscus salvage. *Clin Sports Med* 1990;9:567–576.
11. Cannon WD, Morgan CD. Meniscal repair part II: arthroscopic repair techniques. *J Bone Joint Surg* 1994;76-A:294–311.
12. Keene GCR, Paterson RS, Teague DC. Advances in arthroscopic surgery. *Clin Orthop Rel Res* 1987;224:64–66.
13. DeHaven KE. Rationale for meniscus repair or excision. *Clin Sports Med* 1985;4:267–273.
14. DeHaven KE. Meniscus repair in the athlete. *Clin Orthop Rel Res* 1985;198:31–35.
15. Lanzer WL, Komenda G. Changes in articular cartilage after meniscectomy. *Clin Orthop Rel Res* 1990;252:41–48.
16. Krause WR, Pope MH, Johnson RJ, Wilder DG. Mechanical changes in the knee after meniscectomy. *J Bone Joint Surg* 1976;58-A:599–604.
17. Hede A, Larsen E, Sandberg H. Partial versus total meniscectomy: a prospective, randomised study with long-term follow-up. *J Bone Joint Surg* 1992;74-B:118–121.
18. Abdon P, Turner MS, Pettersson H, Lindstrand A, Stenstrom A, Swanson JG. A long-term follow-up study of total meniscectomy in children. *Clin Orthop Rel Res* 1990;257:166–170.
19. Burr DB, Radin EL. Meniscal function and the importance of meniscal regeneration on preventing late medial compartment osteoarthrosis. *Clin Orthop Rel Res* 1982;171:121–126.
20. Limbird TJ. Application of laser Doppler technology to meniscal injuries. *Clin Orthop Rel Res* 1990;252:88–91.
21. Arnoczky SP, Warren RF, Spivak JM. Meniscal repair using an exogenous fibrin clot: an experimental study in dogs. *J Bone Joint Surg* 1988;70-A:1209–1217.
22. Arnoczky SP, Warren RF, Kaplan N. Meniscal remodeling following partial meniscectomy—an experimental study in the dog. *J Arthroscop Rel Surg* 1985;1:247–252.
23. Henning CE, Lynch MA, Yearout KM, Stallbaumer RJ, Vequist SW, Decker KA. Arthroscopic meniscal repair using an exogenous fibrin clot. *Clin Orthop Rel Res* 1990;252:64–72.
24. Gershuni DH, Skyhar MJ, Danzig LA, Camp J, Hargens AR, Akeson WH. Experimental models to promote healing of tears in the avascular segment of canine knee menisci. *J Bone Joint Injury* 1989;71-A:1363–1370.
25. Moon M, Woo Y, Kim Y. Meniscal regeneration and its effects on articular cartilage in rabbit knees. *Clin Orthop Rel Res* 1988;227:298–304.
26. Raunest J, Oberle K, Loehnert J, Hoetzinger H. The clinical value of

magnetic resonance imaging in the evaluation of meniscal disorders. *J Bone Joint Surg* 1991;73-A:11–16.
27. Applegate GR, Flannigan BD, Tolin BS, Fox JM, Del Pizzo W. MR diagnosis of recurrent tears in the knee: value of intraarticular contrast material. *AJR* 1993;161:821–825.
28. De Boer HH, Koudstaal J. The fate of meniscus cartilage after transplantation of cryopreserved nontissue-antigen-matched allograft. *Clin Orthop Rel Res* 1991;266:145–151.
29. Patten RM, Rolfe BA. MRI of meniscal grafts. *J Comput Assist Tomogr* 1995;19(2):243–246.
30. Stone KR, Rodkey WG, Webber RJ, McKinney L, Steadman JR. Future directions: collagen-based prostheses for meniscal regeneration. *Clin Orthop Rel Res* 1990;252:129–135.
31. Kohn D, Wirth CJ, Plitz W, Maschek H, Erhardt W, Wulker N. Medial meniscus replacement by a tendon autograft. *J Bone Joint Surg* 1992; 74-B:910–917.
32. Odensten M, Hamberg P, Nordin M, Lysholm J, Gillquist J. Surgical or conservative treatment of the acutely torn anterior cruciate ligament. *Clin Orthop Rel Res* 1985;198:87–93.
33. Straub T, Hunter RE. Acute anterior cruciate ligament repair. *Clin Orthop Rel Res* 1988;227:238–250.
34. Gollehon DL, Warren RF, Wickiewicz TL. Acute repairs of the anterior cruciate ligament—past and present. *Orthop Clin North Am* 1985; 16:111–125.
35. Marshall JL, Warren RF, Wickiewicz TL, Reider B. The anterior cruciate ligament: a technique of repair and reconstruction. *Clin Orthop Rel Res* 1979;143:97–106.
36. McDaniel J Jr, Dameron TB Jr. Untreated ruptures of the anterior cruciate ligament. *J Bone Joint Surg* 1980;62A:696–705.
37. Barrack RL, Bruckner JD, Kneisl J, Inman WS, Alexander AH. The outcome of nonoperatively treated complete tears of the anterior cruciate ligament in active young adults. *Clin Orthop Rel Res* 1990;259: 192–199.
38. Andersson C, Odensten M, Good L, Gillquist J. Surgical or nonsurgical treatment of acute rupture of the anterior cruciate ligament. *J Bone Joint Surg* 1989;71A:965–974.
39. Sherman MF, Warren RF, Marshall JL, Savatsky G. A clinical and radiographical analysis of 127 anterior cruciate insufficient knees. *Clin Orthop Rel Res* 1994;227:229–237.
40. Warren RF. Meniscectomy and repair in the anterior cruciate ligament-deficient patient. *Clin Orthop Rel Res* 1990;252:55–63.
41. Hazel WA, Rand JA, Morrey BF. Results of meniscectomy in the knee with anterior cruciate ligament deficiency. *Clin Orthop Rel Res* 1993;292:232–238.
42. Fu FH, Harner CD, Johnson DL, Miller MD, Woo SL-Y. Biomechanics of knee ligaments. *J Bone Joint Surg* 1993;75-A:1716–1727.
43. Simonet WT, Sim FH. Repair and reconstruction of rotatory instability of the knee. *Am J Sports Med* 1984;12:89–97.
44. Zarins B, Rowe CR. Combined anterior cruciate–ligament reconstruction using semitendinosus tendon and iliotibial tract. *J Bone Joint Surg* 1986;68-A:160–177.
45. Odensten M, Gillquist J. Functional anatomy of the anterior cruciate ligament and a rationale for reconstruction. *J Bone Joint Surg* 1985; 67-A:257–262.
46. Clancy WG, Nelson DA, Reider B, Narechana R. Anterior cruciate ligament reconstruction using one-third of the patellar ligament, augmented by extra-articular tendon transfers. *J Bone Joint Surg* 1982; 64-A:352–359.
47. Paterson FWN, Trickey EL. Anterior cruciate ligament reconstruction using part of the patellar tendon as a free graft. *J Bone Joint Surg* 1986;68-B:453–457.
48. Strum GM, Fox JM, Ferkel RD, et al. Intraarticular versus intraarticular and extraarticular reconstruction for chronic anterior cruciate ligament instability. *Clin Orthop Rel Res* 1989;245:188–198.
49. Kohn D. Arthroscopic evaluation of anterior cruciate ligament reconstruction using a free patellar tendon autograft. *Clin Orthop Rel Res* 1990;254:220–224.
50. Roth JH, Kennedy JC, Lockstadt H, McCallum CL, Cunning LA. Polypropylene braid augmented and nonaugmented intra-articular anterior cruciate ligament reconstruction. *Am J Sports Med* 1985;13: 321–336.
51. Harter RA, Osternig LR, Singer KM. Instrumented Lachman tests for the evaluation of anterior laxity after reconstruction of the anterior cruciate ligament. *J Bone Joint Surg* 1989;71-A:975–983.
52. Anderson C, Odensten M, Gillquist J. Knee function after surgical or nonsurgical treatment of acute rupture of the anterior cruciate ligament: a randomized study with a long-term follow-up period. *Clin Orthop Rel Res* 1991;264:255–263.
53. Amis AA, Scammell BE. Biomechanics of intra-articular and extra-articular reconstruction of the anterior cruciate ligament. *J Bone Joint Surg* 1993;75-B:812–817.
54. Dempsy SM, Tregonning JA. Nine-year follow-up results of two methods of MacIntosh anterior cruciate ligament reconstructions. *Clin Orthop Rel Res* 1993;294:216–222.
55. Moeser P, Bechtold RE, Clark T, Rovere G, Karstaedt N, Wolfman N. MR imaging of anterior cruciate ligament repair. *J Comput Assist Tomogr* 1989;13:105–109.
56. Kennedy JC, Stewart R, Walker DM. Anterolateral rotatory instability of the knee joint. *J Bone Joint Surg* 1978;60-A:1031–1039.
57. Radford WJP, Amis AA, Heatley FW. Immediate strength after suture of a torn anterior cruciate ligament. *J Bone Joint Surg* 1994;76-B: 480–484.
58. Moyen BJL, Jenny J, Mandrino AH, Lerat J. Comparison of reconstruction of the anterior cruciate ligament with and without a Kennedy ligament-augmentation device. *J Bone Joint Surg* 1992;74-A: 1313–1319.
59. Gomez-Castresana FB, Bastos MN, Sacristan CG. Semitendinosus Kennedy ligament augmentation device anterior cruciate ligament reconstruction. *Clin Orthop Rel Res* 1992;283:21–33.
60. Noyes FR, Barber SD. The effect of a ligament-augmentation device on allograft reconstruction for chronic ruptures of the anterior cruciate ligament. *J Bone Joint Surg* 1992;74-A:960–973.
61. Rak KM, Gillogly SD, Schaefer RA, Yakes WF, Liljedahl RR. Anterior cruciate ligament reconstruction: evaluation with MR imaging. *Radiology* 1991;178:553–556.
62. Autz G, Goodwin C, Singson RD. Magnetic resonance evaluation of anterior cruciate ligament repair using the patellar tendon double bone block technique. *Skeletal Radiol* 1991;20:585–588.
63. McFarland EG, Morrey BF, An KN, Wood MB. The relationship of vascularity and water content to tensile strength in a patellar tendon replacement of the anterior cruciate in dogs. *Am J Sports Med* 1986; 14:436–448.
64. Mott HW. Semitendinosus anatomic reconstruction for cruciate ligament insufficiency. *Clin Orthop Rel Res* 1983;172:90–92.
65. Lipscomb AB, Johnston RK, Synder RB, Brothers JC. Secondary reconstruction of anterior cruciate ligament in athletes by using the semitendinosus tendon. *Am J Sports Med* 1979;7:81–84.
66. Puddu G. Method for reconstruction of the anterior cruciate ligament using the semitendinosus tendon. *Am J Sports Med* 1980;8:402–404.
67. Alm A, Gillquist J. Reconstruction of the anterior cruciate ligament by using the medial third of the patellar ligament. *Acta Chir Scand* 1974;140:289–296.
68. Eriksson E. Reconstruction of the anterior cruciate ligament. *Orthop Clin North Am* 1976;7:167–179.
69. McMaster JH, Weinert CR, Scranton P. Diagnosis and management of isolated anterior cruciate ligament tears: a preliminary report on reconstruction with gracilis tendon. *J Trauma* 1974;14:230–235.
70. Franke K. Clinical experience in 130 cruciate ligament reconstructions. *Clin Orthop Rel Res* 1992;283:215–222.
71. Horne JG, Parsons CJ. The anterior cruciate ligament: its anatomy and a new method of reconstruction. *Can J Surg* 1977;20:214–220.
72. Buss DD, Warren RF, Wickiewicz TL, Galinat BJ, Panariello R. Arthrosopically assisted reconstruction of the anterior cruciate ligament with use of autogenous patellar-ligament grafts. *J Bone Joint Surg* 1993;75-A:1346–1355.
73. Dahlstedt L, Dalen N, Jonsson U. Gortex prosthetic ligament vs Kennedy ligament augmentation device in anterior cruciate ligament reconstruction. *Acta Orthop Scand* 1990;61:217–224.
74. Amis AA, Camburn M, Kempson SA, Radford WJP, Stead AC. Anterior cruciate ligament replacement with polyester fibre: a long-term study of tissue reactions and joint stability in sheep. *J Bone Joint Surg* 1992;74-B:605–613.
75. Good L, Odensten M, Pettersson L, Gillquist J. Failure of a bovine xenograft for reconstruction of the anterior cruciate ligament. *Acta Orthop Scand* 1989;60:8–12.
76. Yamato M, Yamagishi T. MRI of patellar tendon anterior cruciate ligament autografts. *J Comput Assist Tomogr* 1992;16:604–607.
77. Munk PL, Vellet AD, Fowler PJ, Miniaci T, Crues III JV. Magnetic

resonance imaging of reconstructed knee ligaments. *Can Assoc Radiol J* 1992;43:411–419.

78. Cheung Y, Magee TH, Rosenberg ZS, Rose DJ. MRI of anterior cruciate ligament reconstruction. *J Comput Assist Tomogr* 1992;16: 134–137.
79. Howell SM, Berns GS, Farley TE. Unimpinged and impinged anterior cruciate ligament grafts: MR signal intensity measurements. *Radiology* 1991;179:639–643.
80. Schutzer SF, Christen S, Jakob R. Further observations on the isometricity of the anterior cruciate ligament. *Clin Orthop Rel Res* 1989; 242:247–255.
81. Montgomery RD, Milton JL, Terry GC, McLeod WD, Madsen N. Comparison of over-the-top and tunnel techniques for anterior cruciate ligament replacement. *Clin Orthop Rel Res* 1988;231:144–153.
82. Shellock FG, Mink JH, Curtin S, Friedman MJ. MR imaging and metallic implants for anterior cruciate ligament reconstruction: assessment of ferromagnetism and artifact. *J Magn Reson Imag* 1992;2: 225–228.
83. Smith A, Pope CF, Dillon E, et al. Serial MR images of anterior cruciate ligament autografts during the initial 2 years after surgery. *Radiology* 1991;181(P):303. Abstract.
84. Totterman SM, Adams MJ, Langhans MJ, et al. MR imaging of knee after reconstruction of anterior cruciate ligament. *Radiology* 1991; 181(P):303. Abstract.
85. Sanchis-Alfonso V, Martinez-Sanjuan V, Gastaldi-Orquin E. The value of MRI in the evaluation of the ACL deficient knee and in the post-operative evaluation after ACL reconstruction. *Eur J Radiol* 1993;16:126–130.
86. Arendt EA, Hunter RE, Schneider WT. Vascularized patella tendon anterior cruciate ligament reconstruction. *Clin Orthop Rel Res* 1989; 244:222–232.
87. Paulos LE, Butler DL, Noyes FR, Grood ES. Intra-articular cruciate reconstruction II: replacement with vascularized patellar tendon. *Clin Orthop Rel Res* 1983;172:78–84.
88. Lambert KL. Vascularized patellar tendon graft with rigid internal fixation for anterior cruciate ligament insufficiency. *Clin Orthop Rel Res* 1983;172:85–89.
89. Odensten M, Gillquist J. A modified technique for anterior cruciate ligament (ACL) surgery using a new drill guide for isometric positioning of the ACL. *Clin Orthop Rel Res* 1986;213:154–158.
90. Howell SM, Clark JA. Tibial tunnel placement in anterior cruciate ligament reconstructions and graft impingement. *Clin Orthop Rel Res* 1992;283:187–195.
91. Howell SM, Taylor MA. Failure of reconstruction of the anterior cruciate ligament due to impingement by the intercondylar roof. *J Bone Joint Surg* 1993;75-A:1044–1055.
92. Manaster BJ, Remley K, Newman AP, Mann FA. Knee ligament reconstruction: plain film analysis. *AJR* 1988;150:337–342.
93. Tosch U, Sander B, Lais E, et al. MR follow-up of Gd-DTPA-enhanced autologous patellar ligament transplants for anterior crucial ligament repair. *Radiology* 1991;181(P):303. Abstract.
94. Barton TM, Torg JS, Das M. Posterior cruciate ligament insufficiency: a review of the literature. *Sports Med* 1984;1:419–430.
95. Covey DC, Sapega AA. Injuries of the posterior cruciate ligament. *J Bone Joint Surg* 1993;75-A:1376–1386.
96. Torg JS, Barton TM, Pavlov H, Stine R. Natural history of the posterior cruciate ligament-deficient knee. *Clin Orthop Rel Res* 1989;246: 208–216.
97. Dandy DJ, Pusey RJ. The long-term results of unrepaired tears of the posterior cruciate ligament. *J Bone Joint Surg* 1982;64-B:92–94.
98. Parolie JM, Bergfeld JA. Long-term results of nonoperative treatment of isolated posterior cruciate ligament injuries in the athlete. *Am J Sports Med* 1986;14:35–38.
99. Burks RT, Schaffer JJ. A simplified approach to the tibial attachment of the posterior cruciate ligament. *Clin Orthop Rel Res* 1990;254: 216–219
100. Hughston JC, Bowden JA, Andrews JR, Norwood LA. Acute tears of the posterior cruciate ligament: results of operative treatment. *J Bone Joint Surg* 1980;62-A:438–450.
101. Cross MJ, Powell JF. Long-term followup of posterior cruciate ligament rupture: a study of 116 cases. *Am J Sports Med* 1984;12: 292–297.
102. Moore HA, Larson RL. Posterior cruciate ligament injuries: results of early surgical repair. *Am J Sports Med* 1980;8:68–78.
103. Bianchi M. Acute tears of the posterior cruciate ligament: clinical study and results of operative treatment in 27 cases. *Am J Sports Med* 1983;11:308–314.
104. Loos WC, Fox JM, Blazina ME, Del Pizzo W, Friedman MJ. Acute posterior cruciate ligament injuries. *Am J Sports Med* 1981;9:86–92.
105. Skyhar MJ, Warren RF, Oritz GJ, Schwartz E, Otis JC. The effects of sectioning of the posterior cruciate ligament and the posterolateral complex on the articular contact pressures within the knee. *J Bone Joint Surg* 1993;75-A:694–699.
106. Castle TH, Noyes FR, Grood ES. Posterior tibial subluxation of the posterior cruciate-deficient knee. *Clin Orthop Rel Res* 1992;284: 193–202.
107. Clendenin MB, DeLee JC, Heckman JD. Interstitial tears of the posterior cruciate ligament of the knee. *Orthopedics* 1980;3:764–772.
108. Torisu T. Isolated avulsion fracture of the tibial attachment of the posterior cruciate ligament. *J Bone Joint Surg* 1977;59-A:68–72.
109. Hughston JC, Degenhardt TC. Reconstruction of the posterior cruciate ligament. *Clin Orthop Rel Res* 1982;164:59–77.
110. Indelicato PA, Hermansdorfer J, Huegel M. Nonoperative management of complete tears of the medial collateral ligament of the knee in intercollegiate football players. *Clin Orthop Rel Res* 1990;256: 174–177.
111. Fleming RE, Blatz DJ, McCarroll JR. Lateral reconstruction for anterolateral rotatory instability of the knee. *Am J Sports Med* 1983;11: 303–307.
112. Markolf KL, Wascher DC, Finerman GAM. Direct in vitro measurements of forces in the cruciate ligaments. Part II: the effect of section of the posterolateral structures. *J Bone Joint Surg* 1993;75:387–394.
113. Carpenter JE, Kasman R, Matthews LS. Fractures of the patella. *J Bone Joint Surg* 1993;75-A:1550–1561.
114. Wootton JR, Cross MJ, Wood DG. Patellofemoral malalignment: a report of 68 cases treated by proximal and distal patellofemoral reconstruction. *Injury* 1990;21:169–173.
115. Pihlajamaki H, Bostman D, Hirvensalo E, Tormala P, Rokkanen P. Absorbable pins of self-reinforced poly-L-lactic acid for fixation of fractures and osteotomies. *J Bone Joint Surg* 1992;74-B:853–857.
116. Smith DS, Sharp DC, Resendes M. MRI of healing osteochondritis dissecans fragment with absorbable pins. *J Comput Assist Tomogr* 1994;18:832–833.

Subject Index

Subject Index

Page numbers in italics refer to figures.

N

O

ISBN 0-397-51642-8
9 780397 516421